Bonnie Stance Cleveland

17th Edition

Handbook of Pediatrics

GERALD B. MERENSTEIN, MD, FAAP
Professor
Department of Pediatrics
University of Colorado Health Sciences Center:
  The Children's Hospital
Denver, Colorado

DAVID W. KAPLAN, MD, MPH
Associate Professor
Head, Adolescent Medicine
Department of Pediatrics
University of Colorado Health Sciences Center:
  The Children's Hospital
Denver, Colorado

ADAM A. ROSENBERG, MD
Associate Professor
Department of Pediatrics
University of Colorado Health Sciences Center:
  The Children's Hospital
Denver, Colorado

APPLETON & LANGE
Norwalk, Connecticut

Copyright © 1994 by Appleton & Lange
Paramount Publishing Business and Professional Group
Copyright © 1991, 1987 by Appleton & Lange

94 95 96 97 98 / 10 9 8 7 6 5 4 3 2 1

Prentice Hall International (UK) Limited, *London*
Prentice Hall of Australia Pty. Limited, *Sydney*
Prentice Hall Canada, Inc., *Toronto*
Prentice Hall Hispanoamericana, S.A., *Mexico*
Prentice Hall of India Private Limited, *New Delhi*
Prentice Hall of Japan, Inc., *Tokyo*
Simon & Schuster Asia Pte. Ltd., *Singapore*
Editora Prentice Hall do Brasil Ltda., *Rio de Janeiro*
Prentice Hall, *Englewood Cliffs, New Jersey*

ISBN 0-8385-3657-3
ISBN 0440-1921

Acquisitions Editor: Shelley Reinhardt
Production Editor: Christine Langan
Designer: Kathy Hornyak

PRINTED IN THE UNITED STATES OF AMERICA

Table of Contents

The Authors

Steven H. Abman, MD
Associate Professor, Pediatric Pulmonary Medicine, University of Colorado Health Sciences Center/The Children's Hospital, Denver.

Mark J. Abzug, MD
Assistant Professor of Pediatrics, University of Colorado Health Sciences Center/The Children's Hospital, Denver.

F. Keith Battan, MD
Assistant Professor of Pediatrics, University of Colorado Health Sciences Center/The Children's Hospital, Denver.

Stephen Berman, MD
Professor of Pediatrics, University of Colorado Health Sciences Center/The Children's Hospital, Denver.

David W. Boyle, MD
Assistant Professor of Pediatrics, Indiana University, School of Medicine, Indianapolis.

David Burgess, MD
Associate Professor, Department of Pediatrics, University of Colorado Health Sciences Center, Denver.

Nancy Cohen Carlson, MD
Assistant Professor of Pediatrics, University of Colorado Health Sciences Center/The Children's Hospital, Denver.

Richard C. Dart, MD, PhD
Director, Rocky Mountain Poison and Drug Center, Denver.

Robert E. Eilert, MD
Clinical Professor of Orthopedic Surgery, University of Colorado Health Sciences Center/The Children's Hospital, Denver.

Wendy Frieling, MD
Chief Resident, Department of Pediatrics, University of Colorado Health Sciences Center/The Children's Hospital, Denver.

Benjamin A. Gitterman, MD
Associate Professor of Pediatrics & Preventive Medicine, University of Colorado Health Sciences Center; Director, Ambula-

tory Pediatric Services, Denver Health & Hospitals, Denver, Colorado.

Ronald W. Gotlin, MD
Professor of Pediatrics, University of Colorado Health Sciences Center/The Children's Hospital, Denver.

K. Michael Hambidge, MD
Professor of Pediatrics, and Director, University of Colorado Center for Human Nutrition, University of Colorado Health Sciences Center/The Children's Hospital, Denver.

Taru Hays, MD
Professor of Pediatrics, University of Colorado Health Sciences Center/The Children's Hospital, Denver.

Joanne Janas, MD
Fellow, Department of Neurology, Texas Scottish Rite Hospital, Dallas.

Alan Kamada, PharmD
Clinical Pharmacology Division, Department of Pediatrics, National Jewish Center for Immunology and Respiratory Medicine, Denver, Colorado.

David W. Kaplan, MD
Professor of Pediatrics, and Head, Section of Adolescent Medicine, University of Colorado Health Sciences Center/The Children's Hospital, Denver.

Nancy Krebs, MD
Instructor/Fellow, Department of Pediatrics, University of Colorado Health Sciences Center/The Children's Hospital, Denver.

Carol Ledwith, MD
Assistant Professor of Pediatrics, University of Colorado Health Sciences Center/The Children's Hospital, Denver.

Gary M. Lum, MD
Professor of Pediatrics, University of Colorado Health Sciences Center/The Children's Hospital, Denver.

Kathleen A. Mammel, MD
Assistant Professor of Pediatrics, University of Colorado Health Sciences Center/The Children's Hospital, Denver.

Gerald B. Merenstein, MD
Professor, Department of Pediatrics, University of Colorado Health Sciences Center/The Children's Hospital, Denver.

Joseph G. Morelli, MD
Assistant Professor of Dermatology and Pediatrics, University of Colorado Health Sciences Center, Denver.

John W. Ogle, MD
Associate Professor and Vice Chairman of Pediatrics, University of Colorado Health Sciences Center, Denver.

Lee Ann Pearse, MD
Assistant Professor of Clinical Pediatrics, University of Miami, School of Medicine, Miami, Florida.

David S. Pearlman, MD
Clinical Professor of Pediatrics, University of Colorado Health Sciences Center, Denver.

David F. Raney, MD
Assistant Clinical Professor of Psychiatry, University of Colorado Health Sciences Center, Denver.

Adam A. Rosenberg, MD
Associate Professor, Department of Pediatrics, University of Colorado Health Sciences Center/The Children's Hospital, Denver.

Barry H. Rumack, MD
Clinical Professor of Pediatrics, University of Colorado Health Sciences Center; Director Emeritus, Rocky Mountain Poison Center, Denver.

Robert A. Sargent, MD
Associate Clinical Professor of Ophthalmology, University of Colorado Health Sciences Center/The Children's Hospital, Denver.

Michael S. Schaffer, MD
Associate Professor of Pediatrics, University of Colorado, School of Medicine Health Sciences Center/The Children's Hospital, Denver.

Barton D. Schmitt, MD
Professor of Pediatrics, University of Colorado Health Sciences Center/The Children's Hospital, Denver.

Alan R. Seay, MD
Associate Professor of Pediatrics and Neurology, University of Colorado Health Sciences Center/The Children's Hospital, Denver.

Elizabeth M. Shaffer, MD
Assistant Professor, University of Colorado Health Sciences Center/The Children's Hospital, Denver.

Judith M. Sondheimer, MD
Professor of Pediatrics, University of Colorado Health Sciences Center/The Children's Hospital, Denver.

Steven B. Spedale, MD
Co-Medical Director of Neonatology, Woman's Hospital, Baton Rouge, Louisiana.

Dale William Steele, MD
Instructor of Pediatrics, Brown University; Pediatric Emergency Medicine, Rhode Island Hospital, Providence.

Linda C. Stork, MD
Assistant Professor of Pediatrics, University of Colorado Health Sciences Center/The Children's Hospital, Denver.

Eva Svjansky, MD
Associate Professor of Pediatrics, Biochemistry, Biophysics and Genetics, University of Colorado Health Sciences Center/The Children's Hospital, Denver.

Stanley Szefler, MD
Professor of Pediatrics and Pharmacology, University of Colorado Health Sciences Center; Director of Clinical Pharmacology, National Jewish Center for Immunology & Respiratory Medicine, Denver.

Suzanne M. Tanner, MD
Assistant Professor, Departments of Orthopedics and Pediatrics, CU Sports Medicine Center, Denver.

James K. Todd, MD
Professor of Pediatrics and Microbiology/Immunology, University of Colorado Health Sciences Center/The Children's Hospital, Denver.

Elaine Van Gundy, MD
Assistant Professor, Creighton University, School of Medicine, Omaha, Nebraska.

William L. Weston, MD
Professor of Dermatology and Pediatrics, University of Colorado Health Sciences Center, Denver.

NOTICE

Not all of the drugs mentioned in this book have been approved by FDA for use in infants or in children under age 6 or age 12. Such drugs should not be used if effective alternatives are available; they may be used if no effective alternatives are available or if the known risk of toxicity of alternative drugs or the risk of nontreatment is outweighed by the probable advantages of treatment.

Because of the possibility of an error in the article or book from which a particular drug dosage is obtained, or an error appearing in the text of this book, our readers are urged to consult appropriate references, including the manufacturer's package insert, especially when prescribing new drugs or those with which they are not adequately familiar.

—The Authors

Preface

Handbook of Pediatrics offers a convenient, up-to-date source of practical information on the care of children from infancy through adolescence. Focusing on the clinical aspects of pediatric care, the seventeenth edition covers a wide range of topics, including development and growth of the healthy child, ambulatory care, preventive medicine, and diagnosis and treatment of common pediatric disorders. Pertinent physiologic and pharmacologic principles support the wealth of clinical information.

Audience

Handbook of Pediatrics serves the needs of all health professionals involved in the day-to-day care of pediatric patients. **Medical students and house officers** working in hospitals or ambulatory care facilities will appreciate the concise descriptions of diseases and the accessibility of information. **Nurses and practicing physicians,** particularly those in primary care, will find the Handbook a ready reference for a broad spectrum of information; chapters are included on dermatology, cardiology, otolaryngology, and other relevant pediatric subspecialties.

New to This Edition

The seventeenth edition of *Handbook of Pediatrics* represents a significant revision and reorganization of this classic. Reflecting the original intent of Drs. Silver, Kempe, and Bruyn, the book provides an up-to-date digest of pediatric information. The team of editors and contributors has continued to revise, reorganize, and update the book to enhance its usefulness in today's practice. The latest medical advances and therapeutic recommendations are included. The editors continue to strive to present as much information as possible in the form of tables and figures for ready access to information. The order of the chapters has been reorganized to provide a more fluent presentation. Drug Therapy and Formulary, Pediatric Emergencies, Pediatric Procedures, and the Appendices containing normal laboratory values are all grouped at the back of the book.

New chapters included the following:
- Sports Medicine
- Behavioral, Psychosocial & Psychiatric Pediatrics

- Genetics
- Care of the Newborn
- The Newborn Infant: Diseases & Disorders
  Many chapters have important revisions, including extensive changes in:
- Fluid & Electrolytes
- Neurologic & Muscular Disorders

Continuing Features
- Normal values of blood chemistry, urine, bone marrow, peripheral blood, feces, sweat, and cerebrospinal fluid.
- Descriptions of the most commonly used laboratory tests.
- Extensive pediatric drug formulary
- Chapters on pediatric emergencies and pediatric procedures

Acknowledgements
We wish to thank the authors who contributed to this edition and all those whose work on previous editions.

We wish to express our gratitude to our readers throughout the world who have provided us with helpful suggestions. Comments and suggestions for future editions can be sent to us in care of Appleton & Lange, P.O. Box 5630, Norwalk, CT 06856-5630.

Gerald B. Merenstein
David W. Kaplan
Adam A. Rosenberg

Denver, Colorado
August 1993

Pediatric History & Physical Examination | 1

Benjamin A. Gitterman, MD

HISTORY

For many pediatric problems, the history is the single most important factor in arriving at a correct diagnosis. The physician's interaction with the patient and the parents during the history-taking process is also the first stage in the psychotherapeutic management of the patient. Socioeconomic, cultural, and educational factors may influence the caregiver–patient communication process. Assurance of confidentiality should be part of the process.

The outline in Figure 1–1 should be modified and adapted as appropriate for the age of the child and the reason for the consultation.

Source of History and Reason for Referral

The history and reason for the consultation should be obtained from the parent or whoever is responsible for the care of the child. Much valuable information can also be obtained from the child. Adolescents should be interviewed alone when possible; they may be uncomfortable discussing sensitive information in the presence of their parents.

Identifying Inforamtion

Name, address, and telephone number; sex; date and place of birth; race, religion and nationality; referred by whom; parent's names, occupations, and business telephone numbers.

Chief Complaint (CC)

Patient's or informant's own brief account of the complaint and its duration.

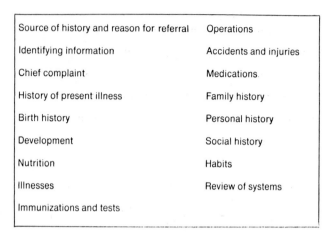

Figure 1–1. Taking a pediatric history.

History of Present Illness (HPI)

(1) When was the patient last entirely well?

(2) How and when did the condition begin?

(3) Progress of disease; order and date of onset of new symptoms.

(4) Specific symptoms and physical signs that may have developed.

(5) Pertinent negative data obtained by direct questioning.

(6) Aggravating and alleviating factors.

(7) Significant medical attention and medications or home therapies given, and over what period of time.

(8) In acute infections, statement of type and degree of exposure, and interval since exposure.

(9) For the well child, factors of significane and general condition since last visit.

(10) Examiner's opinion about the reliability of the informant.

Birth History

A. Antenatal: Health of mother during pregnancy, prenatal care, diet, infections (eg, rubella) and other illnesses, vomiting, bleeding, preeclampsia-eclampsia and other complications. Rh typing and serologic tests, pelvimetry, medications, x-ray procedures, amniocentesis.

B. Natal: Duration of pregnancy, kind and duration of labor, type of delivery, sedation and anesthesia (if known), birth weight, state of infant at birth, resuscitation required, onset of respiration, first cry, special procedures.

C. Neonatal: Apgar score, color (cyanosis, pallor, jaundice), cry, twitching, excessive mucus, paralysis, convulsions, fever, hemorrhage, congenital abnormalities, birth injury. Difficulty in sucking, rashes, feeding difficulties. Length of hospital stay, discharge weight.

Development

(1) Milestones: age when first raised head, rolled over, sat alone, pulled up, walked with help, walked alone, talked (meaningful words, sentences). A standardized developmental screening test (Denver II, etc) should be used if possible (see Chapter 2).

(2) Urinary continence during night; during day.

(3) Control of defecation.

(4) Comparison of development with that of siblings and parents.

(5) Any period of failure to grow or unusual growth.

(6) School grade, quality of work.

Nutrition

A. Breast or Formula Feeding: Type, duration, major formula changes, time of weaning, difficulties.

B. Supplements: Vitamins (type, amount, duration), iron, fluoride.

C. Solid Foods: When introduced, how taken, types, unusual family dietary habits (vegetarian, etc), balancing of food groups.

D. Appetite: Food likes and dislikes, idiosyncrasies, allergies, attitude of child to eating.

Illnesses

A. Hospitalizations.

B. Infections: Age, types, number, severity.

C. Contagious Diseases: Age, measles, rubella, chickenpox, mumps, pertussis, diphtheria, scarlet fever. Complications of any of above.

D. Other Serious Noninfectious Illnesses.

Immunizations & Tests

Indicate type, number, reactions, age of child.

A. Inoculations: Diphtheria, tetanus, pertussis, measles, rubella, mumps, *Haemophilus influenzae*, hepatitis B, others.

B. Oral Immunizations: Poliomyelitis.

C. Serum Injections: Passive immunizations.

D. Tests: Tuberculin, serology, anemia, lead, sickle cell, others.

Operations

Type, age, complications; reasons for operations; apparent response of child.

Accidents & Injuries

Nature, severity, sequelae.

Medications

Chronic use of medications; allergies to medications.

Family History

(1) Father and mother (age and condition of health).

(2) Siblings (age, condition of health, significant previous illnesses and problems).

(3) Stillbirths, miscarriages, abortions; age at death and cause of death of members of immediate family.

(4) Tuberculosis, allergy, blood dyscrasias, mental or nervous diseases, diabetes, cardiovascular diseases, kidney diseases, hypertension, rheumatic fever, neoplastic diseases, congenital abnormalities, convulsive disorders, others.

(5) Health of contacts.

Personal History

A. Relations with Other Children: Independent or clinging to mother; negativistic, shy, submissive; separation from parents; hobbies; easy or difficult to get along with. How is child similar to or different from siblings? How does child relate to others?

B. School Progress: Preschool activity (child care, Head Start, preschool, etc), academic performance, special aptitudes or problems, reaction to school.

Social History

    A. Family Structure: Adults in the home and their relationship to child; stability of family situation; sources of income; home (size, number of rooms, living conditions, sleeping facilities), type of neighborhood, access to play facilities. Who cares for child if parents work outside of home?

    B. Family Support Systems: Relatives nearby or close friends to provide support and give parents "time off."

    C. Child Care Arrangements and Satisfaction.

    D. School: Public or private, students per classroom, satisfaction with school.

    E. Insurance: Type of health coverage, if any.

Habits

    A. Sleeping: Hours, disturbances, snoring, restlessness, dreaming, nightmares.

    B. Recreation: Exercise and play.

    C. Elimination: Urinary, bowel.

    D. Behavioral Concerns: Excessive bed-wetting, masturbation, thumb-sucking, nail-biting, breath-holding, temper tantrums, tics, nervousness, undue thirst, others. Similar disturbances among members of family. School problems (learning, perceptual).

    E. Adolescent Habits: Smoking, alcohol or substance abuse, sexual activity, use of birth control, knowledge regarding STDs, involvement in gangs, use of guns. These questions need not be asked immediately but should be routine if appropriate to the patient's age.

    F. Dental Hygiene: Self-care habits (brushing, flossing), most recent preventive check.

    G. Safety: Use of infant or child restraining devices in automobiles, bicycle helmets, careful storage of medicines and toxic substances, covering of electrical outlets, other (age-appropriate) safety measures.

    H. Family Health Habits as Models: Smoking, alcohol, exercise, safety, diet.

Review of Systems

    A. General Review: Unusual weight gain or loss, fatigue, fevers, pattern of growth, recent behavioral changes.

    B. Skin: Rashes, lumps, itching, dryness, color changes, changes in hair or nails, easy bruising.

C. Eyes: Vision, last eye examination, glasses or contact lenses, pain, redness, excessive tearing, double vision, lazy eye.

D. Ears, Nose, and Throat: Frequent colds, sore throat, sneezing, stuffy nose, nasal discharge or postnasal drip, mouth breathing, snoring, otitis, hearing, adenitis, allergies.

E. Dental: Age at eruption of deciduous and permanent teeth; bleeding gums, condition of teeth, other concerns.

F. Cardiorespiratory System: Frequency and nature of disturbances. Dyspnea, chest pain, cough, sputum, wheezing, history of pneumonia, cyanosis, syncope, tachycardia.

G. Gastrointestinal System: Swallowing problems, spitting, vomiting, diarrhea, constipation, type of stools, abdominal pain or discomfort, jaundice, changes in bowel movements, blood in stools.

H. Genitourinary System: Enuresis, dysuria, frequency, polyuria, pyuria, hematuria, character of stream, vaginal discharge, menstrual history, bladder control, abnormalities of genitalia.

I. Neuromuscular System: Headache, nervousness, dizziness, tingling, convulsions, habit spasms, ataxia, muscle or joint pains, postural deformities, exercise tolerance, gait. Screening for scoliosis.

J. Endocrine System: Disturbances of growth, excessive fluid intake, polyphagia, goiter, thyroid disease, age of onset of pubertal changes.

PHYSICAL EXAMINATION

Every child should have a complete systematic examination at regular intervals (Fig. 1–2). The examination should not be restricted to those portions of the body considered to be involved on the basis of the presenting complaint.

Approaching the Child

Adequate time should be allowed for the child and the examiner to become acquainted. The child should be treated as an individual whose feelings and sensibilities are well developed, and the examiner's conduct should be appropriate to the age of the child. A friendly manner, quiet voice, and slow and easy approach will help to facilitate the examination. If the examiner is not able to establish a friendly relationship but feels that it is important to proceed with the examination, this should be done

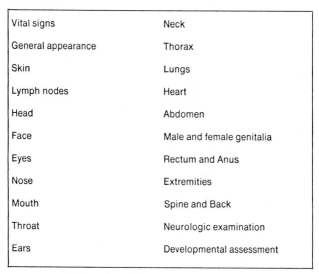

Vital signs	Neck
General appearance	Thorax
Skin	Lungs
Lymph nodes	Heart
Head	Abdomen
Face	Male and female genitalia
Eyes	Rectum and Anus
Nose	Extremities
Mouth	Spine and Back
Throat	Neurologic examination
Ears	Developmental assessment

Figure 1–2. The physical examination.

in an orderly, systematic manner in the hope that the child will then accept the inevitable.

The examiner's hands should be washed in warm water before the examination begins and should be warm.

Observing the Child

Although the very young child may not be able to speak, much information can be obtained by an observant and receptive examiner. The total evaluation of the child should include impressions obtained from the time the child first enters the room; it should not be based solely on the period during which the patient is on the examining table. This is also the best time to assess the interaction between parent and child; the examiner's impressions should be recorded.

In general, more information is obtained by careful inspection than by any other method of examination.

Holding the Child for Examination

Much of the examination can be performed while the child is held in the parent's lap or over the parent's shoulder. Certain parts of the examination can sometimes be done more easily with the child prone or held against the parent so that the examiner cannot be seen.

Removal of Clothing

Clothes should removed gradually to prevent chilling and to avoid resistance from a shy child. To save time and to avoid creating unpleasant associations with the caregiver in the child's mind, undressing the child and taking the temperature are best performed by the parent. The marked degree of modesty that some children exhibit should be respected.

Sequence of Examination

In most cases, it is best to begin the examination of the young child with an area that is least likely to be associated with pain or discomfort. The ears and throat should usually be examined last. The examiner should develop a regular sequence of examination that can be adapted to each child as required by special circumstances.

Painful Procedures

Before performing a disagreeable, painful, or upsetting examination, the examiner should tell the child (1) what is likely to happen and how the child can assist, (2) that the examination is necessary, and (3) that it will be performed as rapidly and as painlessly as possible.

Vital Signs

Record temperature, pulse rate, and respiratory rate (TPR); blood pressure (see Chapter 16); weight; and height. The weight should be recorded at each visit; the height should be determined at regular intervals. The height, weight, and head circumference of the child should be plotted on standardized growth curves and the approximate percentiles recorded. Multiple measurements at intervals are of more value than single ones, since they give information regarding the pattern of growth. The blood pressure should also be compared with standard percentiles.

General Appearance

Does the child appear well or ill? Degree of prostration; degree of cooperation; state of comfort, nutrition, and consciousness; abnormalities; gait, posture, and coordination; estimate of intelligence; reaction to parents, physician, and examination; nature of cry and degree of activity; facies and facial expression.

Skin

Color (cyanosis, jaundice, pallor, erythema), texture, eruptions, hydration, edema, hemorrhagic manifestations, scar, dilated vessels and direction of blood flow, hemangiomas, café au lait areas and nevi, mongolian spots, pigmentation, turgor, elasticity, subcutaneous nodules, sensitivity, hair distribution, character, desquamation, capillary refill.

Practical notes:

(1) Loss of turgor, especially of the calf muscles and skin over the abdomen, is evidence of dehydration.

(2) The soles and palms are often bluish and cold in early infancy; this finding is of no significance.

(3) The degree of anemia cannot be determined reliably by inspection, since pallor (even in the newborn) may be normal and not due to anemia.

(4) To demonstrate pitting edema in a child, it may be necessary to exert prolonged pressure.

(5) A few small pigmented nevi are commonly found, particularly in older children.

(6) Spider nevi occur in about one-sixth of children under age 5 years and almost half of older children.

(7) "Mongolian spots" (large, flat, black or blue-black areas) are frequently present over the lower back and buttocks; they have no pathologic significance.

(8) Cyanosis will not be evident unless at least 5 g of reduced hemoglobin is present; therefore, it develops less easily in an anemic child.

(9) Carotenemia is usually most prominent over the palms and soles and around the nose and spares the conjunctiva.

(10) Striae and wrinkling may indicate rapid weight gain or loss.

Lymph Nodes

Location, size, sensitivity, mobility, consistency. One should routinely attempt to palpate suboccipital, preauricular, anterior cervical, posterior cervical, submaxillary, sublingual, axillary, epitrochlear, and inguinal lymph nodes.

Practical notes:

(1) Enlargement of the lymph nodes occurs much more readily in children than in adults.

(2) Small inguinal lymph nodes are palpable in almost all healthy young children. Small, mobile, nontender shotty nodes are commonly found as residua of previous infection.

Head

Size, shape, circumference, asymmetry, cephalhematoma, bossae, craniotabes, control, molding, bruits, fontanelles (size, tension, number, abnormally late or early closure), sutures, dilated veins, scalp, hair (texture, distribution, parasites), face, transillumination.

Practical notes:

(1) The head is measured at its greatest circumference; this is usually at the mid forehead anteriorly and around to the most prominent portion of the occiput posteriorly. The ratio of head circumference to circumference of the chest or abdomen is usually of little value.

(2) Fontanelle tension is best determined with the child quiet and in the sitting position.

(3) Slight pulsations over the anterior fontanelle may occur in normal infants.

(4) Although bruits may be heard over the temporal areas in normal children, the possibility of an existing abnormality should be ruled out.

(5) Craniotabes may be found in normal newborn infants (especially premature infants) and for the first 2–4 months of life.

(6) A positive Macewen sign ("cracked pot" sound when skull is percussed with one finger) may be present normally as long as the fontanelle is open.

(7) Transillumination of the skull can be performed by means of a flashlight with a sponge rubber collar so that it fits tightly when held against the head.

Face

Symmetry, paralysis, distance between nose and mouth, depth of nasolabial folds, bridge of nose, distribution of hair, size of mandible, swellings, hypertelorism, Chvostek's sign, tenderness over sinuses.

Eyes

Photophobia; visual acuity; muscular control and conjugate gaze; nystagmus; mongolian slant; Brushfield's spots; epicanthic folds; lacrimation; discharge; lids; exophthalmos, or enoph-thalmos; conjunctiva; pupillary size, shape, and reaction to light and accommodation; color of iris; media (corneal opacities, cata-racts); fundi; visual fields (in older children).

Practical notes:

(1) Newborn infants usually will open their eyes if placed prone, supported with one hand on the abdomen, and lifted over the examiner's head.

(2) Not infrequently, one pupil is normally larger than the other. This sometimes occurs only in bright or subdued light.

(3) Examination of the fundi should be part of every com-plete physical examination.

(4) Dilation of the pupils may be necessary for adequate visualization of the eyes.

(5) A mild degree of strabismus may be present during the first 6 months of life but should be considered abnormal after that time.

(6) To test for strabismus in a very young or uncooperative child, note where a distant source of light is reflected from the surface of the eyes; the reflection should be present on corre-sponding portions of the 2 eyes.

(7) Small areas of capillary dilatation are commonly seen on the eyelids of normal newborn infants.

(8) Most infants produce visible tears during the first few days of life.

Nose

Exterior, shape, mucosa, patency, discharge, bleeding, pressure over sinuses, flaring of nostrils, septum.

Mouth

Lips (thinness, downturning, fissures, color, cleft), teeth (number, position, caries, mottling, discoloration, notching, mal-occlusion or malalignment), mucosa (color, redness of Stensen's duct, enanthems, Bohn's nodules, Epstein's pearls), gums, pal-ate, tongue, uvula, mouth breathing, geographic tongue (usually normal).

Practical note: If the tongue can be extended as far as the alveolar ridge, there will be no interference with nursing or speaking. Frenectomy is not a preventive measure for being "tongue-tied."

Throat

Tonsils (size, inflammation, exudate, crypts, inflammation of the anterior pillars), epiglottis, mucosa, hypertrophic lymphoid tissue, postnasal drip, voice (hoarseness, stridor, grunting, type of cry, speech).

Practical notes:

(1) Before examining a child's throat, it is advisable to examine the mouth. Permit the child to handle the tongue blade, nasal speculum, and flashlight in order to overcome fear of the instruments. Then ask the child to stick out the tongue and say "Ah," louder and louder. In some cases, this may allow an adequate examination. In others, a child who is cooperative enough may be asked to "pant like a puppy"; while this is being done, the tongue blade is applied firmly to the rear of the tongue. Gagging need not be elicited in order to obtain a satisfactory examination. In still other cases, it may be expedient to examine one side of the tongue at a time, pushing the base of the tongue first to one side and then to the other. This may be less unpleasant and is less apt to cause gagging.

(2) Young children may have to be restrained to obtain an adequate examination of the throat. Eliciting a gag reflex may be necessary if the oropharynx is to be adequately seen.

(3) The small child's head may be restrained satisfactorily by the parent's hands placed at the level of the child's elbows while the arms are held firmly against the sides of the child's head.

(4) A child who can sit up can be held on the parent's lap, back against the parent's chest. The child's left hand is held in the parent's left, the right hand in the right, and the hands are placed against the child's groin or lower thighs to prevent slipping. If the throat is to be examined in natural light, the parent faces the light. If artificial light and a head mirror are used, the light should be behind the parent. In either case, the physician uses one hand to hold the head in position and the other to manipulate the tongue blade.

(5) Young children seldom complain of sore throat even in the presence of significant infection of the pharynx and tonsils.

Ears

Pinnas (position, size), canals, tympanic membranes (landmarks, mobility, perforation, inflammation, discharge), mastoid tenderness and swelling, hearing.

Practical notes:

(1) A test for hearing is an important part of the physical examination of every infant and child. If a parent says that the child does not hear well, this must be investigated until disproved.

(2) The ears of all sick children should be examined.

(3) When actually examining the ears, it is often helpful to place the speculum just within the canal, remove it and place it lightly in the other ear, remove it again, and proceed in this way from one ear to the other, gradually going farther and farther, until a satisfactory examination is completed.

(4) In examining the ears, use as large a speculum as possible and insert it no farther than necessary, both to avoid discomfort and to avoid pushing wax in front of the speculum so that it obscures the field. The otoscope should be held balanced in the hand by holding the handle at the end nearest the speculum. One finger should rest against the child's head to prevent injury resulting from sudden movement.

(5) Pneumatic insufflation to test mobility of the tympanic membrane should always be part of the examination.

(6) The child may be restrained most easily if lying prone.

(7) Low-set ears are present in a number of congenital syndromes, including several associated with mental retardation. The ears may be considered low-set if they are below a line drawn from the lateral angle of the eye to the external occipital protuberance.

(8) Congenital anomalies of the urinary tract are frequently associated with abnormalities of the pinnas.

(9) To examine the ears of an infant, it is usually necessary to pull the auricle backward and downward; in the older child, the external ear is pulled backward and upward.

Neck

Position (torticollis, opisthotonos, inability to support head, mobility), swelling, thyroid (size, contour, bruit, isthmus, nodules, tenderness), lymph nodes, veins, position of trachea, sternocleidomastoid (swelling, shortening), webbing, edema, auscultation, movement, tonic neck reflex.

Practical note: In the older child, the size and shape of the thyroid gland may be more clearly defined if the gland is palpated from behind.

Thorax

Shape and symmetry, veins, retractions and pulsations, beading, Harrison's groove, flaring of ribs, pigeon breast, funnel shape, size and position of nipples, breasts, length of sternum, intercostal and substernal retraction, asymmetry, scapulas, clavicles, scoliosis.

Practical note: At puberty, in normal children, one breast usually begins to develop before the other. Tenderness of the breast is relatively common in both sexes. Gynecomastia is not uncommon in boys.

Lungs

Type of breathing, dyspnea, prolongation of expiration, cough, expansion, fremitus, flatness or dullness to percussion, resonance, breath and voice sounds, rales, wheezing.

Practical notes:

(1) Breath sounds in infants and children normally are more intense and more bronchial, and expiration is more prolonged, than in adults.

(2) Most of the young child's respiratory movement is produced by abdominal movement; there is very little intercostal motion.

(3) If the stethoscope is placed over the child's mouth and the sounds heard by this route are subtracted from the sounds heard through the chest wall, the difference usually represents the amount produced intrathoracically.

Heart

Location and intensity of apex beat, precordial bulging, pulsation of vessels, thrills, size, shape, auscultation (rate, rhythm, force, quality of sounds—compare with pulse with respect to rate and rhythm; friction rub—variation with pressure), murmurs (location, position in cycle, intensity, pitch, effect of change of position, transmission, effect of exercise) (see Chapter 16).

Practical notes:

(1) Many children normally have sinus dysrhythmia. The child should be asked to take a deep breath to determine its effect on the rhythm.

(2) Extrasystoles are not uncommon in childhood.

(3) The heart should be examined with the child erect, recumbent, and turned to the left.

Abdomen

Size and contour, visible peristalsis, respiratory movements, veins (distention, direction of flow), umbilicus, hernia, musculature, tenderness and rigidity, rebound tenderness, tympany, shifting dullness, pulsation, palpable organs or masses (size, shape, position, mobility), fluid wave, reflexes, femoral pulsations, bowel sounds.

Practical notes:

(1) The abdomen may be examined with the child prone in the parent's lap, held over the shoulder, or seated or the examining table facing away from the doctor. These positions may be particularly helpful where tenderness, rigidity, or a mass must be palpated. In the infant, the examination may be aided by having the child suck at a ''sugar tip'' or nurse at a bottle.

(2) Light palpation, especially for the spleen, often will give more information than deep palpation.

(3) Umbilical hernias are common during the first 2 years of life. They usually disappear spontaneously.

Male Genitalia

Circumcision, meatal opening, hypospadias, phimosis, adherent foreskin, size of testes, cryptorchidism, scrotum, hydrocele, hernia, pubertal changes. Tanner stage should be noted.

Practical notes:

(1) In examining a suspected case of cryptorchidism, palpation for the testicles should be done before the child has fully undressed or become chilled or had the cremasteric reflex stimulated. In some cases, examination while the child is in a warm bath may be helpful. The boy should also be examined while sitting in a chair holding his knees with his heels on the seat; the increased intra-abdominal pressure may push the testes into the scrotum.

(2) To examine for cryptorchidism, one should start above the inguinal canal and work downward to prevent pushing the testes up into the canal or abdomen.

(3) The penis of an obese boy may be so obscured by fat as to appear abnormally small. If this fat is pushed back, a penis of normal size is usually found.

Female Genitalia

Vagina (imperforate, discharge, adhesions), size of vaginal opening (in prepubertal children), hypertrophy of clitoris, pubertal changes. Tanner stage should be noted (I–V).

Practical note: Digital or speculum examination is rarely indicated before puberty.

Rectum & Anus

Irritation, fissures, prolapse, imperforate anus. Note muscle tone, character of stool, masses, tenderness, sensation.

Practical note: The rectal examination should be performed with the little finger (inserted slowly). Examine the stool on glove finger (gross, microscopic, culture guaiac) as indicated.

Extremities

A. General: Deformity, hemiatrophy, bowleg (common in infancy), knock-knee (common at age 2–3 years), paralysis, edema, temperature, posture, gait, stance, asymmetry.

B. Joints: Swelling, redness, pain, limitation, tenderness, motion, rheumatic nodules, carrying angle of elbows, tibial torsion.

C. Hands and Feet: Extra digits, clubbing, simian lines, curvature of little finger, deformity of nails, splinter hemorrhages, flatfeet (feet commonly appear flat during first 2 years of life), abnormalities of feet, dermatoglyphics, width of thumbs and big toes, syndactyly, length of various segments, dimpling of dorsa, temperature.

D. Peripheral Vessels: Presence, absence, or diminution of arterial pulses.

Practical note: Normal femoral arterial pulsations during the newborn period do not definitely exclude coarctation.

Spine & Back

Posture; curvatures; rigidity; webbed neck; spina bifida; pilonidal dimple or cyst; tufts of hair; mobility; mongolian spots; tenderness over spine, pelvis, and kidneys.

Neurologic Examination (after Vazuka)

A. Cerebral Function: General behavior, level of consciousness, intelligence, emotional status, memory, orientation, illusions, hallucinations, cortical sensory interpretation, cortical motor integration, ability to understand and communicate, auditory-verbal and visual-verbal comprehension, visual recognition of object, speech, ability to write, performance of skilled motor acts.

B. Cranial Nerves:

1. I (olfactory)–Identification of odors; disorders of smell.

2. II (optic)–Visual acuity, visual fields, ophthalmoscopic examination.

3. III (oculomotor), IV (trochlear), and VI (abducens)–Ocular movements, strabismus, ptosis, dilatation of pupil, nystagmus, pupillary accommodation, pupillary light reflexes.

4. V (trigeminal)–Sensation of face, corneal reflex, masseter and temporal muscle reflexes, maxillary reflex (jaw jerk).

5. VII (facial)–Wrinkling forehead, frowning, smiling, raising eyebrows, asymmetry of face, strength of eyelid muscles, taste on anterior portion of tongue.

6. VIII (vestibulocochlear)–

a. Cochlear–Hearing, lateralization, air and bone conduction, tinnitus.

b. Vestibular–Caloric tests.

7. IX (glossopharyngeal) and X (vagus)–Pharyngeal gag reflex; ability to swallow and speak clearly; sensation of mucosa of pharynx, soft palate, and tonsils; movement of pharynx, larynx, and soft palate; autonomic functions.

8. XI (accessory)–Strength of trapezius and sternocleidomastoid muscles.

9. XII (hypoglossal)–Protrusion of tongue, tremor, strength of tongue.

Practical note: Cranial nerve function is usually observed in young children. Formal testing is not realistic in most cases.

C. Cerebellar Function: Finger to nose; finger to examiner's finger; rapidly alternating pronation and supination of hands; ability to run heel down other shin and to make a requested motion with foot; ability to stand with eyes closed, walk normally, walk heel to toe; tremor; ataxia; posture; arm swing when walking; nystagmus; abnormalities of muscle tone and speech.

D. Motor System: Muscle size, consistency, and tone; muscle contours and outlines; muscle strength; myotonic contraction; slow relaxation; symmetry of posture; fasciculations; tremor; resistance to passive movement; involuntary movement.

E. Reflexes:

1. Deep–Bicep, brachioradialis, tricep, patellar, and Achilles reflexes; rapidity and strength of contraction and relaxation.

2. Superficial–Abdominal, cremasteric, plantar, and gluteal reflexes.

3. Neonatal–Babinski, Landau, Moro, rooting, suck, grasp, and tonic neck reflexes.

Developmental Assessment

Both a history for "milestones" and developmental screening tests are part of the routine physical evaluation.

Practical note: Screening devices are not diagnostic of particular problems but merely indicate a need for further developmental evaluation.

Development & Growth | 2

David Burgess, MD

Development and growth are continuous dynamic processes occurring from conception to maturity and taking place in an orderly sequence that is approximately the same for all individuals. At any particular age, however, wide variations can be found among normal children; these variations reflect the active response of the growing individual to numerous hereditary and environmental factors.

Development signifies maturation of organs and systems, acquisition of skills, ability to adapt more readily to stress, and ability to assume maximum responsibility and to achieve freedom in creative expression. Growth signifies increase in size.

DEVELOPMENTAL SCREENING & SURVEILLANCE

To provide comprehensive pediatric care, the physician and other health care providers should be aware of normal development at all ages and should be particularly familiar with development during the earliest years. Systematic screening and surveillance are 2 approaches to monitor development and identify developmental deviations.

Screening Tests

In accordance with the guidelines for health supervision put forth by the American Academy of Pediatrics, a 2-stage developmental screening program was devised for use in the primary health care setting to detect developmental delays in infancy and the preschool years. The first stage consists of the Revised Prescreening Developmental Questionnaire (R-PDQ) (Fig. 2–1) and is followed by the Denver II (the 1990 revision of the Denver Developmental Screening Test [DDST]) (Fig. 2–2) as a second stage screening for children identified as suspect.

A. First Stage Screening: The R-PDQ is a parent-answered questionnaire designed to achieve 3 goals:

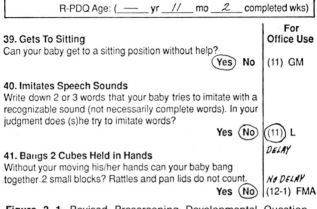

Figure 2–1. Revised Prescreening Developmental Questionnaire.

(1) To make parents more aware of the development of their children.

(2) To document systematically the developmental progress of individual children.

(3) To facilitate early identification of children whose development may be delayed.

Administration of the R-PDQ consists of the following steps (the appropriate R-PDQ form must be used depending on the age of the child):

(1) The child's R-PDQ age is calculated.

(2) The R-PDQ is given to the child's care-giver, who completes it based on available instructions. All appropriate questions must be answered.

(3) Delays are identified. A delay is an item passed by 90% of children (in the original DDST norming studies) at a younger age than that of the child being screened.

Children who have no delays on the R-PDQ are considered developmentally normal. If a child has one or more delays, second stage screening with the Denver II should be considered.

B. Second Stage Screening: The use of the R-PDQ will identify between 15 and 30% of the population as being suspect. Those children who are suspect on first stage screening should be considered for second stage screening using the Denver II.

A child who receives a suspect result on the Denver II (1 or more delays, defined above, and/or 2 or more cautions, an item passed by 75% of children in the Denver II norming sample at a younger age than the child being tested) should be considered for further medical/developmental evaluation.

To use the Denver II effectively, individual examiners must be trained to administer and interpret the test properly. Denver II training consists of an introductory video tape, the Denver II training manual, a written proficiency test accompanied by a video test, practice testing, and administration of the Denver II for a trained observer. Completion of this training insures that the Denver II will be administered in a standardized, reliable manner. A free catalog describing the training materials, the Denver II, and the R-PDQ is available from Denver Developmental Materials, P.O. Box 6919, Denver, CO 80206-0919, (303) 355–4729.

C. Developmental Surveillance: Developmental surveillance is a concept whereby knowledgeable professionals perform skilled observations of children throughout all encounters during child health care. Components include a relevant developmental history, accurate and informative observations, and listening and attending to parental concerns. Developmental surveillance is a process of ongoing monitoring of a child's development rather than a static view of development at one point in time. Within this context, the R-PDQ and/or the Denver II can be used to improve the accuracy of this process. Regardless of whether the R-PDQ/Denver II is used to perform systematic screening of a defined population or within the concept of developmental surveillance, the results from a single screen should not be interpreted in isolation but rather within the context of the overall assessment of each child including the medical history, developmental history, physical findings, and parental concerns.

GROWTH

General Considerations

A. Fetal Growth: During fetal life, the rate of growth is extremely rapid. During the early months, the fetal rate of gain in length is greater than the rate of gain in weight when expressed as percentage of value at birth. By the eighth month, the fetus has achieved 80% of the birth length and only 50% of the birth weight (Table 2–1).

Date

Name

Birthdate

Hosp. No.

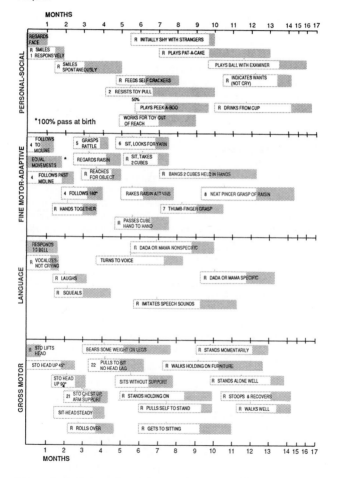

Figure 2–2. Denver Developmental Screening Test.

SCREENING TEST

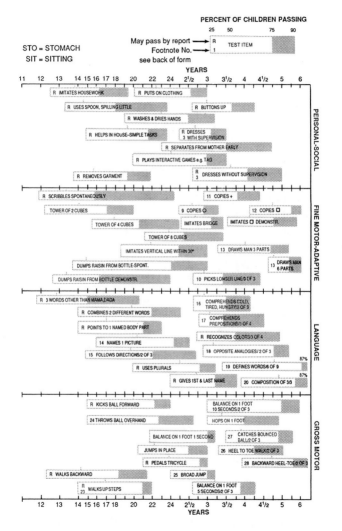

Figure 2–2 (cont'd). Denver Developmental Screening Test.

Table 2–1. Fetal and newborn dimensions and weights of the body and its organs.[1]

Fetal Age (wk)[2]	Crown-heel (cm)	Crown-rump (cm)	Head Circumference (cm)	Body Weight (g)	Adrenal (g)	Brain (g)	Heart (g)	Kidney (g)	Liver (g)	Lungs (g)	Pancreas (g)	Pituitary (g)	Spleen (g)	Thymus (g)	Thyroid (g)
Prenatal and Newborn															
12	9.0	7.5	7.4	18.6	0.087	2.32	0.098	0.163	0.097	0.69	0.013		0.006	0.010	0.026
16	16.7	12.8	12.6	100	0.417	14.40	0.662	0.962	5.94	3.23	0.095	0.011	0.086	0.122	0.133
20	24.2	17.7	17.6	310	1.07	43	2.08	2.77	16.8	8.18	0.314	0.024	0.41	0.553	0.352
24	31.1	21.9	22.3	670	2.02	91	4.47	5.69	34.5	15.2	0.695	0.040	1.16	1.53	0.684
28	37.1	25.5	26.3	1150	3.16	153	7.70	9.43	57.4	23.7	1.22	0.058	2.43	3.14	1.08
30	39.8	27.1	28.1	1400	3.78	189	9.78	11.5	70.3	28.2	1.53	0.067	3.26	4.18	1.33
32	42.4	28.5	29.9	1700	4.44	228	11.6	13.8	84.3	33.0	1.88	0.076	4.25	5.41	1.54
34	44.8	29.9	31.5	2000	5.11	268	13.7	16.2	100.0	37.8	2.24	0.085	5.36	6.77	1.78
36	47.0	31.2	33.1	2450	5.77	309	15.9	18.6	113.0	42.7	2.61	0.094	6.55	8.22	2.01
38	49.1	32.4	34.4	2900	6.45	352	18.2	21.0	129.0	47.5	3.01	0.103	7.86	9.82	2.26
40	51.0	33.5	35.7	3150	7.10	394	20.6	23.5	143.5	52.5	3.40	0.111	9.22	11.5	2.50
Postnatal															
Age (yr)															
1	See Inside Back Cover				4	875	43	62	350	160		0.15	30	23	
5					5	1250	90	110	575	305		0.23	55	28	
10					6	1325	145	150	825	450		0.33	77	31	
15					8	1340	245	220	1275	675		0.48	125	27	
Adult[3]															
Male					6	1375	300	320	1600	1000			165	14	
Female					6	1280	250	280	1500	750			150	14	

[1] Adapted from Edith Boyd. See also inside back cover.
[2] Time from first day of last menstrual period.
[3] Adapted from several sources.

24

B. Organs: At birth, the proportion of the weight of the pancreas and the musculature to that of the entire body is less in the infant than in the adult; that of the skeleton, lungs, and stomach is the same; and that of other organs is greater in the infant than in the adult. Major types of postnatal growth of various parts and organs of the body are shown in Figure 2–3.

C. Trunk/Leg Ratio: At birth, the ratio of the lower to the upper segment of the body (as measured from the pubis) is approximately 1:1.7. The legs grow more rapidly than does the trunk; by age 10–12 years, the segments are approximately equal.

D. Height: Rate of growth is generally more important than actual size. For more accurate comparisons, data should be recorded both as absolute figures and as a percentile for that particular age, and the rate of growth should be determined. Birth length is doubled by approximately age 4 years and tripled by age 13 years. The average child grows approximately 10 inches (25 cm) in the first year of life, 5 inches (12.5 cm) in the second, 3–4 inches (7.5—10 cm) in the third, and approximately 2–3 inches (5–7.5 cm) per year thereafter until the growth spurt of puberty appears (Fig. 2–4).

E. Weight: Body weight is probably the best index of nutri-

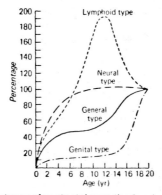

Figure 2–3. Major types of postnatal growth of various parts and organs of the body. Redrawn and reproduced, with permission, from Holt LE, McIntosh R, Barnett HL: *Pediatrics*, 13th ed. Appleton-Century-Crofts, 1962, as redrawn from Harris JA et al: *Measurement of Man*. University of Minnesota Press, 1930.

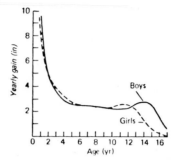

Figure 2–4. Yearly gain in height. Redrawn and reproduced, with permission, from Holt LE, McIntosh R, Barnett HL: *Pediatrics*, 13th ed. Appleton-Century-Crofts, 1962, as redrawn from Harris JA et al: *Measurement of Man.* University of Minnesota Press, 1930.

tion and growth. The average infant weighs approximately 7 lb 5 oz (3.33 kg) at birth. Within the first few days of life, the newborn loses up to 10% of the birth weight. Birth weight is doubled between 4 and 5 months of age, tripled by the end of the first year, and quadrupled by the end of the second year. Between ages 2 and 9 years, the annual increment in weight averages about 5 lb (2.25 kg) per year (Fig. 2–5).

F. Growth at Puberty: See Chapter 9.

G. Growth Charts: Standard growth charts are available that allow height, weight, and head circumference to be plotted longitudinally during well child care.

Specific Considerations

A. Head & Skull: At birth the head is approximately two-thirds to three-fourths of its total mature size, whereas the rest of the body is only one-fourth its adult size.

Six fontanels (anterior, posterior, 2 sphenoid, and 2 mastoid) are usually present at birth. The anterior fontanel normally closed between 10 and 14 months of age, but may be closed by age 3 months or remain open until age 18 months. The posterior fontanel usually closes by age 4 months, but in some children may not be palpable at birth. Cranial sutures do not ossify completely until later childhood. Growth of the skull, as determined by increasing head circumference, is a much more accurate index of brain growth than is the presence or size of the fontanel.

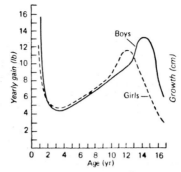

Figure 2–5. Yearly gain in weight. Redrawn and reproduced, with permission, from Holt LE, McIntosh R, Barnett HL: *Pediatrics,* 13th ed. Appleton-Century-Crofts, 1962, as redrawn from Harris JA et al: *Measurement of Man.* University of Minnesota Press, 1930.

B. Sinuses: Maxillary and ethmoid sinus are present at birth, but are not usually aerated for approximately 6 months. The sphenoid sinuses are not usually visible on x-ray until after the third year of life. Frontal sinuses usually become visible by x-ray between 7 and 9 years of age, but seldom before age 5.

The mastoid process at birth is relatively large and has a relatively wide communication with the middle ear. Its cellular structure gradually appears between birth and age 3 years.

C. Respiration & Heart Rate: The respiratory rate decreases steadily during childhood, averaging approximately 30 breaths per minute during the first year of life, 25 during the second year, 20 during the eighth year, and 18 by the 15th year.

The heart rate falls steadily throughout childhood, averaging about 150 bpm in utero, 130 bpm at birth, 105 bpm during the second year of life, 90 bpm during the fourth year, 80 bpm during the sixth year, and 70 bpm during the tenth year.

D. Abdomen: The abdomen tends to be prominent in infants and toddlers. In the infant, the ascending and descending portions of the colon are short compared with the transverse colon, and the sigmoid extends higher in the the abdomen than during later life.

Gas may be roentgenographically visualized in the stomach almost immediately after birth, in the ileum within 2 hours and, on the average, in the rectum in 3–4 hours.

E. Muscle: At birth, muscle constitutes 25% of total body weight, as compared with 43% in the adult.

F. Ossification Centers: At birth, the average full-term infant has 5 ossification centers demonstrable by x-ray: distal end of femur, proximal end of tibia, calcaneus, talus, and cuboid. The clavicle is the first bone to calcify in utero, calcification beginning during the fifth fetal week.

G. Senses: At birth, the newborn infant has mature sensory receptors for pressure, pain, and temperature over the entire body surface, in the mouth, and in the external genitalia; there are also mature pain receptors in the viscera and proprioceptive receptors in muscles, joints, and tendons.

1. Taste–The ability to taste is present in the newborn infant, who is capable of distinguishing the 4 basic tastes.

2. Olfaction–The human infant is born with fully mature receptors for olfaction.

3. Hearing–Normal infants can hear almost immediately after birth, but they respond to sounds at a subcortical level.

4. Vision–About 80% of newborn infants are hyperopic. At birth, the infant demonstrates an awareness of light and dark, possesses peripheral vision, and is capable of rudimentary fixation on near objects. At age 4 months, vision is 20/300–20/200; at age 10 months, 20/200; and by age 2–3 years may reach 20/30–20/20.

Strabismus may be present, normally for the first 4–6 months of life, but persistent deviation requires evaluation.

Susceptibility to amblyopia, subnormal visual acuity in one or both eyes despite correction of refractive error, is greatest during the first 2–3 years of life and lasts until full visual stability has been achieved by the age of 5–6 years. The key to successful treatment of amblyopia is early detection.

H. Water Content: The water content of the body is approximately 95% by weight during early fetal life, 65–75% at birth, and 55–60% at maturity.

I. Blood: At birth, 5% of all red blood cells may be reticulocytes; this percentage drops to less than 1% after the second week of life. Nucleated red cells (up to 5% as a percentage of total number of nucleated cells) and immature lymphocytes may be present in the newborn, but disappear within the first week of life. Fetal hemoglobin accounts for 80% of total hemoglobin at birth, 70% of the total at age 2 weeks, and 45% at age 5 weeks; it falls to less than 10% by age 20 weeks.

The leukocyte count is high at birth, rises slightly during

Table 2-2. Dental growth and development.

Primary or Deciduous Teeth

	Calcification		Eruption		Shedding	
	Begins At	Complete At	Maxillary	Mandibular	Maxillary	Mandibular
Central incisors	4th fetal mo	18–24 mo	6–10 mo	5–8 mo	7–8 yr	6–7 yr
Lateral incisors	5th fetal mo	18–24 mo	8–12 mo	7–10 mo	8–9 yr	7–8 yr
Cuspids	6th fetal mo	30–39 mo	16–20 mo	16–20 mo	11–12 yr	9–11 yr
First molars	5th fetal mo	24–30 mo	11–18 mo	11–18 mo	9–11 yr	10–12 yr
Second molars	6th fetal mo	36 mo	20–30 mo	20–30 mo	9–12 yr	11–13 yr

Secondary of Permanent Teeth

	Calcification		Eruption[1]	
	Begins At	Complete At	Maxillary	Mandibular
Central incisors	3–4 mo	9–10 yr	7–8 yr (3)	6–7 yr (2)
Lateral incisors	Maxilla 10–12 mo Mandible 3–4 mo	10–11 yr	8–9 yr (5)	7–8 yr (4)
Cuspids	4–5 mo	12–15 yr	11–12 yr (11)	9–11 yr (6)
First premolars	18–24 mo	12–13 yr	10–11 yr (7)	10–12 yr (8)
Second premolars	24–30 mo	12–14 yr	10–12 yr (9)	11–13 yr (10)
First molars	Birth	9–10 yr	5½–7 yr (1)	5½–7 yr (1a)
Second molars	30–36 mo	14–16 yr	12–14 yr (12)	12–13 yr (12a)
Third molars	Maxilla 7–9 yr Mandible 8–10 yr	18–25 yr	18–25 yr (13)	17–30 yr (13a)

[1] Figures in parentheses indicate order of eruption. Many otherwise normal infants do not conform strictly to the stated schedule.

the first 48 hours after birth, falls for the next 2–3 weeks, and then rises again. The lymphocyte count is highest during the first year of life, and then falls progressively during the remainder of childhood.

J. Urine: The average infant secretes 15–50 mL of urine per 24 hours during the first 2 days of life, 50–300 mL per day during the next week, and 400–500 mL per day by the latter half of the first year. There is subsequently a gradual increase in urinary output; 700–1500 mL per day secreted between the ages 8 and 14 years.

K. Tears: Tears often are not present with crying until after 1–3 months of age.

L. Teeth: Stages of dental growth and development are shown in Table 2–2.

Ambulatory Pediatrics | 3

Barton D. Schmitt, MD

HEALTH MAINTENANCE VISITS

Health maintenance or health supervision visits are the key to preventive pediatrics. The visit has several purposes: responding to the parent's or child's current concerns, presenting age-appropriate anticipatory guidance, assessing growth and development (Chapter 2), performing a physical examination (Chapter 1), obtaining laboratory screening tests, and administering immunizations (Chapter 6).

PARENTAL CONCERNS

The first part of each well-child visit should be directed toward dealing with the current concerns of the parent, usually the mother. Most expectant mothers have many questions that should be discussed with their pediatrician several weeks prior to delivery. The most frequent concerns include arguments for and against breast-feeding and circumcision, hospital policies about rooming-in and parent–infant contact in the delivery room, essential baby equipment, and ways of decreasing sibling jealousy. It was traditional for the first newborn office visit to take place at 6 weeks. However, a 2-week postpartal office visit is much more logical. First-time mothers who are breast-feeding should bring the baby in for a weight check at 1 week.

A health maintenance visit without parental concerns is uncommon. Some mothers bring a list of questions, ''How much should babies cry?'' ''How do I know he's getting enough to eat?'' ''Can I spoil her by picking her up too much?'' ''Is it all right to spank children?'' ''How old should Johnny be before I let him cross the street alone?'' Many of the questions have no clear-cut answers. The seasoned pediatrician usually enjoys the challenge of these discussions and the satisfaction that comes with reassuring an anxious parent.

ANTICIPATORY GUIDANCE

Anticipatory guidance usually includes nutritional counseling, accident prevention, behavioral counseling, suggestions for developmental stimulation, sex education, dental recommendations, medical information, etc. Special counseling is in order for adolescents (see Chapter 9). A list of suggested topics to be discussed at particular ages is found on the health maintenance forms presented in Figure 3–1. A blank space or line on these forms indicates that a comment is required following that item. All anticipatory guidance advice is followed by the optimal age for discussion in parentheses. A check mark that follows each of these advice items indicates that this counseling was done.

INJURY PREVENTION

Injuries kill more children than the 6 other leading causes of childhood deaths combined. Between ages 1 and 14, over 50% of deaths are due to injuries; between ages 15 and 23, over 80% are due to injuries. Each year 100,000 children under 15 years of age are left with permanent disabilities owing to injuries. During the first 3 years of life, children have little sense of danger or self-preservation. They are totally dependent on adults to look after their safety.

Injury prevention advice should be an integral part of medical care provided for all infants and children. Several years ago, the American Academy of Pediatrics put together The Injury Prevention Program (TIPP), which includes parent questionnaires for assessing risk and information sheets to prevent accidents. The main thrust of the program was to advise parents in the 5 following areas:

  (1) Approved child car restraints.
  (2) Smoke detectors.
  (3) Hot water heater set to less than 130°F.
  (4) Guards for windows and gates for stairways.
  (5) Syrup of Ipecac.

PEDIATRIC HEALTH MAINTENANCE
Birth through 3 months

Parent's concerns

Newborn data base
  Birth weight _____ Gestational age _____
  Pregnancy or delivery problems Neonatal problems

Growth (comment on growth curve)

Feeding advice
  Formula _____ oz/24 hours_____
  Breast-feeding: Frequency _____ min/feeding _____
  Vitamins _____ Iron _____
  Solids _____ Fluoride drops _____
  Feeding problems
  Advice: Introduce bottle in breast fed (2m) ❑; Introduce fluids other than milk (2m) ❑

Developmental status
  Stimulation advice: Hold baby (2m) ❑ Talk to baby (2m) ❑

Childrearing advice
  Sleep pattern _____
  Crying or colic _____
  Mother-child interaction _____
  Sibling rivalvy (2w) _____

Family status
  Advice: Paternal involvement, family planning (2w) ❑ Utilize sitter (2m) ❑

Accident prevention advice
  Car seat, crib safety (2w) ❑ Rolling over (2m) ❑ Smoke detector ❑

Medical advice
  Demonstrate use of suction bulb for nose (2w) ❑ Foreskin or circumcision care ♂
  2w ❑ Temperature taking, Tylenol and fever handout (2m) ❑ Discuss when to call
  doctor (2m) ❑

Intercurrent illness

Figure 3–1. Pediatric health maintenance record.

PEDIATRIC HEALTH MAINTENANCE
4 months through 14 months

Parent's concerns

Growth (comment on growth curve)

Feeding advice
  Formula _____   oz/24 hours_____
    Breast-feeding: Frequency _____   min/feeding _____
  Vitamins _____   Iron _____
  Solids _____   Fluoride drops _____
  Feeding problems_____
  Advice: No bottles in bed; introduce solids, spoon, cup (4m) ❏
  Confirm intake of iron-rich solids (6m) ❏
  Introduce finger foods, confirm on 3 meals/day (9m) ❏
  Entirely on table foods. Phase out bottle by 18 mo (12m) ❏

Developmental status
  Stimulation advice: Toys for reaching (4m) ❏ Avoid confining baby equipment (6m) ❏
  Repeat baby's sounds (9m) ❏ Name objects and pictures for baby (12m) ❏

Childrearing advice
  Sleep pattern _____
  Behavior problems _____
  Advice: Sleeps through the night (4m) ❏ Normal separation anxiety (6m) ❏
  Discipline: Use negative voice and eye contact rather than physical punishment (9m) ❏
  Don't punish for normal exploratory behavior, discuss positive strokes for good
    behavior (12m) ❏

Family status

Accident prevention advice
  Safe toys (4m) ❏ Stairs and gates, drowning in bathtub (9m) ❏
  Electrical cords (6m) ❏ Ipecac and poison talk (12m) ❏

Medical Advice
  Teething myths (6m) ❏ Avoid expensive shoes (9m) ❏ Use of 911 (12m) ❏

Intercurrent Illness

Figure 3–1. Pediatric health maintenance record. (*Continued*)

PEDIATRIC HEALTH MAINTENANCE
15 months through 3 years

Parent's concerns

Growth (comment on growth curve)

Diet
  Milk _____ oz/24 hours
  Eating problems _____
  Advice: Entirely on table foods, off all bottles (18m) ❏
  Normal decreased appetite, iron intake (2y) ❏

Developmental status
  Advice: Read to child (1¹⁄₂, 2) ❏ Listen to child (2) ❏ TV rules (3) ❏

Childrearing advice
  Sleep problems _____
  Behavior problems _____
  Frequency of spanking _____
  Advice: Don't punish for normal negativism, ignore temper tantrums (1¹⁄₂) ❏
  Discuss toilet training and readiness (1¹⁄₂, 2, 3) ❏
  Discuss positive "strokes" for good behavior (2) ❏
  Emphasize consistency in discipline and use of time-out room (2, 3) ❏

Family status

Injury prevention advice
  Scalds, aspiration foods (1¹⁄₂) ❏ Street/garage safety (2) ❏
  Drowning in ditch and pools (3) ❏

Dental advice
  Brushing frequency _____ Fluoride intake _____
  Advice: Avoid snacks that cause cavities (1¹⁄₂) ❏ Benefits of fluoride toothpaste (2) ❏
  Brushing techniques (3) ❏

Intercurrent Illness

Figure 3–1. Pediatric health maintenance record. (*Continued*)

PEDIATRIC HEALTH MAINTENANCE
4 years thorough 5 years

To be completed by parent	Check correct answer	
School readiness:		
1. Does your child pay attention when being read to?	Yes	No
2. Can your child play quietly for over $\frac{1}{2}$ hour?	Yes	No
3. Does your child mind adults and follow instructions?	Yes	No
4. Does your child speak clearly enough for others to understand?	Yes	No
5. Does your child object to being left with a sitter?	No	Yes
6. Can your child dress without help?	Yes	No
7. Does your child ever wet or soil him/herself during the day?	No	Yes

To be completed by physician or nurse

Parent's concerns

Growth (comment on growth curve)

Diet

School readiness
  Problems detected by above questions _____
  Development: PDQ (4, 5) Score _____ Weak category _____
    DDST (if fails PDQ) Result _____
    Articulation: DASE (4) Score _____ Percentile _____
  Advice: Preschool if any problems (4) ☐

Injury prevention advice
  Adult seat belts, petting dogs (4) ☐ Crossing street, trampoline (5) ☐

Dental advice
  No daytime thumb-sucking (4) ☐ No nighttime thumb-sucking (5) ☐
  Frequency of brushing _____ Type of toothpaste _____Fluoride intake _____

Intercurrent Illness

Figure 3–1. Pediatric health maintenance record. (*Continued*)

PEDIATRIC HEALTH MAINTENANCE
6 years through 11 years

Parent's concerns

Diet

School
　Name of school ＿＿＿＿＿＿＿＿＿＿＿＿＿＿＿＿　Grade ＿＿＿＿＿＿
　Academic performance ＿＿＿＿＿＿＿＿＿＿＿＿＿＿＿＿＿＿＿＿＿
　Attendance ＿＿＿＿＿＿＿＿＿＿＿＿＿＿＿＿＿＿＿＿＿＿＿＿＿
　Behavior ＿＿＿＿＿＿＿＿＿＿＿＿＿＿＿＿＿＿＿＿＿＿＿＿＿＿
　Advice: Child's responsibility for schoolwork (6) ❑
　　Adult at home before and after school (6–10) ❑

Behavior
　Behavior problems ＿＿＿＿＿＿＿＿＿＿＿＿＿＿＿＿＿＿＿＿＿＿
　Chores ＿＿＿＿＿＿＿＿＿＿＿＿＿＿＿＿＿＿＿＿＿＿＿＿＿＿＿
　Friends ＿＿＿＿＿＿＿＿＿＿＿＿＿＿＿＿＿＿＿＿＿＿＿＿＿＿
　Advice: TV less than 2 h/d (6) ❑ Understanding of death (6) ❑
　　One sport or club (8–10) ❑ Smoking (10) ❑

Family status

Sex education
　Discuss puberty and menarche before junior high school (10) ❑
　Menstrual status (10 ♀) ＿＿＿＿＿＿＿＿＿＿＿＿＿＿＿＿＿＿＿

Injury prevention advice
　Bicycle safety (6) ❑ Swimming lessons (8) ❑
　Fires, matches (10) ❑

Dental advice
　Frequency of brushing ＿＿＿＿ Type of toothpaste ＿＿＿＿ Fluoride intake ＿＿＿＿
　Dental referral (6) ❑

Intercurrent Illness

Figure 3–1. Pediatric health maintenance record. (*Continued*)

PEDIATRIC HEALTH MAINTENANCE
12 years through 18 years

Parent's concerns

Adolescent's concerns

Growth (comment on growth curve)

Diet

School
 Name of school _____ Grade _____
 Academic performance _____
 Attendance _____
 Behavior _____
 Career plans _____

Behavior
 Free time/friends _____
 Chores/job _____
 Person to confide in _____
 Predominant mood _____
 Advice: Discuss values of babysitting (12) ❑ Discuss drugs and alcohol (12–16) ❑
  Discuss smoking (14) ❑

Family status
 Advice: Discuss independence and parent's trust (16) ❑

Sex education
 Dating, masturbation (14) ❑ Marriage (18) ❑
 Sexual activity, preventing pregnancy, STD (14, 16, 18)_____

Injury prevention advice
 Firearms (12) ❑ Cycling safety (14) ❑ Driving safety, water safety (16) ❑
 Motorcycles, seat belts, riding with driver who drinks (18) ❑

Dental advice
 Frequency of brushing _____ Type of toothpaste _____

Medical advice
 Acne ❑ Personal hygiene (14) ❑ Teach self-examination of breasts (16♀) ❑

Intercurrent Illness

Figure 3–1. Pediatric health maintenance record. (*Continued*)

38

Motor Vehicle Crashes

The number one killer and crippler of children in the United States is motor vehicle crashes. Proper use of car safety seats can reduce fatalities and hospitalizations by at least 70%. Laws have been passed in all 50 states that require children to be sitting in an approved safety seat. The type of safety seat depends on the child's weight. In general, the smaller seats are more protective and should be used as long as they are appropriate. The following are guidelines for selecting a seat based on weight: less than 20 pounds, rear-facing infant seat; 20 to 40 pounds: forward-facing toddler seat; 40 to 60 pounds: booster seat; over 60 pounds: regular lap belt; over 48 inches (4 feet): the shoulder strap can be safely used.

Prevention of Burns

(1) Never drink anything hot while holding a baby.

(2) Keep hot substances away from the edge of a table or stove.

(3) Don't let your child touch the faucet handles in the bathtub.

(4) Set your hot water heater to less than 130°F.

(5) Use flame-resistant sleepwear.

(6) Install smoke detectors in your home.

(7) Keep cigarette lighters and matches away from children.

(8) Keep electric cords unplugged or out of the reach of children.

Prevention of Choking

(1) Don't allow your children to have foods that are commonly aspirated into the lungs until they are old enough to chew them (usually 4 years of age): nuts of any kind, sunflower seeds, orange seeds, cherry pits, raw carrots, raw peas, raw celery.

(2) Carefully chop up any foods that might block the windpipe, such as hot dogs, grapes, and caramels.

(3) Warn babysitters and siblings not to share these foods with small children.

(4) Don't allow children to run or play with food in their mouth.

(5) Avoid toys with small detachable parts that could enter the windpipe.

(6) Dispose of button batteries carefully.

Prevention of Drowning

(1) Never leave a child less than 3 years old unattended in the bathtub or a wading pool.

(2) Never leave children who can't swim unattended near a swimming pool—more children drown in backyard swimming pools than at beaches or public pools.

(3) Remember that infant water programs are for fun, not for learning how to swim. (Children cannot be made water safe before age 3.)

(4) Try to arrange swimming lessons for your child between ages 3 and 8.

Prevention of Head Trauma

(1) Never leave an infant of any age alone on a high place.

(2) Always leave the side rails on the crib up.

(3) Avoid bunk beds before age 6.

(4) Avoid baby walkers. (Over 35% of infants using them have an accident requiring emergency care. The most serious accidents occur when children fall down a stairway in a walker. Keep a sturdy gate at the top of all stairways.)

(5) Teach your child how to cross the street safely at age 5 or 6.

(6) Don't teach your child to ride a bicycle until age 7 or 8.

(7) Forbid trampolines.

Prevention of Poisoning

(1) Keep chemicals and drugs locked up and out of reach. Drain cleaners, furniture polish, and insecticides are the most dangerous of the common household poisons.

(2) Use the safety cap on all drug containers.

(3) Have some syrup of Ipecac handy.

(4) Know the telephone number of your nearest poison control center.

PHYSICAL EXAMINATION

A complete physical examination should be performed during most health maintenance visits (see Chapter 1). Height, weight, and head circumference should be measured and plotted on growth curves (see Chapter 2). During childhood, most chronic diseases will affect growth. Although physical examinations are usually normal, they serve as a point of reference in evaluating future illnesses. Therefore, the extent of the examination should be carefully recorded. To save time, the checklist shown in Table 3–1 can be used. Elaboration is required only for the abnormal findings.

Some physical findings are silent—ie, they are not noticee-

Table 3–1. Checklist for physical examination.

	Normal	Abnormal
1. GENERAL APPEARANCE: well nourished, hydrated, alert		
2. SKIN: color, rash, swelling, hair, nails		
3. HEAD: shape, anterior fontanelle		
4. EYES: conjunctiva, cornea, pupils, extraocular movement		
5. EARS: pinnae, canals; tympanic membrane appearance, mobility		
6. NOSE: nares, turbinates		
7. MOUTH: tongue, teeth, oral mucosa, tonsils, pharynx		
8. NECK: thyroid, range of motion		
9. NODES: cervical, axillary, inguinal, other		
10. CHEST: symmetry, expansion, breasts		
11. LUNGS: rate, auscultation, percussion		
12. HEART: rate, rhythm, S_1, S_2, murmur, femoral pulses		
13. ABDOMEN: contour; palpation of liver, spleen, and kidney; mass; tenderness		
14. GENITALIA: ♀ external; ♂ penis, meatus, testes, hernia		
15. SPINE: curvature (scoliosis), sacral area		
16. EXTREMITIES: range of motion, tenderness, edema, clubbing, cyanosis		
17. NEUROLOGIC (SCREEN): cranial nerves 3, 4, 6, 7, and 12; gait; cerebellar function; motor system (strength, tone)		
18. NEUROLOGIC (COMPLETE): above plus other cranial nerves: sensory and motor systems (deep tendon reflexes, clonus)		

able to parents and cause few if any symptoms. Of greatest concern are disorders that are treatable if detected early but potentially serious when not detected. A routine examination will diagnose most such conditions (eg, congenital heart disease). A few conditions are detected only by a detailed examination (eg, retinoblastoma [red fundus reflection test], strabismus [corneal light reflection test], congenital hip dislocation [Ortolani maneuver, or restricted abduction], scoliosis, coarctation of the aorta [femoral pulses], hypertension, lower urinary tract obstruction [inquire about urine stream], imperforate hymen, and labial adhesions). Visual deficits (eg, refractive errors or color blindness) and hearing deficits can also be missed if appropriate testing is not included. Dental caries may be overlooked by physicians who assume, not always rightly, that their patients are receiving periodic dental examinations. Baby bottle caries of the upper incisors should be looked for in any child over age 1 who still receives a bottle. Early cancer detection can be improved by teaching self-examination of the breasts or testes.

THE SCHOOL READINESS EXAMINATION

The preschool examination of the 4- or 5-year-old child should be designed to answer the basic question, "Is the child ready for school?" Auscultation of the heart and lungs at this time is probably far less important than noting any abnormalities of speech, hearing, or vision and determining if developmental age is commensurate with chronologic age, if attention span is adequate for learning, and if parents have adequately prepared the child for separation when entering school. These problems should also be investigated earlier, but they are of greatest significance at the preschool examination. A school readiness screening questionnaire is included in Figure 3–1.

Vision

Five to 10% of preschool children have some kind of visual impairment. The illiterate E chart, Snellen chart, STYCAR test, or Allen picture cards can be used for checking visual acuity, and each eye should be tested separately. Testing should be attempted at age 3. The 5-year-old child should have a visual acuity of 20/30 (6/9) or better in both eyes, and there should be no more than a 1-line difference between the 2 eyes. Suppression amblyopia affects 3% of children and must be detected early before permanent loss of vision occurs. Amblyopia is often secondary to strabismus, which can be detected by noting the position where light is reflected off both corneas or by the cover test. Alignment can be tested by 6 months of age.

Hearing

Fixed hearing deficits occur in approximately 1% of young school children, and in 10% the loss is profound and bilateral. More children have a temporary hearing loss from recurrent purulent otitis media or serious otitis media. Although the losses are generally not too severe, if they occur at an inopportune time they may be sufficient to prevent an early school-age child from learning phonics; hence, the effect of the loss may be carried on and magnified throughout much of the school years (see Chapter 13). If such losses are detected before entry into school, some of the learning, behavior, and discipline problems that occur secondary to poor attention might be averted. Audiologic screening tests can be performed by nonprofessional technicians and should be a part of the preschool examination.

Speech

The child entering school should be able to speak distinctly and clearly without difficulty; should be able to answer questions; and, after a period of getting acquainted, should be able to carry on a conversation with the physician about recent events. Poor speech may impair performance in school. An easily administered screening articulation test—the Early Language Milestone Scale—has been developed to identify children who should be referred to a speech pathologist for definitive evaluation.

LABORATORY SCREENING TESTS

A health maintenance flow sheet (Fig. 3–2) is a helpful reminder to the nurse and physician that certain procedures, laboratory tests, developmental evaluations, and immunizations need to be done. All these items can be initiated by the nurse or aide if the physician establishes the routine to be followed.

Blood

Iron deficiency anemia (see Chapter 19) is found more often in lower socioeconomic populations and has its highest incidence

Title: _____   Hosp. No.: _____   Date of Birth: _____

Name: _____

Directions: Record date only for all immunizations.
Record value for head circumference, height, weight, BP, and Hct.
Record N (normal) or ABN (abnormal) for all other items.

	NB	2 wk	2 mo	4 mo	6 mo	9 mo	12 mo	15 mo	18 mo	2 yr	3 yr	4 yr	5 yr	6 yr	8 yr	10 yr	12 yr	14 yr	16 yr	18 yr
Today's date																				
Head circumference																				
Height (cm)																				
Weight (kg)																				
BP																				
Dental caries screen																				
DTP (Td after 6 years)																				
OPV																				
Measles, mumps, rubella																				
Haemophilus influenzae type b conjugated vaccine																				

Figure 3–2. Health maintenance flow sheet.

TB test[6]																					
PDQ or DDST = R[7]																					
Speech (ELM)																					
Hearing[1]																					
Vision[2]																					
Metabolic screen[3]																					
Hct																					
Sickle cell test for black patients[4]																					
Pap smear/GC[5]																					

LEGEND:

[1] High-risk inquiry (NB)
Listens to soft sounds (2m)
Turns to sound (6m)
Audiometrics (4y and thereafter)

[2] Red reflex (NB or 2w)
Regards smiling face (2m)
Follows past midline (4m)
Corneal light reflections test (6m)
Visual acuity (3y and thereafter)
Color vision once (6y)

[3] PKU, thyroid, galactosemia (newborn nursery)
PKU retest (2w) if first test done before 48 hours
Perform according to state law.

[4] If not performed in newborn, perform at 2 months of age

[5] Sexually active patients

[6] High risk groups; TB test yearly

[7] Screen with PDQ if high school graduate. Screen with
DDST=Revised if parent did not complete high school.
If child fails PDQ or DDST=R, perform complete DDST.

Figure 3-2. Health maintenance flow sheet. (*continued*)

in infants between 9 and 24 months of age. A routine hemoglobin or hematocrit is recommended in this age group and is particularly important in the child who received a low iron formula or whose diet is low in iron-containing foods. The American Academy of Pediatrics (1991) continues to recommend routine hematocrits at 9 months and at 2, 8, and 18 years.

Children with sickle cell disease (see Chapter 19) must be diagnosed before 6 months of age to prevent death due to sepsis or splenic sequestration (10–20% mortality rate). Do not wait for the routine hematocrit at age 9 months. Prophylactic antibiotics should be started by 3 months of age. It is strongly recommended that all black newborns have hemoglobin electrophoresis performed on cord blood or in conjunction with heel-stick testing for phenylketonuria. If it is not done then, the test should be performed at the 2-month check-up.

All states now require screening for phenylketonuria (see Chapter 7) by blood test in the hospital nursery prior to the infant's discharge. An infant with this disorder who failed to ingest sufficient milk protein may have a negative test in the first few days of life. Therefore, most centers recommend a repeat test at 10–14 days of age if the first test was performed before 48 hours of age. Screening newborns for other treatable causes of mental retardation, congenital hypothyroidism, and galactosemia is required in most states and should be performed in all newborns regardless of the state law. A T_4 or TSH assay can be done by using cord blood.

Screening for lead poisoning (see Chapter 30) is extremely important in areas where the child has access to lead-based paint or soil contaminated by lead. Children living in such neighborhoods should have a routine blood lead level performed at 18–24 months of age. This test should be repeated at 6-month intervals until age 3 years in children with pica or where there is an index case in their building.

Universal cholesterol testing of all children is controversial. For now, the AAP recommends testing of those children who have a family history of hyperlipidemia (cholesterol > 240) or early myocardial infarction (< 50 years of age in men and < 60 in women). Testing should be performed at 2 to 3 years of age.

Urine

Routine urinalysis has a low yield in the asymptomatic patient. In contrast to the adult population, it is unusual for a child to have asymptomatic diabetes, and proteinuria is a rare presenting sign for renal abnormality in an asymptomatic child. Transient orthostatic proteinuria is common in adolescents but benign. While many physicians recommend that the urine dipstick test be performed only on symptomatic children, testing once at age 3 or 4 is not unreasonable. The American Academy of Pediatrics (1991) continues to recommend routine urinalysis at 6 months and at 2, 8, and 18 years.

In screening for asymptomatic urinary tract infection, microscopic examination of the urinary sediment is time-consuming and not reliable. Several inexpensive methods are available to screen a first-morning specimen for bacteriuria (eg, nitrite or glucose detection strips), followed by a urine culture if the dipstick test is positive. Since untreated asymptomatic bacteriuria usually clears spontaneously and does not lead to renal damage, screening should be reserved for high-risk groups (eg, children with diabetes). On the other hand, the clinician must not hesitate to check the urine for bacilluria in any child with unexplained fevers, unexplained abdominal pain, enuresis, foul-smelling urine, or other vague symptoms.

Teenage girls who are sexually active will benefit from annual gonococcal cultures, chlamydia cultures, and Papanicolaou smears. Birth control counseling and sexuality counseling can also be offered at this time.

IMMUNIZATIONS

A child's immunization status can be easily monitored on the health maintenance flow sheet (Fig. 3–2). A record of the child's immunizations should also be given to the parents and updated by the nurse as additional immunizations are given. The details of routine immunization of children are presented in Chapter 6.

ACUTE ILLNESS VISITS

ASSESSING ACUTE ILLNESS

Optimal management of an acute illness mainly includes telephone triaging, office triaging, diagnosis, assessment of the need for hospitalization, home therapy, and a follow-up plan.

1. TELEPHONE TRIAGING & ADVICE

Does the Patient Need to Be Seen?

The physician is the person best qualified to give medical advice, both in the office and over the phone. However, because talking with parents on the phone may take up too much of the physician's time, this function is usually delegated to another member of the office team. Most of the questions are routine ones that require only routine answers. An office nurse specifically trained for the role is probably the best person to take routine calls. Office policies about medical advice over the phone should be standardized. Routine instructions for handling minor infections, minor injuries, reactions to immunizations, infant feeding problems, newborn care, and prescription refills are easy to communicate to parents if they are written down in an office protocol book. The protocol book should also specify the point at which each problem requires an office visit. This decision depends on (1) the type of symptom, (2) the duration of the symptom, (3) the age of the patient, (4) whether or not the patient acts "very sick," (5) an assessment of the parents' anxiety, and (6) the presence of any underlying chronic disease. (For example, most patients under 1 year of age with diarrhea and vomiting need to be examined.) After telephone baseline data are gathered, the nurse must be able to decide whether the child needs to be seen immediately, by appointment, or can safely be cared for at home. The nurse should err on the side of giving an appointment when in doubt. For patients not seen, any pertinent telephone data should be entered on a temporary log sheet.

2. OFFICE TRIAGING & PROCEDURES

How Sick Is the Patient?

The nurse should screen all sick patients as soon as possible after they arrive at the office. They can be thought of in terms of 3 general groups: emergency, contagious, and minor illness. Most patients have a minor illness (eg, cold, accident, earache) and can be seen at their appointed time. Some patients are contagious until proved otherwise and should quickly be moved from the waiting room to an isolated examining room (eg, febrile illnesses with rashes, lice, jaundice, possible pertussis). An attempt should be made to keep children with bronchiolitis or croup away from infants. When an office emergency (eg, febrile seizures, respiratory distress) is recognized by the nurse, the physician should be notified immediately. The physician can take appropriate emergency action, stabilize the patient, and arrange for transfer to the hospital if necessary (eg, an acidotic, dehydrated infant).

Preparation of the Patient for the Physician

The office aide can record the sick patient's temperature, height, and weight. The office nurse can record the chief complaint. Depending upon the symptom, the nurse can take vital signs and initiate the office's standing orders on laboratory procedures and symptomatic treatment listed below.

Initial Treatment & Laboratory Workup

Steps in initial management are listed below. Details of procedures are outlined elsewhere in the text.

A. Abodominal Pain: Take samples for urinalysis and urine culture; save stool specimen for occult blood testing.

B. Animal Bite: Wash out immediately with liquid soap and water for 10 minutes. Initiate the official reporting form, and call the county health department. Delay irrigation if the wound is infected and a culture is needed.

C. Cough: If present over 1 month, apply a tuberculin skin test.

D. Diarrhea: Take a sample for stool culture if the stool contains blood or mucus or if diarrhea has persisted for more than 1 week at any age. For children under age 2, give 180 mL (6 oz) of an oral electrolyte solution, and record the naked weight on each visit. If a child appears dehydrated, collect urine for specific gravity.

E. Earache: Give acetaminophen if in obvious pain. If there is a possibility of mumps, isolate the patient.

F. Eye Injury: Test visual acuity if child is over age 3. Place eye tray in the examining room.

G. Fever: In children, the degree of fever may not reflect the severity of the disease process. Extremes of temperature may occur without relation to the significance of the infection. A small infant may have a very serious illness with normal or subnormal temperatures, whereas a 2- to 5-year-old child may have a fever above 40°C (104°F) with a minor respiratory infection. In children over age 8 years, temperature response is similar to that in adults.

Some children with high temperatures may convulse ("febrile convulsions"). Therefore, rapid elevation of temperature should receive prompt care in the form of antipyretic therapy. Fever and convulsions may be the presenting findings of a central nervous system infection, and the patient may require a spinal tap for diagnostic evaluation. In general, fever as high as 41°C (105.8°F) is not in itself harmful.

For a fever over 39°C (102.2°F), give acetaminophen at 15 mg/kg per dose. Put the child in an examining room and assist with undressing. Give a sponge bath if the temperature exceeds 40°C (104°F) despite drugs and if the child is uncomfortable. Provide a bag for urine if the child is not toilet trained. If unexplained fever has been present over 24 hours, order a white count and differential. If the infant is under 2 months of age, notify the physician immediately.

H. Fractures: Notify physician immediately, obtain equipment to immobilize the site, and fill out the x-ray request.

I. Head Injury: Record vital signs and level of consciousness, and check pupils for equal size and reaction to light.

J. Infectious Hepatitis Exposure: Record weights of persons who have had close contact with the patient, and anticipate giving immune serum globulin, 0.03 mL/kg intramuscularly.

K. Lacerations: Wash thoroughly for at least 10 minutes. Check date of last tetanus shot and record. Shave around the wound edges if necessary (but never shave eyebrows). Have parents sign consent for suturing.

L. Nosebleed: Instruct the parent or child on how to compress the bleeding site for 10 minutes. Check blood pressure. If a chronic problem, perform fingerstick for hematocrit.

M. Painful Urination (Burning or Frequency): Take sample for urinalysis, urine culture, nitrite dipstick, and a gram-stained smear of unspun drop.

N. Pinworms: Record the approximate weights of all family members if the infection is a recurrent one (see Chapter 11).

O. Sore Throat: Take material for throat culture (contraindicated if the patient has croup).

P. Streptococcal Sore Throat (Culture Positive): Inquire about penicillin allergy and record. Arrange for symptomatic family contracts to have throat cultures taken.

Q. Vomiting: Record exact weight. Give patient emesis basin and sips of ice water while waiting. If patient appears dehydrated, collect urine for specific gravity.

3. THE WORKING DIAGNOSIS

The physician makes the final decision about the diagnosis and the severity of the disease. Emergency conditions (eg, shock or meningitis) may be noted and emergency intervention begun. A history of recent contact with persons with contagious diseases is often important. Severity can be partially assessed by inquiries about playfulness, energy, ability to sleep, and the parent's feelings about how sick the child is this time compared with other times. If a family of sick children is brought in, the physician should ask the mother which children she considers the sickest. The physical examination should be mainly directed toward the chief complaint. A patient with a dog bite does not require a complete examination, but a patient with an earache must be checked for mastoid swelling and meningeal signs in addition to otoscopic examination. A child with a fever usually requires a complete exam.

Utilizing the conventional techniques of history, physical examination, and laboratory tests, the physician will correctly diagnose most acute chief complaints. However, a vigilant clinical mind is necessary in order not to miss a diagnosis of septicemia. Septic children usually present with unexplained fever, but (unlike children with acute viral fevers) they often will not smile or play, even with their parents. They frequently are physically exhausted and too weak to resist the physical examination, constantly irritable and unable to sleep, and respond paradoxically to cuddling by the mother. Irritability usually stems from pain or hypoxia. A less common finding in the toxic child is constant lethargy or sleepiness. This is difficult to assess because most sick children sleep more than normally.

4. INDICATIONS FOR HOSPITALIZATION

For every acute problem, the physician must decide whether to treat the child at home or in the hospital.

The 3 major indications for hospitalization are major emergencies, potentially life-threatening illnesses, and psychosocial problems.

Major Emergencies

Some examples of obvious life-threatening conditions are shock, severe dehydration, coma, meningitis (bacterial or of unknown cause), respiratory distress, congestive heart failure, symptomatic hypertension, acute renal failure, status epilepticus, and surgical emergencies.

Potentially Life-Threatening or Crippling Illnesses

Some patients are not in critical condition when first seen but require hospitalization because their problem may be rapidly progressive during treatment. If deterioration occurs in the hospital, emergency therapy can be rapidly instituted. Most of the entities in this group are caused by infection or trauma. Endogenous diseases rarely change this rapidly. Although absolute rules cannot be formulated for every situation, the following guidelines can be applied to most cases of acute illness. Obviously, these recommendations will have some exceptions, such as when the emergency room has an 8-hour observation area.

The following sections list problems that may require hospitalization, according to body systems:

A. Skin:

1. Cellulitis if the patient is less than 2 months old; if there is buccal involvement or the cavernous sinus drainage area is involved; if underlying sinusitis or osteomyelitis is suspected; if cellulitis is secondary to a puncture wound in the foot; or if there is no response after 2 days of therapy.
2. Erysipelas, toxic empidermal necrolysis, or acute necrotizing fasciitis. Omphalitis if the patient is less than 2 months old.
3. Suspected thrombophlebitis.
4. Burns (second- or third-degree) involving more than 10% of surface area (> 15% if the patient is more than 1 year old); burns of perineal area, hand, or face if they might need grafting; all inhalation burns; and most electrical burns.
5. Purpura or petechiae with fever, without fever but unexplained, or without fever but progressive.

B. Eyes:

1. Gonococcal conjunctivitis or bacterial keratitis.
2. Eye injury if visual activity is decreased.
3. Papilledema.

C. Ears, Nose, and Throat:

1. Acute otitis media if the patient is less than 1 month old with fever, systemic symptoms, or no response after 2 days of therapy.
2. Mastoiditis.
3. Sinusitis if overlying redness or edema is present.

4. Nasal obstruction if the patient is less than 6 months old and an apneic episode has occurred.

5. Epistaxis if uncontrolled; if hypertension is present; if there is bleeding elsewhere; or if severe anemia is present.

6. Fluctuant tonsillar abscess.

7. Retropharyngeal abscess.

8. Diphtheria (any symptoms at any age).

9. Cervical adenitis if the patient is toxic, dehydrated, dysphagic, dyspneic, or less than 6 months old and needs treatment by incision and drainage.

   D. Respiratory System:

1. Epiglottis (all cases).

2. Croup if there is stridor at rest, dyspnea, or drooling; if the child has repeatedly awakened from sleep with stridor; if there is a history of a previous bout with rapid progression; if there are apneic or cyanotic episodes; or if the patient is less than 1 year old and the stridor is easily provoked (eg, occurs with any crying).

3. Pertussis if symptomatic and the patient is less than 1 year old; pertussis at any age if accompanied by apnea, respiratory distress, a whoop, or weight loss.

4. Bronchiolitis if the patient is dyspneic, has a resting respiratory rate greater than 60, has apneic or cyanotic episodes (Po_2 < 50), has poor fluid intake, or is unable to sleep.

5. Asthma if respiratory distress persists after 2 injections of epinephrine or 2 nebulized doses of a beta-agonist.

6. Pneumonia if the patient is less than 1 month old; if bacterial pneumonia is suspected and the patient is less than 6 months old; if there is a history of dyspnea (any age); if there is pleural effusion; if staphylococcal pneumonia is suspected (any age); if aspiration pneumonia is present; if fluid intake is poor; if there is underlying cystic fibrosis or congenital heart disease; or if there is no response after 2 days of therapy.

7. Suspected foreign body of the airway.

8. Hemoptysis if unexplained; if there is bleeding elsewhere; or if anemia is present.

9. Apnea in all cases except periodic breathing, breath-holding spells, or mild choking on food.

   E. Cardiovascular System:

1. Suspected subacute bacterial endocarditis.

2. Any myocarditis or pericarditis.

3. Acute hypertension or shock.

4. Unexplained dysrhythmias.
   F. Gastrointestinal System:
1. Vomiting with dehydration, delirium, or persistent abdominal pain.
2. Hematemesis if documented and not caused by swallowed blood.
3. Diarrhea if explosive in character; if accompanied by abdominal distention or associated Kussmaul repirations; if typhoid fever is suspected in a patient of any age; if acute *Shigella* infection is suspected in a patient less than 1 year old; or in a patient who has moderate or mild dehydration with vomiting or fluid refusal.
4. Melena or unexplained bright-red blood mixed in the stools.
5. Suspected appendicitis, peritonitis, or intussusception.
6. Abdominal trauma if penetrating injury has occurred or if damage to the spleen, liver, kidneys, pancreas, or intestines is suspected.
7. Toxic ileus.
   G. Urinary System:
1. Pyelonephritis if the patient is less than 2 months old, toxic, or unimproved after 2 days of therapy; if gram-negative sepsis is suspected; if underlying renal disease is present; or if recurrences have been frequent.
2. Acute edema, oliguria, or azotemia.
3. Hematuria with symptoms listed in (2), renal colic, and unexplained or posttraumatic gross hematuria.
4. Acute urinary retention.
   H. Genitalia:
1. Vaginitis if associated with salpingitis.
2. Vaginal injury with sharp object.
3. Suspected testicular torsion.
4. Priapism.
   I. Skeletal System:
1. Suspected osteomyelitis.
2. Arthritis if possibly septic or acute rheumatic fever.
3. Wringer injury if above the elbow; if a hematoma or avulsed skin is present; if a fracture or nerve injury is present; or if the peripheral pulse is diminished.
   J. Nervous System:
1. Aseptic meningitis if the level of consciousness is depressed or there is a motor deficit.
2. Suspected tetanus.
3. Suspected epidural spinal abscess or brain abscess.

4. Febrile or afebrile seizures if they continue more than 30 minutes; if there are persistent neurologic signs; if the level of consciousness is decreased; or if serious underlying disease cannot be ruled out.
5. Head injury if the patient has been unconscious longer than 5 minutes; if there are persistent neurologic signs; if the level of consciousness is decreased; if a seizure has occurred; if cerebrospinal fluid rhinorrhea or otorrhea is present; if there is significant swelling over the middle meningeal artery; if there are retinal hemorrhages or progressive headaches; or if abnormal or irregular vital signs are present.
6. Skull fractures that are depressed or compound (ie, into air sinuses or overlying scalp laceration), fractures across the middle meningeal artery or venous sinus, occipital fracture into the rim of the foramen magnum, or any fracture with an underlying bleeding disorder.
7. Suspected spinal cord trauma.
8. Acute muscle weakness.
9. Acute cognitive deterioration (altered mental status), including delirium that is unexplained or persists longer than 2 hours.
10. Suspected increased intracranial pressure.

K. General:

1. Fever if the patient is less than 2 months old; if toxicity is evident and serious underlying disease cannot be ruled out; or if fever is due to heat stroke.
2. Poisoning if the patient is symptomatic (eg, respirations slow or irregular, drowsiness, etc); the agent or dosage is unknown; or the dosage is a potentially fatal one.
3. Suspected lead poisoning.
4. Unexplained mass.
5. Failure to thrive if severe or unexplained or if serious neglect is suspected.
6. Unexplained hypoglycemia.
7. Suspected anaphylactic reaction with laryngeal reaction, bronchospasm, hypotension, or dysrhythmias.
8. Inconsolable crying or irritability lasting several hours.

Psychosocial Problems

Patients with acute psychosocial problems now comprise a larger proportion of hospitalized children than was formerly the case. In many cities, the child can be placed in an emergency receiving home or an acute psychiatric ward. Sometimes the child can temporarily stay with a relative. Psychosocial indications for hospitalization fall into 3 general groups: parent, child, and disease problems.

A. Parent Problems:

1. Child abuse (eg, physical abuse, failure to thrive secondary to neglect, or incest).

2. Incipient battering (eg, the parent has made a homicidal threat against a child).

3. Absent parents (eg, abandonment, emancipated minors without caretakers, or the parents themselves are hospitalized).

4. Physically exhausted parents (eg, no sleep for 2 nights).

5. Severely overanxious parents (eg, if the parents remain immobilized and extremely anxious after a careful explanation of their child's illness).

6. Neglectful parents who seem uninterested in their child's illness or therapy (eg, neglected eczema). This is a rare situation compared with overly anxious parents.

7. Intellectually incompetent parents (eg, a mentally retarded mother who cannot reliably follow verbal or written instructions).

8. Emotionally disturbed parents who need psychiatric hospitalization and treatment for their own problems (eg, a floridly psychotic mother).

9. Parent who is an alcoholic or drug abuser.

B. Child Problems:

1. Suicide attempt—a short hospital admission allows time for the mental health worker to make an evaluation and for the family to look seriously at their problems.

2. A destructive, dangerous child can be held on a pediatric ward pending placement. A dangerous adolescent will require a psychiatric care facility.

3. An incapacitating emotional symptom (eg, a severe conversion reaction such as paraplegia or blindness).

C. Disease Problems:

1. An incapacitating (but not life-threatening) physical disease (eg, severe Syndenham's chorea).

2. Initial diagnosis of a disease with a complex treatment regimen. The parents and patient deserve a careful, unhurried, and organized introduction to the complex home management of some chronic diseases (eg, diabetes mellitus).

3. Initial diagnosis of a life-threatening disease—this gives the family time to work through the impact phase (eg, leukemia).

4. Terminal care if the family does not want the child to die at home.
5. Chronic diseases that are exacerbated by family conflicts (eg, ulcerative colitis).
6. Hazardous home (eg, carbon monoxide or lead poisoning).

5. TREATMENT OF THE NONHOSPITALIZED PATIENT

Words are as necessary as drugs in the treatment of a sick child. The parents expect to be told their child's diagnosis and its causes, prognosis, and treatment. They also need to have their special concerns acknowledged and clarified. If this communication does not take place, the parents will often be dissatisfied with the quality of care being given, and their compliance with regard to medications, advice, and follow-up will probably be less than optimal.

If the child has a mild acute illness (eg, viral nasopharyngitis), the parent would be reassured by the following general types of comment.

Diagnosis

"David has a cold." The diagnosis should be conveyed in plain English, not in medical jargon. If the physician does not specifically state the diagnosis, the parents may assume none has been arrived at.

Etiology

"It's due to a virus." This means to most parents that the infection is not serious. Some parents need an added statement that there was nothing they could have done to prevent it—eg, "Everyone is coming down with this."

Parents' Concerns

Mothers often do not listen to their physician's instructions until their own main concerns have been discussed. These concerns are easily elicited by Korsch's 3 questions: (1) "Why did you bring David to the clinic today?" (2) "What worried you most about him?" (3) "Why did that worry you?" After these concerns are out in the open, the physician is in a position to clarify misconceptions. Reassurance can be specific—eg, "He doesn't have meningitis, appendicitis, dehydration, etc."

Treatment

In self-limited disease, the goal of medication is to keep the patient comfortable. A list of useful approaches to management (sometimes overlooked) is as follows: (1) An antipyretic is useful if the patient's fever causes discomfort. (2) Dextromethorphan can be used for an acute cough that interferes with sleep. (3) Teaching the parent how to suction the nose properly can turn a restless baby into a sleeping one. (4) Advice about diet and bed rest is also appreciated by the parent. In general, free choice and frequent small feedings at intervals of 1–2 hours are sufficient to maintain optimal water, electrolyte, and sugar intake during the acute phase of the illness. Enforced bed rest should be avoided since it usually leads to crying and distress. In addition, it's unnecessary and not enforceable. (5) Isolation within the family structure is rarely indicated, since exposure has usually preceded the diagnosis. (6) Parents can be reassured about temporary moodiness and emotional regression during an acute illness. A return to the previous level of maturity need not be encouraged until good health returns.

Prognosis

"David will probably feel better in 2 or 3 days. This is not a serious infection. If his fever lasts over 3 days or he gets worse, give me a call." Nothing is gained by mentioning all the possible complications. Without promoting anxiety, the door to additional medical evaluation is quietly left open for any new problems that might arise.

Closing

"You're doing a fine job with David. Just hold the fort and he will be his old self in a few days." The visit should close on a positive note, even a compliment if possible. If David is older, an attempt can be made to boost his morale as well—eg, "This won't keep *you* out of action for long."

6. FOLLOW-UP OF THE NONHOSPITALIZED PATIENT

Many children seen in an emergency room have conditions that require following up (eg, asthma, bronchiolitis, croup, pneumonia, otitis media, burns, and seizures). If a child has an ambiguous diagnosis (eg, high fever of unknown origin) or an unpredictable course (eg, vomiting), daily follow-up is necessary. This protects both the patient and the physician. Follow-up can be accomplished by revisits, telephone calls, or a visiting nurse.

Revisits

Daily office visits are the best approach to the more serious problem. The weight of an infant with diarrhea and the degree of respiratory distress in a child with croup cannot be estimated over the phone. If a scheduled appointment is not kept, the office clerk should immediately notify the physician, and a phone call or home visit should be made on that same day. If transportation is a problem for the parent, a community service agency can usually help. If the late results of laboratory tests indicate that an illness is quite serious (eg, stool culture growing *Salmonella* in a 2-month-old infant) and reasonable attempts to locate the parents fail, the police may be asked to find and bring the patient to the clinic or office.

Telephone Calls

A daily telephone call will suffice for milder problems when only historical follow-up data are needed (eg, vomiting or lethargy). Since these calls are essential to proper management, the physician or nurse should make them. A daily telephone list can be kept and the charts pulled prior to calling. If the follow-up is felt to be important, parents should not be depended upon to initiate these calls. Telephone calls become the realistic choice of follow-up when long distances and cost are a factor.

THE PREVENTION OF MALPRACTICE SUITS

The management of acute illness offers the greatest potential for malpractice litigation in pediatrics. Physicians are legally liable for injuries caused not only by their own mistakes but by the mistakes of their employees as well. Errors can be made in any of the areas previously discussed. An error in telephone triaging can result in a delay in diagnosis (eg, calling meningococcemia a viral exanthem, or arranging an appointment for the next day for scrotal pain that turns out to be a testicular torsion). An error in underhospitalization can lead to death (eg, epiglottitis being treated on an outpatient basis). Errors in therapy may result in sciatic nerve palsy if an injection is given into an inappropriate quadrant of the buttocks or may result in acute rheumatic fever if penicillin is not given for streptococcal sore throat because it was not cultured. Errors in follow-up can result in undiagnosed abdominal pain silently progressing to ruptured appendix.

To improve patient care and decrease your risk for malpractice suits, consider the following suggestions:

(1) Stay up-to-date in your field. Read journals, attend conferences, and discuss cases with your colleagues. Understand the changing standards of care for the various conditions you treat.

(2) Maintain accurate, complete, and legible medical records. Consider common complications of the conditions you diagnose, and record their absence.

(3) Document all telephone advice. Telephone triage by office staff should be linked to written protocols.

(4) Don't prescribe prescription drugs without examining the patient first.

(5) Avoid excessive waiting time in your office, since this is a leading cause of parent dissatisfaction.

(6) Seek consultation whenever you are uncertain about what is happening with an acutely and perhaps seriously ill patient.

(7) Obtain parent written consent (eg, for lumbar punctures) or verbal consent (eg, for suturing) unless an emergency exists.

(8) Base all medical decisions on what is best for the patient.

MEDICAL CARE COMPLIANCE

One aspect of quality of care not easy to assess by chart review is patient compliance. Superb recommendations do not guarantee implementation. Medical care does not become effective until the parent accepts the diagnosis and carries out the therapeutic recommendations. Compliance is improved by providing written instructions, including the parent in treatment planning, simplifying the treatment regimen, linking medication-taking with daily routines, explaining the reason for each treatment, and clarifying misconceptions. Strong parent–physician rapport also enhances compliance. The physician must make an effort to find out why appointments are not kept, medications are not given, etc; otherwise, even the best-conceived therapeutic goals will often not be achieved.

Nutrition & Feeding | 4

K. Michael Hambidge, MD, ScD,
& Nancy F. Krebs, MD, MS

The act of feeding is important to the young child not only because of the nutritive substances obtained from the food but also because of the emotional and psychologic benefits derived. Drinking and eating are intense experiences to an infant and can and should be sources of great satisfaction. From these experiences and from the persons who feed them, infants obtain many of their early ideas about the nature of life and people.

Parents must be made to understand that there is much individual variation in the nutritional needs and desires of infants and that differences occur in the same child at various times.

The feeding of children is constantly being made more flexible and simple as knowledge of their nutritional requirements increases; however, certain basic information and data are necessary for a practical understanding of the subject.

Neither strict adherence to a time schedule nor feeding when the infant cries is necessary for successful and satisfactory feeding. For most parents and infants, a flexible schedule with reasonable regularity is most satisfactory, but in some cases either a strict routine or complete "demand" feeding gives better results.

BREAST-FEEDING

Advantages & Disadvantages

Apart from considerations of economy and convenience (temperature, asepsis, automatic adjustment in most instances to infant's needs), breast-feeding is superior to bottle-feeding because the composition of breast milk is ideal for nearly all infants; because breast milk has specific antibacterial and antiviral activities that protect infants from gastrointestinal disease; because breast-feeding produces less infantile allergy; and because breast-feeding can be psychologically beneficial to both mother and infant.

In the past decade, breast-feeding has been reestablished as the predominant mode of feeding the young infant in the United States. Unfortunately, breast-feeding rates remain low among several subpopulations of women, including low-income, minority, and young mothers. Many mothers face unique obstacles to maintaining lactation once they return to work. Skilled use of the breast pump may help to maintain lactation in this circumstance.

Breast-feeding may be temporarily impossible for a weak, ill, or premature infant or one with a cleft palate, although in such cases breast milk may be expressed and fed in another way.

Absolute contraindications to breast-feeding (eg, galactosemia) are rare. Maternal infection with human immunodeficiency virus and untreated tuberculosis are other contraindications.

Infants weighing less than 1500 g are likely to benefit from the addition of an infant milk fortifier to increase the density of energy, protein, calcium, and phosphorus. Some breast-fed infants with cystic fibrosis also will need a supplement.

Menstruation is not a contraindication to breast-feeding.

Transmission of Drugs & Toxins in Breast Milk

Virtually all drugs consumed by the mother will appear in her milk to some degree, usually in homeopathic amounts. Drug excretion into milk is affected by the drug's ionization, lipid solubility, protein binding, and molecular size, as well as other factors. Effects on the infant also depend upon the route of administration, the dosage, and the mother's timing in taking the drugs as well as the drug's metabolites and whether it is absorbed in the gastrointestinal tract. It is believed that the amount of drugs present in breast milk is least just before the mother takes medications.

Maternal use of illicit or recreational drugs is a contraindication to breast-feeding.

While it is wise to observe carefully a nursing infant whose mother is taking medications, very few drugs are actually contraindicated. Those that are include radioactive compounds, antimetabolites, lithium, diazepam (Valium), chloramphenicol, and tetracycline. A regional drug center should be consulted for up-to-date information on which drugs are contraindicated. When a course of therapy of a potentially hazardous drug will be brief, the mother can temporarily interrupt breast-feeding and maintain her supply by expressing and discarding her milk.

Composition of Breast Milk (Table 4–1)

Favorable features of human milk include an optimal amino acid and protein content for the normal infant; a generous, but not excessive, quantity of essential fatty acids; an adequate but relatively low sodium content; a low solute load compared with cow's milk; and very favorable absorption of iron, calcium, and zinc, which results in the provision of adequate quantities of these nutrients to the infant fully breast-fed for 4–6 months.

Breast-fed infants do require standard neonatal prophylactic vitamin K and may require vitamin D supplements if not exposed to any sunlight or if maternal vitamin D status is suboptimal. Breast milk will be low in vitamin B_{12} if the mother is an unsupplemented vegetarian; low in thiamine if the mother abuses alcohol; and low in folate if the mother is generally malnourished.

Management of Breast-Feeding

Because today's grandmothers predominantly bottle-fed their children, the "art" of breast-feeding is no longer automatically passed from mother to daughter. Hence, the role of the health professional in supporting and promoting breast-feeding is of utmost importance.

Perinatal hospital routines and follow-up pediatric care have a great impact on the successful initiation of breast-feeding. Breast-feeding is promoted by prenatal and postpartum education, frequent mother/baby contact after delivery, one-on-one advice about breast-feeding technique, demand feeding, rooming in, avoidance of bottle supplements, early follow-up after delivery, maternal confidence, family support, adequate maternity leave, and accurate advice for common problems such as sore nipples.

Before discharge, individualized assessment should identify those mother/baby pairs needing additional support. In all such cases, there should be early follow-up after discharge. The onset of copious milk secretion between the second and fourth postpartum day is a critical time in the establishment of lactation.

A. Prelactation (Colostrum) Phase: Colostrum is an alkaline, yellow, breast secretion that may be produced during the last few months of pregnancy and for the first 2–4 days after delivery. It has a higher specific gravity (1.040–1.060); a higher content of protein, fat-soluble vitamins, and minerals; and a lower content of carbohydrate and fat than does breast milk.

Colostrum contains secretory IgA, leukocytes, and other

Table 4-1. Comparison of composition of milk and commercial formula (per 100 mL).[1]

Component	Unit	Human Milk	Typical Commercial Formula	Whole Cow's Milk
Osmolality	mosm/kg water	282	290	275
Energy	kcal	67	67	61
Carbohydrate (lactose)	g	7.3	7.2	4.7
Fat	g	4.2	3.8	3.3
Minerals				
Calcium	mg	25	51	119
Chloride	mg (meq)	40 (1.1)	53 (1.5)	102 (2.9)
Copper	μg	35	41	30
Fluorine	μg	7	20	15
Iodine	μg	7	10	5
Iron	μg	40	150 (1200 w/Fe)	50
Magnesium	mg	3	4.1	13
Manganese	μg	0.4	3	2–4
Phosphorus	mg	15	39	93
Potassium	mg (meq)	58 (1.5)	78 (2)	152 (3.9)
Sodium	mg (meq)	15 (0.8)	25 (1.1)	49 (2.1)

64

		100–300	500	300
Zinc	µg			
Proteins				
Casein	mg	187	1185	2700
Lactalbumin	mg	161	52	400
Total proteins	g	0.9	1.5	3.3
Vitamins				
A (retinol equivalents)	µg (IU)	47 (155)	75 (250)	31 (126)
B_6 (pyridoxine)	µg	28	40	42
B_{12} (cyanocobalamin)	ng	26	150	357
C (ascorbic acid)	mg	4	5.5	0.9
D	µg (IU)	0.04 (1.6)	1 (40)	1 (42)
E (total tocopherols)	µg (IU)	315 (0.32)	1700 (1.7)	80 (0.08)
K	µg	0.21	3	6
Folic acid	µg	5.2	5	5
Niacin	µg	200	790	84
Pantothenic acid	µg	225	300	314
Riboflavin	µg	35	100	162
Thiamine	µg	16	65	30

¹ Adapted from various sources.

immune substances that play a part in the immune defenses of the newborn. Colostrum has a natural laxative action and is an ideal starter food.

Although the milk may not "come in" until 2–4 days after delivery, prelactation nursing is very important because of the value of colostrum, the effect of the nursing stimulus to increase milk supply and lessen engorgement, and the opportunity nursing provides for the mother and infant to become accustomed to one another. While some infants nurse irregularly the first few days, others demand feeding as often as every 2 hours. Nursing is commonly limited to 5 minutes per breast per feeding the first day, 10 minutes per breast per feeding the second day, and 15 minutes or longer per breast per feeding thereafter.

There is no need for routine supplementation for the full-term, healthy infant who appears satisfied, but when the infant is persistently hungry or has an underlying condition (eg, hypoglycemia) requiring increased caloric intake, then formula may be offered after nursing until the milk comes in. Once milk is in, further supplements should not be given.

B. Lactation Phase: Forty-eight to 96 hours postpartum, the mother's breasts change from soft to firm and full as engorgement (lactogenesis) occurs. The infant may be fed at each hungry period, day and night, which is usually every 2–3 hours during the first month with longer intervals (4–5 hours) at night. The infant should nurse at the first breast for approximately 10 minutes and then be put to the other breast and allowed to suckle as long as required (unless the nipples are sore). At the next feeding, the last breast nursed should be offered first. During the early weeks of lactation, the milk supply seems to be more sensitive to negative stimuli such as maternal fatigue, anxiety, and lack of suckling. The infant will usually have frequent, somewhat loose bowel movements (often with each feeding) during this period.

The let-down reflex, by which milk is actively ejected through the duct system for easy access to the infant, is usually conditioned and evident by 2 weeks. The mother feels "tightening," "stinging," "tingling," or "burning" circumferentially in both breasts shortly after the infant begins nursing. The nursing mother should eat a well-balanced diet with additional intake of protein, calcium, and fluids. Drinking a glass of liquid with each nursing is helpful. Additional rest, with several naps each day, should be encouraged.

"Frequency days," or "appetite spurts" when infants desire to nurse more often than their established routine, typically occur for several days at approximately 3 weeks, 6 weeks, 3 months, and 6 months of age. Increased frequency of nursing increases the milk supply and allows resumption of the former nursing schedule.

A woman with activities outside the home should feel free to take her nursing infant with her and breast-feed discreetly when the infant is hungry.

Problems with Breast-Feeding

A. Failure to Thrive: Some breast-fed infants fail to thrive. The most common cause of early failure to thrive is poorly managed mammary engorgement, which will rapidly decrease milk supply. Unrelieved engorgement can result from inappropriately long intervals between feeding, improper infant suckling, a nondemanding infant, sore nipples, maternal or infant illness, nursing from only one breast, and latching difficulties. Poor maternal knowledge and lack of maternal fluids and rest can all be factors. Some infants are too sleepy to do well on an ad libitum regimen and, in particular, may need waking to feed at night. Primary lactation failure is rare but does occur. Some decline in weight for age percentiles after 3 months should not necessarily be taken as an indication of inadequate nutrition, since the commonly used percentile charts have been constructed from data on infants who have been primarily formula-fed. However, if there is a decline in weight-for-length of more than 20 percentile points, solids should be introduced earlier than may otherwise be intended and formula supplement may be indicated for individual infants.

B. Breast-Feeding Jaundice: Breast-feeding jaundice is exaggerated physiologic jaundice associated with inadequate intake of breast milk, infrequent stooling, and unsatisfactory weight gain. Where possible, this condition should be managed by increasing the frequency of nursing and, if necessary, augmenting the infant's suckling with regular breast pumping. Supplemental feedings may be necessary but care should be taken not to decrease breast-milk production further.

C. Breast-Milk Jaundice: In a small percentage of breast-fed infants, breast-milk jaundice occurs as the result of an unidentified property of the milk that inhibits conjugation of bilirubin or deconjugates bile in the lumen of the small intestine. In severe cases, interruption of breast-feeding for 24–36 hours may be necessary. The mother's breast should be emptied with an electric breast pump during this period.

D. Sore Nipples: Mild nipple tenderness requires attention to proper positioning of the infant and correct latch-on. Ancillary measures include nursing for shorter periods, beginning feeds on the less sore side, air drying the nipples after nursing, and the application of lanolin cream. Severe nipple pain and cracking usually indicate improper infant attachment. Temporary pumping, which is well tolerated, may be needed.

E. Mastitis: Maternal mastitis should be suspected when a nursing mother complains of a "flu-like" illness, with local breast tenderness. Antibiotic therapy providing coverage against beta-lactamase–producing organisms should be given for 10 days. Analgesics may be necessary but breast-feeding should be continued. Breast pumping may be a helpful adjunctive therapy.

FORMULA FEEDING

The standard milk-based infant formulas (Table 4–2) contain heat-treated protein (at reduced concentration), lactose and minerals from cow's milk, vegetable oils, minerals, and vitamin additives. Iron-fortified formulas are recommended after 2 months. Standard formulas contain 20 kcal/oz and 0.45 g protein/oz.

Evaporated milk formula can be used as an alternative to proprietary infant formulas. It is prepared as follows: To make 32 oz of formula, mix 1 can (13 oz) of whole evaporated milk, 1½ cans (19 oz) of water, and 2 tablespoons of corn syrup. To make 5 oz, mix 2 oz of evaporated milk, 3 oz of water, and 1 teaspoon of corn syrup.

Infants should be fed formula for a minimum of 6 months—or, ideally, for the entire first year of life. Low-fat and skimmed milk are inappropriate for use in the first year of life.

Lactose intolerance is the main indicator for a soy-based formula. Semi-elemental formulas have a wide range of uses in intestinal disease, including malabsorption syndromes, chronic diarrhea, and short-bowel syndrome. They are also used in infants who are intolerant of cow's protein and soy protein. Elemental formulas also find some applications in infancy, for example, when continuous drip feeding is indicated in infants with cystic fibrosis. Special formulas are marketed for several inborn metabolic diseases and for a variety of disease states. Polycose and medium-chain triglycerides are used as formula supple-

Table 4–2. Selected normal and special infant formulas.[1]

Product	Protein Source, Amount	CHO Source, Amount	Fat Source, Amount	Indications for Use	Comments (Nutritional Adequacy)
Milk-based formulas					
Enfamil (Mead Johnson)†	Nonfat cow's milk, reduced mineral whey, 1.5 g/dL	Lactose, 6.9 g/dL	Coconut, soy oils, 3.8 g/dL	For full-term and premature infants with no special nutritional requirements	Available fortified with iron, 12 mg/L; whey:casein ratio 60:40
Similac (Ross)[2]	Nonfat cow's milk, 1.5 g/dL	Lactose, 7.2 g/dL	Coconut, soy oils, 3.6 g/dL	Same as Enfamil	Available fortified with iron, 12 mg/L
SMA (Wyeth)[2]	Nonfat cow's milk, demineralized whey, 1.5 g/dL	Lactose, 7.2 g/dL	Oleo, coconut, oleic, soy oils, 3.6 g/dL	Same as Enfamil	Supplemented with iron, 12 mg/L; whey:casein ratio 60:40
Soy-protein formulas					
Isomil (Ross)	Soy protein isolate, 1.8 g/dL	Sucrose, corn syrup,[3] 6.8 g/dL	Coconut, soy oils, 3.7 g/dL	For infants with lactose intolerance or milk-protein allergy	Supplemented with iron, 12 mg/L
Nursoy (Wyeth)	Soy protein isolate, 2.1 g/dL	Sucrose, 6.9 g/dL	Oleo, coconut, oleic, soy oils, 3.6 g/dL	Same as Isomil	Same as Isomil
ProSoBee (Mead Johnson)	Soy protein isolate with added L-methionine, 2.0 g/dL	Corn syrup solids, 6.6 g/dL	Soy, coconut oils, 3.5 g/dL	Same as Isomil	Same as Isomil

(continued)

Table 4–2. Selected normal and special infant formulas[1] (*continued*).

Product	Protein Source, Amount	CHO Source, Amount	Fat Source, Amount	Indications for Use	Comments (Nutritional Adequacy)
Products for premature infants					
Enfamil Premature Formula (Mead Johnson)	Nonfat cow's milk demineralized whey, 2.4 g/dL	Lactose, corn syrup solids, 7.5 g/dL	MCT,[4] (coconut source), corn, coconut oils, 3.4 g/dL	For rapidly growing low-birth-weight infants	Protein, 3 g/100 kcal; Ca:P ratio, 2:1; E:PUFA ratio,[5] 2.8:1
Preemie SMA (Wyeth)	Nonfat cow's milk, whey protein concentrate, 2.0 g/dL	Lactose, glucose polymers, 7.0 g/dL	MCT,[4] oleo, oleic, soy, coconut oils, 3.5 g/dL	Same as Enfamil Premature Formula	Protein, 2.5 g/100 kcal; osmolality, 268 mosm/kg water; E:PUFA ratio,[5] 3.0:1
Similac 24 Special Care (Ross)	Nonfat cow's milk, whey protein concentrate, 2.2 g/dL	Lactose, glucose polymers, 8.5 g/dL	MCT,[4] coconut, soy oils, 4.3 g/dL	Same as Enfamil Premature Formula	Protein, 2.7 g/100 kcal; E:PUFA ratio[5] 2.5:1, osmolality, 280 mosm/kg water
Partially demineralized whey formulas					
Similac PM 60/40 (Ross)	Whey, caseinate, 1.6 g/dL	Lactose, 6.8 g/dL	Coconut, soy oils. 3.7 g/dL	For newborns predisposed to hypocalcemia and infants with renal or heart disease	Ca:P ratio, 2:1; low phosphorus; relatively low solute load: Na = 7 meq/L E:PUFA ratio,[5] 1.0:1

	Protein	Carbohydrate	Fat	Indications	Comments
Semi-elemental formulas					
Nutramigen (Mead Johnson)	Casein hydrolysate, 1.9 g/dL	Modified corn starch, corn syrup solids, 9.0 mg/dL	Corn oil, 2.6 g/dL	For infants and children intolerant of food proteins and for galactosemic patients	
Pregestimil (Mead Johnson)	Casein hydrolysate, 70% amino acids, 30% peptides, 1.9 g/dL	Corn syrup solids, dextrose 6.9 g/dL	60% MCT,[4] 20% corn oil, 20% high oleic safflower, 3.8 g/dL	For infants with malabsorption syndromes	
Alimentum (Ross)	Casein hydrolysate 1.8 g/dL	71% sucrose, 29% modified tapioca starch, 6.9 g/dL	50% MCT,[4] 40% safflower oil, 10% soy oil, 3.8 g/dL	Same as Pregestimil	
Other formulas for malabsorption syndromes					
Portagen (Mead Johnson)	Sodium caseinate, 2.3 g/dL	Sucrose, corn syrup solids, 7.7 g/dL	88% MCT,[4] (coconut source), corn oil, 3.2 g/dL	For management of chyluria, intestinal lymphangiectasia, various forms of steatorrhea, biliary atresia	88% MCT[4] oil, low in essential fatty acids
Elemental formula					
Tolerex (Norwich Eaton)	Free amino acids, 2.1 g/dL	Glucose, oligosaccharides, 22.6 g/dL	Safflower oil, 0.5 g/dL	Use limited in infants; eg, nocturnal tube feeding in cystic fibrosis	Osmolality 550 mosm/kg water at 1 kcal/ml. Use at $\leq \frac{2}{3}$ strength for infants

(continued)

Table 4-2. Selected normal and special infant formulas[1] (continued).

Product	Protein Source, Amount	CHO Source, Amount	Fat Source, Amount	Indications for Use	Comments (Nutritional Adequacy)
Products for infants with inborn errors					
Lofenalac (Mead Johnson)	Casein hydrolysate, L-amino acids	Corn syrup solids, modified tapioca starch	Corn oil	For infants and children with phenylketonuria	*Must be* supplemented with other foods or infant formula to provide minimal phenylalanine
MSUD Diet (Mead Johnson)	L-Amino acids	Corn syrup solids, modified tapioca starch	Corn oil	For children with branched-chain ketoaciduria	Leucine-, isoleucine-, and valine-free; *must be* supplemented
Phenyl-Free (Mead Johnson)	L-Amino acids	Sucrose, corn syrup solids, modified tapioca starch	Corn and coconut oils	For children over 1 year of age with phenylketonuria	Phenylalanine-free. Permits increased supplementation with normal foods

72

Product	Protein	Carbohydrate	Fat	Use	Characteristics
Analog XP (Ross Laboratories)	L-Amino acids	Corn syrup solids	Peanut oil, animal fat (pork), coconut oil	For infants and children with phenylketonuria	Phenylalanine-free; must be supplemented with other milk, formula or foods.
Product 3232A (Mead Johnson)	Enzymatically treated casein	Modified tapioca starch	MCT,[4] corn oil	Protein hydrolysate formula base for use in diagnosis and nutritional management of infants with disaccharidase deficiencies	Monosaccharide- and disaccharide-free powder
Product 80056 (Mead Johnson)	None	Corn syrup solids, modified tapioca starch	Corn oil	For formulation of special diets for infants requiring specific mixtures of amino acids	Protein-free; carbohydrate, fat, vitamin, and mineral mix

[1] Committee on Nutrition. American Academy of Pediatrics: Commentary on breast feeding and infant formulas including proposed standards for formulas. *Pediatrics* 1976;**57**:278. Committee on Nutrition. American Academy of Pediatrics: Nutritional needs of low-birthweight infants. *Pediatrics* 1977,**60**:519.
[2] Ready-to-use, concentrated liquid, and powder forms.
[3] Composed of glucose, maltose, and dextrins.
[4] Medium-chain triglycerides (MCT).
[5] Ratio of vitamin E (E) to polyunsaturated fatty acids (PUFA).

ments. Increasing the concentration of the formulas to provide
> 24 kcal/oz is preferable if the aim is an overall increase in
nutrient density.

Infants who are fed most complete proprietary infant formulas require no additional vitamin supplements. Those fed evaporated milk formula should have daily supplements of vitamins
C and D. Supplemental vitamin D, generally recommended for
breast-fed infants, is most conveniently given as a multivitamin
liquid preparation.

"SOLID" FOODS

(1) Solid foods can be introduced gradually starting at age
4–6 months. Solids should not be introduced until the infant can
sit with support and show good control of the head and neck.
The infant should be able to indicate a desire for food by opening
the mouth and leaning forward and to indicate disinterest by
leaning back and turning away.

Start with an iron-fortified cereal, preferably rice. This may
be followed by pureed vegetables, fruits, strained meat, and egg
yolks. Junior-type foods can be introduced at age 7–8 months.

(2) There is no exact order for starting solid foods. The
first physiologic requirement for foods other than milk occurs
at about age 4–6 months, when a need for iron develops. When
solid foods are started, they should initially be given in small
amounts for several consecutive days to determine the infant's
reaction and any adverse response. The amount should be gradually increased if the food is well tolerated.

(3) Many infants can learn to take semisolid food from a
small spoon by age 4 months. If the infant cannot master spoon-feeding, postpone the attempt for a few weeks; otherwise, undesirable behavior may result and may make spoon-feeding difficult
for months.

(4) The transition from strained to chopped foods should
be gradual and may be started when the infant begins to make
chewing motions.

(5) Egg white, wheat, orange juice, corn, and other allergenic foods should not be given (especially when there is a family
predisposition to allergy) until the child is in the latter part of
the first year of life.

(6) Infants should be allowed to feed themselves with fingers or a spoon when they wish to do so.

(7) Avoid feeding nuts, popcorn, and other foods that are easily aspirated to all children under age 4 years.

NUTRIENT REQUIREMENTS

Recent estimates of energy requirements for infants, based on measurements of energy expenditure and energy intakes of breast-fed infants, are lower than earlier figures (Table 4–3). The components of energy expenditure are given in Table 4–4. There are wide individual variations in energy requirements. In general, appetite, and, especially, growth provide useful guides. Protein requirements for infants are also given in Table 4–3. These have also recently undergone downward revision. Infants require 43% and children 36% of their protein as essential amino acids. Cysteine, tyrosine, and taurine are considered partially essential in the premature infant.

Infants should receive 45–50% of their calories as fat until age 2 years, after which fat consumption should be reduced to < 30% of calories. At least 2% of calories should be provided as essential fatty acids of the ω6 series, and up to 1% as the ω3 series.

Medium-chain triglycerides (MCTs), energy density 7.6 kcal/g, are not essential in the normal diet but are invaluable in malabsorption syndromes. MCTs are especially useful when bile secretion is diminished or absorption and transport of long-chain fatty acids is impaired by other mechanisms. MCTs are very readily absorbed without mycelle formation and are transported via the portal circulation directly to the liver where they undergo rapid beta-oxidation (without the need for carnitine) or ketogenesis.

Recommended dietary allowances (RDAs), which exceed the actual requirements of most individuals, can be found in the reference *Recommended Dietary Allowances,* 10th edition (National Academy Press, 1989). The utility of the RDAs is especially limited for young infants because recommendations cover a wide age range at a time when physiolgic changes are occurring rapidly. It should be emphasized that the RDAs are not designed to provide guidelines for individual requirements.

Table 4-3. Guide to protein, energy, and fluid requirements of infants and frequency of feeds.[1]

Age (mo)[2]	0	1	2	3	4	5	6	7	8	9	10	11	12
Calories (kcal/kg/d)	120	115	105		95				90				
Protein (g/kg/day)	2.25 0–3 months			2.0 3–4 months			1.7 4–6 months				1.5 6–12 months		
Fluid	130–200 mL/kg/d (2–3 oz/lb/d)				130–165 mL/kg/d (2–2.5 oz/lb/d)			130 mL/kg/d (2 oz/lb/d)					
Number of feedings (per day)	6–7		5–7		4–5				3–4				3
Amount (oz) per feeding	2.5–4	3.5–5	4–6	5–7	6–8					7–9			

[1] Some prepared milk formulas may be deficient in vitamins C and D and need to be supplemented with vitamins (25–50 mg of vitamin C and 400 units of vitamin D daily). Iron supplementation of formulas is recommended after 2 months.

[2] Underweight or overweight infants generally have the same food requirements as do infants of the same age with a normal weight. Undiluted whole milk or formulas of equal parts of evaporated milk and water should not be used for young infants, since their kidneys do not have a range of safety in the event of high environmental or body temperature.

Table 4–4. Approximate daily expenditure of calories during the first year of life.

Use	Amount (kcal/kg/d)
Basal metabolism	50
Thermic effect of foods	5
Caloric loss in the excreta	10
Allowance for bodily activity[1]	2–20
Growth	50 → 10
Total	120 → 90

[1] Range is for infants up to 1 month old to those 6–12 months old.

NUTRIENT DEFICIENCIES AND EXCESSES

Failure to Thrive

Failure to thrive (FTT) is a term that is commonly applied to mild or moderate undernutrition. Errors in diet or feeding technique (eg, wrong dilution of formula, inadequate breast-feeding, too-small holes in bottle nipples) account for about 20% of cases of FTT. Thirty percent are secondary to organic disease, and 50% result from nutritional deprivation. Whatever the primary event, malnutrition is the final common pathway and the pattern of impaired growth is "wasting," that is, a low weight-for-length percentile with the weight-age declining earlier and more severely than the length-age. However, the end result, if not effectively treated at an early stage, is "stunting," which is characterized by a low height-for-age percentile and relatively normal weight-for-height percentile. "Stunting" of nutritional origin is usually seen only after infancy in the United States but frequently occurs before 6 months of age in less developed countries. Stunting must be distinguished from endocrinopathy and structural dystrophia. If the head circumference is severely affected, the differential diagnosis includes primary central nervous system disease, severe intrauterine growth retardation, or very severe and early FTT.

For malnourished infants, requirements can be based on ideal body weight (ie, 50th percentile weight-for-height age) or by calculating energy required for the desired "catch-up" growth (5 kcal/g new tissue). Protein requirements also increase during "catch-up" growth (0.2 g protein/g new tissue). Weight velocity during rehabilitation of wasted infants is up to 20 times normal, but in stunting does not exceed 3 times normal.

Marasmus & Kwashiorkor

Marasmus is the end result of severe undernutrition in which there has been successful adaptation to prolonged lack of energy and nutrients. Body weight is less than 60% median for age.

Kwashiorkor is edematous malnutrition with body weight 60–80% median for age. In kwashiorkor, hepatic protein synthesis is depressed at an early stage. Adaptation to malnutrition is poor, and a life-threatening disease develops despite the presence of some energy reserves and skeletal muscle. The etiology of this complex state of malnutrition remains controversial. Lack of protein in the diet appears to be a contributory factor in at least some cases. The features of kwashiorkor and marasmus are compared in Table 4–5.

Whereas FTT can be managed with aggressive nutritional rehabilitation from the outset, great care and patience are required in the initial management of kwashiorkor. Small, frequent, oral feeds should be given to avoid hypoglycemia. During the acute phase, provide only maintenance energy (95 kcal/kg/d) and protein (less than 1.5 g/kg/d), a very generous supply of

Table 4–5. Comparison of clinical and laboratory features of marasmus and kwashiorkor.

Clinical Features	Marasmus	Kwashiorkor
Weight loss	+ + + +	+ +
Loss of muscle	+ + + +	+
Loss of fat	+ + + +	+
Edema	– – –	+ + + +
Psychological impairment	+ +	+ + + +
Anorexia	+	+ + + +
Hepatomegaly	– – –	+ +
Associated infections	+ +	+ + + +
Diarrhea	+ + +	+ + +
Skin lesions	– – –	+ +
Hair changes	+	+ +
Laboratory Features		
Anemia	+	+ + +
Low serum albumin, transferrin, etc.	+	+ + + +
Impaired sodium homeostasis	+	+ + + +
Total body potassium deficiency	+ +	+ + + +
Prothrombin time	Normal	Prolonged
Immune system	Depressed	Depressed

potassium to replace intracellular losses, and a minimal amount of sodium (avoiding intravenous sodium completely). (Intracellular sodium levels and total body sodium are abnormally high.) Infections must be treated aggressively. Initial progress over the first 1–2 weeks is characterized by loss of weight as the edema resolves. During the recovery phase provide 3.5 g protein and 150–200 kcal/kg/d with abundant minerals, vitamins, and trace elements.

Obesity

Obesity is a rapidly increasing problem in the United States; weight problems are evident in children as young as 6 years of age. Obesity results from an imbalance between energy intake and expenditure. However, it frequently involves more than simply overeating. For example, energy expenditure is probably low in preobese and definitely low in postobese states.

For nutritional management, obtain a diet history and focus on reducing or eliminating specific items. For example, encourage intake of skim milk, nonsugared cereals, and diet soda, and avoidance of high-energy snacks, mayonnaise, and salad dressing. Even without counting calories, these measures are likely to reduce energy intake by about one-third. A reduction of 500 kcal/d will result in the loss of 1 pound of fat per week, provided the same rate of energy expenditure is maintained as weight is lost. Exercise and behavioral modification are important components of weight management.

Essential Fatty Acids

Clinical features of ω6 deficiency include growth failure, abnormal scaliness of the skin, erythematous skin lesions, decreased capillary resistance, increased fragility of erythrocytes, thrombocytopenia, poor wound healing, and increased susceptibility to infection. Deficiency of ω3 fatty acids (linolenic) has been less clearly documented but recent evidence shows that visual acuity is compromised by feeding premature infants formulas that lack docosohexanoic acid (22:6 ω3). Excess ω6 fatty acids may lead to an undesirable increase in the production of leukotrienes and thromboxane.

Carbohydrates

A high intake of complex carbohydrates (more than 55–60% of calories) and of fiber is a key feature of the diet now recommended for children more than 2 years of age. Ketosis develops with diets containing less than 10% carbohydrates.

Sucrose is currently consumed in large quantities by children and adolescents in North America in such items as soda, candy, syrups, and sweetened breakfast cereals. A high intake of sucrose predisposes to obesity and is a major risk factor for dental caries.

Vitamins, Minerals, & Micronutrients

See Table 4–6 for a discussion of nutrient sources, deficiency states, and toxicity.

INTRAVENOUS NUTRITION

Indications

The principal indication for total parenteral nutrition (TPN) is loss of ability to absorb nutrients from the gastrointestinal tract. If it is apparent in a newborn that the loss is permanent, TPN should not be started. Supplemental intravenous nutrition, which can be administered via a peripheral vein, is useful as a temporary measure in the premature neonate or, for example, in the malnourished postoperative surgical patient.

Catheter Selection & Placement

The Broviac is the catheter of choice. Use a double-line catheter if required for multiple purposes. If TPN will be needed for less than a month, a Perq catheter can be inserted into a peripheral vein. The tip of the central venous catheter should be located in the superior vena cava or right atrium. Check placement radiologically before using.

Complications

Because of the cost and the risk of complications, TPN should be used only with adequate indication. Complications include mechanical complications that result from problems with insertion; thrombosis of a major vessel; metabolic complications including TPN liver disease and bone disease; and, most commonly, septic complications. The latter, in particular, underlie the need for rigid protocols for nurses and physicians and the advantage of an effective nutrition support team.

Central catheters may be lost owing to sepsis; lack of response to therapy; thrombosis; composition of the infusate (ex-

Table 4-6. Deficiency states and toxicity of vitamins and minerals.

Nutrient	Examples of Good Food Sources	Etiology	Deficient States		Treatment	Toxicity
			Clinical Features	Diagnosis		
Vitamin A	Dairy products, fortified margarine, eggs, liver, carotene (from vegetables)	Fat malabsorption, prematurity, TPN, protein–energy malnutrition, cultural (lack of vegetables)	Night blindness → xerophthalmia & Bitot's spots, keratomalacia → ulceration & perforation of cornea → prolapse of lens and iris → blindness, follicular hyperkeratosis & pruritus. ?predisposes to BPD in the premature	Serum retinol < 10 μg/dL, retinol: RBP < 0.7	Fat malabsorption: 2,500–500 IU/day, eye changes: 50,000 IU orally or IM. preparation: aquasol A (water soluble), [0.1 mL = 5000 IU = 1.6 mg]	>20,000 IU/day vomiting, increased intracranial pressure: irritability, headaches, emotional lability, insomnia, dry desquamating skin, myalgia and arthralgia, abdominal pain, hepatosplenomegaly, cortical thickening of bones of hands and feet
Vitamin D	Ultraviolet light synthesis of D3 in skin; fortified milk & formulas, fish oils	Lack of adequate sunlight coupled with low dietary intake, fat malabsorption syndromes, decreased by hepatic and renal disease and by P450 stimulating drugs, inborn errors of metabolism	Rickets (children), osteomalacia (adults)	Skeletal radiologic abnormalities, high alk phos and PTH, low serum P, low 25-OH D	Fat malabsorption: may need calciferol (vit D3) 800–1200 IU/day or 25-OH D (Rocaltrol) 5–7 μg/kg/day; rickets: D3 1600–5000 IU/day (1 mg = 8000 IU): renal disease: + 1.25 OH2D 0.5–0.2 μg/kg/day	>40,000 IU/day: hypercalcemia, vomiting, constipation, nephrocalcinosis

(continued)

Table 4-6. Deficiency states and toxicity of vitamins and minerals (continued).

Nutrient	Examples of Good Food Sources	Deficient States				Toxicity
		Etiology	Clinical Features	Diagnosis	Treatment	
Vitamin E	Vegetable oils, wheat germ, nuts, seeds	Fat malabsorption syndromes, esp. cholestatic liver disease, abetalipoproteinemia, isolated inborn error of Vit E metabolism, increased utilization during oxidant stress, premature infant	Decreased red cell half life may cause hemolytic anemia; progressive neurologic disorders (loss of deep tendon reflexes, loss of coordination, weakness, scoliosis, etc); ?predisposes to oxidant injury to retina, lung, and brain in premature infant	Serum Vit E < 3 μg/mL < 0.8 mg Vit E/ 1 g total lipids; increased H_2O_2 induced hemolysis	Fat malabsorption: 20 mg/kg/day (< 200 mg); abetalipoproteinemia: 100–200 mg/day	25–100 mg/kg/day IM in premature infants associated with necrotizing enterocolitis and liver toxicity but probably due to polysorbate 80 solubilizer
Vitamin K	Vit K1: leafy vegetables, soybean oil, fruits, seeds; Vit K2: cows milk; intestinal bacteria	Newborn (esp breast fed), fat malabsorption syndrome, anticoagulant drugs (eg, warfarin)	Hemorrhagic disease of newborn, hemorrhage into skin, GI and GU tracts, gingiva, lungs, joints, CNS	Plasma levels of PIVKA, prothrombin time	Newborn: 0.5–1.0 mg IM; children: 3–10 mg IM or IV; malabsorption: 2.5 mg × 2 weekly or 5 mg/day orally; warfarin reversal: 50–100 mg IV	
Vitamin C	Fruits: citrus, strawberries, melons; vegetables: broccoli, green pepper, tomato, potato	Prematurity, no dietary fruits or vegetables	Anorexia, apathy, fever, failure-to-thrive; anemia; increased susceptibility to infections; petechiae; long bone tenderness (severe deficiency: scurvy)	Serum ascorbate < 0.2 mg/dL, low leukocyte ascorbate	Scurvy: 5–10 mg/kg/day IV or PO	Interferes with copper absorption; decreased tolerance to hypoxia; decreased oxalic acid excretion

	Sources	Causes of Deficiency	Deficiency Signs/Symptoms	Lab Test	Dose	Toxicity
Folic acid	Orange juice, whole grains, green leafy vegetables, legumes and meats (heat labile; easily destroyed in cooking)	Prematurity; term breast fed infants whose mothers are folate deficient; term infants fed whole cow's or goat milk; kwashiorkor; dependence on foods cooked for long periods; malabsorption due to sprue, celiac disease; drugs including phenytoin, sulfasalazine	Megaloblastic anemia; hypersegmented neutrophils; delayed maturation of CNS in infants; maternal deficiency in 1st trimester may cause neural tube defects	Serum erythrocyte folate, urinary excretion of FIGLU	0.5–1.0 mg/day of pteroylglutamic acid (PO)	None, (except masking B12 deficiency)
Thiamine	Whole grains, pork, legumes	Alcoholism, hemodialysis, inborn errors of metabolism; breast fed infant of deficient mother	Beri-beri: muscle tenderness, weakness; foot/wrist drop, sensory neuropathy; cardiomyopathy → congestive heart failure → edema. Wernicke-Korsakoff Syndrome: Confusion, ataxia, ophthalmoplegia, psychosis	Erythrocyte transketolase	0.3–1 mg/day (PO)	Very low
Riboflavin	Dairy products, eggs, liver, wheat germ	Diabetes, oral contraceptive use (subclinical), phototherapy for hyperbilirubinemia in newborns on IV nutrition	Cheilosis, angular stomatitis, seborrheic dermatitis, photophobia	Erythrocyte glutathione reductase	0.4–1.0 mg/day (PO)	Very low

(continued)

Table 4–6. Deficiency states and toxicity of vitamins and minerals (continued).

| Nutrient | Examples of Good Food Sources | Deficient States | | | Toxicity |
		Etiology	Clinical Features	Diagnosis	Treatment	Toxicity
Niacin	Meats, poultry, fish, legumes; *precursor*: tryptophan (sources include milk, eggs); 60 mg tryptophan equivalent to 1 mg niacin	Chronic low intake; associated with predominantly corn-based diets	Pellagra: severe diarrhea, dermatitis (aggravated by sun exposure), dementia	Urine N1-methyl-niacinamide (N1-ME) and N1-methyl-6-pyridone-3-carboxamide; random urine N1-ME to creatinine ≤ 0.5 mg/1 g creatinine suggestive of deficiency	6 mg (PO)	Relatively non-toxic: doses at 2–6 g/day associated with peripheral vasodilation, increase uric acid, hepatotoxicity, glucose intolerance
Pyridoxine	Meat, fish, poultry; broccoli; whole grains	Drug interactions: isoniazid, penicillamine, oral contraceptives; historically, heat destruction in processing of infant formula; inborn errors of metabolism; infants fed goat's milk	Seborrheic dermatitis; peripheral neuropathy, seizures, hyperoxaluria, anemia	Erythrocyte glutamic pyruvic transaminase index > 1.25; urine xanthurenic acid after tryptophan load (2–5 g)	Ratio ≥ 0.02 mg B6 per gram protein ingested	Sensory neuropathy in adults associated with 2–6 g/day doses
Biotin	Organ meats, egg yolks, legumes, nuts	Ingestion of raw egg whites (binding by avidin); prolonged antibiotic therapy; inborn errors of metabolism; hemodialysis	Seborrheic dermatitis; alopecia, glossitis, pallor	Plasma biotin and urinary excretion	20 mg/day IV	Very low

Cobalamin (B12)	Animal foods	Poor absorption from deficient intrinsic factor secretion, gastrectomy, Crohn's disease, ileal resection; strict vegetarians	Hypersegmented neutrophils, megaloblastic anemia, posterior and lateral column demyelinization in spinal cord, paresthesias, sensory deficits, loss of deep tendon reflexes, confusion, memory defects Note: Neurologic changes may be irreversible	Serum B12 level, serum folate, erythrocyte folate, schilling test	30–50 mg IM; 1 mg/day IV	Low
Carnitine	Red meats, dairy products	Infants (esp premature) who are fed implemented soy formulas or fed IV, dialysis patients, inherited defects in carnitine synthesis, organic acidemics, valporic acid	Fatty liver hypoglycemia, progressive muscle weakness, cardiomyopathy	Serum carnitine	Oral or IV carnitine, oral doses = 50–300 mg/kg/day	None recognized
Iron	Animal meats, breast milk, iron-fortified formula, iron-fortified infant cereal, whole grains, legumes (absorption enhanced with concurrent ascorbate)	Dietary deficiency, blood loss, prematurity, generalized malnutrition	Microcytic anemia, impaired cognitive development, decreased exercise tolerance, anorexia, failure-to-thrive	Complete blood count, serum ferritin, serum iron/total iron binding capacity, erythrocyte protoporphyrin	3 mg iron/kg/day; avoid accidental overdose	Acute hemorrhagic gastroenteritis, shock; acidosis; defects; coma: coagulation hepatic failure and death

(continued)

85

Table 4–6. Deficiency states and toxicity of vitamins and minerals (continued).

Nutrient	Examples of Good Food Sources	Etiology	Clinical Features	Diagnosis	Treatment	Toxicity
			Deficient States			
Iodine	Milk, green leafy vegetables	Geochemical deficiency	Goiter, hypothyroidism, cretinism (fetus), deafness (fetus)	Thyroid function tests and urine iodine	Iodized salt or water, iodized oil orally or intravenously (2–4 mL)	Thyrotoxicosis, goiter
Zinc	Animal meats, shellfish, legumes, whole grains	Dietary deficiency; generalized malnutrition, prematurity, intravenous nutrition, diarrhea, renal disease, chelation therapy, inborn metabolic diseases	Acro orifacial skin lesions, diarrhea, alopecia, growth retardation, anorexia, immune dysfunction, impaired wound healing, personality changes, impaired taste perception	Plasma zinc < 60 μg/dL	1 mg Zn^{2+}/kg body wt/day	*Chronic*: copper deficiency, depressed HDL cholesterol; *acute*: diarrhea, vomiting, irritability, headache and lethargy
Copper	Animal meats, shellfish, nuts, whole grain, legumes, some water supplies	General malnutrition, diarrhea, prematurity, intravenous nutrition, excess zinc intake, inborn metabolic disease, chelation therapy, cow's milk diet	Anemia (microcytic unresponsive to iron), neutropenia, osteoporosis, fractures, seborrheic skin lesions, failure-to-thrive, impaired CNS function, connective tissue defects	Plasma copper, plasma ceruloplasmin, red cell superoxide dismutase	Infants: 0.2–0.6 mg Cu/day as 1% solution of copper sulfate; children < 1–2 mg Cu/day	*Chronic*: ?Cirrhosis, ?recurrent diarrhea and vomiting, ?prooxidant mediated CNS damage; *acute*: gastrointestinal disfunction, hepatic central lobular necrosis, intravascular hemolysis, renal tubular damage, cardio toxicity

Selenium	Animal meats, fish, whole grain, cereals	Geochemical, intravenous nutrition, low-selenium synthetic diets, premature infants, generalized malnutrition	Cardiomyopathy, skeletal myopathy, macrocytosis and hair depigmentation	Plasma selenium, whole blood selenium, hair selenium, plasma glutathione peroxidase	0.1 mg sodium selenite/ day	*Chronic:* loss of hair, rough finger nails, fatigue; *acute:* vomiting and diarrhea, paresthesias and irritability
Manganese	Whole grain cereals, legumes, nuts, tea	None confirmed				Extrapyramidal central nervous system dysfunction, ?cholestatic liver damage
Calcium	Dairy products, vegetables, canned salmon/sardines	Prematurity; milk-free diet; lactating adolescent; vitamin D deficiency; diuretics	Osteoporosis/ rickets, increased blood pressure	Hypocalcemia (rarely due to calcium deficiency), dietary history most useful	Calcium supplement for the very low birth weight infant, adequate intake of diary products and calcium supplement	Primarily iatrogenic, associated with excessive infusion, infiltration
Phosphorus	Meat, fish, poultry, eggs, cow's milk, cheese, whole grains, nuts, legumes	Protein energy malnutrition, prematurity (human milk), intravenous feeding, severe burns, acidosis, phosphate binding antacids; hypophosphatemia triggered by: glucose loading, insulin, nutritional rehabilitation	Respiratory insufficiency, decreased cardiac contractility, hematologic abnormalities, osteomalacia, bone pain, behavioral changes, peripheral neuropathy, muscle weakness, myalgia	Hypophosphatemia, elevated creatine phosphokinase	Phosphate salts, skimmed milk	Neonatal tetany; if due to renal failure: hyperparathyroidism, metabolic bone disease

(continued)

Table 4–6. Deficiency states and toxicity of vitamins and minerals (continued).

| Nutrient | Examples of Good Food Sources | Deficient States | | | Toxicity |
		Etiology	Clinical Features	Diagnosis	Treatment	
Magnesium	Vegetables (chlorophyll), cereals, nuts	Protein energy malnutrition, renal magnesium wasting, impaired magnesium absorption	Muscle fasciculation/ tremors, muscle weakness, cardiac arrhythmias (depressed S-T & T), personality changes, neurologic abnormalities, rickets (2° to impaired calcium metabolism)	Hypomagnesemia, decrease in muscle Mg	Magnesium salts	Lethargy, respiratory arrest
Sodium	*High*: many processed foods including bread, cured meats, cheese, butter, margarine; *low*: fruits, vegetables, nuts (unsalted), grains, human milk	Diarrhea, excessive sweating, cystic fibrosis	Dehydration, anorexia, vomiting, mental apathy, muscle cramps, seizures	Serum sodium (may be misleadingly low in protein energy malnutrition and in hypermetabolic states)	Oral or parenteral saline	With insufficient water → hypernatremic dehydration; with adequate water → edema; hypertension; increase in intracellular sodium impairs cellular metabolism

Potassium	Unprocessed foods (meat, fish, potatoes, beans, bananas, apricots, prunes, raisins, whole grains)	Protein energy malnutrition, any catabolic state, acidosis, diarrhea, loop diuretics	Muscle weakness, mental confusion, cardiac arrhythmias, sudden death	Hypokalemia, muscle K	High intake of potassium salt (PO) if kidney functioning	Muscle weakness, mental apathy
Chloride	Closely linked to sodium	Chloride inadvertently low in infant formulas, cystic fibrosis, severe vomiting, diarrhea, loop diuretics, Bartter's syndrome	Hypochloremic, hypokalemic alkalosis, failure-to-thrive (including impaired head growth), anorexia, lethargy, muscle weakness, vomiting	Hypochloremia: urine chloride depends on the cause of chloride depletion	Sodium/potassium chloride	

PEDIATRIC PARENTERAL NUTRITION (PN) ORDER FORM

Imprint Patient Plate

Weight of patient _____ kg   Central line _____   Peripheral line _____

Rate _____

	Standard Order	Modifications To Standard Order
Protein (as amino acid)*	g%	
Dextrose	g%	
Na	30 meq/L	
K	25 meq/L	
Cl	20 meq/L	
Acetate	45 meq/L	
Ca (as gluconate) (10 mM Ca/L)	20 meq/L	
Mg (as sulfate)	3 meq/L	

Adjustments for Neonates and Premature Infants (Circle these when required and cross out corresponding items under "standard order").

*Use trophamine and cysteine for patients in level II and III nurseries who have a central line or are on day 6 of peripheral therapy.

P .... 10 mM/L
MVI Pediatric .... *5.0 mL/d
Zinc .... *1.0 mg/L
Copper .... 200 µg/L
Manganese .... 5.0 µg/L
Chromium .... 2.0 µg/L
Selenium .... 20.0 µg/L
Iodide .... 10 µg/L
Heparin .... 1000 Units/L
Cysteine (40 mg/g trophamine)* _____ mg/L

Pharmacy will automatically account for electrolytes provided in amino acid preparation.
Changes in Na or K to be made as: Cl only ___, or Acetate only ___, or Cl: Acetate 1:1 ___, or other
Cl: Acetate ratio (specify _____).

*2 mL/kg/d for patients < 2.5 kg
*Zn: 400 µg/kg/d < 2 kg body weight
250 µg/kg/d others < 3 mo old

*Use only with trophamine

Date: _____ Signature: _____ M.D.

Figure 4-1. Pediatric parenteral nutrition (PN) order form. (Modified from the pediatric parenteral nutrition order form of the University of Colorado Health Sciences Center Department of Pharmacy.)

cessive concentrations of calcium and phosphorus); incompatible medications administered with the infusate; or slipping, kinking, or breaking of the catheter. Most breaks are exterior to the skin and can be repaired with kits, which must be kept readily available. Urokinase is effective in dissolving recently formed clots in the catheter.

Nutrient Requirements & Administration

Energy requirements are approximately 10% lower than those for enteral feeding. At least 60% of energy is provided as dextrose monohydrate (3.4 kcal/g). Dextrose concentrations greater than 12.5% (630 mosm/kg water) cannot be administered via peripheral vein. With a central catheter, start with D10 and advance by approximately 2.5% per day as tolerance (owing to decreased endogenous glucose production) increases, up to 20% or higher if needed. The rate of advance and final concentration will depend on flow rates.

Tolerance to IV dextrose is especially limited in premature infants and hypermetabolic ICU patients. Excess administration of dextrose will cause hyperglycemia, osmotic diuresis, fatty liver and elevated $Paco_2$. If unexpected hyperglycemia occurs, check for error in dextrose concentration, uneven flow rate, sepsis, stress, or pancreatitis. Intravenous insulin may not be metabolically desirable. When the infusate is discontinued either temporarily or during cyclic IV feeding, taper glucose delivery over at least 2 hours to avoid hypoglycemia. A minimum of about 5% of total calories per week should be provided as an intravenous fat emulsion (2.7% calories as essential fatty acids) to avoid risk of essential fatty acid deficiency; there are potential advantages in providing up to 40% of calories as lipid according to individual tolerance. Advantages include the high energy density, low osmolality, low CO_2 production, and negligible energy cost of storage. However, administration of fat emulsions beyond tolerance will impair leukocyte function, cause coagulation defects, decrease pulmonary oxygen diffusion, and compete with bilirubin and drugs for albumin binding sites. Commence fat emulsion with 1 g/kg/day and, as tolerated, advance by 0.5 g/kg/d up to a maximum of 3 g/kg/d.

Provide nitrogen (1 g N = 6.25 g protein) as an amino acid solution, usually 1–3% depending on flow rate and requirements (the same as for enteral feeding). Trophamine (McGaw) may currently be the best source of nitrogen for the premature infant with added cysteine (40 mg/g trophamine). Optimal N (g):kcal ratios are usually 1:150–300. When energy intake is low, administration of nitrogen will improve but not correct negative nitrogen balance. When nitrogen intake is low, provision of energy (< 70 kcal/kg/day in an infant) will improve negative nitrogen balance.

One vial (5 mL) of MVI Pediatric (Armour) meets the vitamin guidelines for term infants. Administer 2 mL (40% of a single-dose vial) per kg to premature infants. Additional supplements of vitamins A (250 μg) and E (10 mg) may be beneficial.

Mineral and trace element recommendations are given in Figure 4–1.

Ordering

See sample order form in Figure 4–1. Orders should be reviewed each morning.

Monitoring

Maintain PN flow chart at bedside or in hospital chart.

(1) Weight daily; height and head circumference weekly.

(2) Urine glucose, specific gravity: Dipstick once each shift while changing concentrations of dextrose.

(3) Blood glucose: 4 hours after starting or changing infusion rate or changing glucose concentration; then daily for 2 days; then every third day.

(4) Serum Na-K-Cl-CO_2-BUN: Daily for 2 days after starting or changing infusion rate or changing composition of infusate; then every third day.

(5) Serum Ca-Mg-P: Every third day initially then once weekly when flow rate and composition of infusate are stabilized.

(6) Total protein, albumin, bilirubin, AST, GGT, alkaline phosphatase, CBC: Initially and then weekly. Zinc and copper: Initially, then monthly.

(7) Serum triglycerides (monitor if IV fat emulsion is used): 1 day after starting or changing quantity of fat, then weekly. (Draw level just prior to starting daily infusion of fat emulsion.)

Note: These assays will have to be performed more frequently in some patients according to their clinical status and the results of previous assays.

5 | Fluids & Electrolytes

Carol A. Ledwith, MD

Children differ from adults in their fluid and electrolyte requirements. Children have: (1) a greater percentage of total body weight that is water, (2) a higher basal metabolic rate, and (3) a higher body surface area-to-weight ratio. These features lead to greater water turnover per kilogram of body weight when compared with adults.

Fluid and electrolyte therapy for children may be approached by considering four major components: rapid volume expansion to treat shock and restore perfusion, continuation of deficit replacement, provision of maintenance requirements, and replacement of ongoing losses.

MAINTENANCE REQUIREMENTS

Calculations of water requirements are based on caloric expenditure. One mL of water is required for every kcal burned. Electrolyte needs are based on water requirements, and electrolyte losses occur primarily through the urine with smaller amounts lost through the skin and stool. During short-term intravenous hydration, enough glucose must be provided in the solution to prevent ketosis and minimize protein breakdown. Table 5–1 shows how to calculate maintenance requirements based on body weight.

Special Considerations

Maintenance requirements may differ depending on the clinical situation. Maintenance requirements may need to be adjusted upward for premature and low-birthweight infants, fever (increase water by 12% per 1°C rise), sweating, respiratory distress, skin disease, diabetes insipidus, high-output renal failure, burns, and phototherapy.

Requirements need to be adjusted downward for syndrome

Table 5–1. 24-hour maintenance requirements.

Water	100 mL/kg for first 10 kg 50 mL/kg for next 10 kg 20 mL/kg for each kg above 20 kg
Sodium	3 mEq/100 mL H_2O = 30 mEq/L
Potassium	2 mEq/100 mL H_2O = 20 mEq/L
Glucose	5 g/100 mL H_2O = 5% dextrose solution

Example: A 23 kg patient requires:

$$[(10 \times 100) + (10 \times 50) + (3 \times 20)] \text{ mL/24 h} = 1560 \text{ mL/24 h}$$

Therefore, appropriate maintenance solution is $D_5\frac{1}{4}NS$[1] with 20 mEq/L KCl at 65 mL/h

[1] NS (Normal Saline) = 154 mEq/L Na^+; $\frac{1}{2}$NS = 77 mEq/L; $\frac{1}{4}$NS = 38 mEq/L.

of inappropriate ADH secretion, increased intracranial pressure, congestive heart failure, and oliguric renal failure.

DEHYDRATION

General Considerations

Children are at high risk for the development of dehydration. The reasons for this are many. (1) Children have an increased incidence of gastrointestinal disease, especially gastroenteritis. (2) Gastrointestinal symptoms occur with many nongastrointestinal diseases. (3) Children suffer relatively greater gastrointestinal losses than do adults. (4) Infants cannot respond to thirst independently. All sick children, not merely those with gastroenteritis, should be assessed for their hydration status.

One of the main consequences of dehydration is acidosis. Acidosis is the result of inadequate tissue perfusion, decreased O_2 delivery, lactic acid and keto-acid production, and decreased renal perfusion.

History

A detailed history must be taken to determine the child's fluid intake and the exact type of fluid that the child has been drinking. History should include frequency and amount of vomiting, diarrhea, and urine output. If a previous recent weight is known, it can be extremely useful in calculating the degree of dehydration. Weight loss with an acute illness represents water loss and is the most accurate measure of the water deficit. (1 mL H_2O = 1 g). Degree and duration of fever, underlying medical conditions, and medications given must also be noted.

Clinical Assessment

Table 5–2 shows trends in physical findings and laboratory values with increasing levels of dehydration. In general, the most reliable signs and symptoms of dehydration in children are prolonged capillary refill time (Table 5–3), decreased urine output, altered mental status/decreased level of consciousness, and tachycardia. Low or falling blood pressure is a late sign of shock in pediatrics. Children are able to maintain their blood pressure even in the face of severe hypovolemia. Shock is defined by inadequate tissue perfusion and not by hypotension. Do not be reassured by a normal blood pressure.

Types of Dehydration

The type of dehydration is based on the serum sodium (Na^+) concentration. Isotonic dehydration is defined as a loss

Table 5–2. Estimating the severity of dehydration.[1]

Physical Signs	Mild	Moderate	Severe
Weight loss			
Infant	5%	10%	15%
Older child	3%	6%	9%
Vital Signs			
Pulse	± ↑	↑	↑ ↑
Blood pressure	normal	normal	normal or ↓
Eyes	± tearing	↓ tearing	↓ tearing
		± sunken	sunken
Mucous membranes	± tacky	tacky/dry	parched
Skin			
Turgor	± ↓	↓	↓ ↓
Perfusion	normal	± mottled	poor/mottled
Laboratory Findings			
Urine output	↓	↓ ↓	↓ ↓ ↓
Urine specific gravity	↑	↑	↑
BUN	normal	± ↑	↑
CO_2	↓	↓ ↓	↓ ↓ ↓

[1] Adapted from Barkin RM (editor): *Emergency Pediatrics*, Mosby, 1986, p 44.

Table 5–3. Estimating level of dehydration.

Capillary Refill Time	Level of Dehydration
<2 sec	Normal
2–3 sec	Mild 3–5%
3–4 sec	Moderate 6–10%
>4 sec	Severe 9–15%

of total body water while maintaining a serum sodium of 130–150 mEq/L. This is the most common form of dehydration. See Tables 5–4 and 5–5 for management. Hypertonic (hypernatremic) dehydration is characterized by a serum sodium of > 150 mEq/L in the presence of a total body water deficit. Hypotonic (hyponatremic) dehydration is defined as a loss of water and sodium with a serum sodium < 130 mEq/L. See algorithms in Tables 5–6 and 5–7 for management guidelines. Additional etiologies of hypo- and hypernatremia are included in Table 5–8.

Table 5–4. Acute hypovolemic dehydration: principles of initial management.

Volume expansion for *ALL* types of dehydration

Always bolus with isotonic fluid
(NS, LR [Lactated Ringers]) 20 mL/kg
↓
Bedside rapid glucose check
Bolus with glucose as indicated
D_{10} 2–4 mL/kg if < 3 mo
D_{25} 2 mL/kg if > 3 mo
↓
Obtain serum electrolytes,[1] urea nitrogen, glucose
↓
Continue to treat with isotonic fluid in 20-mL/kg boluses until perfusion is restored and patient is hemodynamically stable
↓
Calculate and begin deficit replacement (see Table 5–5) when adequate tissue perfusion has been demonstrated (such as improved capillary refill, urine output, or improved mental status)
↓
If, after 40 mL/kg of isotonic fluid, perfusion has not been restored, must consider other etiology such as hemorrhagic shock, septic shock, cardiogenic shock

[1] *Electrolytes = sodium (Na^+), potassium (K^+), chloride (Cl^-), bicarbonate (HCO_3^-).*

Table 5-5. Isotonic dehydration: management guidelines.[1]

Procedure	Example
Calculate fluid deficit based on weight loss, if known, or based on estimated percent dehydration	Known 10 kg previous (hydrated) weight. Now weighs 9 kg = 1 kg (1000 mL) deficit *or* Current weight 9 kg with estimated 10% dehydration; therefore, current weight is 90% of hydrated weight $\Rightarrow$ 9 kg = 90% × (hydrated weight). 9 ÷ 9 = 10 kg = hydrated weight. 10 kg − 9 kg = 1 kg (1000 mL) deficit.
$\Downarrow$	$\Downarrow$
Subtract bolus fluids from total deficit	If 200 mL bolus fluids given, remaining deficit is 800 mL
$\Downarrow$	$\Downarrow$
Replace ½ of total deficit over the first 8 h, and ½ of total deficit over the next 16 h	400 ÷ 8 = 50 mL/h × 8 h; then 400 ÷ 16 = 25 mL/h × 16 h
$\Downarrow$	$\Downarrow$
Add in maintenance fluid requirements (based on hydrated weight)	1000 mL/24 h = 40 mL/h maintenance; therefore, 40 + 50 = 90 mL/h × 8 h; then 40 + 25 = 65 mL/h × 16 h
$\Downarrow$	$\Downarrow$
For isotonic dehydration, appropriate electrolyte solution is same as maintenance solution	D_5 ¼ NS with 20 mEq/L KCl[2]
$\Downarrow$	$\Downarrow$
Replace ongoing losses: diarrhea; nasogastric, duodenal or jejunal tube secretions; vomiting; urine (such as with diabetic patient)	For most accurate assessment when output is high, send the fluid of concern for electrolyte concentrations and order additional solutions accordingly. Output may be calculated every 8 h and replaced mL per mL.

[1] Treat shock as in Table 5-4 with isotonic solution.
[2] K acetate rather than KCl may be used in acidotic patient. Do not add K^+ until serum potassium is documented and patient has produced urine.

Table 5–6. Hypotonic dehydration and deficit replacement.[1]

Hypotonic dehydration

Seizures secondary to hyponatremia (usually not seen with serum Na$^+$ ≥ 120 mEq/L)	No seizures—go directly to deficit replacement

⇓

Administer 3% NaCl intravenously over 1 h (3% NaCl = 0.5 mEq NaCl/mL)

Correct with this formula:
(Desired Na$^+$ − measured Na) × 0.6[2] × weight (kg) = mEq NaCl required

General rule: 6 mL/kg of 3% NaCl raises Na$^+$ by 5 mEq/L

Note: Desired Na$^+$ = 135 mEq/L

⇓

Deficit replacement

Procedure	Example
Calculate fluid deficit as in isotonic dehydration	For the 10 kg (hydrated weight) infant with 10% dehydration = 1000 mL deficit
⇓	⇓
Calculate Na$^+$ deficit with desired Na$^+$ = 135 mEq/L	For Na$^+$ = 115 mEq/L (135 − 115) × 0.6 × 10 kg = 120 mEq Na$^+$ deficit
⇓	⇓
Replace ½ of total water and Na$^+$ deficit over the first 8 h, and ½ over the next 16 h. Add in maintenance fluid and Na$^+$ requirements.	**Water** **Na$^+$** Deficit 1000 mL 120 mEq Maintenance 30 mEq/24 h 1000 mL/24 h 1st 8 h: 500 mL deficit + 320 mL maintenance (water) 60 mEq deficit + 10 mEq maintenance (Na$^+$) Total = 70 mEq Na$^+$ in 820 mL water or D$_5$½NS at 100 mL/h for 8 h. Then D$_5$½NS at 70 mL/h for next 16 h.

Note:
- If 3% NaCl given, subtract this from total Na$^+$ deficit
- Remember to subtract bolus fluids from total fluid deficit
- Replace ongoing losses as in isotonic dehydration
- Add potassium as indicated
- Follow Na$^+$ carefully: Na$^+$ should correct over 24 h; rate of rise should not exceed 2 mEq/L/h
- Too rapid correction may lead to central pontine myelinolysis

[1] Treat shock as in Table 5–4 with isotonic solution.

[2] 0.6 = volume of distribution for Na$^+$.

Table 5–7. Hypertonic dehydration.[1]

Procedure	Example
Calculate fluid deficit as in isotonic dehydration	For the 10 kg infant with 10% dehydration = 1000 mL deficit
⇓	⇓
Replace this deficit evenly over 48 h; add maintenance fluids	1000 mL deficit + 2000 mL maintenance (48 h) = 3000 mL at 60 mL/h. Use $D_5\frac{1}{4}NS$ as higher Na^+ concentration will not allow serum Na^+ to decrease
⇓	⇓
If serum Na^+ is not correcting, may need to replace free water portion of deficit as D_5W. Formula to calculate free water deficit: 4 mL/kg free water for each mEq of Na^+ that serum Na^+ exceeds 145.	If serum Na^+ = 160: (160 − 145) × 4 mL/kg × 10 kg = 600 mL (free water deficit). Replace with D_5W over 48 h at 12 mL/h. Give maintenance and remainder of total fluid deficit as $D_5\frac{1}{4}NS$.

Note:
- Goal is to drop serum Na^+ slowly (0.5 mEq/L/h); follow every 2 h
- Too rapid correction may cause cerebral edema and refractory seizures
- Remember to subtract bolus fluids from total fluid deficit
- Replace ongoing losses as in isotonic dehydration
- Add potassium as indicated

[1] Treat shock as in Table 5–4 with isotonic solution.

SPECIFIC ELECTROLYTE DISTURBANCES

1. HYPERKALEMIA

Clinical Findings

Causes of hyperkalemia include renal failure, hemolysis, rhabdomyolysis, adrenal insufficiency, tumor cell lysis during induction chemotherapy, tissue destruction seen with burns and crush injuries, and excess administrations (usually IV). Always document serum potassium (K^+) with a nonhemolyzed specimen.

Clinical effects of hyperkalemia include listlessness, confusion, parasthesias, peripheral vascular collapse, bradycardia, and asystole. The most important clinical effects of hyperkalemia are cardiac. Electrocardiographic changes include peaked T waves, widened QRS complex, increased P-R interval, heart

Table 5–8. Hyponatremia and hypernatremia: classification and etiologies.

Hyponatremia
↓ total body sodium > ↓ total body water (as in hypovolemic dehydration):
  Commonly seen in infants and children with gastroenteritis who are rehydrated with water, weak tea, or other no sodium or low sodium fluids
↑ total body sodium < ↑ total body water (conditions associated with edema):
  Congestive heart failure, renal failure, hepatic failure
Normal total body sodium with ↑ total body water:
  SIADH, water intoxication
↓ total body sodium with normal or ↓ total body water:
  Seen in patients with excessive sodium losses such as in cystic fibrosis, adrenal insufficiency.
Factitious:
  Hyperglycemia, mannitol, hyperlipidemia
Hypernatremia
↑ total body sodium:
  Seen most commonly secondary to excessive sodium administration, such as through inadequately diluted powdered or concentrated formula
↓ total body water:
  Diabetes insipidus
↓ total body sodium < ↓ total body water:
  Osmotic diuretics
  Gastroenteritis and dehydration with excessive sodium in oral rehydration solution

---

block, and ventricular tachycardia or fibrillation. Symptoms often will not be manifest until the potassium rises above 7 mEq/L. (Normal potassium ranges are higher for premature and newborn infants.) See algorithm in Table 5–9 for management guidelines.

2. HYPOKALEMIA

Clinical Findings
  Causes of hypokalemia include vomiting, diarrhea, nasogastric suction, inadequate intake, diuretics, correction of metabolic acidosis, and renal tubular acidosis. The clinical effects include weakness, hypotonia, decreased deep tendon reflexes, ileus, and respiratory depression and failure. ECG changes consistent with

Table 5–9. Treatment of hyperkalemia.

Serum potassium > 6 mEq/L but < 7 mEq/L.
⇓
Repeat serum potassium.
⇓
Continuously monitor ECG.
⇓
Withhold all potassium.
⇓
Kayexalate exchange resin 1 g/kg PO or PR.
⇓
Note: If serum potassium is > 7 mEq/L or cardiovascular instability is present, follow algorithm as above then proceed.
⇓
Calcium gluconate (10% solution) .5 mL/kg IV over 3 min (maximum 10 mL) (.5 mL/kg = 50 mg/kg of 10% solution). Best emergency treatment for dysrhythmias.
⇓
Sodium bicarbonate 1–2 mEq/kg IV. This transiently moves potassium intracellularly.
⇓
Glucose 0.5 g/kg/h and insulin 1 U regular for each 3 g glucose.
⇓
Dialysis is indicated for refractory symptomatic hyperkalemia.
⇓
Treat the underlying condition.

hypokalemia include flattened T waves, the presence of U waves, S-T segment depression, and AV block. AV block may be exacerbated if the patient is taking digitalis.

Treatment

(1) Obtain serum and urine electrolytes, urinalysis, ECG.

(2) Establish adequate urine output before giving potassium.

(3) Correct if serum potassium is less than 3.5 mEq/L.

(4) Parenteral correction can be done with 20–40 mEq/L potassium added to peripheral IV fluids. Higher concentrations require a central venous line and ICU monitoring. A rapid infusion up to 0.5 mEq/kg/h can be done with ECG monitoring.

(5) Correction with 3 mEq/kg/d can also be done orally. Potassium irritates the gastrointestinal tract and should be given on a full stomach.

5. ACID–BASE DISTURBANCES

The normal pH range is 7.38–7.42. pH changes 0.15 units for every 10 mEq/L change in serum bicarbonate HCO_3^- and 0.08 units for every 10 torr change in P_{CO_2}.

The laboratory findings in acute acid–base disturbances are given in Table 5–10.

Metabolic Acidosis

Metabolic acidosis is caused by a gain in hydrogen ion or a loss of bicarbonate. Calculation of the anion gap can help determine the cause (Table 5–11). Anion gap = $Na^+ - (CL^- + HCO_3^-)$. A normal anion gap is 8–16 mEq/L. An increased anion gap suggests accumulation of organic acids.

Treatment of acidosis involves identification of the underlying cause. Bicarbonate therapy is rarely indicated. Bicarbonate therapy may be considered when a metabolic acidosis with pH less than 7.2 is documented, and if adequate ventilation is established. The vast majority of lactic acidosis associated with dehydration will resolve with rehydration. The dose of bicarbonate is calculated as weight (kg) × base deficit × 0.6. The base deficit is the desired HCO_3^- − the measured HCO_3^-. Half the calculated dose can be given immediately with the remainder given over the next 1–2 hours.

Respiratory Acidosis

Respiratory acidosis occurs as a result of hypoventilation due to pulmonary disease or central respiratory depression. Treatment involves adequate ventilation. Bicarbonate therapy is not indicated and will exacerbate the acidosis.

Metabolic Alkalosis

This condition results from loss of hydrogen ion (vomiting), excess intake of bicarbonate, or as compensation for excess

Table 5–10. Laboratory findings in acute acid–base disturbances.

	pH	P_{CO_2}	HCO_3^-
Metabolic acidosis	↓	↓	↓
Respiratory acidosis	↓	↑	Normal or ↑
Metabolic alkalosis	↑	↑	↑
Respiratory alkalosis	↑	↓	Normal or ↓

Table 5–11. Causes of metabolic acidosis.

Normal anion gap
GI losses: diarrhea, enterostomies, fistulas
Renal tubular acidosis
Hyperalimentation
Increased anion gap
Lactic acidosis
Diabetic ketoacidosis
Inborn errors of metabolism
Uremia
Ingestions (ethanol, methanol, ethylene glycol, salicylates, paraldehyde)

renal loss of chloride (Cl^-) (diuretics). The underlying cause must be treated and adequate chloride supplements provided.

Respiratory Alkalosis

The presence of a respiratory alkalosis suggests hyperventilation or salicylate intoxication. Treatment involves identification of the underlying cause.

ORAL REHYDRATION THERAPY

Oral rehydration should be considered for pediatric patients with mild to moderate dehydration secondary to gastroenteritis. Vomiting is not an absolute contraindication to oral rehydration; in fact, many children with a history of vomiting will tolerate oral rehydration solutions quite well.

An oral glucose-electrolyte solution containing 50–90 mEq of sodium per liter and 20–25 g of glucose per liter should be used. Small aliquots are given ad libitum to provide approximately 50 mL/kg over a 4-hour period to the child with mild dehydration. For moderate dehydration, the dose should be increased to 100 mL/kg over 6 hours.

Inability to tolerate oral rehydration suggests the need for intravenous therapy.

Immunization Procedures, Vaccines, Antisera, & Skin Tests | 6

John W. Ogle, MD

Active immunity to infectious diseases occurs following inoculation of bacterial, viral, and parasitic antigens, either in a live attenuated form, as inactivated whole organisms, or as portions or products of organisms. New vaccines are being developed and tested and are introduced periodically. In addition, vaccine composition, recommended schedules, and contraindications continue to change. Readers are advised to consult the recommendations of the Advisory Committee for Immunization Practices (ACIP) and the *Report of the Committee on Infectious Diseases* of the American Academy of Pediatrics (the *Red Book*) to supplement the information given in this chapter.

Passive immunity, administered in the form of intravenous gamma globulin (IVIG) or as one of several specific immune globulins or animal serum, provides temporary protection against infection or disease. Only a limited number of infectious agents are susceptible to passive antibody; in general, it is preferable to use a vaccine for a disease (if available) to provide active immunity than to provide passive protection.

PROCEDURES FOR ACTIVE IMMUNIZATION

General Principles

A. Sources of Information: *Always* consult authoritative sources before using any of the vaccines, sera, or immune globulins. Among these sources are (1) the CDC's *Morbidity and Mortality Weekly Report* (MMWR), (2) the American Academy of Pediatrics' periodic updates of the *Report of the Committee on Infectious Diseases* (the *Red Book*), (3) the manufacturer's package insert that accompanies each biologic product, and (4) the CDC's *Health Information for International Travel*. The package inserts are reasonably complete, but the recommendations may contain conflicting information (usually occasioned by legal considerations), in which case it is best to follow the advice of the CDC or the American Academy of Pediatrics.

B. Informed Consent: Providers are required to provide detailed information to parents on the risks and benefits of immunization. Providers may use brochures developed by the CDC and available through local health departments, or may develop and use their own materials provided they conform to the requirements of the law. Signed informed consent must be obtained prior to immunization.

C. Storage and Administration of Vaccines: Scrupulous attention should be paid to proper handling and storage of vaccines and other biologic products. Consult the package insert for specifications for each product, as instructions vary for different types of products and manufacturers.

Aseptic technique should be used in removing vaccine from a vial, preparing the injection site, and administering the vaccine. Intramuscular injections are best given to children in either the lateral thigh or, in older children, the deltoid muscle. Administration in the gluteal region can cause injury to the sciatic nerve and therefore should be avoided. The tissue at the injection site should be compressed and the needle should be inserted in the upper lateral quadrant of the thigh with the syringe directed inferiorly at a 45-degree angle to the long axis of the leg and posteriorly at a 45-degree angle to a line parallel to the table top. Before injecting the vaccine, the syringe plunger should be pulled back; if blood appears, the needle should be withdrawn, new vaccine drawn up into a new syringe, and injected into a different site. To decrease the likelihood of local reactions to vaccines, a needle long enough to enter the muscle—2.5 cm or 1 inch—is recommended for intramuscular injections in children of all ages. When injecting an irritating material, the injection site should be rotated at subsequent inoculations and the injection site noted in the chart. Two vaccines should never be injected into the same site, and separate vaccines should never be mixed in one syringe.

D. Monitoring and Reporting Adverse Reactions: Parents should be informed of any possible adverse reactions and given specific instructions for reporting such reactions. Severe reactions require a physical assessment of the child and appropriate therapeutic intervention. The parents should be given an immunization record, which should be updated each time a vaccine is given. The National Childhood Vaccine Injury Act, which went into effect on March 21, 1988, requires health care providers to record certain information and events. The health care provider who administers the vaccine should enter into the permanent medical record the following information: date of vaccine administration; vaccine manufacturer and lot number; and the name, address, and title of the person administering the vaccine. Certain reportable adverse events after vaccination are listed in Table 6–1. Adverse events due to vaccines must be reported to the Vaccine Adverse Events Reporting System (VAERS). Forms may be requested by calling (800) 822–7967. Adverse events that must be reported are found in Table 6–1.

The National Childhood Vaccine Injury Act of 1988 provides compensation to families in the form of "no fault" compensation adjudicated by a panel of special masters appointed to hear evidence and decide on compensation. Compensation forms are available by calling (800) 338–2382. Claims for compensation through the National Vaccine Injury Compensation Program must be filed within 3 years of the first symptom or within 2 years after death.

E. General Precautions and Contraindications: The physician should be aware of the recommended precautions and contraindications for each vaccine. The following are general guidelines: (1) Avoid giving live vaccines to women during pregnancy. (2) Do not administer a live vaccine to any person suspected or proved to be immunodeficient (eg, a patient with a known or suspected congenital defect, a patient with an acquired immunodeficiency disease, or a patient receiving immunosuppressive therapy or corticosteriods). (3) Vaccines are generally given only to healthy children; however, minor illness, whether there is fever or not, is not a contraindication to live viral vaccine administration. DTP should not be given to children who have a febrile illness because the symptoms may be attributed to the vaccine. However, if a child has a nonfebrile upper respiratory tract infection, DTP vaccine can be administered as scheduled, to prevent multiple visits or a delay in completing the immunization schedule.

PRIMARY IMMUNIZATION OF CHILDREN IN THE FIRST YEAR OF LIFE

The recommended schedule of immunizations is listed in Table 6–2. Adequate protection against diphtheria, pertussis,

Table 6-1. Reportable events following vaccination.[1]

Vaccine/toxoid	Event	Interval from Vaccination
DTP, P, DTP/polio combined	A. Anaphylaxis or anaphylactic shock	24 hours
	B. Encephalopathy (or encephalitis)[2]	7 days
	C. Shock-collapse or hypotonic-hyporesponsive collapse[2]	7 days
	D. Residual seizure disorder[2]	(See Aids to Interpretation[2])
	E. Any acute complication or sequela (including death) of above events	No limit
	F. Events in vaccinees described in manufacturer's package insert as contraindications to additional doses of vaccine[2] (such as convulsions)	(See package insert)
MMR, DT, Td, tetanus toxoid	A. Anaphylaxis or anaphylactic shock	24 hours
	B. Encephalopathy (or encephalitis)[2]	15 days for MMR vaccines; 7 days for DT, Td, and T toxoids
	C. Residual seizure disorder[2]	(See Aids to Interpretation†)
	D. Any acute complication or sequela (including death) of above events	No limit
	E. Events in vaccinees described in manufacturer's package insert as contraindications to additional doses of vaccine[2]	(See package insert)
Oral polio vaccine	A. Paralytic poliomyelitis: in a nonimmunodeficient recipient in an immunodeficient recipient in a vaccine-associated community case	30 days 6 months No limit
	B. Any acute complication or sequela (including death) of above events	No limit

108

	C. Events in vaccinees described in manufacturer's package insert as contraindications to additional doses of vaccine[2]	(See package insert)
Inactivated polio vaccine	A. Anaphylaxis or anaphylactic shock	24 hours
	B. Any acute complication or sequela (including death) of above event	No limit
	C. Events in vaccinees described in manufacturer's package insert as contraindications to additional doses of vaccine[2]	(See package insert)

[1] From Centers for Disease Control. Vaccine adverse event reporting system—United States; requirements. *MMWR* 1990;**39**:730–732.

[2] **Aids to interpretation:** Shock-collapse or hypotonic-hyporesponsive collapse may be evidenced by signs or symptoms such as decrease in or loss of muscle tone, paralysis (partial or complete), hemiplegia, hemiparesis, loss of color or turning pale white or blue, unresponsiveness to environmental stimuli, depression of or loss of consciousness, prolonged sleeping with difficulty arousing, or cardiovascular or respiratory arrest.

Residual seizure disorder may be considered to have occurred if no other seizure or convulsion unaccompanied by fever or accompanied by a fever of less than 102 °F occurred before the first seizure or convulsion after the administration of the vaccine involved.

and, if in the case of measles-, mumps-, or rubella-containing vaccines, the first seizure or convulsion occurred within 15 days after vaccination *or* in the case of any other vaccine, the first seizure or convulsion occurred within 3 days after vaccination.

and, if 2 or more seizures or convulsions unaccompanied by fever or accompanied by a fever of less than 102 °F occurred within 1 year after vaccination.

The terms *seizure* and *convulsion* include grand mal, petit mal, absence, myoclonic, tonic–clonic, and focal motor seizures and signs. *Encephalopathy* means any significant acquired abnormality of, injury to, or impairment of function of the brain. Among the frequent manifestations of encephalopathy are focal and diffuse neurologic signs, increased intracranial pressure, or changes in level of consciousness lasting at least 6 hours, with or without convulsions. The neurologic signs and symptoms of encephalopathy may be temporary with complete recovery, or they may result in various degrees of permanent impairment. Signs and symptoms, such as high-pitched and unusual screaming, persistent inconsolable crying, and bulging fontanel are compatible with an encephalopathy, but in and of themselves are not conclusive evidence of encephalopathy. Encephalopathy usually can be documented by slow wave activity on an electroencephalogram.

The health-care provider must refer to the CONTRAINDICATION section of the manufacturer's package insert for each vaccine.

Table 6-2. Recommended schedule for active immunization of normal infants and children.[1,2]

Recommended Age[3]	Immunizations[4]	Comments
Birth	HBV[5]	HBV should be given within 12 hours of birth to infants of HBSAg-positive mothers or those with an unknown HBSAg status; and as soon as possible after birth to infants of HBSAg-negative mothers.
1 month	HBV[5]	HBV should be given at 1 month to infants of HBSAg-positive mothers and between 1 and 2 months to all others.
2 months	DTP, HbCV,[6] OPV	DTP and OPV can be initiated as early as 4 weeks after birth in areas of high endemicity or during epidemics.
4 months	DTP, HbCV,[6] OPV	2-month interval (minimum of 6 weeks) desired for OPV to avoid interference from previous dose.
6 months	DTP, HbCV,[6] HBV[6,7]	Third dose of OPV is not indicated in the USA but is desirable in geographic areas where polio is endemic.
15 months	MMR,[6] HbCV[9]	Tuberculin testing may be done at the same visit.
15–18 months	DTP,[10,11] (DTaP),[12] OPV[13]	(See footnotes.)
4–6 years	DTP,[14] (DTaP),[12] OPV (MMR)[15]	At or before school entry.

Age	Vaccine	Notes
11–12 years	MMR	At entry to middle school or junior high school unless second dose previously given.
14–16 years	Td	Repeat every 10 years throughout life.

[1] Reproduced with permission from: Immunization. In: *Current Pediatric Diagnosis and Treatment*, 11th ed. Norwalk, CT: Appleton & Lange; 1993, p 214.

[2] For all products used, consult manufacturer's package insert for instructions for storage, handling, dosage, and administration. Biologicals prepared by different manufacturers may vary, and package inserts of the same manufacturer may change from time to time. Therefore, the physician should be aware of the contents of the current package insert.

[3] These recommended ages should not be construed as absolute. For example, 2 months can be 6–10 weeks. However, MMR usually should not be given to children younger than 12 months. (If measles vaccination is indicated, monovalent measles vaccine is recommended, and MMR should be given subsequently, at 15 months.)

[4] DTP = diphtheria and tetanus toxoids with pertussis vaccine; HbCV = *Haemophilus* b conjugate vaccine; HBV = hepatitis V vaccine; HBsAg = hepatitis B surface antigen; DTaP = diphtheria and tetanus toxoids and acellular pertussis vaccine; OPV = oral poliovirus vaccine containing attenuated poliovirus types 1, 2, and 3; MMR = live measles, mumps, and rubella viruses in a combined vaccine; Td = adult tetanus toxoid (full dose) and diphtheria toxoid (reduced dose) for adult use.

[5] See section on hepatitis B virus vaccine for details.

[6] See section on *Haemophilus influenzae* vaccination for details.

[7] HBV should be given at 6 months in infants of HBsAg-positive mothers but can be given between 6 and 18 months to all others.

[8] May be given at 12 months of age in areas with recurrent measles transmission.

[9] Any licensed *Haemophilus* b conjugate vaccine may be given.

[10] Should be given 6–12 months after the third dose.

[11] May be given simultaneously with MMR at 15 months.

[12] DTaP is recommended only if 3 doses of DTP have already been administered. See section on pertussis and acellular pertussis vaccine for details.

[13] May be given simultaneously with MMR and HbCVF at 15 months or at any time between 12 and 24 months; priority should be given to administering MMR at the recommended age.

[14] Can be given up to the seventh birthday.

[15] The ACIP recommends MMR at this time.

tetanus, *Haemophilus influenzae* type b, hepatitis B, and polio-myelitis should be initiated early in infancy and carried through with the recommended "booster" doses of vaccine. A combination product containing measles, mumps, and rubella vaccines (MMR) is administered at 15 months of age with a second dose recommended for school-aged children. By the time of school entry, the healthy child should have received all vaccines in the primary series and thereafter need only be given booster doses of the adult preparation of diphtheria-tetanus toxoid (Td) at 10-year intervals. Pertussis vaccine should not be given after 7 years of age, and no additional doses of poliovirus vaccine are required.

The following guidelines pertain to variations from the schedule shown in Table 6–2.

(1) If a child misses any of the DTP doses, ignore the interval and proceed with completion of the schedule.

(2) If pertussis vaccine is contraindicated in a child under 7 years of age, the pediatric preparation of diphtheria-tetanus toxoid (DT) should be substituted for DTP.

IMMUNIZATION OF CHILDREN NOT IMMUNIZED IN INFANCY

The schedule for immunization of persons not immunized in infancy is shown in Table 6–3. The following guidelines should be observed:

(1) Pediatric DT is used only for children 7 years of age. Adult Td is used for primary immunization of older children and adults (Table 6–3).

(2) Live oral poliovirus vaccine (OPV) should not be given to persons over 18 years of age. Inactivated (killed, Salk) poliovirus vaccine (IVP) should be used instead. Follow the manufacturer's instructions for dosage and booster intervals.

(3) MMR can be administered to persons of any age.

(4) *Haemophilus influenzae* b conjugate vaccine should be given to all children between the ages of 2 months and 5 years. Only those children at high risk (eg, splenectomized children, children with sickle cell disease or immunodeficiency) should receive the vaccine after the fifth birthday if they have never received it before.

IMMUNIZATION OF INSTITUTIONALIZED CHILDREN

Children who are residents of institutions, particularly institutions for the mentally retarded, may be at high risk of acquiring contagious diseases. Each resident should be immunized either before admission to the institution or at entry. The vaccines and schedule to be used will depend on the age of the resident (Tables 6–2 and 6–3).

All residents should be protected against measles, mumps, and rubella. Previous immunization documented by a physician is the only acceptable reason for not administering MMR on or shortly before admission.

Influenza vaccine should be given annually as recommended.

Poliovirus immunization should be up-to-date or should be initiated at entry if none has been given previously. For residents 18 years or older, only the inactivated vaccine (IPV) should be used.

If the child is between 2 months old and 5 years old, *Haemophilus influenzae* type b PRP-D vaccine should be administered.

Because hepatitis may pose special risks to institutionalized children, it is recommended that immune globulin be given to all residents and staff if an outbreak of hepatitis A occurs. Hepatitis B vaccine should be administered in the prescribed regimen to all individuals who enter custodial institutions.

IMMUNIZATIONS FOR ALL CHILDREN

Diphtheria

Immunization against diphtheria is effected by administration of toxoid to stimulate antitoxin production. Levels of antitoxin are related to immunity against disease, but they do not protect against the carrier state.

A. Diphtheria-Tetanus-Pertussis (DTP): This vaccine is used routinely in infants and children. It combines diphtheria and tetanus toxoids with a suspension of killed *Bordetella pertussis* organisms. Three doses of 0.5 mL each are given intramuscularly at 2-month intervals; the first dose is usually given when the infant is 2 months of age (Table 6–2). Booster doses may be given 6–12 months after the third DTP dose; at the 15-month examination along with MMR and OPV, if compliance is a con-

Table 6–3. Recommended immunization schedule for normal children not immunized in the first year of life.[1]

Recommended Time/Age	Immunizations[4]	Comments
		YOUNGER THAN 7 YEARS
First visit	DTP, OPV, MMR	MMR if child ≥ 15 months old; tuberculin testing may be done at same time.
	HbCV[3]	For children aged 15–59 months, can be given simultaneously with DTP and other vaccines (at separate sites).[4]
Interval after first visit		
2 months	DTP, OPV (HbCV)[5]	Second and third dose of HbCV is indicated only in children whose first dose was received when younger than 15 months.
4 months	DTP (HbCV)	Third dose of OPV is not indicated in the USA but is desirable in other geographic areas where polio is endemic.
10–16 months	DTP, (DTaP)[6] OPV	OPV is not necessary if third dose was given earlier.
4–6 years (at or before school entry)	DTP (DTaP),[6] OPV (MMR)[5]	DTP is not necessary if the fourth dose was given after the fourth birthday; OPV is not necessary if the third dose was given after the fourth birthday.
11–12 years	MMR	At entry to middle school or junior high.
10 years later	Td	Repeat every 10 years throughout life.

7 YEARS AND OLDER[7,6]

First visit	Td, OPV, MMR[9]	
Interval after first visit		
2 months	Td, OPV	
8–14 months	TD, OPV	
11–12 years	MMR	
10 years later	Td	Repeat every 10 years throughout life. At entry to middle school or junior high.

[1] Reproduced with permission from: Immunization. In: *Current Pediatric Diagnosis and Treatment*, 11th ed, Norwalk, CT: Appleton & Lange; 1993, p 215.

[2] Abbreviations are explained in footnote 4 to Table 6–2.

[3] See *Haemophilus influenzae* vaccination section.

[4] The initial 3 doses of DTP can be given at 1- to 2-month intervals; hence, for the child in whom immunization is initiated at age 15 months or older, one visit could be eliminated by giving DTP, OPV, and MMR at the first visit; DTP and HBV at the first visit). Subsequent doses of DTP and OPV 10–16 visit (1 month later); and DTP, HBV, and OPV at the third visit (2 months after the first visit). Subsequent doses of DTP and OPV 10–16 months after the first visit are still indicated. HbCV, MMR, DTP, and HBV can be given simultaneously at separate sites if failure of the patient to return for future immunizations is a concern.

[5] Please see section on hepatitis B vaccine for discussion of recommendations by the AAP and ACIP.

[6] DTaP is recommended only if 3 prior doses of DTP have been administered.

[7] The ACIP recommends MMR at this time.

[8] If person is ≥ 18 years old, routine poliovirus vaccination is not indicated in the USA.

[9] Minimal interval between doses of MMR is 1 month.

cern; or at the 18-month visit along with PRP-D and OPV. The fifth dose of DTP is given between 4 and 6 years of age. Thereafter, the pertussis component of the vaccine is not used. DTP and live virus vaccines can be given at the same time. If pertussis is prevalent in the community, immunization may be started as early as 2 weeks of age and doses may be given 4 weeks apart. Reduced or split doses of vaccine may not be efficacious and are not recommended. Premature infants should be appropriately immunized according to the schedule given in Table 6-2. Altered dosages or schedules should not be used with the exception that administration of OPV should be delayed, in hospitalized newborns, until hospital discharge.

B. Diphtheria-Tetanus-Acellular Pertussis (DTaP): Acellular pertussis vaccine combined with diphtheria and tetanus toxoids may be substituted for DTP at the fourth and fifth doses only. Acellular vaccines contain the following antigens: pertussis toxin, filamentous hemagglutinins, agglutinogens, and a 69 Kd outer-membrane protein. Several different acellular vaccines were developed and used in Japan with estimated vaccine efficacy of 90%. A Swedish trial with 2 of these vaccines demonstrated vaccine efficacy of 54 to 95%.

DTaP is licensed only as the fourth or fifth dose for children previously immunized with 3 doses of DTP. DTaP is administered intramuscularly in a dose of 0.5 mL.

C. Diphtheria-Tetanus (DT) (Pediatric): This preparation contains full amounts of diphtheria and tetanus toxoids and is used in children for whom pertussis vaccine is contraindicated. Three doses of 0.5 mL each are given intramuscularly at 4–8 week intervals, with a booster injection 6–12 months later. DT toxoid should not be given to anyone older than 7 years.

D. Diphtheria-Tetanus (Td) (Adult): This preparation contains less diphtheria toxoid than does the DT preparation and should be used for booster doses in older children and adults. The dose is 0.5 mL intramuscularly, given at the intervals shown in Table 6-3.

E. Diphtheria (D): This toxoid is used only when combined preparations are contraindicated.

Pertussis

Immunization with suspensions of phase I *Bordetella pertussis* prepared as vaccine can effectively reduce the risk of clinical pertussis. Infants are immunized with DTP; children over 7 years of age do not receive the pertussis component. Common adverse effects to pertussis vaccine include redness, pain or swelling at vaccination site, fever, drowsiness, fretfulness, anorexia, and vomiting. These reactions occur shortly after the vaccine and subside within 24–48 hours; however, the tendency of these reactions to occur increases with subsequent doses of the vaccine. Children who experience these reactions should receive other doses of the vaccine as scheduled; the administration of acetaminophen (15 mg/kg per dose) given at the time of vaccination and every 4 hours for 3 doses may decrease side effects to the pertussis vaccine.

More serious adverse reactions, including encephalopathy, have been reported after pertussis vaccine, but experts disagree whether the vaccine causes the reactions. None of the reported reactions are unique to pertussis vaccine; all the reactions also occur in young children who have not received pertussis vaccine. Nonetheless, future administration of pertussis vaccine is contraindicated in children who have any of the following reactions: encephalopathy within 7 days; convulsion, with or without seizure, within 3 days; persistent unconsolable screaming or crying for 3 or more hours; a high-pitched cry within 48 hours; collapse or shock-like state within 48 hours; unexplained temperature of 40.5°C (104.9°F) or higher within 48 hours; and an immediate severe or anaphylactic allergic reaction. Future administration of pertussis vaccine is contraindicated in children who have any of these more serious reactions.

Children with a neurologic disorder who have a progressive developmental delay or changing neurologic findings have an increased risk of seizures after receiving pertussis vaccine. Therefore, it may be prudent to defer pertussis vaccine because the risk of seizures after pertussis vaccine in these children may be greater than the risk of contracting pertussis itself. The decision to defer pertussis immunization should be reassessed at each visit based on the risk of postvaccine seizure compared with the risk of complications due to pertussis disease. Infants and children with well-controlled seizures may be vaccinated with pertussis because, in these children, the risk of complications owing to pertussis disease may be increased. The risk of contracting pertussis is increased in children who may travel to areas where pertussis is endemic and in children in daycare centers, special clinics, or residential care institutions. Children with neurologic conditions that predispose to seizures should not receive pertussis vaccine. These conditions include tuberous sclerosis and metabolic or degenerative disease. Such children should be observed for a time to determine the course of their neurologic involvement, and the decision whether to vaccinate should be re-evaluated at each visit. Children whose disease is controlled, resolved, or corrected may be vaccinated. A family history of seizures, SIDS, or severe reaction to pertussis vaccine by a family member is not a contraindication to pertussis immunization. All families should be informed of the risks and benefits of pertussis vaccine and given advice about appropriate medical care in the event of a seizure.

Acellular pertussis vaccines are associated with a decreased frequency of minor adverse events compared to vaccines containing whole cell pertussis. Fever, local reactions, and minor systemic reactions occur in 10–33% of children. Hyperpyrexia (temperature > 40.5°C), febrile seizures, persistent inconsolable crying, and hypotonic-hyporesponsive events have not been reported following DTaP. Severe neurologic events such as encephalopathy and prolonged seizures are rare following DTP, and no data are available on the incidence of temporal association with DTaP.

Tetanus

Tetanus toxoid is an excellent immunizing agent. Every child should receive adsorbed tetanus toxoid during infancy, usually administered in the form of DTP vaccine (see under Diphtheria, above, and Table 6–2). Older children and adults receive Td or booster injections of purified tetanus toxoid (T) every 10 years unless wound management dictates otherwise. More frequent boosters may be accompanied by local hypersensitivity reactions.

Poliomyelitis

Live, trivalent oral poliovirus vaccine (OPV) provides effective immunity and is the choice for immunization of infants in most countries. Inactivated poliovirus vaccines (IPV) are used increasingly because of the rare cases of poliomyelitis associated with OPV.

A. Live Polio Vaccine: Attenuated strains of virus types I, II, and III are grown in cell culture. Standardized suspensions of virus are stored frozen until they are administered orally. OPV is commonly administered to infants 2–3 times at 2-month intervals. This schedule usually ensures development of antibodies and immunity to all 3 types of viruses. Boosters are frequently given at 15–18 months and at 4–6 years of age; they may be given later in life under special circumstances (eg, travel to endemic regions, an outbreak of poliomyelitis).

OPV is contraindicated in children with immunodeficiency diseases, including HIV infection (Table 6–4). Children who have household contacts with immunodeficiency diseases, or who are immunosuppressed because of pharmacologic or radiation therapy should receive IPV because of the risk of paralytic disease following OPV. Vaccine-associated paralysis in vaccines or contacts have been reported to occur at a rate of one in 7.8 million. Parents and vaccinees should be informed of this rare adverse reaction.

B. Inactivated Polio Vaccine: Enhanced-potency inactivated polio vaccine (IPV-E) has a higher antigen content than previous IPV vaccine, and contains antigens of all 3 polio virus strains. IPV-E is administered in a dose of 0.5 mL subcutaneously. IPV-E is given in 2 doses 4–8 weeks apart with a final dose 6–12 months later. The necessity for 5-year booster doses, which were recommended for IPV, has not been established for IPV-E. IPV-E is the polio vaccine of choice for patients with HIV infection or other immunodeficiencies, transplant recipients, and for partially immunized adults. Family members and

Table 6–4. Recommendations for routine immunization of HIV-infected children—United States, 1988.[1]

| | HIV Infection | |
Vaccine	Known Asymptomatic	Symptomatic
DTP[2]	Yes	Yes
OPV[3]	No	No
IPV[4]	Yes	Yes
MMR[5]	Yes	Yes[6]
PRP-D[7]	Yes	Yes
Pneumococcal	No	Yes
Influenza	No	Yes

[1] Reprinted with permission from *MMWR* 1988:**37**:181–183.
[2] DTP = diphtheria and tetanus toxoids and pertussis vaccine.
[3] OPV = oral, attenuated poliovirus vaccine; contains poliovirus types 1, 2, and 3.
[4] IPV = inactivated poliovirus vaccine; contains poliovirus types 1, 2, and 3.
[5] MMR = live measles, mumps, and rubella viruses in a combined vaccine.
[6] Should be considered.
[7] PRP-D = *Haemophilus influenzae* type b conjugate vaccine.

other close contacts of patients with impaired immunity should also receive IPV-E.

Measles

Live attenuated measles virus vaccine is grown in cell culture and given subcutaneously in combination with MMR. MMR may be inactivated by heat and light, so the vaccine must be kept at 35.6–46.5°C or colder and must be protected from light.

The number of reported cases of measles in the United States decreased from 500,000 per year to a nadir of 1497 in 1983. An increase to 18,000 cases occured in 1989, and over 27,000 cases occured in 1990. Measles cases occur most frequently in unvaccinated preschool-aged children and previously vaccinated school-aged children. Both children in junior high school and college students have been infected during measles outbreaks in schools.

The increase in measles cases in school-aged children prompted the ACIP and American Academy of Pediatrics to recommend a 2-dose schedule for administration of MMR vaccine. The new 2-dose schedule attempts to protect the estimated 5% of children who do not respond to the initial dose of MMR.

The first dose of MMR is usually given at 15 months of age but can be given at any age thereafter. If vaccine is given earlier than 15 months, a significant number of individuals will fail to become immune, presumably as a result of persistent transplacental antibody. The ACIP recommends a second dose of MMR upon entrance to kindergarten (4–6 years of age). This recommendation was made to fit into the pre-existing immunization schedule for children. In contrast, the Red Book Committee recommends the second dose of MMR at the time of entry to middle or junior high school (11–12 years of age).

State or local health departments may require the second dose of MMR at school entry. Practitioners should be familiar with current local requirements.

Colleges, technical schools, and post-high school educational programs should require students who were born after 1957 to provide documentation of 2 doses of measles-containing vaccine, documentation of physician-diagnosed measles disease, or laboratory evidence of measles immunity. Students who lack documentation of measles immunity should receive 1 dose of MMR at the time of school entry and a second dose of MMR no less than 1 month after the first dose. Similar recommendations apply to medical personnel.

During local measles outbreaks or in areas with recurrent measles transmission among preschool-aged children (a county with 5 cases of measles among preschool children during each of the previous 5 years, a county with a recent outbreak among unvaccinated preschool-aged children, and cities with large unvaccinated populations), monovalent measles vaccine may be recommended as early as 6 months of age or the first visit thereafter. Children vaccinated with MMR before 12 months of age should have a repeat vaccination at 15 months of age and a third dose at the time of entry to junior high or middle school.

During school outbreaks of measles, all children and their siblings born after January 1, 1957, who have not received 2 doses of measles-containing vaccine after 12 months of age should be revaccinated.

The "further attenuated" measles virus vaccine (Moraten strain) is the only vaccine currently available in the USA. In 5% of children, the live MMR vaccine may produce a transient rash 6–14 days after vaccination. Five to 15% of children develop a fever of 39.4°C (103°F) or higher beginning 6–14 days postvaccination and lasting 1–2 days. Children with febrile seizures may be given antipyretic prophylaxis realizing that the treatment should begin before the expected onset of fever and continued for 1 week. Postvaccine encephalitis has been reported in 1 per 3 million doses of MMR.

Contraindications to measles vaccine include pregnancy, immunodeficiency, immunosuppression, recent administration of immune globulin, and known anaphylactic reaction to materials in the vaccine (ie, eggs, neomycin).

Although immunodeficiency is a contraindication to the administration of live virus vaccines, children with pediatric HIV infection should receive MMR (Table 6–4). Measles is a severe disease with frequent mortality in children with HIV infection. The risk of adverse reactions to MMR in children with symptomatic HIV is small, and must be weighed against the likelihood of acquiring severe measles infection.

Mumps

Mumps is usually benign but can be accompanied by aseptic meningitis, pancreatitis, orchitis, or oophoritis. Live vaccine confers immunity.

Live attenuated mumps vaccine is a chick embryo-adapted virus that is usually given together with live measles and rubella vaccines (MMR). Mumps vaccine is dispensed as a freeze-dried powder that must be reconstituted before subcutaneous administration. (Follow manufacturer's directions for reconstitution.)

Contraindications to mumps vaccine are listed in the manufacturer's package insert and include immunodeficiency, hypersensitivity to eggs, and all contraindications to measles vaccine (listed above).

Rubella

Rubella is a benign disease in children, but infection in pregnant women and the resulting fetal infection can have catastrophic consequences. Maternal antibodies can fully protect the fetus. Live attenuated rubella vaccine (strain RA 27/3, grown in diploid cells) is recommended for all infants, usually in combination with live measles and mumps vaccines. The contraindications are the same as for measles and mumps vaccines.

Rubella vaccine may be given to prepubertal girls and to nonpregnant, susceptible women (ie, those with negative serologic test results). Such persons should be advised not to become pregnant for at least 3 months after receiving vaccine. The vaccine strain occasionally has been isolated from placental tissues of women inadvertently vaccinated during pregnancy, but no fetal abnormalities have been definitely associated with such an occurrence. Inadvertent administration of rubella vaccine to more than 250 pregnant women has not resulted in congenital rubella syndrome. Efforts should be made to ensure that other groups, such as college students, military recruits, and postpubertal males and females, are immunized. Prenatal and antepartum screening for rubella is recommended and the vaccine should be administered to susceptible women in the immediate postpartum period prior to discharge. Protection of daycare workers, school employees, and health care workers, both male and female, should be ensured either with a history of immunization or actual disease.

Adverse reactions, which may occur 5–12 days after immunization, include fever, rash, and lymphadenopathy in a small number of children. Postpubertal females may have pain in small peripheral joints 7–21 days postvaccination, but arthritis is uncommon.

Haemophilus influenzae Type b Conjugate Vaccine

Haemophilus influenzae type b (HIB) is the cause of severe infections in young infants including sepsis, epiglottitis, and meningitis. The initial vaccine directed against HIB, the PRP vaccine, was poorly immunogenic, particularly in infants less than 1 year of age. Conjugate vaccines composed of capsular polysaccharide linked to protein molecules are far more immunogenic and have been used to successfully immunize infants beginning at 2 months of age.

Three different conjugate vaccines are available. PRP-D is manufactured by Connaught Laboratories and is composed of capsular polysaccharide covalently linked to diphtheria toxoid. This vaccine is indicated only for infants older than 15 months. This vaccine conferred only limited protection in a study in Alaskan native infants and therefore is not licensed for infants younger than 15 months.

HBOC vaccine (manufactured by Lederle-Praxis) is composed of capsular polysaccharide directly linked to a mutant diphtheria toxoid (CRM-197). This vaccine was shown 100% protective (95% confidence, interval 68–100%) in a large study in Northern California where infants were vaccinated at 2, 4, and 6 months of age.

PRP-OMP vaccine is composed of capsular polysaccharide linked with a spacer molecule to an outer membrane protein of *Neisseria meningiditis*. PRP-OMP was shown effective in a large study conducted in Navajo children. Children immunized at 2 and 4 months were protected for disease with an estimated efficacy of 93% (95% confidence, interval 45–99%). This vaccine is manufactured by Merck, Sharpe and Dohme.

HBOC and PRP-OMP were approved for administration on different schedules. HBOC is usually administered at 2, 4, and 6 months, with a booster dose at 15–18 months. PRP-OMP is usually administered at 2 and 4 months with a third dose at 12 months. It is preferable to complete the schedule of immunization with the vaccine initially used. HBOC, PRP-OMP, and PRP-D are considered to be equally safe and efficacious when used in children older than 15 months.

All infants should receive immunization against HIB using HBOC or PRP-OMP beginning at 2 months. The schedule for immunization is complex and is summarized in Tables 6–2 and 6–5. Unimmunized children older than 5 years who are at risk for invasive disease due to sickle cell anemia or asplenia should be immunized with a single dose of any of the 3 conjugate vaccines.

The dose and route for all 3 conjugate vaccines is 0.5 mL intramuscularly. Adverse effects are uncommon with these vac-

Table 6–5. Summary of recommended regimens for use of *H influenzae* type b vaccines.[1]

Age Immunization Initiated (Months)	Vaccine Product Used at Initiation	Total Number of Doses to Be Administered	Currently Recommended Vaccine Regimens (see Text)
2–6	HbOC	4	a. Initial 3 doses at 2-month intervals b. Fourth dose at 15 months of age[2] c. HbOC for doses 1–3 d. HbOC, PRP-OMP, or PRP-D for dose 4[2]
	PRP-OMP	3	a. Initial 2 doses at 2-month intervals b. Third dose at 12 months of age c. PRP-OMP for all 3 doses[3]
7–11	HbOC	3	a. Initial 2 doses at 2-month intervals b. Third dose at 15–18 months of age[2] c. HbOC, for doses 1–2 d. HbOC, PRP-OMP, or PRP-D for dose 3[2]
	PRP-OMP	3	a. Initial 2 doses at 2-month intervals b. Third dose at 15–18 months of age[2] c. PRP-OMP for doses 1–2 d. PRP-OMP, PRP-D, or HbOC for dose 3[2]

12–14	HbOC	2	a. 2–3 month interval between doses b. If the second dose is given at or after 15 months HbOC, PRP-OMP, or PRP-D may be given[2]
	PRP-OMP	2	a. 2–3 month interval between doses b. If the second dose is given at or after 15 months, PRP-OMP, PRP-D, or HbOC may be given[2]
15–59	HbOC PRP-OMP PRP-D	1	HbOC, PRP-OMP, or PRP-D[2]
60 and older[4]	HbOC PRP-OMP PRP-D	1	HbOC, PRP-OMP, or PRP-D[2]

[1] Reproduced with permission from The American Academy of Pediatrics. Committee on Infectious Diseases. *Haemophilus influenzae* type b conjugate vaccines: Recommendations for immunization of infants and children 2 months and older: Update. *Pediatrics* 1991;**88**:169.

[2] The Academy considers that safety and efficacy are likely to be equivalent for PRP-OMP, PRP-D, and HbOC for use in children 15 months of age or older.

[3] If the third dose is inadvertently delayed until the child is 15 months of age or older, the Academy considers that the safety and efficacy are likely to be equivalent for PRP-OMP, PRP-D, and HbOC for this third dose.

[4] Only for children with chronic illness known to be associated with an increased risk for *H influenzae* type b disease (see text).

cines, consisting of fever, local reactions, or mild systemic reactions in fewer than 5% of vaccinees.

Hepatitis B Vaccine

Universal immunization against hepatitis B is now recommended for all infants. Although hepatitis B vaccination has been available since 1982, the policy of selective immunization of high risk populations has not appreciably diminished morbidity and mortality due to hepatitis B. Patients at high risk for hepatitis B often do not seek immunization. Furthermore, 40% or more of patients with hepatitis B infection lack identifiable risk factors. Universal immunization in childhood is recommended rather than immunization at an older age because of the success of childhood immunization programs, and the decreased cost of immunization during infancy. Although universal immunization is recommended, this program is both controversial and expensive, due to the high price of vaccine. Antibody levels correlate with protection against hepatitis B. Antibody is known to persist for 5–8 years following immunization in the majority of patients, and protection may be more long lived. The longevity of protection from immunization in infancy is not known, but currently, booster doses are not recommended.

Two recombinant vaccines are currently available. Plasma derived HBsAg vaccine is no longer available. Recombivax HB (Merck, Sharpe and Dohme) containing 10 μg/mL and Engerix-B (Smith-Kline) containing 20 μg/mL are available for routine use, although the dosage and schedule vary with the age of the patient (Table 6–6).

All women should be tested for hepatitis B during pregnancy. Infants born to chronically infected women should receive hepatitis B immune globulin (HBIG) 0.5 mL intramusularly and hepatitis B vaccine at a different site as soon as practical and within 12 hours following birth. Infants born to HBsAg negative women should be immunized at 0–2 days, 1–2 months, and 6–18 months.

Adolescents at high risk of hepatitis B infection due to sexual activity or intravenous drug abuse should also receive immunization. Many other patient populations should be offered vaccination: hemodialysis patients, individuals likely to be exposed occupationally to blood, and caregivers of chronically infected patients. Postexposure prophylaxis following percutaneous or mucosal exposure to an HBsAg individual is also recommended.

The rate of adverse events following immunization is very

Table 6–6. Recommended schedule for immunization
with hepatitis B vaccine

	Dose of Vaccine	
	Recombivax (mL)	Engerix-B[1] (mL)
Infants[2]		
Mother HBsAg-negative[3]	0.25	0.50
Mother HBsAg-positive[4]	0.50	0.50
Children[5] < 11 years	0.25	0.50
Children[5] 11–19 years	0.50	1.00
Adults[5] > 20 years	1.00	1.00
Immunosuppressed and dialysis	1.00	2.00

[1] Engerix-B also licensed on schedule of 0, 1, 2, and 12 months.

[2] All pregnant women should be screened. Infants born to HBsAg-positive women should receive 0.5 mL HBIG at birth or within 12 hours. The schedule for immunization consists of 3 doses at 0–2 days, 1–2 months, and 6–18 months.

[3] An alternative schedule (2, 4, and 6–18 months) for infants born to HBsAg-negative mothers is acceptable but not preferred. The preferred schedule is 0–2 days, 1 month, 6 months.

[4] Infants born to HBsAg-positive women should be tested at 9 months for HBsAg and anti-HBs. An additional dose of vaccine should be administered to infants who are HBsAg-negative to infants who are HBsAg-negative and anti-HBs < 10 IU.

[5] Older children not vaccinated at birth and adults are immunized at 0, 1, and 6 months.

low and usually limited to minor local reactions and fever (less than 5%).

IMMUNIZATION FOR CHILDREN WITH SPECIAL INDICATIONS

Cholera

For children traveling to or residing in areas where cholera is endemic (or for travel to countries that require a certificate of cholera vaccination), suspensions of killed *Vibrio cholerae* vaccine give only partial protection from disease and must be repeated at 6-month intervals. The vaccine is not recommended in the control of cholera outbreaks nor for infants less than 6 months of age. The vaccination is used primarily to satisfy the requirements of several countries for vaccination prior to travel. Newer subunit or recombinant live vaccines appear safer and more efficacious in several trials and will probably replace currently available killed vaccines. Control of sanitation and use of chemoprophylaxis are also necessary.

Influenza

Epidemic influenza A or B may cause serious respiratory disease in infants or children with cardiac, pulmonary, metabolic, renal, or neurologic disease, including those with immunodeficiency and immunosuppression. Institutionalized children or those in child-care centers are at special risk. For these individuals, influenza vaccines may reduce the risk of serious illness or complications. Routine immunization is recommended *only* for children at increased risk—not for normal healthy infants and children.

The subtypes of influenza A and B to be incorporated into vaccines are selected every year, based on the strains expected to circulate during the next season. Viruses are grown in embryonated chicken eggs, purified, chemically inactivated, and made into "split" virus products. To avoid severe febrile reactions, *only* the split virus form of vaccine should be given to children less than 12 years old. More than one injection, given 4 or more weeks apart, is usually required for primary immunization. For children previously vaccinated, boosters are indicated every year. Each year, the CDC issues recommendations for influenza vaccine usage in children. Hypersensitivity to eggs is a contraindication.

Meningococcal Meningitis

Polysaccharide preparations derived from meningococcus groups A, C, Y, and W-135 are available. The type A polysaccharide is immunogenic in children 3 months of age and older, but the other types are poorly immunogenic in infants less than 2 years of age. Meningococcal vaccine is indicated during meningococcal outbreaks, if an individual plans to visit or reside in a country with endemic meningococcal disease, for children with asplenia, and for individuals with increased susceptibility to disease owing to absence of the terminal components of the complement cascade. The dose is 0.5 mL subcutaneously. The vaccine is well tolerated.

Plague

Killed *Yersinia pestis* vaccine may be used in children traveling in or residing in areas where plague is highly endemic, but is not recommended for routine use in plague enzootic areas of the country. The vaccine should be given in doses recommended by the manufacturer. Control of exposure to vectors and use of chemoprophylaxis for exposed individuals are necessary.

Pneumococcal Vaccine

A mixture of capsular polysaccharides from 23 types of pneumococci, including those that account for about 80% of bacteremic infections, is available. This preparation is not recommended for routine immunization. It should be considered for use in children at high risk of death from pneumococcal infection and in children over 2 years of age who suffer from sickle cell disease, asplenia, nephrosis, and B cell immunodeficiencies. Vaccination of children with recurrent otitis media is controversial, but the vaccine may be beneficial. The vaccine is well tolerated in children, but some children 2 years of age or older fail to develop adequate antibody responses. Children in high-risk groups must receive penicillin prophylaxis against life-threatening pneumococcal infections. The dose is 0.5 mL given intramuscularly or subcutaneously, and the vaccine is generally given only once. Routine revaccination is not indicated. However, some centers revaccinate children with sickle cell anemia, nephrotic syndrome, renal failure, transplant recipients, and asplenia 3–5 years after initial vaccination because of their very high risk of pneumococcal infection.

Rabies

Rabies develops following bites by rabid animals. It is almost always fatal. Because the disease is so feared, many persons receive rabies treatment after contact with an animal even when the chance may be very small that the animal was rabid.

The risk of rabies is dependent on the species of animal, the nature of the bite or exposure, and the geographic locale. Local health authorities are usually very knowledgeable regarding the risk of rabies and should be consulted prior to beginning vaccination.

Two vaccines are licensed for use in the United States. Rabies vaccine, adsorbed (RVA) was developed and is distributed by the Michigan Department of Health. The vaccine is supplied in liquid rather than lyophilized form and is available only from the Biologics Products Program, Michigan Department of Health ([517] 335–8050). The vaccine is a cell culture-derived vaccine that is used for either preexposure or postexposure use.

Human diploid cell rabies vaccine (HDCV) is supplied in

lyophilized form for either preexposure or postexposure use. Preexposure immunization requires three 1 mL doses of vaccine given intramuscularly on days 0, 7, and 21 or 28. Intradermal administration of HDCV only (RVA cannot be used) can be recommended as an alternative to intramuscular immunization. 0.1 mL of HDCV is given intradermally on days 0, 7, and 21 or 28. Postexposure vaccination in previously unimmunized individuals consists of five 1-mL intramuscular doses on days 0, 3, 7, 14, and 28. The vaccine should not be given in the buttock; the deltoid muscle is the preferred site in adults, and the anterolateral thigh should be used in children. For postexposure vaccination, 20 IU/kg of rabies immune globulin (RIG) is recommended. One half the dose is infiltrated around the wound and the remainder is given intramuscularly at a site separate from the vaccine. Persons with previous vaccination need only 1 mL of RVA given intramuscularly on days 0 and 3. Adverse reactions to RVA are similar to those to HDCV and include pain, redness, and swelling at injection site in 85–90% of vaccinees, and include fever, nausea, and arthralgia in 10%. Approximately 6% of persons vaccinated with HDCV developed a serum sickness-like allergic reaction.

Tuberculosis

Bacille Calmette-Guérin (BCG) is an attenuated strain of *Mycobacterium bovis*; different substrains of the organism are produced as vaccine in different countries. These substrains exhibit marked differences in invasiveness and immunogenicity. Studies of the effectiveness of BCG vary significantly, and therefore, use of BCG is controversial. Administration of BCG is limited to individuals who have a negative tuberculin skin test and who are at very high risk of infection because of (1) intimate and prolonged contact with persons untreated or ineffectively treated for pulmonary tuberculosis, or (2) exposure to persons with isoniazid- or rifampin-resistant tuberculosis and who cannot be removed from the source of exposure. BCG is also recommended for infants and children who live in areas where the rate of new infections exceeds 1% per year and where usual treatment programs have failed. The manufacturer's recommendations must be followed. BCG is not recommended for health care workers. These workers should be monitored by periodic tuberculin skin testing and isoniazid therapy for skin test-positive workers. Use of BCG varies widely in different countries, depending on socioeconomic conditions and on available measures for medical and public health control of active tuberculosis. Any form of immune deficiency is an absolute contraindication to the administration of BCG because of the possibility of disseminated and fatal BCG infection. The tuberculin skin test in a child injected with BCG will yield positive results, at least temporarily. The PPD should be repeated 2–3 months after immunization; immunization should be repeated if the child remains PPD negative. Immunization with BCG should not supplant isoniazid prophylaxis, which is of proved efficacy. The dose of vaccine is 0.05 mL intradermally in neonates and 0.1 mL in older individuals.

Typhoid

Immunization against *Salmonella typhi* infection is possible, but currently available vaccines are of moderate efficacy. Immunization is indicated for travelers to endemic areas, individuals with close contact to typhoid carriers such as household contacts, and laboratory workers with frequent contact with *S typhi*.

An inactivated vaccine has been available for many years and is associated with a high rate of systemic and local reactions. The dose is 0.25 mL subcutaneously for children < 10 years, and 0.5 mL subcutaneously in older children and adults. The vaccine is given twice separated by at least 4 weeks.

An oral, live attenuated vaccine derived from *S. typhi*, Ty21a, is available for adults and children 6 years and older. The dose of oral vaccine is one capsule per day every other day for a total of 4 capsules. Vomiting and diarrhea are infrequent reactions following oral immunization.

Booster doses are given every 3 years when parenteral vaccine is used. The manufacturer recommends revaccination after oral vaccine in 5 years.

Varicella-Zoster

A vaccine of live attenuated varicella-zoster, OKA strain, has been used extensively in normal children in Japan; in this country, similar vaccines have been tested extensively in susceptible immunosuppressed children receiving chemotherapy for neoplasia. This vaccine appears to be protective and safe, but is not currently licensed.

Yellow Fever

For children 9 months of age or older living in or visiting areas where yellow fever is endemic, a single injection of live attenuated vaccine (consisting of the 17D strain of yellow fever virus) is indicated. Infants younger than 4 months are at higher risk of encephalitis that is temporally associated with yellow fever vaccine. The vaccine is administered only by certain public health officials and may be repeated 6–8 years later. Yellow fever and cholera vaccines should be administered at least 3 weeks apart if both are required because of poor immune response to both when simultaneously administered. A valid certificate for yellow fever vaccination is required for travel to some countries.

MATERIALS USED FOR PASSIVE IMMUNIZATION

IMMUNE GLOBULINS

Standard immune globulin (IG) is prepared from pooled plasma and contains sufficient antibodies against measles, hepatitis, and other pathogens to be used as follows:

(1) For **measles prophylaxis** in unimmunized individuals exposed to the disease, give 0.25 mL/kg intramuscularly as a single dose; the maximum dose is 15 mL. For immunocompromised susceptible individuals, the dose is 0.5 mL/kg. Prophylaxis should be given within 6 days of exposure.

(2) For **hepatitis A prophylaxis** in individuals exposed to hepatitis A virus, give 0.02 mL/kg intramuscularly. Susceptible individuals include family contacts of the index case and daycare workers and children in the same classroom as the index case. If the daycare setting involves children who are not yet toilet trained and HAV infection is identified in an employee or child, or if household contacts of 2 children in a daycare setting contract HAV, all employees and enrolled children should receive IG. If the exposure is continuous, such as occurs in endemic areas of the world, this dose should be repeated in 5 months.

Recent studies have shown that intravenous immunoglobulin (IVIG) is more effective than intramuscular immune globulin. Several preparations of IVIG are now available for use in a number of conditions, yet its use in other conditions remains controversial. There is good evidence that IVIG is efficacious in the following conditions: primary hypogammaglobulinemia, selected cases of idiopathic thrombocytopenic purpura, Kawasaki disease, bone marrow and renal transplant recipients at risk for cytomegalovirus infections, and patients with lymphocytic leukemia.

Several special immune globulins are available: tetanus (TIG), rabies (RIG), varicella-zoster (VZIG), and hepatitis B (HBIG). Consult the product brochure, and follow the advice of the CDC and the Infectious Diseases Committee of the American Academy of Pediatrics for their use in specific situations.

SKIN TEST

Tuberculin Skin Test (Mantoux Test)

The Mantoux Test (0.1 mL of intermediate strength purified protein derivative containing 5 TU and inoculated intradermally) is read at 48 to 72 hours. False-negative reactions are seen in malnourished and immunocompromised patients, and in those with overwhelming disease. Temporary suppression is associated with viral infections (measles, mumps, influenza, varicella) after live virus immunization, and when corticosteroid or other immunosuppressive agents are given. A control antigen that is expected to yield a positive result in children with normal immunity should be given (tetanus, *Candida antigens*).

Tine tests consist of old tuberculin (OT) or PPD on multiple puncture metal tines. Tine tests are not recommended for screening high risk populations or patients with suspected tuberculosis due to frequent false-negative results. Positive tine tests need to be confirmed by Mantoux tests. As such, tine testing is usually not useful.

Mantoux testing is recommended in persons with suspected tuberculosis. Family members and other close contacts should also be tested. High risk populations should be screened annually.

The interpretation of a Mantoux test depends on the estimated risk of tuberculosis. Usually ≥ 10 mm of induration is considered a positive reaction. In patients at high risk of tuberculosis due to contact with an active case, chest radiograph consistent with tuberculosis, or immunocompromise, induration of ≥ 5 mm should be considered positive.

False-positive Mantoux tests (usually 5–10 mm) are often due to nontuberculous mycobacterial infection. False-negative Mantoux tests are often due to subcutaneous injection of PPD.

7 | Care of the Newborn

David W. Boyle, MD, and Steven B. Spedale, MD

ASSESSMENT & CARE OF THE NEWBORN

Assessment and care of the newborn can be divided into 3 distinct phases: antenatal evaluation, delivery room management, and postnatal care.

ANTENATAL EVALUATION

The antenatal evaluation begins with a thorough history that includes the medical history of both the mother and father, previous obstetric history, and the history of the current pregnancy. Many of the medical problems presented by an ill neonate may be anticipated from a complete history. Particular attention should be paid to chronic illnesses in the mother, maternal use of medications, illicit drugs including alcohol and tobacco, and acute medical problems (Tables 7–1 and 7–2). High-risk pregnancies should be identified early and monitored carefully for evidence of fetal distress. Whenever possible, arrangement should be made to deliver mothers with high-risk pregnancies at perinatal centers, thus avoiding transport of an ill neonate after delivery.

DELIVERY ROOM MANAGEMENT

Transition from Fetus to Newborn

The fetal circulation is shown in Figure 7–1. In utero, oxygenated blood is delivered from the placenta to the fetus by the umbilical vein. Most of this is preferentially shunted through the right atrium into the left atrium via the foramen ovale and then into the left ventricle for distribution to the myocardium, brain, and upper body. The remaining blood in the right atrium (includ-

Table 7–1. Maternal drugs and effects in the fetus and newborn.

Drug	Effect
Progestins, testosterone, and other hormones	Virilization and advanced bone age of female fetus
Thalidomide	Phocomelia
Nitrofurantoin	Hemolysis
Sulfonamides, novoblocin, oxacillin, cephalothin, sodium benzoate, and salicylates	Competitive binding with albumin in serum with resultant hyperbilirubinemia due to displacement of bilirubin
Chloramphenicol	Cardiovascular collapse and the "gray baby syndrome"
Aminopterin, methorexate, and chlorambucil	Anomalies and abortions
Dicumarol	Hemorrhage and fetal death
Heroin, morphine, and other narcotics	Tremors, neonatal death, and neonatal withdrawal symptoms in maternal addiction
Smoking	Intrauterine growth retardation
Streptomycin	Deafness
Cancer chemotherapeutic agents and phenothiazines	Parkinsonism-like syndrome
Mepiracaine and lidocaine	Central nervous system depression or seizures and irritability
Thiazides	Electrolyte imbalance, thrombocytopenia, and leukopenia
Inorganic mercury	Brain damage with cerebral palsy
Reserpine	Nasal congestion, bradycardia, hypothermia, and drowsiness
Tetracyclines	Retarded bone growth and mottled and stained teeth
Magnesium sulfate	Depression or convulsions (rare)
General anesthetics	Respiratory distress
Spinal anesthetics	Maternal hypotension with fetal distress
Paracervical block	Fetal bradycardia
Oxytocin induction	Water intoxication in the mother and hyponatremia, hypotension, and hypotonia in the infant
Vitamin K_3	Hyperbilirubinemia
Salicylates	Coagulation defects with neonatal bleeding
Quinine	Thrombocytopenia and deafness
Ganglionic blocking agents	Paralytic ileus

(*continued*)

Table 7–1. Maternal drugs and effects in the fetus and newborn.
(*continued*)

Drug	Effect
Phenobarbitol	Increase the rate of neonatal drug metabolism; a large dose may depress the infant; barbiturate withdrawal; neonatal hemorrhage due to depletion of vitamin K-dependent factors
Hexamethonium	Ileus
Atropine	Tachycardia
Prochlorperazine	Depression
Chloroquine	Retinal damage
Corticosteroids	Adrenal insufficiency
Oral hypoglycemic agents	Hypoglycemia
Radioiodine	Fetal thyroid destruction
Thiouracil derivative, potassium iodide, and potassium perchlorate	Congenital goiter
Phenytoin	Congenital anomalies (fetal hydantoin syndrome); neonatal hemorrhage due to depletion of vitamin K-dependent factors

ing superior vena cava blood) flows preferentially through the right atrium into the right ventricle and out the main pulmonary artery. As the pulmonary vascular resistance of the fetus is higher than the systemic circulation (reflecting low resistance of placenta), most of the right ventricular output is shunted across the ductus arteriosus into the aorta, which supplies the lower body. Blood returns to the placenta via the umbilical arteries.

With the onset of spontaneous respirations at birth, pulmonary vascular resistance falls and pulmonary blood flow increases secondary to the uncoiling of pulmonary vessels and vasodilation as a result of increasing Pao_2. Pressures decrease in the pulmonary artery, right ventricle, and right atrium, while left atrial pressure rises because of an increase in pulmonary venous return and in systemic vascular resistance owing to the removal of the placenta from the circulation. Left atrial pressure exceeds right atrial pressure, thus closing the foramen ovale. Systemic pressure exceeds pulmonary pressures and shunting through the ductus arteriosus is reversed. Increasing arterial oxygen tension leads to constriction of the ductus arteriosus.

Successful transition also requires that the neonate remove fetal lung fluid present in the lung prior to birth and establish

Table 7-2. Factors that increase neonatal morbidity and mortality.

Maternal Conditions	Labor and Delivery Conditions	Fetal Conditions
Previous neonatal death	Premature/prolonged rupture of membranes	Multiple gestation
Previous congenital anomalies	Prolapsed umbilical cord/cord compression	Premature delivery
Incompetent cervix	Abnormal presentation (face, brow, breech, transverse, lie, dystocia)	Fetal distress (abnormal heart rate or rhythm; passage of meconium; acidosis, fetal scalp capillary pH < 7.20)
Antepartum hemorrhage (placenta previa, abruptio placenta)	Prolonged labor	Oligo/polyhydramnios
Blood type or group isoimmunization	Mid or high forceps delivery	Intrauterine growth retardation
Maternal infection (rubella, cytomegalovirus, human immunodeficiency virus, hepatitis B virus, varicella-zoster, chlamydia, herpes simplex virus, gonorrhea, group B streptococcus, listeria, syphilis, tuberculosis, toxoplasmosis, etc)	Cesarean section	Macrosomia
	Complications of analgesia or anesthesia	Fetal malformations
	Maternal hypotension	Evidence of immaturity of pulmonary sufactant system (low lecithin: sphingomyelin ratio/absence of phosphatidylglycerol in amniotic fluid)
	Chorioamnionitis	
Chronic maternal illness (hypertension, diabetes [including gestational], renal disease, thyroid disease, cardiovascular disease, anemia, collagen or vascular disease, convulsive disorders, etc)		
Maternal age < 16 or > 35 years		
No prenatal care		
Ethanol or other substance abuse		
Smoking		

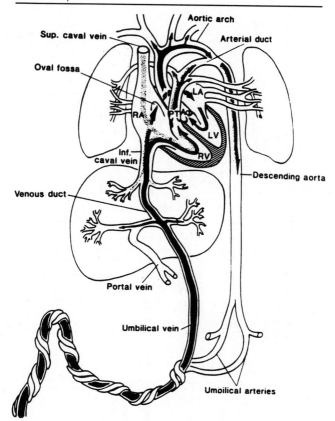

Figure 7–1. Diagram of the course of the fetal circulation.

the neonatal lung volume. As much as 30 mL of fetal lung fluid is removed during passage through the birth canal as a result of the ''physiologic squeeze.'' Additional fluid removal via absorption by alveolar epithelial cells, as well as increases in pulmonary blood and lymphatic flows, occurs in the first few hours after vaginal delivery. Initial lung inflation may require pressures of 30–40 cm H_2O. Subsequent breaths usually only require 15–20 cm H_2O. During the first 24 hours of life, the Pao_2 increases from about 55 torr to 90 torr.

The goal of high-risk obstetrics and neonatal resuscitation

is to prevent asphyxia, a condition where hypoxemia and metabolic acidosis are present in the fetus or newborn infant, which may result in end-organ damage. The physiology of asphyxia is illustrated in Figure 7–2. Primary apnea is defined as the period following hypoxia when respiration ceases as the heart rate and blood pressure begin to fall. At this point, tactile stimulation and oxygen are adequate to induce respirations. However, if asphyxia continues, the infant develops gasping respiration followed by secondary or terminal apnea, a period where there

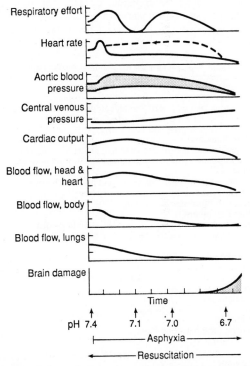

Figure 7–2. Schematic sequence of cardiopulmonary changes with asphyxia and resuscitation. (Adapted from Dawes G: *Feotal and Neonatal Physiology.* Year Book, 1968.) (Reproduced, with permission, from Avery GB: *Neonatology: Pathophysiology and Management of the Newborn.* Lippincott, 1987.)

is continued decline in heart rate and blood pressure. Positive pressure ventilation is often required for resuscitation. This sequence may occur in utero; therefore, one must assume that an infant who is apneic at birth is in secondary apnea and resuscitative efforts should proceed quickly.

Neonatal Resuscitation

Preparation and anticipation are the keys to successful neonatal resuscitation. Personnel attending deliveries should be certified in neonatal resuscitation as demonstrated by participation in the American Heart Association and American Academy of Pediatrics Neonatal Resuscitation Course. The supplies and equipment necessary for a successful resuscitation are listed in Table 7–3. The algorithm for neonatal resuscitation is presented in Figure 7–3.

Table 7–3. Equipment for neonatal resuscitation.[1]

Suction Equipment
  Bulb syringe
  DeLee mucus trap with #10 French catheter and mechanical suction
  Suction catheters #5 or #6, #8, #10 French
  #8 French feeding tube and 20-mL syringe
Ventilation Equipment
  Infant resuscitation bag connected to a pressure manometer or with a
    pressure-release valve; bag should be capable of delivering 90–100%
    oxygen
  Soft-rimmed face masks—newborn and premature sizes
  Oral airways—newborn and premature sizes
  Oxygen with flowmeter and tubing
Intubation Equipment
  Neonatal laryngoscope with #0 and #1 straight blades
  Endotracheal tubes—sizes 2.5, 3.0, 3.5, 4.0 mm OD
  Stylet
Administration of Medications
  Sterile umbilical catheterization tray
  Umbilical catheters—#3.5 and #5.0 French
  Sterile syringes and needles
  Medications (as listed in text)
  Betadine and alcohol sponges
Miscellaneous
  Clock with sweep second hand
  Radiant warmer
  Gloves, gown, mask, goggles (universal precautions)
  Stethoscope
  Adhesive tape ($\frac{1}{2}$- or $\frac{3}{4}$-inch width) and benzoin
  Scissors

[1] Modified and reproduced, with permission, from American Heart Association, American Academy of Pediatrics: *Textbook of Neonatal Resuscitation.* AHA, 1987.

Table 7–4. Mechanical causes of failed resuscitation.[1]

Cause	Examples
Equipment failure	Malfunctioning bag, oxygen not connected or running
Endotracheal tube malposition	Esophagus, right main stem bronchus
Occluded endotracheal tube	
Insufficient inflation pressure to expand lungs	
Space-occupying lesions in the thorax	Pneumothorax, pleural effusions, diaphragmatic hernia
Pulmonary hypoplasia	Extreme prematurity, oligohydramnios

[1] Reproduced, with permission, from Rosenberg AA, Battaglia FC: The newborn infant. Chapter 4 in: *Current Pediatric Diagnosis and Treatment,* 10th ed. Hathaway WE et al (editors). Lange, 1990.

Most neonates will respond to positive-pressure ventilation with 100% oxygen. Rarely should a neonate require cardiac massage or drugs. Mechanical causes for a failed resuscitation are listed in Table 7–4. Medications for resuscitation are shown in Table 7–5.

Apgar scores (Table 7–6) should be assigned at 1 and 5 minutes and every 5 minutes thereafter until 20 minutes have passed or until consecutive scores of 7 or higher are obtained. A brief screening examination should be performed in the delivery room. Special emphasis should be placed on identifying dysmorphic features, adequate chest expansion and air exchange, heart tones, abdominal masses, torsion of testes, birth trauma, and perfusion of the skin. The umbilical cord should be checked for the number of vessels present.

Indications for Endotracheal Intubation

Endotracheal intubation should be considered:

1. When the amniotic fluid is stained with meconium (see below)
2. In the preterm infant, especially those below 1000 g
3. When a diaphragmatic hernia is suspected
4. When bag and mask ventilation is ineffective
5. For prolonged positive-pressure ventilation

Management of Infants with Meconium-Stained Amniotic Fluid

Careful obstetric monitoring of fetal well being is required for these infants. The following steps should be undertaken in the delivery room:

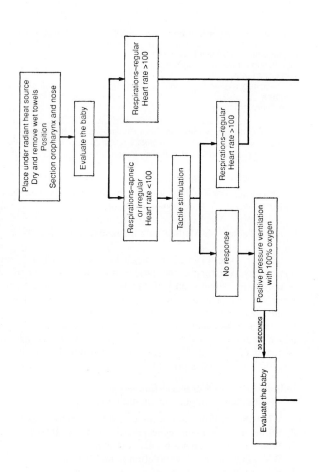

Place under radiant heat source
Dry and remove wet towels
Position
Section oropharynx and nose

Evaluate the baby

Respirations–regular
Heart rate >100

Respirations–apneic
or irregular
Heart rate <100

Tactile stimulation

Respirations–regular
Heart rate >100

No response

Positive pressure ventilation
with 100% oxygen

30 SECONDS

Evaluate the baby

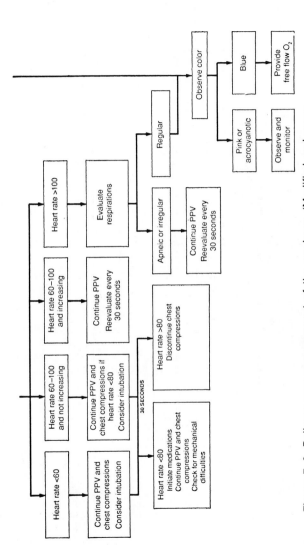

Figure 7–3. Delivery room management of the newborn. (Modified and reproduced, with permission, from American Heart Association and American Academy of Pediatrics: *Textbook of Neonatal Resuscitation.* AHA, 1987.)

Table 7-5. Medications for neonatal resuscitation.

Drug or Volume Expander	Concentration to Administer	Preparation (Based on Recommended Concentration)	Dosage	Route/Rate
Epinephrine	1:10,000	1 mL in a syringe Can dilute 1:1 with normal saline if giving IT	0.1–0.3 mL/kg	IV or IT Give rapidly
Volume Expanders	• Whole blood • 5% albumin/Saline Solution • Normal Saline • Ringer's Lactate	40 mL to be given by syringe or IV drip	10mL/kg	IV Give over 5–10 minutes
Sodium Bicarbonate	0.5 mEq/mL (4.2% solution)	20 mL in a syringe or Two 10-mL prefilled syringes	2 mEq/kg	IV Give slowly over at least 2 minutes (1 mEq/kg/min)
Naloxone Hydrochloride	NARCAN 1 mg/mL	1 mL in a syringe	0.1 mg/kg	IV, IM, SQ, or IT Give rapidly

Table 7–6. Apgar score of newborn infant.[1]

Sign	Score		
	0	**1**	**2**
A Appearance (color)	Blue; pale	Body pink; extremities blue	Completely pink
P Pulse (heart rate)	Absent	< 100	> 100
G Grimace (reflex irritability in response to stimulation of sole of foot)	No response	Grimace	Cry
A Activity (muscle tone)	Limp	Some flexion of extremities	Active motion
R Respiration (respiratory effort)	Absent	Slow; irregular	Good strong cry

[1] Practical epigram of Apgar Score. (Reproduced, with permission, from Butterfield J, Covey M: *JAMA* 1962;**181**:353. Copyright American Medical Association.)

1. As soon as the baby's head is delivered, pass a DeLee catheter or #10 French suction catheter attached to wall suction through the nares to the level of the nasopharynx and aspirate any meconium. Suction the mouth and hypopharynx.
2. If the meconium is thin or watery, complete delivery in the usual manner and provide routine resuscitation of the infant.
3. If the meconium is thick or particulate, immediately hand the baby to the pediatrician with minimal stimulation. Position the baby appropriately on the warmer and dry his or her face lightly. Suction out any residual meconium in the oropharynx using a #10 French catheter attached to wall suction.
4. If obstetric suctioning has been good and the baby already has vigorous respiratory efforts, no further intervention is indicated.
5. If obstetric suction has not been done (eg, precipitous delivery) or if the infant has not had respiratory efforts, perform direct laryngoscopy and endotracheal suctioning via an endotracheal tube and wall suction. When the airway is cleared of meconium, complete resuscitation in the usual manner.

POSTNATAL CARE

Immediate Care of the Newborn

Place the infant in a heated crib or under a radiant warmer and maintain a stable axillary temperature between 36.3 and

NEUROMUSCULAR MATURITY

	0	1	2	3	4	5
Posture						
Square window (wrist)	90°	60°	45°	30°	0°	
Arm recall	180°		100°–180°	90°–100°	<90°	
Popliteal angle	180°	160°	130°	110°	90°	<90°
Scarf sign						
Heel to ear						

Apgar _____ 1 min _____ 5 min

Age at exam _____ (hr)

Race _____ Sex _____

B.D. _____

LMP _____

EDC _____

Gestational age by dates _____ (wk)

Gestational age by exam _____ (wk)

Birth weight _____ (g)

Length _____ _____ percentile (cm)

Head circum. _____ _____ percentile (cm)

Clin. dist. _____ None _____ Mild _____ Mod. _____ Severe

Figure 7-4. Assessment of neonatal maturity. (Reproduced, with permission, from American Academy of Pediatrics and American College of Obstetricians and Gynecologists: *Guidelines for Perinatal Care*, 2nd ed. AAP and ACOG, 1988.)

PHYSICAL MATURITY

	0	1	2	3	4	5
Skin	gelatinous red, transparent	smooth pink, visible veins	superficial peeling and/or rash, few veins	cracking pale areas, rare veins	parchment, deep cracking, no vessels	leathery, cracked, wrinkled
Lanugo	none	abundant	thinning	bald areas	mostly bald	
Plantar creases	no creases	faint red marks	anterior transverse crease only	creases anterior two-thirds	creases cover entire sole	
Breast	barely perceptible	flat areola, no bud	stippled areola. 1–2 mm bud	raised areola. 3–4 mm bud	full areola, 5–10 mm bud	
Ear	pinna flat, stays folded	Slightly curved pinna, soft with slow recoil	well-curved pinna, soft but ready recoil	formed and firm with instant recoil	thick cartilage, ear stiff	
Genitals ♂	scrotum empty, no rugae		testes descending, few rugae	testes down, good rugae	testes pendulous, deep rugae	
Genitals ♀	prominent clitoris and labia minora		majora and minora equally prominent	majora large, minora small	clitoris and minora completely covered	

MATURITY RATING

Score	Weeks
5	26
10	28
15	30
20	32
25	34
30	36
35	38
40	40
45	42
50	44

36.9°C. Avoid heat loss by drying the baby thoroughly and postponing the initial bath until the infant has stabilized and the temperature is normal. Assess gestational age based on the maternal menstrual history, obstetric milestones, and gestational age assessment and physical examination of the neonate (Fig 7–4). Plot growth parameters (weight, length, head circumference) versus gestational age to determine if the infant is appropriate-size-for-gestational-age (AGA), small-for-gestational-age (SGA), or large-for-gestational-age (LGA) (Fig 7–5). Administer vitamin

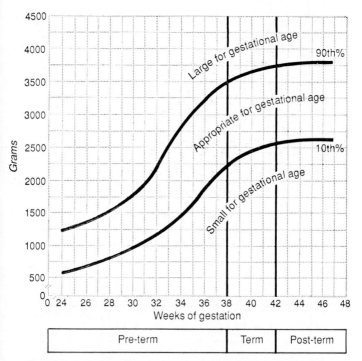

Figure 7–5. University of Colorado Medical Center classification of newborns by birth weight and gestational age. (Adapted from Battaglia FC, Lubchenco LO: *J Pediatr* 1967;**71**:159. (Reproduced, with permission, from Avery GB: *Neonatology: Pathophysiology and Management of the Newborn.* Lippincott, 1987.)

K_1 oxide (phytonadione) in a single parenteral dose of 0.5–1.0 mg within 1 hour of birth to prevent hemorrhagic disease of the newborn. Instill 1% silver nitrate, 0.5% erythromycin, or 1% tetracycline into the eyes for prophylaxis against gonococcal ophthalmia. In areas where chlamydial infection is low, silver nitrate is recommended, especially if penicillianse-producing *Neisseria gonorrhoea* are present. However, in areas where chlamydial conjunctivitis is common, topical erythromycin or tetracycline may be preferable.

Physical Examinations

All infants should have a complete physical examination within 12 hours of birth; sick infants as soon as they are stable. Term newborns have the following characteristics at birth and shortly thereafter.

A. Resting Posture: Extremities are flexed and somewhat hypertonic. Positioning may be reflective of in utero position (eg, thighs flexed on abdomen following breech presentation). Fists are clenched. Asymmetries of skull, face, jaw, or extremities may result from intrauterine pressures.

B. Skin: Skin is usually ruddy and often mottled. Localized cyanosis of hands and feet (acrocyanosis) normally disappears after several days. Skin may appear dry and peeling in the postterm newborn.

1. Lanugo (fine downy growth of hair) may be present over the shoulders and back.

2. Vernix caseosa (whitish or clay-colored, cheesy, greasy material) may cover the body but is usually on the back and scalp and in the creases of the term infant.

3. Milia of the face (distended sebaceous glands producing tiny whitish papules) are especially prominent over the nose, chin, or cheeks.

4. Mongolian spots (benign bluish pigmentation over the lower back, buttocks, or extensor surfaces) may be found in infants of dark-skinned races.

5. Capillary hemangiomas ("flame nevi") are common over the eyelids, forehead, and neck.

6. Petechiae are sometimes present over the head, neck, and back, especially in association with nuchal cord. If generalized, thrombocytopenia should be suspected.

7. Miliaria, caused by blocked sweat gland ducts, are pustules without a red base.

8. Newborns of 32 weeks or more gestational age may perspire when too warm. The forehead is usually the first site noted.

9. Erythema toxicum is characterized by erythematous raised areas with a pustule filled with eosinophils.

10. Pustular melanosis is a pustular rash that has pigment when the pustule ruptures. The pustules are noninfectious but may contain neutrophils.

C. Head: The head is large in relation to the rest of the body; it may exhibit considerable molding with overriding of the cranial bones.

1. Caput succedaneum (localized or fairly extensive ill-defined soft tissue swelling) may be present over the scalp or other presenting parts. It usually extends over a suture line.

2. Cephalhematoma (see birth injuries).

3. Anterior and posterior fontanelles may measure 0.6–3.6 cm in any direction and are soft. They may be small initially. A third fontanelle between these 2 is present in approximately 6% of infants and is more likely to occur in children with various abnormalities.

4. Transillumination normally produces a circle of light no greater than 1.5 cm beyond the light source in term infants.

5. Craniotabes (slight indentation and recoil of parietal bones elicited by lightly pressing with the thumb) is normal in newborns.

D. Face: Unusual facies occur with syndromes. Check face for bruising or forceps marks and facial nerve palsy.

1. Eyes–The irises are slate gray except in dark-skinned races. Tears may or may not be present. Most term infants look toward a light source and transiently focus on a face. Subconjunctival, scleral, and retinal hemorrhages occur with birth trauma. The pupillary light reflex is present. Lens opacities are abnormal. A red reflex can be seen on ophthalmoscopic examination. The infant will turn to follow a face more than other stimuli.

2. Ears–Eardrums may be difficult to visualize but have a characteristic opaque appearance and decreased mobility. Severe malformation of the pinnas may be associated with abnormalities of the genitourinary tract. Normal newborns respond to sounds with a startle, blink, head turning, or cry.

3. Nose–The newborn, a preferential nosebreather, experiences respiratory distress in bilateral choanal atresia. Patency should be confirmed by passage of a nasogastric tube if obstruction is suspected.

4. Mouth–Small, pearl-like retention cysts at the gum margins and in the midline of the palate (Bohn's and Epstein's pearls) are common and insignificant. Natal teeth should be removed. Rule out clefts of the lip and of the hard and soft palate. Examine the size of the tongue and mandible. The tonsils are quite small. Excessive drooling occurs with esophageal atresia.

5. Cheeks–The cheeks are full because of sucking pads.

E. Neck: Check for webbing, sinus tracts, and masses.

F. Chest: Check for fractured clavicles.

1. Breasts–Breasts are palpable in most mature males and females: size is determined by gestational age and adequacy of nutrition.

2. Lungs–Breathing is abdominal and may be shallow and irregular; rate is usually 40–60 breaths per minute, with a range of 20–100 breaths per minute. Breath sounds are harsh and bronchial. Faint rales may be heard immediately following birth and normally clear in several hours.

3. Heart–Rate averages 130 beats per minute, but rates from 90–180 may be present for brief periods in normal infants. Sinus dysrhythmia may be present. Transient murmurs are common. Check brachial and femoral pulses to rule out coarctation of the aorta. Blood pressure is a function of birth weight (Fig 7–6).

G. Abdomen–The abdomen is normally flat at birth but soon becomes more protuberant; a markedly scaphoid abdomen suggests diaphragmatic hernia. Two arteries and one vein are usually present in the umbilical cord. The liver is palpable. The tip of the spleen can be felt in 10% of newborns. Both kidneys can and should be palpated. Bowel sounds are audible shortly after birth.

H. Genitalia: Appearance in both sexes is dependent on gestational age (Fig 7–4). Edema is common, particularly after breech delivery. Rule out ambiguous genitalia. In females, an imperforate hymen may be visible. Females may develop a whitish, with or without bloody, discharge. In males the prepuce is adherent to the glans of the penis. White epithelial pearls 1–2 mm in diameter may be present at the tip of the prepuce.

I. Anus: Patency should be checked. An anteriorly displaced anus may be associated with stenosis.

J. Skeleton: Check for bony abnormalities (eg, absence of a bone, clubfoot, syndactyly, polydactyly). Examine for hip dislocation by attempting to dislocate the femur posteriorly and then abducting the legs to relocate the femur. Examine for ex-

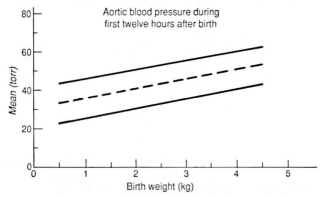

Figure 7–6. Mean aortic blood pressure versus birth weight. The solid lines are the 95% confidence limits. (Adapted from Versmold HT, Kitterman JA, Phibbs RH et al: *Pediatrics* 1981;**67**:607, copyright American Academy of Pediatrics, 1981.) (Reproduced, with permission, from Avery GB: *Neonatology: Pathophysiology and Management of the Newborn.* Lippincott, 1987.)

tremity fractures, palsies, and arthrogryposis (limited joint movement). Rule out myelomeningocele and other spinal deformities (eg, scoliosis).

   K. Neurologic Examination:

   1. Neurologic development is dependent on gestational age.

   2. Assess muscle tone and strength.

   3. Assess character of cry.

   4. Most reflexes, including the Moro, tonic neck, grasp, sucking, rooting, stepping, Babinski, deep tendon, abdominal, cremasteric, and Chvostek reflexes, are normally present at birth.

Routine Care of the Term Infant

   A. Observation: Following stabilization, observation should be made and recorded every 8 hours. Most importantly, this includes vital signs, overall well being, voiding and stooling patterns, and feeding patterns. The normal full-term neonate passes meconium in the first 24 hours of life and voids within the first 12 hours. Delays beyond 48 and 24 hours, repectively, may indicate obstruction. Daily weights should be obtained and a weight loss of 5–10% over the third to fifth day may be expected.

B. Feedings: Both breast and bottle feeding can be started immediately if the infant is stable. For infants in whom a difficult delivery and resuscitation have occurred, feedings should be delayed. Feedings may be initiated with breast milk or formula. Sterile water feedings are not necessary. The normal term infant should feed every 2–4 hours with volumes of feeding increasing from ½ to 1 ounce per feed to 1½ to 2 ounces per feed on day 3. Breast-fed infants will also feed every 2–3 hours, increasing from 4 to 10 minutes on each side. Bottle-fed babies receiving a standard iron-containing formula need no further supplementation except fluoride (0.25 mg/d) if they do not live in an area with fluoridated water supply. Breast-fed infants should receive supplemental fluoride.

C. Laboratory Screening: Cord blood is used for blood typing, Rh determination, and Coombs antibody testing. Most states have mandatory screening programs for inborn errors of metabolism (eg, phenylketonuria, maple syrup urine disease, homocystinuria, galactosemia, etc) and for congenital hypothyroidism. Samples of blood for screening tests should be taken only after the infant has had adequate intake of milk (protein) for 24 hours. Hematocrit may be done at 4 hours of age and blood glucose checked where indicated (stressed, LGA, SGA infants).

D. Circumcision: The decision to circumcise an infant should be an individual decision by parents after consultation with the pediatrician.

E. Length of Hospitalization: Neonates and their mothers are routinely being discharged after 12–48 hours. Nurseries should provide good parental education on both routine newborn care and signs and symptoms of concern to watch for (eg, jaundice, lethargy, poor feeding, vomiting, and fever).

Care of the Small-for-Gestational-Age (SGA) Infant

Regardless of gestational age, the SGA infant's weight is less than the tenth percentile for that age (Fig 7–5). The infant often appears malnourished. With increasing severe growth retardation, the infant's length and head circumference are compromised. Asymmetric growth retardation (sparing of growth in length and head circumference) implies a problem late in pregnancy (placental insufficiency of any etiology), whereas symmetric growth retardation (weight, length, and head circumference < 10%) implies an early pregnancy event (chromosomal abnormality, drug or alcohol use, congenital viral infection).

SGA infants have a higher morbidity and mortality rate than

do AGA infants. SGA infants may present with severe asphyxia in the delivery room and should be carefully examined for congenital anomalies and evaluated for intrauterine infections. Approximately two-thirds of preterm SGA and one-third of term SGA infants develop neonatal hypoglycemia (blood glucose < 40 mg/dL). SGA infants are also more likely to develop polycythemia/hyperviscosity and feeding difficulties.

Care of the Large-for-Gestational-Age (LGA) Infant

An LGA neonate is one whose birth weight is greater than the 90th percentile for gestational age. Only a portion of LGA neonates are infants of diabetic mothers. These infants are more likely to have birth injuries and hypoglycemia.

Infants of diabetic mothers have a characteristic macrosomic appearance. They are obese and plethoric and have round, full faces. In addition to the above problems, they also have an increased incidence of renal vein thrombosis (manifested by flank mass and hematuria), congenital anomalies (especially skeletal and frequently below the waist), and cardiomyopathy, as well as an increased incidence of respiratory distress syndrome, polycythemia/hyperviscosity, hypocalcemia, and hyperbilirubinemia.

Care of the Premature Infant

Initial support and resuscitation of the premature infant is the same as that for a term infant. However, he or she may need extra support owing to the functional and anatomic immaturity of various organs. In the immediate newborn period, this includes support of respiration (mechanical ventilation and oxygen), thermoregulation (radiant warmer or isolette), and fluid intake (often increased secondary to water loss through the skin). Intravenous glucose and subsequently parenteral nutrition are often necessary. Enteral feedings will need to be through a tube until after 34–36 weeks gestation.

DISEASES OF THE NEWBORN

DISEASES OF THE RESPIRATORY SYSTEM

Apnea

A. Clinical Findings: Apneic episodes occur mainly in preterm infants and are defined as a respiratory pause > 20 seconds

Table 7–7. Causes of apnea in infants

1. Temperature instability—cold or heat stress
2. Response to passage of a feeding tube
3. Gastroesophageal reflux
4. Hypoxemia: pulmonary parenchymal disease, patent ductus arteriosus, ? anemia
5. Infection: sepsis (viral or bacterial), necrotizing enterocolitis
6. Metabolic: hypoglycemia, hyponatremia
7. Intracranial hemorrhage
8. Posthemorrhagic hydrocephalus
9. Seizures
10. Drugs, eg, morphine
11. Apnea of prematurity

that is accompanied by cyanosis and bradycardia. Prematurity is the most common cause due to the immaturity of central respiratory regulation centers and of protective mechanisms that aid in maintaining airway patency. It must be differentiated from periodic breathing, which is regularly occurring ventilatory cycles interrupted by short pauses not associated with bradycardia or color changes. Various causes are listed in Table 7–7.

B. Treatment: Therapy should be guided toward the underlying cause. If apnea is due to prematurity, prophylactic cutaneous stimulation may relieve mild symptoms. Frequent or severe apnea may require intubation and ventilation or pharmacologic therapy with theophylline (loading dose 5 mg/kg and maintenance dose 1–2 mg/kg every 6–12 h) or caffeine (loading dose 10 mg/kg-base or 20 mg/kg-citrate and maintenance 2.5–5.0 mg/kg every 24 h) are helpful. Drug levels must be followed (normal 5–10 μg/mL).

C. Prognosis: In the majority of premature infants, apnea and bradycardia cease by 34–36 weeks postconception. If persistent at time of discharge, home monitoring should be considered as well as continued use of methylxanthines.

Respiratory Distress in the Newborn

A. Clinical Findings: Respiratory distress is among the most common problems seen in the newborn. Etiologies include both noncardiopulmonary as well as cardiopulmonary causes and are listed in Table 7–8. The most important clinical features include respiratory rate greater than 60/min with or without associated cyanosis, nasal flaring, intercostal and sternal retractions, and expiratory grunting. Most noncardiopulmonary causes can

Table 7-8. Respiratory distress in the newborn.

Non-cardiopulmonary	Cardiovascular	Pulmonary
Hypo- or hyperthermia	Left sided outflow tract obstruction	Upper airway
Hypoglycemia	Hypoplastic left heart	Obstruction
Polycythemia	Aortic stenosis	Choanal atresia
Metabolic acidosis	Coarctation of the aorta	Vocal cord paralysis
Drug intoxications; withdrawal	Cyanotic lesions	Lingual thyroid
CNS insult	Transposition of the great vessels	Meconium aspiration
Asphyxia	Total anomalous pulmonary venous return	Clear fluid aspiration
Hemorrhage	Tricuspid atresia	Transient tachypnea
Neuromuscular disease	Right sided outflow obstruction	Pneumonia
Phrenic nerve injury		Pulmonary hypoplasia
Skeletal abnormalities		Hyaline membrane disease
Asphyxiating thoracic dystrophy		Pneumothorax, pleural effusions
		Mass lesions
		Lobar emphysema
		Cystic adenomatoid malformation

be ruled out by history, physical, and a few simple laboratory tests (eg, glucose chemstrip, blood gas, hematocrit). The evaluation of cardiovascular disorders will be discussed later. The differential diagnosis of common causes of respiratory distress in term infants is presented in Table 7–9.

Hyaline Membrane Disease

A. Clinical Findings: Premature infants represent the largest population of infants with respiratory distress. The most common cause is hyaline membrane disease (HMD) or deficiency of surfactant. Surfactant deficiency results in poor lung compliance and atelectasis. The diagnosis is based on gestational age of infant, clinical presentation, and chest x-ray. Incidence is 5% at 35–36 weeks and rises to 65% at 29–30 weeks. On chest x-ray, the lung fields classically have a "ground glass" appearance with normal to small lung volumes and evidence of atelectasis as shown by the appearance of air bronchograms.

B. Treatment: The overall goal of therapy is to maintain a Pao_2 60–70 mm Hg with a normal pH and $Paco_2$ (35–45 mm Hg). Respiratory assessment includes arterial blood gas sampling and noninvasive oxygen monitoring with pulse oximetry or transcutaneous O_2 monitoring. Arterial access through either a peripheral or umbilical artery catheter should be obtained if the infants require a $FIO_2 > 0.40$. The need for intubation is present if the infant is unable to maintain a $Pao_2 > 60$ and $Paco_2 < 50$ mm Hg in $FIO_2 > 0.60$. Infants greater than 30 weeks gestation may benefit from a trial of CPAP alone.

The clinical availability of exogenous surfactant replacement has significantly reduced the mortality and morbidity from HMD. Commercially available surfactant preparations from lung extracts (bovine: Survanta, Infasurf; porcine: Curosurf) as well as a synthetic surfactant (Exosurf) have undergone widespread clinical testing. Each of these surfactants have demonstrated the ability to decrease mortality from HMD. Additionally, benefits such as decreased air leaks (pneumothorax, pneumomediastinum) and lower ventilator settings and FIO_2 over the first 3 days of life have been demonstrated. It has yet to be shown that exogenous surfactant replacement can decrease the incidence of BPD.

C. Prognosis: Mortality from HMD is less than 10% for infants greater than 28 weeks gestation. The major long-term sequelae is the development of chronic lung disease in 20% of the survivors, but this may change with the administration of surfactant.

Table 7–9. Common causes of respiratory distress in the term infant

Condition	Presentation	Diagnosis	Course
Delayed absorption of amniotic fluid (TTN)[1]	Slightly preterm infant or term infant delivered by C-section; tachypnea, cyanosis, grunting, retractions soon after birth	CXR—hyperexpansion, perihilar infiltrates, fluid in fissures	Usually require < 40% FIO_2; resolves 12–24 h
Clear fluid aspiration, or	Tachypnea, cyanosis, grunting, retractions soon after birth	CXR—hyperexpanded; patchy infiltrates	Protracted course of 4–7 d; may require FIO_2 30–60%
Meconium aspiration	As for clear fluid aspiration; barrel chest, fetal distress	CXR—hyperexpansion, course irregular infiltrates	Resolves 4–7 d, may require high FIO_2, at risk for PPHN[2] and air leaks; $\approx 25\%$ mortality
Pneumonia	Onset of respiratory symptoms within 6–12 h of birth, history of prolonged rupture of membranes, ± chorioamnionitis, associated shock, absolute neutropenia on CBC	CXR—variable—can mimic TTN, aspiration syndromes, HMD[3]	Variable; 10–15% mortality rate
Pneumothorax	Tachypnea, shifted heart sounds, cyanosis	CXR—transillumination	Usually resolve within 24–48 h; rarely require drainage; FIO_2 requirement usually < 40%

[1] TTN, transient tachypnea of newborn.
[2] PPHN, persistent pulmonary hypertension of the newborn.
[3] HMD, hyaline membrane disease.

158

Diseases of the Cardiovascular System

Cardiovascular causes of respiratory distress in the neonatal period can be divided into two major groups: those with structural heart disease (present with cyanosis or congestive heart failure) and those with shunting through fetal pathways and a structurally normal heart.

STRUCTURAL HEART DISEASE

A. Clinical Findings: Examples of cyanotic lesions are transposition of the great vessels, total anomalous pulmonary venous return, tricuspid atresia certain types of truncus arteriosus, and right heart obstruction (pulmonary/tricuspid atresia). Cyanosis presents early and may not be associated with any respiratory distress. However, over time many infants will develop respiratory symptoms due to increased pulmonary blood flow or secondary to metabolic acidosis from hypoxia. Diagnostic aids include failure of an infant's Pao_2 to increase significantly when placed in 100% oxygen (all lesions), decreased pulmonary lung markings on chest x-ray (right heart obstruction), and left-sided forces predominating on ECG (tricuspic atresia). Diagnosis can be confirmed with echocardiography.

Infants presenting with congestive heart failure usually have some form of left outflow obstruction (aortic stenosis, aortic atresia, coarctation). Lesions involving left to right shunting (VSD) do well until the pulmonary vascular resistance drops (3–4 weeks) and shunting becomes significant leading to heart failure. Infants with obstructive lesions do well until the patent ductus arteriosus closes (1–2 days), which previously had provided for most or all of the systemic flow. At this time heart failure and metabolic acidosis develop. Diagnostic aids include abnormal pulses on physical exam. Chest x-ray shows a large heart with pulmonary edema. Arterial blood gases are remarkable for profound metabolic acidosis.

Each infant with the various structural lesions may require basic stabilization. Specific therapy includes infusion of prostaglandin E_1, 0.05–0.1 μg/kg/min to maintain ductal patency. In some cyanotic lesions, this will improve pulmonary blood flow and Pao_2 by allowing shunting through the ductus to the pulmonary artery. In left-sided outflow tract obstruction, systemic blood flow is ductal dependent, so this will improve systemic perfusion and resolve the baby's acidosis. Further specific therapies are covered in Chapter 16.

Prognosis for structural heart lesions is dependent on the type lesion and is reviewed in Chapter 16.

SHUNTING THROUGH FETAL PATHWAYS

A. Clinical Findings:

1. Persistent Pulmonary Hypertension of the Newborn (PPHN)–This occurs in full or post-term infants who have experienced perinatal asphyxia and represents a failure of the postnatal decrease in pulmonary vascular resistance normally seen. It is also associated with hypothermia, meconium aspiration, hyaline membrane disease, polycythemia, sepsis, chronic intrauterine hypoxia, and pulmonary hypoplasia. Clinical syndrome is characterized by (1) onset 1st day, usually from birth; (2) respiratory distress; (3) poor response in PaO_2 in 100% O_2; (4) ± myocardial depression with hypotension; and (5) right to left shunting at level of PDA or foramen ovale.

2. Patent Ductus Arteriosus (PDA)–This is the most frequent cardiovascular disorder seen in the preterm infant. Presentation may occur on day 1–2 in small prematures, but most often becomes clinically significant on days 3–7 as the infant is recovering from HMD. Clinical findings include a hyperdynamic precordium, increased peripheral pulses, widened pulse pressure, and ± systolic murmur. Respiratory support may need to be increased. Echocardiogram may be confirmatory.

B. Treatment: Therapy of PPHN involves supportive therapy for related postasphyxial problems (eg, anticonvulsants for seizures, fluid and electrolyte management for renal failure). Specific therapy is designed to raise systemic pressure higher than pulmonary pressure in order to reverse the right to left shunting through fetal pathways. These include (1) O_2 and ventilation, which lowers the pulmonary vascular resistance; (2) colloid infusions (10–30 mL/kg) to improve systemic pressure; (3) systemic vasopressors to aid compromised cardiac function (Dopamine 5–20 µg/kg/min and/or Dobutamine 5–20 µg/kg/min); (4) alkalosis to raise pH 7.55–7.65 (done by hyperventilation with systemic bicarbonate administration if necessary); and (5) pulmonary vasodilators (Isuprel 0.1–1.0 µg/kg/min, Tolazoline 1–2 mg/kg IV push followed by an infusion of 0.2 µg/kg/h). Caution should be exercised with the use of vasodilators as they may cause severe systemic hypotension and worsen some infants.

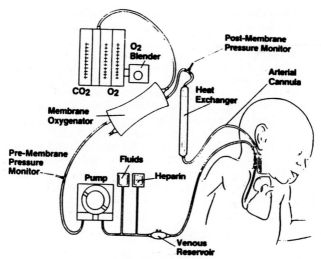

Figure 7-7. Venoarterial extracorporeal membrane oxygenation (ECMO) circuit and its components.

Recent trials with inhaled nitric oxide as a selective pulmonary vasodilator have shown promising preliminary results.

Term and near-term infants with PPHN who fail the above conventional therapy may benefit from extracorporeal membrane oxygenation (ECMO) (Fig 7-7). ECMO is the establishment of cardiopulmonary artery bypass, which provides lung "rest" for infants thought to have a *reversible* form of pulmonary hypertension commonly seen with meconium aspiration. Blood is drained from the right atrium through a catheter placed in the right internal jugular vein with the tip of the catheter in the right atrium. Blood is then passed through a membrane oxygenator where the exchange of O_2 and CO_2 takes place. The oxygenated blood is then warmed and returned to the infant via a catheter in the right common carotid artery. This procedure has had a significant impact in decreasing the mortality rate from pulmonary hypertension secondary to meconium aspiration. Risks to the patients include (1) permanent ligation of the carotid artery and internal jugular vein and (2) hemorrhage (including intraventricular) secondary to anticoagulation. Long-term sequelae are as yet unknown.

Management of PDA is both medical and if needed, surgical. Indomethacin (0.2 mg/kg IV) in a schedule dependent on the infant's age may close the ductus in about two-thirds of the cases. If the ductus reopens, a second trial may be undertaken. If this fails, surgical ligation is indicated. A major side effect of indomethacin is a transient oliguria, which can be treated by fluid restriction until urine output improves. Indomethacin does not increase the incidence and severity of intracranial hemorrhage. It should not be used if the infant is hyperkalemic, the creatinine is > 2.0 mg/dL, or the platelet count is $< 50,000/mm^3$.

C. Prognosis: PPHN carries a mortality of approximately 10–15% with long-term neurologic morbidity approximately 10%. The other major long term morbidity is chronic lung disease secondary to the extensive ventilator support required by many of these infants.

BIRTH INJURIES

Birth injuries occur during both labor and delivery. Factors predisposing the infant at risk include macrosomia, cephalopelvic disproportion, prematurity, dystocia, prolonged labor, and abnormal presentation.

Soft tissue injury consisting of petechiae, erythema, and ecchymosis is common. It usually involves the presenting part of the infant and, most often, requires no treatment. It should be noted that petechiae away from the presenting part may represent signs of an underlying hemorrhagic disorder.

Cephalhematoma is present in 0.4–2.5% of live births and represents a subperiosteal collection of blood caused by localized trauma. Cephalhematoma presents as a lump on day 1 that does not cross suture lines. Most commonly the lump is over the parietal bone. Rarely there can be enough bleeding to cause shock or anemia. Subgaleal bleeds occur beneath the scalp and are not restricted by sutures. This type of injury is rare, but can result in significant blood loss. Subdural and subarachnoid bleeds can also be seen as the result of a traumatic delivery.

The most common fracture resulting from birth trauma is to the clavicle. It may be clinically palpable or suspect in an infant who does not move an upper extremity. Therapy is usually not necessary; healing occurs with good callus formation in 7–10 days. The most common long bone fracture is to the humerus.

Nerve injuries most often involve the brachial plexus or facial nerves. Three types of brachial plexus injuries are described. (1) Duchenne-Erb: upper-arm paralysis resulting from damage to the fifth and sixth cervical nerves; (2) Klumpke's (lower arm): damage to the eighth cervical and first thoracic nerves; and (3) entire arm. Treatment involves physical therapy to prevent contractures. Most infants will recover good arm function, although 15% will suffer significant handicap. Phrenic nerve injuries, like brachial plexus injuries, occur during deliveries where the neck is severely stretched. Eighty to 90% of phrenic injuries are associated with brachial plexus damage. The clinical presentation of a phrenic nerve injury is tachypnea and cyanosis. Facial nerve injuries occur at the point where the nerve emerges from the stylomastoid foramen. Unilateral facial muscle weakness will be seen with complete resolution over several days in most cases.

NEONATAL HYPERBILIRUBINEMIA

Bilirubin Metabolism

The two sources of bilirubin in the neonate are from breakdown of circulating RBCs (75%) and ineffective erythropoiesis and tissue heme proteins (25%). Heme is converted to unconjugated (lipid-soluble) bilirubin in the reticuloendothelial system and is transported by albumin to the liver. In the liver it is conjugated with glucuronic acid in a reaction catalyzed by glucuronyl transferase. The conjugated bilirubin (water soluble) is secreted into the bilary tree for excretion via the GI tract. The enzyme B-glucuronidase is present in the small bowel and hydrolyzes some of the conjugated bilirubin. This unconjugated bilirubin can then be reabsorbed into the circulation, adding to the total load of unconjugated bilirubin (enterohepatic circulation).

Physiologic Hyperbilirubinemia
(Physiologic Jaundice)

This is a transient hyperbilirubinemia in the first week of life seen in most newborns (average 5–7 mg/dL). It is secondary to low levels of glucuronyl transferase and increased bilirubin load from an increased RBC volume with decreased survival, increased ineffective erythropoiesis, and enterohepatic circulation. Clinically, physiologic jaundice should (1) not present on day 1; (2) total bilirubin should rise by less than 5 mg/dL/d peaking at less than 12.9 mg/dL on days 3–4 (term infant) and 15 mg/dL on days 5–7 (preterm infant); (3) conjugated fraction should be less than 2 mg/dL; and (4) jaundice should persist no longer than 1 week in the term infant and 2 weeks in the preterm infant.

Nonphysiologic Hyperbilirubinemia

If criteria are not met for a diagnosis of physiologic jaundice, the cause of the jaundice needs to be investigated. Appropriate laboratory tests at this time include CBC, platelets, reticulocyte count, Coombs' test, and peripheral blood smear. The various etiologies are as follows:

A. Overproduction of Bilirubin:

1. Increased rate of Hemolysis–Increased unconjugated bilirubin and reticulocyte count.

a. Positive Coombs'–Rh incompatibility, ABO incompatibility, other blood group sensitization.

b. Negative Coombs'–RBC membrane defects (spherocytosis, elliptocytosis, pyknocytosis, stomatocytosis) and RBC enzyme defects (glucose-6-phosphate deficiency, pyruvate kinase deficiency, hexokinase deficiency).

2. Nonhemolytic Causes–Increased unconjugated bilirubin, normal reticulocyte count.

a. Extravascular Hematoma–Cephalhematoma, bruising, CNS hemorrhage.

b. Polycythemia:

c. Exaggerated Enterohepatic Circulation–GI obstruction, ileus.

B. Decreased Rate of Conjugation: Increased unconjugated bilirubin, normal reticulocyte count.

1. Physiologic Jaundice:

2. Criggler-Najjar–Type I glucuronyltransferase deficiency, autosomal recessive.

3. Type II Glucuronyltransferase Deficiency–Autosomal dominant.

4. Breast Milk Jaundice:

C. Excretion or Reabsorption Abnormalities: Increased conjugated and unconjugated bilirubin, Coombs' negative, normal reticulocyte count.

1. Hepatitis–Viral, bacterial, parasitic, toxic.

2. Metabolic–Galactosemia, glycogen storage disease, cystic fibrosis, hypothyroidism.

3. **Biliary Atresia:**
4. **Choledochal Cyst:**
5. **Obstruction of the Ampulla of Vater:**
6. **Sepsis:**

Bilirubin Toxicity

The importance of monitoring serum bilirubin is to prevent kernicterus (staining of basal ganglia and hippocampus). It occurs when unconjugated bilirubin enters nerve cells and produces cell death. Mortality is high. Clinical symptoms include lethargy, refusal to feed, high-pitched cry, hypertonicity, opisthotonos, seizures, and apnea. Sequelae include athetoid cerebral palsy, high frequency hearing loss, paralysis of upward gaze, and dental dysplasia. The risk of kernicterus in a given infant is not well-defined. The only group in which a specific bilirubin level (20 mg/dL) has been associated with an increased risk of kernicterus is infants with Rh hemolytic disease. This observation has been extended to the management of other neonates with hemolytic disease, although no definitive data exist for these infants. The risk is likely negligible for term infants without hemolytic disease, even at levels > 20 mg/dL. Prematures of 32 to 38 weeks gestation are probably safe up to levels of 20 mg/dL, while meaningful data for infants of < 32 weeks gestation are not available.

Treatment

Two modalities are in use today for treatment of hyperbilirubinemia. In phototherapy, unconjugated bilirubin in the skin is converted to a water soluble photoisomer and excreted in the bile and urine. The infant's eyes should be shielded and fluid administration should be increased to compensate for evaporative losses. Other side effects are loose stools, skin rashes, and problems with thermoregulation. In term and near-term infants, phototherapy is started at levels 4–5 mg/dL below exchange transfusion level. In babies with hemolytic disease, phototherapy can be instituted earlier (eg, level of 5–10 mg/dL on day 1 and 10 mg/dL on day 2). In very immature babies, many centers institute ''prophylactic'' phototherapy.

Double-volume exchange transfusions are utilized when the bilirubin level approaches toxic ranges to rapidly decrease serum bilirubin. As discussed above, it is difficult to specify a precise bilirubin level at which exchange transfusion should be performed. Term infants with erythroblastosis should be exchanged as the bilirubin approaches 20 mg/dL. This level can also be extrapolated to the management of infants with other hemolytic diseases. Well term infants are probably safe with levels as high as 25 mg/dL. In well preterm infants of more than 32 weeks, a level of 20 mg/dL can be used, whereas sick infants in this age range are usually exchanged at lower levels (15–18 mg/dL). In infants of less than 32 weeks, exchange transfusions are performed for levels of 12–15 mg/dL in most settings. In addition, exchange transfusions are also utilized for other indications in the care of erythroblastic infants. A partial isovolemic exchange done with packed red cells (35 mL/kg) corrects the anemia and adjusts blood volume. An early double-volume exchange with whole blood will remove the sensitized cells, hopefully decreasing the number of subsequent exchange transfusions to remove bilirubin. Indications for early double-volume exchange are cord hematocrit < 40% and/or bilirubin > 6.0 mg/dL.

Specific Causes of Hyperbilirubinemia

A. Breast Milk Jaundice: Breast milk jaundice is an unconjugated hyperbilirubinemia that peaks late (usually by days 6–14). The infant is well, and bilirubin levels are approximately 12–20 mg/dL. It can be distinguished from other causes by a prompt reduction in bilirubin upon substituting formula feeds for 1–2 days. This entity is to be distinguished from jaundice in the breast-fed infant during the first week of life. Breast-fed infants, when compared to formula-fed infants, have higher bilirubin levels due to decreased intake over the first several days of life. The treatment is not to stop breast feeding, but to increase the frequency of feedings.

B. ABO Incompatibility: ABO incompatibility is an indirect hyperbilirubinemia secondary to destruction of neonatal RBCs by maternal IgG, which crosses placenta into the fetal circulation (mother O, infant A or B). The infants may have anemia with or without jaundice, jaundice with or without anemia, or neither. Since the amount of circulating IgG antibody varies, it is not possible from one pregnancy to another to predict the severity of the process. Guidelines for phototherapy for term infants are day 1 bilirubin levels > 10, day 2 level > 13, day 3 and later level > 15 mg/dL. Exchange transfusions should be considered at levels > 20 mg/dL.

C. Erythroblastosis: Erythroblastosis is caused by isoimmunization to Rh antigens (D, C, E, d, c, or e), Kell, Duffy, Lutheran, or Kidd. Most commonly, D antigen is involved. Fetal blood may enter the maternal circulation as an initiating event. The problem worsens with subsequent pregnancies. Clinically, some infants are more affected than others. Those more severely affected will have hydrops (pleural effusions, ascites) secondary to intrauterine high output failure from anemia and hypoproteinemia. Less severe cases are characterized by hepatosplenomegaly, anemia, or jaundice.

D. Extravascular Hemorrhage: Extravascular hemorrhage within the body (eg, cephalhematoma, bruising, CNS hemorrhage) may result in an unconjugated hyperbilirubinemia secondary to a extra bilirubin load for the liver. The jaundice peak tends to peak at 3–4 days of age.

E. Gastrointestinal Tract Obstruction: Gastrointestinal tract obstruction (functional or structural) can result in unconjugated hyperbilirubinemia due to enhanced enterohepatic circulation of bilirubin.

INFECTION OF THE NEWBORN

A. Clinical Findings: There are 3 major routes of perinatal infection: (1) blood-borne transplacental infection of the fetus (eg, CMV, rubella, syphilis); (2) ascending infection with disruption of the barrier provided by the amniotic membranes (eg, bacterial infection after ruptured membranes); and (3) infection upon passage through an infected birth canal or exposure to infected blood at delivery (eg, herpes simplex, hepatitis B infections).

Early onset bacterial infections are related to perinatal risk factors and usually present on the first day of life. Symptoms include respiratory distress (most common), poor perfusion, and hypotension. Late onset disease is more subtle and may present with poor feeding, lethargy, hypotonia, temperature instability, altered perfusion, new or increased oxygen requirement, and apnea. Laboratory findings may include an abnormal CBC (decreased total count, neutropenia, increased immature/mature neutrophil ratio, thrombocytopenia), hyperglycemia, and an unexplained metabolic acidosis. Latex agglutination on a urine sample may be helpful in the diagnosis of group B streptococcus. Definitive diagnosis is made from positive blood and CSF cultures. Signs suggestive of congenital viral infection include small size for gestational age, petechiae, jaundice, and hepatosplenomegaly. A review of specific neonatal infections is presented in Table 7–10.

Table 7–10. Characteristics of specific neonatal infections.

Infection	Etiologies	Clinical Tips	Treatment
Bacterial sepsis	GBS[1], Gram negative enteric (E coli), S aureus, L monocytogenes, Enterococcus, S epidermidis	Early onset: shock, pneumonia; late onset: meningitis, local infection. Maternal diarrhea may be associated with listeria. S epidermidis is increased with indwelling lines.	Ampicillin plus aminoglycoside or third-generation cephalosporin. Vancomycin for S epidermidis. Duration of therapy 10–14 d. Intrapartum penicillin/ampicillin has had some success against early GBS.
Fungal sepsis	C Albicans	High-risk group: VLBW infants with indwelling lines.	Amphotericin B.
Meningitis	GBS, gram-negative enterics, viral (enterovirus)	High-risk group: Infants with bacterial sepsis.	Appropriate antibiotics for 21 d.
Pneumonia	Bacterial, viral (CMV[2], RSV[3], adenovirus, influenza, parainfluenza), ureaplasma, mycoplasma, chlamydia	Infection in utero or upon passage through birth canal. Older neonates: look for new onset respiratory distress or an increase in FiO_2 or ventilator settings in infants receiving respiratory support.	Specific therapy when known. Ventilatory support as needed.
Urinary tract infection	Gram-negative enterics	Uncommon early onset infection: usually associated with GU anomalies. Obtain urine culture by aspiration or catheterization.	Treat 10–14 d. Evaluate for GU anomalies.
Osteomyelitis	GBS, S aureus	Uncommon in neonates. Usually late onset disease.	See chapter 21.
Otitis	Usual bacterial agents, gram-negatives	Gram-negatives more common in long-term patients. Seen with increased incidence in infants with prolonged endotracheal intubation.	Appropriate antibiotics.

Omphalitis	Group A strep, S aureus, gram-negatives	Some degree of purulent material at the base of cord is common. Diagnosis requires erythema, edema of surrounding soft tissues.	Broad spectrum antibiotics.
Congenital viral infection	CMV[2]	Most common transmitted in utero virus. Clinical disease: SGA, hepatosplenomegaly, petechiae, thrombocytopenia, increased conjugated bilirubin. Mortality 20% with symptomatic CMV, sequelae in 90% of symptomatic survivors and 5–15% asymptomatic infants. Sequelae: hearing loss, mental retardation, delayed motor development, chorioretinitis, optic atrophy, seizures, language delay, learning disabilities. Fetal/neonatal infection increased with primary maternal infection. Can be postnatally acquired (transfusions). Diagnosis: viral cultures (blood, CSF, urine, throat, placenta, amniotic fluid).	Gancyclovir: experimental.
	Rubella	80% of fetal infection during first trimester. Clinical syndrome: adenopathy, bone radiolucencies, encephalitis, cardiac defects, cataracts, retinopathy, IUGR, hepatosplenomegaly, thrombocytopenia, purpura. Sequelae: mental retardation, hearing loss. Diagnosis: compare infant and maternal IgG; specific IgM in infant. Cultures of pharyngeal secretions.	No therapy. Prevention: Prenatal immunization for mother.
	Varicella	Congenital infection (first and second trimester) rare. Findings: limb hypoplasia, cutaneous scars, microcephaly, cortical atrophy, cataracts, chorioretinitis. Perinatal exposure (5 d before, 2 d after delivery) causes severe-fetal disseminated varicella. Diagnosis: rise in maternal IgG. IgM in infant. Culture vesicles.	Prevention: VZIG to baby in perinatal period. Can treat illness with acyclovir.

(continued)

Table 7–10. Characteristics of specific neonatal infections (*continued*).

Infection	Etiologies	Clinical Tips	Treatment
Parasitic	Toxoplasmosis (*Toxoplasma gondii*)	Congenital infection (first and second trimester). 40% children infected (15% severe clinical damage). Exposure to cat feces, raw meat. Sequelae: IUGR, chorioretinitis, seizures, jaundice, hydrocephalus, microcephaly, hepatosplenomegaly, adenopathy, cataracts, thrombocytopenia, pneumonia. Diagnosis: IgG serologies in mother. IgM in infants.	Can potentially treat known cases transplacentally by treating mother.
Perinatal acquired	Herpes simplex	Usually acquired through passage of birth canal. Primary maternal infection carries higher risk to infant. Risk likely low to infant with reactivated disease. Local/disseminated disease (onset 5–14 d); 70% may present with local skin or oral vesicles. Progression of disease common. Disseminated: pneumonia, shock, hepatitis. CNS (onset 14–28 d). Lethargy, instability, seizures. Diagnosis: viral cultures.	Acyclovir prevents progression of local disease. Decreases mortality with disseminated and CNS disease.
	Hepatitis B	Screen mothers with HBsAg[5]. Clinical illness rare at birth. Exposed infants at risk to be chronic carriers.	Maternal HbsAg positive: HBIG[6] at birth followed by vaccination. Vaccine now recommended for all newborns.
	Enterovirus	Late summer/fall: maternal illness (fever, diarrhea, rash) in week prior to delivery. Infant: fever, rash, diarrhea, lethargy. May be more severe with meningoencephalitis, myocarditis, hepatitis, pneumonia, shock DIC. Diagnosis: viral cultures—rectal, CSF, blood.	No therapy. Prognosis good except for disseminated disease.

Human Immunodeficiency Virus (HIV)	Clinical features: IUGR, microcephaly, prominent forehead, flattened nasal bridge, prominence of eyes, blue sclera, hypertelorism, long philtrum, patulous lips. May be transplacental or perinatal. Majority of infected infants present < 2 yr.	See chapter 10.
Syphilis (T pallidum)	Transplacental infection. symptoms: mucocutaneous lesions, lymphadenopathy, hepatitis, bony changes, hydrops. Diagnosis: darkfield identification of organism. Presumptive: rising serologies (VDRL); FTA-IgM. CSF exam.	IV/IM PCN 10 d.
Other congenital diseases	Congenital form rare (mother with hematogenous spread). Women with pulmonary form infect infant after delivery.	
Tuberculosis		Mother with + PPD and neg cxr: treat mother with INH and follow infant with skin tests. Mother with active disease requires separation from infant until mother no longer contagious. Follow with skin tests.
Conjunctivitis		
Neisseria gonorrhoeae	Onset 3–7 d. Gram-negative intracellular diplococci on gram stain.	PCN (systemic).
Chlamydia	Onset 5 days to several wk. Congestion, edema, and discharge	PO erythromycin

---

[1] Group B streptococcus.
[2] Cytomegalovirus.
[3] Respiratory syncytial virus.
[4] Varicella zoster immune globulin.
[5] Hepatitis B surface antigen.
[6] Hepatitis B immune globulin.

171

Table 7–11. Management of bacterial infection in the term infant.

Risk Factor	Clinical Signs[1]	Evaluation and Treatment
24-h rupture of membranes	None	Observation
>24 h rupture of membranes; chorioamnionitis ± maternal antibiotics	None	CBC, blood cultures, 48–72 h broad spectrum antibiotics
None or any of the above	Present	CBC, CSF, and blood culture, ± urine culture, broad spectrum antibiotics[2]

[1] In any infant without signs consistent with infection, it is reasonable just to observe without treatment, provided close observation is possible.

[2] Any infant, irrespective of age of presentation, who appears infected by clinical criteria should have a CSF examination. Urine culture is indicated in the evaluation of infants who were initially well and develop symptoms after 2–3 days in the nursery.

B. Treatment: Guidelines for evaluation and management of term infants are listed in Table 7–11. It must be remembered that respiratory distress in a preterm infant might also be evidence of infection. Preterm infants have a 5-fold risk for infection compared to term infants; each premature infant with respiratory distress should have blood cultures obtained. Empiric antibiotics should be given for 48–72 hours until cultures are negative. Infants with strong clinical signs of sepsis should have their CSF examined. Intravenous gamma globulin (500 mg/kg) may be given to infants with known or clinically suspect infections.

C. Prognosis: The prognosis for neonatal infection is dependent upon the specific agent and type of infection.

DISORDERS OF THE GASTROINTESTINAL SYSTEM

Tracheoesophageal Fistula/Esophageal Atresia

A. Clinical Findings: Tracheoesophageal fistula (TEF) and esophageal atresia consist of a blind esophageal pouch and fistulous connection between either the proximal or distal esophagus and airway. There is often a significant maternal history of polyhydramnios and infant history of copious secretions, choking, cyanosis, and respiratory distress. Chest x-ray following placement of a nasogastric tube will show the tube in the blind proximal pouch. If a TEF is present to the distal esophagus, gas will be present in the abdomen.

B. Treatment: Surgery provides the definitive therapy. It may be staged if initial reanastomosis of esophageal ends is not possible. A gastrostomy may also be performed until reanastomosis heals. Prior to surgery, the goal is to minimize aspiration of gastric fluid through fistula into the lungs. The infant should be supported with IV fluids and glucose, the head of bed elevated, and a nasogastric tube in the proximal pouch attached to continuous suction.

C. Prognosis: Prognosis is determined primarily by the presence or absence of associated anomalies (vertebral, cardiac, limb, and anal).

Obstructive Lesions
    A. Clinical Findings: Obstructive lesions are classified as high or low based on their location with respect to the ligament of Treitz. Clinical findings suggestive of high obstruction include a maternal history of polyhydramnios, and early onset of emesis, often bilious (Table 7–12).

Distal obstructions present with increasing intolerance of feeds, abdominal distension, and decreased or absent stooling. Imperforate anus should be sought out early as it is often missed on a cursory exam. Other causes include meconium ileus, Hirschsprung's disease, meconium plug, small left colon, and ileal and colonic atresia. Plain films will show gaseous distension with air through a considerable portion of the bowel and air fluid

Table 7–12. High intestinal obstruction in the neonate.

Lesion	Clinical Tips
Duodenal atresia	Non-bilious emesis. Abdominal x-ray will show double bubble (stomach/dilated duodenum). May be associated with trisomy 21.
Malrotation with volvulus	Bilious emesis. Abdominal x-ray often needs to be supplemented with contrast studies for diagnosis (contrast enema looking for location of caecum or upper GI study). PROMPT surgical repair necessary to prevent ischemic damage from torsion of intestine and superior mesenteric artery.
High jejunal atresia	Bilious emesis. Diagnosis confirmed with upper GI.

levels. Meconium ileus or plug and small left colon are diagnosed by contrast enema. Contrast enema and rectal biopsy are used to diagnose Hirschsprung's disease.

B. Treatment: Definitive treatment is surgical, with the exception of meconium plug and small left colon. Prior to surgery, infants should have nasogastric suction and administration of IV fluids.

C. Prognosis: Most lesions carry a good prognosis. Ten percent of infants with meconium plug will have cystic fibrosis, while all infants with meconium ileus will have cystic fibrosis. Imperforate anus is associated with other anomalies (vertebral, renal, cardiac, limb), and duodenal atresia is associated with trisomy 21. Otherwise, after surgical repair, most of these infants do well.

Abdominal Wall Defects

Omphaloceles are formed by incomplete closure of the anterior abdominal wall after the return of midgut to the abdominal cavity. The defect is usually covered by a sac, with the umbilical cord insertion into the center of the defect. The size of the defect varies but may contain intestine, stomach, liver, and spleen. There is a high incidence of associated anomalies including cardiac, other gastrointestinal, and chromosomal anomalies. Acute therapy includes covering the defect with sterile warm saline to prevent fluid loss, nasogastric decompression, IV fluids, and glucose. Definitive therapy is surgery.

Gastroschisis is a defect in the anterior abdominal wall lateral to the umbilicus. There is no covering sac, and herniated viscera is limited to intestine. The underlying etiology may be an infarct to the abdominal wall. Other than intestinal atresia, associated anomalies are uncommon. Acute therapy is as for omphalocele and definitive therapy is surgical.

Diaphragmatic Hernia

Diaphragmatic hernia is a herniation of abdominal organs into the hemithorax—usually the left—and is caused by a defect in the posterior lateral diaphragm. Infants present in the delivery room with respiratory distress, cyanosis, decreased breath sounds on the side of the hernia, and shift of the mediastinum to the opposite side of the hernia. Definitive repair is surgical but infants often require extensive resuscitation including intubation and nasogastric decompression. Postoperative course is often complicated by PPHN.

Acquired Conditions

Necrotizing enterocolitis (NEC) is the most commonly seen acquired GI emergency in the newborn period, usually affecting premature infants. The pathogenesis is multifactorial and is related to previous ischemic episodes, bacterial or viral infection, and immunologic immaturity of the infant.

A. Clinical Findings: The primary presenting sign is abdominal distension with or without associated vomiting, increased gastric residual, heme positive stool, abdominal tenderness, temperature instability, increased apnea and bradycardia, decreased urine output, and poor perfusion. CBC may show increased WBC with bandemia and decreased platelets. Diagnosis is confirmed by the presence of pneumatosis intesinalis (air in bowel wall on x-ray).

B. Treatment: Surgery is required if evidence of necrotic bowel (perforation with free air on x-ray, fixed dilated loop on serial films, abdominal wall cellulitis, progressive deterioration) is present. Otherwise, medical management consisting of nasogastric decompression, IV fluids (TPN), withholding feedings, and antibiotics is usually sufficient. Infants should not be refed until disease is resolved, examination of the abdomen is normal, and x-ray reveals resolution of pneumatosis. This usually takes 10–14 days.

C. Prognosis: Mortality rate 10%. Surgery is needed in fewer than 25% of cases. Long-term prognosis depends on the amount of intestine lost.

DISEASES OF THE BLOOD/HEMATOPOIETIC SYSTEM

Bleeding Disorders

A. Clinical Findings: Bleeding in newborns may result from inherited clotting disorders or acquired disorders that include deficiency of vitamin K dependent clotting factors: hemorrhagic disease of the newborn (HDN), disseminated intravascular coagulation (DIC), liver failure, and thrombocytopenia. Clinical features of coagulation disorders are presented in Table 7–13 and the differential diagnosis of thrombocytopenia (platelet count < 150,000) in Table 7–14.

B. Treatment: Treatment for coagulation disorders is presented in Table 7–13. Thrombocytopenia is treated by 10 mL/kg of platelets. Indication for transfusion in the term infant is clinical bleeding or a total count less than $10,000–20,000/mm^3$.

Table 7–13. Features of infants bleeding from HDN, DIC, or liver failure.

	HDN	DIC	Liver Failure
Clinical	Well infant, no prophylactic vitamin K	Sick infant; Hypoxia; sepsis, etc.	Sick infant: hepatitis, inborn errors of metabolism, shock liver
Bleeding	GI tract, umbilical cord, circumcision, nose	Generalized	Generalized
Onset	2–3 d	Anytime	Anytime
Platelet count	Normal	Decreased	Normal or decreased
PT	Prolonged	Prolonged	Prolonged
PTT	Prolonged	Prolonged	Prolonged
Fibrinogen	Normal	Decreased	Decreased
Factor V	Normal	Decreased	Decreased
Therapy	Vitamin K 1 mg	Address underlying condition; replace factors	Similar to DIC

Table 7–14. Differential diagnosis of neonatal thrombocytopenia.

Disorder	Clinical Tips
Immune Passively acquired antibody (ITP, SLE, drug induced) Isoimmune sensentization to PLA-1 antigen	Proper history, maternal thrombocytopenia Positive antiplatelet antibodies in baby's serum, sustained rise in platelets by transfusion of mother's platelets
Infections Bacterial Congenital viral infections	Sick infants with other signs consistent with infection
Syndromes Absent radii Fanconi's anemia	Congenital anomalies, also associated pancytopenia
DIC	Sick infants, abnormalities of clotting factors
Giant hemangioma	
Thrombosis	Hyperviscous infants, vascular catheters
High risk infant with RDS, pulmonary hypertension, etc	Isolated decrease in platelets is not uncommon in sick infants even in the absence of DIC

In the preterm infant at risk for intraventricular hemorrhage, transfusion is indicated for counts less than 40,000–50,000/mm³. Isoimmune thrombocytopenia requires transfusion of maternal platelets. In some cases infants born to mothers with ITP respond to corticosteroids.

Anemia

   A. Clinical Findings: Anemia can be caused by hemorrhage, hemolysis, or failure of RBC production. Evaluation of anemia includes (1) clinical assessment for signs of acute blood loss and (2) laboratory evaluation consisting of CBC, peripheral smear, reticulocyte count, and direct and indirect Coombs' test. Anemia in the first 24–48 hours of life is due to hemorrhage or hemolysis. Kleihauer-Betke on maternal blood should be performed when a fetomaternal bleed is suspected.

   Hemorrhage can occur in utero (fetoplacental, fetomaternal, twin-twin), perinatally (cord rupture, placental previa, placental incision at C-section), or internally (intracranial, rupture of liver or spleen). Infants with chronic blood loss (eg, fetomaternal) will be pale at birth but will compensate without signs of volume loss. Initial hematocrit will be low. Acute bleeding will present with hypovolemia (tachycardia, poor perfusion, hypotension) and a normal or low initial hematocrit. Hemolysis is caused by blood group incompatibility, enzyme/membrane abnormalities, infection and DIC.

   B. Treatment: Acute treatment is provision of volume (10–20 mL/kg) as 5% albumin or with whole blood to restore normovolemia. Later treatment with packed red cells is indicated for symptomatic anemia.

Anemia in the Premature Infant

   Anemia of prematurity is due to decreased erythropoietin production in response to a low red cell mass. Symptoms include poor feeding, lethargy, tachycardia, poor weight gain, and apnea. Transfusion may be indicated if an infant is symptomatic (usually occurs with a hematocrit less than 25%). Trials using human erythropoietin are under way assessing this therapy to decrease the need for late transfusions.

   Preterm infants are also at risk for Vitamin E deficiency which presents at 4–6 weeks with a hemoglobin of 6–10 mg/dL, increased reticulocytes, thrombocytosis, and edema. Prevention is possible with 25 IU Vitamin E given daily.

Table 7–15. Organ-related symptoms of hyperviscosity.

Central nervous system	Irritability, jitteriness, seizures, lethargy
Cardiopulmonary	Respiratory distress secondary to congestive heart failure or persistent pulmonary hypertension
Gastrointestinal	Vomiting, heme-positive stools, distension, NEC
Renal	Decreased urine output, renal vein thrombosis
Metabolic	Hypoglycemia
Hematologic	Hyperbilirubinemia, thrombocytopenia

Supplemental iron should be started in prematures at 2–4 months of age to prevent iron deficiency anemia.

Polycythemia

A. Clinical Findings: Polycythemia occurs in 2–5% of live births. Etiologies include twin-twin transfusion, maternal–fetal transfusion, intrapartum transfusion from the placenta associated with fetal distress, and chronic intrauterine hypoxia. The consequence is hyperviscosity, which decreases effective perfusion of capillary beds in the microcirculation. Clinical consequences can relate to any organ system and are presented in Table 7–15. Venous hematocrits greater than 70% at less than 12 hours of age and greater than 65% after 12 hours of age should be considered indicative of hyperviscosity.

B. Treatment: Treatment with partial exchange transfusion is recommended for symptomatic infants. Whether or not to treat asymptomatic infants based only on hematocrit is controversial. Albumin (5%) is transfused over a constant rate through a peripheral IV while blood is removed through an umbilical venous line. The amount to exchange is as follows:

$$\frac{\text{Peripheral venous Hct} - \text{Desired Hct}}{\text{Peripheral venous Hct}}$$

$$\times \text{ blood volume/kg} \times \text{ body weight}$$

Desired hematocrit 50–55%; Blood volume 80 mL/kg.

C. Prognosis: Followup studies at 1–2 years have revealed that infants with hyperviscosity have more motor problems, more abnormal neurologic exams, and delayed speech development. At 7 years of age, some subtle findings persist. Whether or not this outcome can be improved by treatment is unclear.

METABOLIC DISORDERS

Hypoglycemia

Hypoglycemia is defined as blood glucose less than 40 mg/dL. Although glucose concentration normally decreases in all infants during the postpartum period, most term babies have stable glucose (50–80 mg/dL) by 3 hours of age. Two high risk groups for hyperglycemia are infants of diabetic mothers and infants with intrauterine growth retardation.

In infants of diabetic mothers (IDM), hypoglycemia develops because of an imbalance in insulin-glucagon secretion due to hyperinsulinemia from islet cell hyperplasia. Infants are macrosomic because other sites grow abnormally in utero secondary to an increased flow of nutrients. They may also have asymmetric septal cardiac hypertrophy, small left colon, hypercoaguability, and polycythemia. As these infants are immature for gestational age, there is an increased risk for HMD, hypocalcemia, and hyperbilirubinemia. IDMs are also at increased risk for congenital anomalies likely related to first trimester glucose control.

Intrauterine growth-retarded infants have appropriate endocrine control but low carbohydrate stores in the form of glycogen.

Other causes of hypoglycemia include other disorders with islet cell hyperlasia (Beckwith-Wiedemann, nesidioblastosis, erythroblastosis fetalis), inborn errors (leucine sensitivity, glycogen storage diseases, galactosemia), and endocrine disorders (panhypopituitarism). Hypoglycemia may also be associated with birth asphyxia and sepsis.

A. Clinical Findings: Symptoms can be nonspecific and include lethargy, irritability, poor feeding, and regurgitation. More severe symptoms are cardiorespiratory distress, apnea and seizures. Catecholamine related symptoms may be present and include pallor, sweating, cold extremities and increased heart rate. Hypoglycemia may be detected by commercially available test strips, but these may be unreliable with glucose levels less than 40 mg/dL. All low glucose levels should be supplemented by direct measurement with glucose analyzer.

B. Treatment: A treatment regimen is present in Table 7–16.

C. Prognosis: Prompt therapy improves prognosis. CNS sequelae present with hypoglycemic seizures.

Table 7–16. Hypoglycemia: Suggested therapeutic regimens.

Screening Test	Presence of Symptoms	Action
Test strip 20–40 mg/dL	None	Confirm with blood glucose; if the infant is alert and vigorous, feed; follow frequent test strips. If the baby continues after 1 or 2 feeds to have test strips < 40 mg/dL, provide intravenous glucose at 6 mg/kg/min.
Test strip < 40 mg/dL	Present	Confirm with blood glucose; provide bolus (2 cc/kg) of $D_{10}W$ followed by an infusion of 6 mg/kg/min.
Test strip < 20 mg/dL	±	Confirm with blood glucose; provide bolus (2 mL/kg) of $D_{10}W$ followed by an infusion of 6 mg/kg/min. If IV access cannot be obtained immediately, an umbilical venous line should be utilized.

Hypocalcemia

Hypocalcemia is defined as a total serum concentration less than 7–8 mg/dL (equivalent to calcium activity of 3–3.5 mEq/L). Early onset on day 1–2 is seen in IDM, sepsis, asphyxia, prematurity, and maternal hyperparathyroidism. Late onset (1–2 weeks of age) is seen in infants receiving modified cow's milk with high phosphorus content.

A. Clinical Findings: Clinical signs include a high-pitched cry, jitteriness, tremulousness, and seizures. ECG may show increased QT interval.

B. Treatment: Calcium gluconate (0.5–1 g/kg/d) may be given orally (45–90 mg/kg elemental calcium). It is administered IV for frank tetany and seizures. Cautious IV use is necessary to prevent the right atrial calcium concentration rising too quickly causing bradycardia. Close observation for tissue infiltrates is important. The dosage is 10% calcium gluconate as a 2 mL/kg bolus over 10–20 minutes. Do not add calcium salts to IV solutions with sodium bicarbonate as they will precipitate.

C. Prognosis: Prognosis is excellent.

INFANTS OF MOTHERS WITH DRUG ABUSE

Drug abuse continues to be an increasing problem in all parts of the country. Maternal history of abuse is often difficult to obtain but must be pursued. Withdrawal symptoms are common with many drugs, narcotics and alcohol being most prominent (Table 7–17).

1. RENAL DISORDERS

Renal function is dependent on postconceptional age. Normal renal function and tests are presented in Table 7–18. Normal urine output is 1–3 mL/kg/h.

The most common disorders seen in newborns are (1) renal failure, (2) renal vein thrombosis (RVT), and (3) congenital anomalies.

Renal Failure
A. Clinical Findings: Renal failure is often seen following an asphyxial episode, hypovolemia, or sepsis. Two phases are present: (1) anuria/oliguria (first 2–3 days) associated with hematuria, proteinuria, increased creatinine and (2) polyuria with increased urine losses of sodium and bicarbonate.

B. Treatment: The initial step is fluid resuscitation, if necessary, followed by fluid restriction equal to insensible water losses (40–60 mL/kg/d) plus urine losses. Hyperkalemia must be observed for in the presence of oliguria/anuria. During the polyuric phases, the infant should be allowed to diurese if fluid overloaded with careful attention to water, salt, and acid–base balance.

Renal Vein Thrombosis
RVT is seen most frequently in IDMs and infants with dehydration and polycythemia. Clinically, one might suspect this on basis of new renal mass (usually unilateral), hematuria, and proteinuria. Anuria may be present if RVT is bilateral. Diagnosis can be confirmed with renal ultrasound. Treatment involves correcting predisposing condition, and heparinization. Systemic hypertension has been noted in some infants.

Congenital Anomalies
Abdominal masses in the newborn are most frequently due to renal enlargement (multicystic/dysplastic kidney) and hydronephrosis. Anomalies might also be suspected on the basis of maternal history of oligohydramnios that can be associated with renal agenesis or posterior urethral valves. Diagnosis in most cases is aided by renal ultrasound.

Table 7-17. Common drugs abused during pregnancy.

Drug	Clinical Tips	Treatment and Prognosis
Narcotics (heroin, methadone, propoxyphene, codeine)	Heroin/methadone withdrawal similar with methadone having longer duration. Early onset 1–2 d, although methadone withdrawal may be delayed. Symptoms: irritability, hyperactivity, tremors, high-pitched cry, excessive hunger, salivation, sweating, sneezing, yawning, nasal stuffiness, tachypnea, diarrhea, and seizures.	Supportive care (quiet environment, swaddling) usually sufficient. Medical control: phenobarbital (loading dose 15–20 mg/kg load with maintenance dose 5 mg/kg divided BID) valium, paregoric. Prognosis good but mortality can occur in severe cases. Increased incidence of sudden infant death syndrome.
Ethanol	Fetal/newborn effects proportional to abuse amount. Effects: SGA, dysmorphic features (short palpebral fissures, microcephaly), cardiac and joint anomalies; withdrawal similar to narcotics.	Treat as in narcotic withdrawal. Postnatal growth may be slow, mental retardation hyperactivity in severe cases.
Tobacco	SGA	Education of mother important.
Cocaine	May see abruptio placenta and CNS infarct of infant secondary to vasoconstrictive properties of drug. Genitourinary anomalies also reported.	Screen infant for metabolites with suspected maternal history. Close observation, no specific therapy.

Table 7–18. Summary of neonatal renal function.

Function	Premature	Full-term	2 wk	8 wk	1 yr
Glomerular filtration (mL/min/1.73 m^2)	13–58	15–60	50	63–80	120
Concentrating ability (mOsm/L)	480	800	900	1200	1400
Urine volume (mL/24 h)	24–72/kg	15–60/kg	250–400	250–400	500–600

Tests	Gestational Age			
Creatinine (mg/dL)	< 28 wk	29–32 wk	33–36 wk	36–42 wk
0–2 d	1.2	1.1	1.1	0.8
28 d	0.7	0.6	0.45	0.3

2. BRAIN AND NEUROLOGIC DISORDERS

Hypoxic Ischemic Encephalopathy

Hypoxic ischemia encephalopathy (HIE) occurs in both preterm and term infants. It is often associated with intraventricular hemorrhage in the preterm infant.

A. Clinical Findings: Infants with evidence of fetal distress before and during labor are at risk. Clinical features include (1) birth to 12 hours: decreased level of consciousness, hypotonia, decreased spontaneous movement, periodic breathing or apnea, possible seizures; (2) 12–24 hours: seizures, apnea, jitteriness, weakness; (3) over 24 hours: decreased level of consciousness, progressive apnea, onset of brain stem dysfunction, hypotonia, poor feeding.

The severity of clinical signs and length of time the signs persist correlate with the severity of insult. Other helpful diagnostic tools include EEG, CT scan, evoked potentials, and MRI.

B. Treatment: The mainstay of therapy is to provide adequate oxygen to the injured brain with normal Pao$_2$ and blood pressure. Fluids may be modestly restricted, glucose normalized, and anticonvulsants given for seizures.

C. Prognosis: The best predictor of outcome is the severity of clinical encephalopathy (severe symptoms are correlated with a 75% chance of death and 100% rate of neurologic sequelae). The major sequelae in survivors are cerebral palsy and mental retardation.

Intracranial Bleeding

A. Subdural Hemorrhage: Subdural bleeding is usually related to birth trauma and occurs in 3 locations (tentorial laceration, falx laceration, rupture of superficial cerebral veins). The major complication of the first 2 types is extension of bleeding infratentorially causing brainstem compression requiring immediate surgical drainage. Bleeds in the third location are the most common and may be asymptomatic or cause seizures on days 2–3. Diagnosis can be confirmed with CT scan or MRI. The prognosis is poor for bleeding in first 2 locations; 75% of infants with bleeding of the third type have normal followup.

B. Subarachnoid Hemorrhage: Subarachnoid bleeding is the most common type of hemorrhage. In premature infants, it is associated with germinal matrix bleed and in term infants with birth trauma. The most common presentation is with seizures and irritability on day 2 of life. Diagnosis aided by CT scan and lumbar puncture. Prognosis is good.

C. Periventricular/Intraventricular Hemorrhage: Intraventricular hemorrhage is seen almost exclusively in premature infants. The incidence is 25–35% in infants less than 31 weeks and 1500 g. Other risk factors include birth asphyxia, severe respiratory distress, and pneumothorax. Bleeding is most commonly seen in the subependymal germinal matrix but may extend into the ventricular cavity. Primary parenchymal hemorrhages can be seen as well. Fifty percent of bleeds occur by 24 hours of age and the vast majority by 4 days. Clinically, these bleeds range from asymptomatic to rapid-catastrophic presentations (coma, hypoventilation, acidosis, shock, drop in hematocrit). Diagnosis is by realtime ultrasound. The grading system is as follows: grade I—germinal matrix bleed only (60% of bleeds); grade II—intraventricular bleed without enlargement of the ventricles; grade III—intraventricular bleed with enlargement of the ventricles; and grade IV—any of the above plus intracerebral hemorrhage.

Routine screening is at 4–7 days in infants less than 31 weeks or any "sick" infant 31–35 weeks. Followup for grade I/II at 2 weeks of age; grade III/IV within 1 week of initial screen. Further followups are dictated by progression of ventricular enlargement. One should also seek evidence of periventricular leukomalacia (cystic changes in periventricular white matter), which is usually evident by 17–21 days of age.

1. Treatment–Initial treatment should be based on the infant's status; the more severely affected may require volume resuscitation, transfusion, and increased ventilatory support. If progressive posthemorrhagic hydrocephalus develops, it can be controlled by decreasing CSF production (Lasix 1 mg/kg/d plus

Diamox, increasing doses from 25–100 mg/kg/d) or by removal of CSF with daily lumbar puncture.

2. Prognosis–There is no mortality with grade I/II bleeds, while grade III/IV carry a 10–20% mortality risk. Ventriculomegaly is rare with grade I, but is found in 54–87% of grade II–IV. Long-term neurologic risk in grade I/II is no different from other prematures who experience no bleeding; with grade III/IV, severe sequelae occur in 20–25%, mild 35%, and absent in 40%. The major severe long-term sequelae include hydrocephalus, cerebral palsy, and mental retardation.

Seizures

Organized tonic-clonic seizures in infants are rare due to incomplete cortical organization and a preponderance of inhibitory synapses. The most common type of seizure is characterized by a constellation of findings including horizontal deviation of eyes with or without jerking, eyelid blinking or fluttering; sucking, smacking, drooling; swimming, rowing or paddling movements; and apneic spells. One can also see strictly tonic or multifocal clonic episodes. The differential diagnosis of neonatal seizures is listed in Table 7–19.

Table 7–19. Differential diagnosis of neonatal seizures.

Diagnosis	Comment
Hypoxic-ischemic encephalopathy	Most common etiology (60%); onset first 24 h
Intracranial hemorrhage	Up to 15% of cases: PVH/IVH, subdural, or subarachnoid bleeds
Infection	12% of cases
Hypoglycemia	SGA, IDM
Hypocalcemia, hypomagnesemia	Low-birth-weight infant, IDMs
Hyponatremia	Rare, seen with SIADH (syndrome of inappropriate secretion of antidiuretic hormone)
Disorders of amino and organic acid metabolism, hyperammonemia	Associated acidosis, altered level of consciousness
Pyridoxine dependency	Seizures refractory to routine therapy; cessation of seizures after administration of pyridoxine
Developmental defects	Other anomalies, chromosomal syndromes
Drug withdrawal	—
No cause found	10% of cases

A. Treatment: Supportive therapy to assure adequate ventilation and perfusion should be provided. Hypoglycemia should be promptly treated; other therapy is directed towards specific underlying cause. Phenobarbital (20 mg/kg as a loading dose with supplemental doses of 5 mg/kg/d up to 40 mg/kg) can be utilized. If seizures persist, therapy with dilantin, sodium valproate, lorazepam, and paraldehyde may be tried. A trial of pyridoxine for refractory seizures is indicated.

B. Prognosis: Prognosis is related to the cause of the seizure—the more difficult they are to control, the worse the prognosis. Seizures due to hypoglycemia and CNS infection, some inborn errors of metabolism, and developmental defects also have a high rate of poor outcome.

Behavioral, Psychosocial, & Psychiatric Pediatrics | 8

David F. Raney, MD

Pediatricians are in a unique position to diagnose and treat psychological and behavioral problems in children. These problems are very common and pediatricians have the opportunity to bring a holistic view to assessment and treatment including developmental, physiologic, psychological, and social perspectives. Many patients in a general pediatric practice will have significant psychopathology. Many others will have symptoms that do not define a psychiatric syndrome but are distressing nevertheless. Pediatricians can expect to encounter depression, anxiety disorders, enuresis, failure to thrive, anorexia, bulimia, drug and alcohol abuse, attention deficit hyperactivity disorder, oppositional defiant disorder, mental retardation associated with behavioral problems, etc, with great frequency in their practices. Despite the frequency of psychological and behavioral problems in general pediatric practice, these difficulties are often underdiagnosed.

ASSESSMENT

Just as one develops a structured approach to the investigation of physical complaints that ensures an adequate data base, a similar approach to psychological and behavioral complaints is crucial. Forming a "therapeutic alliance" or therapeutic contract is critical to working with psychological and behavioral problems. The physician must convey an interest in being helpful, noncritical empathy, and respect. The boundaries of confidentiality are often crucial to address, especially with adolescent patients. It is useful to establish early on that life-threatening or potentially life-threatening information will not be kept in confidence, nor will any information that may pertain to child abuse or neglect. It is important to be direct and clear. An interviewer who is comfortable interviewing engenders trust and comfort in patients and their families, which of course leads to better assessment.

INTERVIEWING

Interview of the Patient

With younger children, of course, most of the history will best come from the parents. However, verbal children of any age can often answer simple questions regarding feelings, fears, etc. It should be noted that if child abuse or neglect is suspected, it is imperative to interview the child alone at some point during the course of the evaluation. With younger children, who are nonverbal or only partially verbal, a great deal of data can still be gathered by observing how they interact with you and the environment (the examination room) as well as how they act upon separating and reuniting with family. Language used should be geared to the child's developmental level. It often helps to directly check out with the child if they understand the questions they are asked. Many children can appear to understand language that is actually quite a bit over their heads. It is useful to explain to the child or adolescent what the purpose of the examination is. For younger children, an explanation along the lines of "I'd like to talk to you about how you feel inside and how you behave" may be useful. With older children and adolescents, it is often useful to review the boundaries of confidentiality. It is best to interview adolescents without their parents at some time during the assessment (see also Chapter 9).

Interview of the Family

It is often very useful to see the child and family together. Often they will demonstrate their problem areas right in front of you. For instance, difficulties with limit setting will often be enacted in the examination room. Issues regarding control, parent/child conflict, and differences of opinion regarding how to define the problem are also usually readily apparent. It is sometimes helpful to interview parents separately from the child. This can be particularly useful in situations in which there is considerable conflict between the child and parents. At times it can be useful to understand the parents' own past history and personal experience with the developmental stage that their child is currently going through. Very frequently, parents have difficulty with their children when their children reach the developmental stage at which the parents themselves had difficulty. Exploration of parental past history may seem out of place to some parents and is best done with an adequate alliance.

Emotional Reactions

Patients and families may arouse feelings in the interviewer that can serve as useful data. For example, fear of a patient may be your first tip off to potential violence. Unexplained sadness may clue you into a hidden depression. Your emotional experience of patients or their families is a combination of what you pick up from them filtered through your own unique history. Each of us has a propensity to react in certain ways to certain situations. A working knowledge of major tendencies is often helpful.

Fortunately, most patients and their families have feelings toward caretakers which are positive, with an expectation of benign helpfulness. However, some patients and families may have had strongly negative past experiences with caretakers that can color their experience with clinicians. These patients and families can often be demanding, hostile, argumentative, and undermining of the treatment and treatment relationship. The presence of these feelings in the patient and family can be a useful clue regarding their past experiences with caretakers.

HISTORY

History should include medical/surgical history, current medication, allergies, etc—just as with the investigation of physical symptoms. In addition, *developmental history* can help place the symptoms in an appropriate developmental context as well as clue one in to more pervasive processes, which may significantly effect development over time.

Current symptoms, associated factors, and the history of symptoms over time should be elicited. Major life events/stressors for the family and/or the patient can also be useful contextual information. Both positive and negative life events have been associated with increased psychological and physical illness (e.g., deaths, moves, marriage). *Family history* of psychiatric disorders is critical, as many of these run strongly in families (including mood disorders, schizophrenia, and others).

MENTAL STATUS EXAMINATION

The importance of the mental status examination in assessing serious psychological and behavioral problems cannot be overstated. One should view the mental status examination as the *brain* examination. The mental status examination is an objective, semi-standard organization and recording of observations of the patient. It includes both a formal and a descriptive section. It is very useful to record the mental status examination in a semi-standard way. Many illnesses involve changes in mental status over time. A semi-standardized format will help ensure that your mental status examination will be of use to future clinicians. Clinicians are frequently tempted to omit the formal mental status examination, believing that they can "tell" if the patient's brain is functioning well by informal assessment. However, even relatively large cognitive defects may be missed without direct assessment. A screening mental status exam is detailed in Table 8–1. Interpretation of the mental status exam can be complex. In general, one is looking for gross variance from age/grade-expected norms. Interpretation of the mental status examination is covered in more detail in the emergency assessment section. It is useful to introduce the mental status examination in a matter-of-fact way designed to put the patient at ease. For instance: "I'm going to ask you a series of questions that will help me understand how you think. Some of the questions may not apply to you. Some may seem too easy or too hard. I ask everyone the same questions."

PHYSICAL EXAMINATION

Remember that for any psychological or behavioral symptom there are numerous potential identifiable organic factors that can cause or be associated with the symptom. Tables 8–2 through 8–9 detail some of these.

LABORATORY EVALUATION

This can be tailored to the patient based on the symptoms presented and the results of the mental status examination and physical. Suggested laboratory evaluations will be presented in the discussion of specific disorders later in the chapter.

Table 8–1. Mental status examination.

Descriptive:

A. **Appearance:** Age appropriate? Neat or sloppy? Dysmorphic features?

B. **Mood/Affect:** Older children can usually tell you how they feel. Behavioral observation augments what the patient tells you.

C. **Motor Behaviors:** Look for increased or decreased activity level or abnormal movements.

D. **Thought Form:** Are thoughts logical and coherent?

E. **Thought and Behavior Content:** Are there hallucinations, delusions, loose associations, conflictual themes?

Formal Mental Status Examination:

A. **Level of Consciousness:** Can be increased *or* decreased, or can vary.

B. **Orientation:**
Person:	Verbal children should know their names.
Place:	Young children will know whether or not they are at home. School-aged children should know that they are in a doctor's office.
Time:	A complete sense of time is usually formed by age 8 or 9. Younger children can tell if it is day or night.

C. **General Information:** Tailor to age (sports, music). School-aged children should know their teacher's name.

D. **Memory:**
Immediate:	This involves repeating words or numbers. Standards are available.
Short-Term:	Ask the patient to remember 3 objects, make sure they can repeat them back, then ask again in 3 to 5 minutes.
Long-term:	For example, ask birthday or what they had for breakfast.

E. **Abstracting (Proverbs and Similarities):** In testing similarities, the patient needs to understand that you are looking for the common category the objects are in. Only patients in Piaget's formal operations stage do these tasks well. Many older adolescents have reached this stage.

F. **Calculations:** Age/grade level can guide you.

G. **Judgment:** These questions are not useful, as even patients with very poor judgement can get the standard judgement questions correct.

EMERGENCY ASSESSMENT

The role of emergency assessment is to determine if any action is urgently necessary on your part in order to prevent serious physical or psychological morbidity/mortality. A complete assessment with a complete diagnosis and full treatment plan is not necessary. The assessment needs to be focused on learning enough to make emergency intervention and to *begin*

Table 8–2. Drugs associated with psychosis.[1]

Alcohol	Corticosteroid
Amantadine	Cyclobenzaprine (Flexeril)
Aminocaproic acid	Cycloserine
Amiodarone	Cyclosporine
Amphetamines	Dapsone
Anabolic steroids	Decongestants
Anticonvulsants	Oxymetazoline (Afrin)
Barbiturates	Phenylephrine
Carbamazepine	Pseudoephedrine
Ethosuximide	Phenylpropanolamine
Valproic acid	Deet (Bug Spray)
Primidone	Digitalis
Antidepressants	Disopyramide
Tricyclic antidepressants	Disulfiram
Monoamine oxidase inhibitors	Dronabinol
Bupropion	Ephedrine
Trazodone	H2-Blockers
Antihistamines	Cimetidine
Antimicrobial/antiviral agents	Ranitidine
Acyclovir	Hallucinogens
Cephalosporins	LSD
Quinine derivatives	PCP
Ethionamide	Mescaline
Gentamicin	THC
Isoniazid	Psilocybin
Ketoconazole	Interferon
Metronidazole	Isosorbide Dinitrate
Nalidixic Acid	Levodopa
Procaine penicillin and other	Lidocaine
procaine derivatives	Methyldopa
Tobramycin	Methylphenidate
Trimethoprin-sulfamethoxazole	Methysergide
Zidovudine	Metoclopramide (Reglan)
Asparaginase	Metrizamide (Contrast)
Atropine, anticholinergics	Narcotics
Baclofen	Nonsteroidal Anti-Inflammatory
Benzodiazepines	Drugs
Beta-adrenergic blockers	Podophyllin
Bromocriptine	Prazosin
Caffeine	Promethazine (Phenergan)
Captopril	Quinidine
Chlorambucil	Salicylates
Clomiphene	Thyroid Hormone
Clonidine	Verapamil
Cocaine	Vincristine

[1] Used with permission from Campo J. Medical issues in the care of child and adolescent inpatients. In: Bellack AS, Hersen M, eds. Handbook of Behavior Therapy in the Psychiatric Setting. New York: Plenum; 1993: 378.

Table 8–3. Medical conditions associated with psychosis.[1]

Drugs/withdrawal (*see* Table 8–2)
Toxins
  Heavy metals
  Organic fluorides
  Organic phosphates
  Carbon disulfide
Metabolic
  Electrolyte imbalance
  Hypercalcemia, hypocalcemia
  Hypoglycemia
  Hepatic failure/hyperammonemia
  Inborn errors of metabolism (eg, acute intermittent porphyria, Wilson's
    disease, homocystinuria)
Endocrine
  Hypo or hyperthyroidism
  Hyper or hypoparathyroidism
  Hyperadrenalism
  Hypoadrenalism
Infectious
  CNS Infection (eg, viral meningoencephalitis, parasitosis)
  Neurosyphilis
  HIV infection
  Systemic infection
Neurologic/CNS
  Epilepsy (partial complex epilepsy)
  Cerebrovascular disease (stroke, hemorrhage, hematoma)
  Intracranial mass lesion (tumor, AVM)
  Trauma
  Neurodegenerative disorders (eg, Huntington's chorea, spinocerebellar
    degeneration)
  Multiple sclerosis
Nutritional
  Zinc deficiency
  Thiamine deficiency
  B_{12}, folate deficiency
  Nicotinic acid deficiency (pellagra)
  Pyridoxine deficiency
Systemic illness
  Systemic lupus erythematosus, collagen–vascular disease
  Sleep or sensory deprivation
  Post operative state
  Systemic malignancy

[1] Used with permission from Campo J. Medical issues in the care of child and adolescent inpatients. In: Bellack AS, Hersen M, eds. Handbook of Behavior Therapy in the Psychiatric Setting. New York: Plenum; 1993: 379.

Table 8–4. Drugs associated with depression.[1]

Acyclovir	Interferon
Amphetamines	Isoniazid
Anabolic steroids	Isosorbide dinitrate
Asparaginase	Isotretinoin (Accutane)
Baclofen	Levodopa
Barbiturates	Methyldopa
Benzodiazapines	Metoclopramide (Reglan)
Beta adrenergic blockers	Metrizamide (contrast)
Bromocriptine	Metronidazole
Clonidine	Nalidixic acid
Cocaine	Narcotics
Corticosteroid	Neuroleptics
Cycloserine	Nifedipine (Procardia)
Dapsone	Nonsteroidal anti-inflammatory
Digitalis	agents
Diltiazem	Norfloxacin
Disopyramide	Oral contraceptives, estrogens
Disulfiram	Pergolide
Ethambutol	Phenylephrine
Ethionamide	Prazosin
Etretinate	Procaine derivatives
Halothane	Reserpine
H₂ blockers	Thiazide diuretics
Cimetidine	Thyroid hormone
Ranitidine	Trimethoprim-sulfamethoxazole

[1] Used with permission from Campo J. Medical issues in the care of child and adolescent inpatients. In: Bellack AS, Hersen M, eds. Handbook of Behavior Therapy in the Psychiatric Setting. New York: Plenum; 1993: 381.

the process of treatment. This may involve referrals to other agencies and/or professionals. Remember that you may be the only physician to be involved in the patient's assessment and thus may be crucial in the appropriate evaluation of physical problems. Unfortunately, many mental health professionals may seriously underestimate the possibility of organic pathology and thus do not refer back to the pediatrician for assessment of this as appropriate. If you suspect organic pathology, be sure to communicate this when making a referral for followup. If you are uncertain of organic pathology, or the evaluation is ongoing, do *not* declare the patient "medically cleared". This is often misinterpreted by mental health professionals to mean that all possible contributing physical conditions have been ruled out.

Table 8–5. Medical conditions associated with depression.[1]

Drugs/withdrawal (*see* Table 8–4)	Tuberculosis
Prenatal exposure to	Neurologic/CNS
diethylstilbestrol (DES)	Intracranial mass lesion (tumor,
Toxins	arteriovenous malformation)
Heavy metals	Cerebrovascular disease
Metabolic	(stroke, hemorrhage,
Electrolyte imbalance	hematoma)
Uremia	Trauma
Anemia	Neurodegenerative disorders
Hepatic failure	Epilepsy (especially partial
Hypocalcemia, hypercalcemia	complex epilepsy)
Hypomagnesemia	Migraine
Wilson's disease	Nutritional
Endocrine	B$_{12}$, folate deficiency
Hypo- or hyperthyroidism	Thiamine deficiency
Hypopituitarism	Nicotinic acid deficiency
Adrenal insufficiency (Addison's	(pellagra)
disease)	Iron deficiency
Hyperadrenalism (Cushing's	Malnutrition, protein deficiency
syndrome)	Vitamin C deficiency
Hyperparathyroidism	Zinc deficiency
Hyperaldosteronism	Systemic Disease
Hyperinsulinism	Systemic malignancy (eg,
Infectious	lymphoma)
HIV infection	Carcinoid syndrome
Encephalitis	Sarcoidosis
Neurosyphilis	Systemic lupus erythematosus,
Hepatitis	rheumatoid arthritis, collagen-
Influenza	vascular disease
Infectious mononucleosis	Inflammatory bowel disease
Malaria	Sleep deprivation, obstructive
Brucellosis	sleep apnea

[1] Used with permission from Campo J. Medical issues in the care of child and adolescent inpatients. In: Bellack AS, Hersen M, eds. Handbook of Behavior Therapy in the Psychiatric Setting. New York: Plenum; 1993: 381.

Instead, direct communication of your findings and what you think needs to be looked for in the future and how to approach this is indicated. A psychiatric diagnosis is not by "rule out." If you don't find a known physical cause, this does not necessarily mean that the symptoms are psychiatric. Flexible thinking and collaboration with the mental health professionals involved will ensure proper ongoing evaluation.

Table 8–6. Drugs associated with mania.[1]

Amantadine	Dapsone
Amphetamines	Decongestants
Anabolic steroids	Deet (bug spray)
Anticholinergics, atropine	Hallucinogens
Anticonvulsants	LSD
Antidepressants	PCP
Tricyclic antidepressants	H$_2$ Blockers
Fluoxetine	Cimetidine
Monoamine oxidase inhibitors	Ranitidine
Trazodone	Isoniazid
Bupropion	Levodopa
Antihypertensives	Metoclopramide (Reglan)
Clonidine	Metrizamide (Contrast)
Propranolol	Niridazole
Hydralazine	Nonsteroidal anti-inflammatory
Captopril	agents
Baclofen	Procarbazine
Beta adrenergic blockers	Quinine derivatives
Bromocriptine	Theophylline
Corticosteroid	Thyroid hormones
Cyclobenzaprine (Flexeril)	Yohimbine
Cyclosporine	Zidovudine

[1] Used with permission from Campo J. Medical issues in the care of child and adolescent inpatients. In: Bellack AS, Hersen M, eds. Handbook of Behavior Therapy in the Psychiatric Setting. New York: Plenum; 1993: 382.

The emergency assessment can be focused by answering the following questions:

1. **Is there a physical illness that may be causing or contributing to the emotianal and behavioral symptoms presented?** See Tables 8–2 through 8–9.
2. **Are there serious short-term medical consequences to the behavioral/emotional symptoms?** For example, starvation in anorexia nervosa or poor compliance in a seriously ill child.
3. **Is there potential for violence?** Are the patient or other family members seriously destructive/suicidal or seriously aggressive/homicidal?
4. **Why now?** A complete emergency assessment usually answers the question of why the patient/family are presenting for urgent evaluation at that time. If you cannot clearly answer this question, there is likely some critical missing data.

Table 8–7. Medical conditions associated with mania.[1]

Drugs/withdrawal (*see* Table 8–6)	HIV infection
Toxins	Neurologic/CNS
Manganese	Multiple sclerosis
Copper	Intracranial mass lesion
Vanadium	(especially right-sided
Bromides	lesions)
Metabolic	Cerebrovascular disease
Hypocalcemia	(stroke, hemorrhage,
Hemodialysis encephalopathy	hematoma)
Hepatic failure	Trauma
Wilson's disease	Epilepsy
Endocrine	Neurodegenerative disease
Hyperthyroidism	Myasthenia gravis
Hyperadrenalism (Cushing's	Nutritional
disease)	B_{12} deficiency
Infectious	Nicotinic acid deficiency
Neurosyphilis	(pellagra)
Meningoencephalitis	Systemic illness
Cryptococcal meningitis	Systemic lupus erythematosus
Epstein–Barr virus infection	Multiple lentigines syndrome
Influenza	(leopard syndrome)

[1] Used with permission from Campo J. Medical issues in the care of child and adolescent inpatients. In: Bellack AS, Hersen M, eds. Handbook of Behavior Therapy in the Psychiatric Setting. New York: Plenum; 1993: 383.

Table 8–8. Drugs associated with anxiety.[1]

Amphetamines	Metrizamide (contrast)
Antihistamines	Nabilone
Anticholinergics, atropine	Narcotics
Baclofen	Nifedipine
Bromocriptine	Nonsteroidal anti-inflammatory
Caffeine	agents
Captopril	Norfloxacin
Cocaine	Pergolide
Cycloserine	Procaine derivatives
Decongestants	Promethazine (Phenergan)
Dronabinol	Quinine derivatives
Interferon	Theophylline, bronchodilators
Monoamine oxidase inhibitors	

[1] Used with permission from Campo J. Medical issues in the care of child and adolescent inpatients. In: Bellack AS, Hersen M, eds. Handbook of Behavior Therapy in the Psychiatric Setting. New York: Plenum; 1993: 386.

Table 8–9. Medical conditions associated with anxiety.[1]

Drugs/withdrawal (*see* Table 8–8)	Hepatitis
Prenatal exposure to	Infectious mononucleosis
diethylstilbestrol (DES)	Tuberculosis
Toxins	Malaria
Heavy metals	Brucellosis
Metabolic	CNS/Neurologic
Inborn errors of metabolism	Multiple sclerosis
(acute intermittent porphyria)	Intracranial mass lesion
Electrolyte imbalance	Cerebrovascular disease
Hypoxia	Trauma
Hypoperfusion/anemia	Epilepsy
Hypoglycemia	Neurodegenerative disorders
Wilson's disease	Myasthenia gravis
Endocrine	Nutritional
Hyperthyroidism	B_{12} deficiency
Hyperadrenalism (Cushing's	Nicotinic acid deficiency
syndrome)	(pellagra)
Hypoparathyroidism	Zinc deficiency
Hypoadrenalism (adrenal	Systemic Illness
insufficiency)	Systemic lupus erythematosus,
Pheochromocytoma	collagen–vascular disease
Infectious	Supraventricular tachycardia
Neurosyphilis	Mitral valve prolapse
Encephalitis	Malignancy

[1] Used with permission from Campo J. Medical issues in the care of child and adolescent inpatients. In: Bellack AS, Hersen M, eds. Handbook of Behavior Therapy in the Psychiatric Setting. New York: Plenum; 1993: 387.

EMERGENCY ASSESSMENT OF SPECIFIC EMOTIONAL/ BEHAVIORAL PRESENTATIONS

Self-Destruction/Suicide

The most common reason for missing suicidal ideation or behavior in an emergency assessment is not asking. Asking about this should be a routine part of your emergency assessment. Questions are best presented in a matter-of-fact way. It is useful to begin by asking more general and less emotionally loaded questions such as, "Do you ever feel like you can't go on? Do you ever wish you were dead? More specific questions can follow, such as, "Do you ever feel like hurting yourself? Have you ever hurt yourself? Do you have a current plan to hurt yourself? How?'' Self-destructive/suicidal ideation is very common. Positive answers to the above questions should not surprise you. These questions are designed to let you judge the relative risk of self-destructive or suicidal plans or actions. Information should not be kept in confidence in relationship to serious self-destructive/suicidal ideation or plans. It is appropriately discussed with your consultant and is usually appropriately discussed with parents or guardians in detail.

Suicide risk is increased by many factors. The following is not intended to be a comprehensive list but rather is designed to detail some of the more common and clinically relevant factors:

Suicide risk is higher if:

1. There is a history of prior attempts.
2. There is a specific plan, especially one in which the likelihood that someone can intervene (rescue the patient) is low.
3. There is a family history of attempted or completed suicide.
4. There is an altered mental status with increased impulsivity and thinking difficulties such as in
   a. chronic brain dysfunction (mental retardation or dementia)
   b. Acute brain dysfunction (delirium)
   c. functional (psychiatric) psychosis.
5. Depressive symptoms are present.
6. Firearms are available.
7. The circumstances leading to the attempt or the ideation have not resolved or changed.
8. Certain demographic factors are present. Many demographic factors are known to increase risk in patients. For instance, boys complete suicide more often than girls, though girls attempt more often than boys. However, demographic factors usually are not particularly helpful in evaluating a particular patient.
9. Recent exposure to suicide by a friend or relative or exposure to a well publicized suicide in the media may increase risk (this area of research is still evolving).
10. Alcohol or substance abuse is present, as this may increase impulsivity and adversely effect judgement.

Thoroughly assessing suicide risk requires special training and experience. Your assessment should be for the purpose of screening for self-destructive/suicidal problems enough to know if emergency consultation is required. Any suicide attempt, even those that do not appear serious, should lead to consultation. In the case of suicidal ideation, unless you are clear that the patient is safe in the near future and has adequate followup in place, consultation with a mental health professional before ending the assessment is necessary. If you are concerned about the patient, do not send them home before attaining appropriate consultation. The need for an evaluation by the consultant is best presented to the patient and family in a matter-of-fact way and not as optional.

Aggression/Homicide

The most common reason for missing or inappropriately evaluating aggressive or homicidal symptoms is not asking enough questions. Many clinicians are reluctant to ask about homicidal ideation. It should be a routine part of the emergency assessment. It is useful to begin with screening questions such as, "Do you ever get out of control and hurt other people? Do you worry about getting out of control and hurting someone?" You eventually want to get more specific: For example, "If there has been violence in the past, how severe was it? Did anyone go to the hospital? Do you carry weapons? Are you planning on hurting or killing someone now?" Your assessment should be designed as a screening exam to determine whether or not consultation is needed. Remember that feeling anxious about a patient's potential aggression or feeling threatened by the patient is significant data. There is no need to endanger yourself. If you think there is a chance that a patient or family member will be violent during the assessment, appropriate use of consultation and security personnel is indicated. Similar factors to those that increase the risk of suicide increase the risk of homicide. Past violence is associated with the potential for violence in the present. Any condition that increases impulsivity or alters thinking (drugs, alcohol, delirium, etc) increases risk. If you are concerned about significant violence, consultation is needed.

Child Abuse

Screening for child abuse and neglect is an essential part of the emergency emotional/behavioral assessment. It helps to question the child alone. The questions should be matter-of-fact and direct. For instance, "Has anyone physically hurt you on purpose? Has anyone touched you in ways that made you feel uncomfortable or funny?" Questions will need to be aimed at the child's developmental level. Positive responses will lead you to ask for more detail. In some circumstances, you may suspect abuse without direct verbal confirmation from the patient because of a pattern of injuries or symptoms.

Suspected abuse or neglect must be reported to the local child protective service agency. Consultation about whether to report something or how to further assess the potential for child abuse is often helpful. Most hospitals have social workers or even child protection teams with expertise in this area who are available for consultation. Severe cases may require immediate protective action such as admitting the child.

It is usually best to inform parents of any report you make to child protective services and why you are doing it. It helps to present this in a matter-of-fact way. It often helps to explain that the *law requires you to report suspicion.* Many parents end up displacing their anger about the report onto the law or "system" and this may make it possible to continue an alliance with the parents.

Runaway

A teenager presenting alone in the emergency room may be a runaway. Runaway behavior is often associated with severe family conflict including physical or sexual abuse. Runaways often have severe emotional and behavioral problems including suicidality, violence, drug abuse, frequent victimization, sexual acting out, depression, etc. Many runaways significantly endanger themselves or others such that psychiatric assessment and treatment (even involuntary) may be indicated. Many runaways may already have social services caseworkers or even be in the custody of social services. The caseworker can often be instrumental in obtaining needed services. Consultation with a mental health professional is often useful in planning intervention with runaways. Remember, runners run. You may need to take steps to prevent the patient from eloping during the assessment.

Substance Abuse

Substance abuse or experimentation may or may not constitute an emergency. It does constitute an emergency if (1) The level of intoxication is severe; (2) the likelihood of serious with-drawal symptoms is present; or (3) it is associated with signifi-cant self-destructive or aggressive behavior. Remember that, al-though drug screens may be helpful, they are usually not definitive. It is helpful to discuss the particular screen available with your laboratory to find out what drugs are screened for and how effectively. Some drugs may require separate special screens.

Noncompliance

Noncompliance with important medical care can easily con-stitute an emergency and may represent covert suicidal ideation, serious family discord, or even neglect by parents. Children with chronic illnesses can often easily endanger themselves medi-cally. The extent of the emergency is usually clear based on the medical presentation. Admission for medical stabilization and child psychiatric consultation is often indicated.

Evaluation of Altered Thinking

Children may present with signs and symptoms of seri-ously altered thinking including difficulty with memory, con-centration, hallucinations, paranoia, etc. In some cases it may be the parents or caretakers who have noticed the change and not the patient.

Significantly altered thinking should always be considered as potentially secondary to an acute or chronic medical illness and potential medical illnesses should be appropriately excluded. Physical examination, appropriate laboratory examination, and adequate *mental status examination* are the most crucial parts of the evaluation. Table 8–10 details the important considera-tions in the evaluation of altered thinking.

MENTAL HEALTH CONSULTATION

The appropriate use of mental health consultation is often not as clear-cut as for other specialty consultations. This is due in part to the nature of the field (less concrete scientific knowl-edge) and in part to the variety of practitioners, each with differ-

Table 8–10. General principles in the assessment of altered thinking.\

1. *Abnormal vital signs* may indicate an organic cause.
2. *An altered level of consciousness* is considered a sign of organicity. In some patients this may include a markedly heightened level of arousal. (For instance with PCP intoxication).
3. *Disorientation* (after accounting for developmental level) should be considered organic until proven otherwise.
4. *A waxing and waning mental status* examination indicates organic pathology.
5. *New onset hallucinations* are an emergency requiring medical and psychological assessment. Although auditory hallucinations commonly occur in functional psychosis, they also occur in organic psychosis. Visual hallucinations without auditory hallucinations often signal an organic process. Hallucinations in other senses (for example touch or smell) are usually organically based.
6. *A good neurological examination* is indicated when there is significantly altered thinking.
7. *Cognitive functioning* less than age expectancy on the formal mental status examination raises suspicion of organicity. Even with retarded patients a drop in cognitive functioning can usually be determined by getting information from the parents on baseline mental functioning. Patients with functional psychosis (schizophrenia, mania, depression with psychosis, etc.) usually can still perform adequately on formal mental status examination. Infrequently, the psychotic symptoms are so prominent as to effect attention (such as in manic delirium) and thus give an abnormal mental status examination. Other psychiatric disorders effecting attention or effort (for example, severe depression) may at times effect the formal mental status examination.
8. *Precipitating psychosocial stressors* may mislead one away from organic causes.

ent skills and backgrounds. Consultation on emotional and behavioral problems is available from social workers, psychologists, behavioral pediatricians, behavioral neurologists, child psychiatrists, and others. To get optimal consultation it helps to have a preexisting relationship with the consultant, including knowing in general their areas of expertise. It is much easier to call someone you already know when you are in a crisis situation then someone you don't know. Good consultation should be timely and understandable. Consultants should make sense to you when they give you their findings. If they don't, it is unlikely that they will make much sense to the patient or family.

Indications for Mental Health Consultation:

Mental Health Consultation may be helpful for patients in which:

1. It is unclear if the symptoms are organic, psychological, or both.
2. The patient's emotional/behavioral symptoms constitute an emergency.
3. You suspect serious psychiatric morbidity, ie, the symptoms are more than developmental or a normal adjustment to stress.
4. The symptoms do not respond as expected to your usual treatment.
5. There is noncompliance in a patient with a serious illness that does not respond to an educational approach.
6. Something "doesn't feel right" to you. For example, the patient and the family make you anxious or leave you feeling markedly sad or angry for no apparent reason.

COMMON BEHAVIORAL/EMOTIONAL PROBLEMS

GENERAL PRINCIPLES

The vast majority of emotional and behavioral symptoms presented by patients and families are well managed without referral to mental health professionals. Many patients and families present with problems and questions that can be handled by educating the parents about normal development. Parents often have anxiety about developmental stages which raise conflicts in them based on their own experiences during that stage. Extensive history regarding the parents' own childhood is not indicated, but empathic listening to the parents' experience of the problems goes a long way.

A surprising number of patients and families present with difficulty in limit setting. A pediatrician can be extremely helpful by educating parents on the appropriate use of limits and rewards. When evaluating problems around limit setting, a good approach is to consider the problem as psycho-educational. Exploring the parents' own experience with discipline when they were children is useful as well. Parents' basic knowledge about limit setting, such as how long a time-out should be for a particular-aged child, what rewards need to be, etc, should be assessed. The following are common areas of breakdown in limit setting:

1. There is a lack of knowledge about appropriate limit setting.
2. Parents are uncomfortable when the child is angry at them and thus have difficulty following through with limits.
3. The parents have turned to the child for support and the child gets out of limits by threatening to withdraw support.
4. Parents are uncomfortable with their own anger and become immobilized when the child acts out. This may be due to bad experiences the parents had when they were children.
5. The parent lacks the energy to follow through with limits consistently. This could be because of lack of support for themselves, depression, etc.
6. The child has a psychiatric condition that interferes with the limit setting process, eg, attention deficit hyperactivity disorder, bipolar disorder, depressive disorder, psychotic disorder.

PSYCHIATRIC DISORDERS OF CHILDHOOD AND ADOLESCENCE

The majority of this section follows the *Diagnostic Stastical Manual, 3rd Edition, Revised (DSM-III-R)* system of classification. In addition to following this system of classification, much of the descriptive information and demographic information is adapted from this manual.

Mental Retardation

The essential features of mental retardation are significantly subaverage general intellectual functioning as defined by I.Q. testing (or clinical examinations in the very young child) and significant deficits or impairments of adaptive functioning and onset before age 18 (Table 8–11). Mental retardation is common, occurring in approximately 1% of all children. Definitive etiologic factors, either biologic, psychosocial, or a combination, may be determinable in up to 70% of the cases of mental retardation. Causative factors include hereditary factors, factors effect-

Table 8–11. Mental retardation I.Q. ranges.

Mild Mental Retardation: I.Q. 50–55 to approximately 70

Moderate Mental Retardation: I.Q. 35-40 to 50-55

Severe Mental Retardation: I.Q. 20–25 to 35–40

Profound Mental Retardation: I.Q. Below 20–25

ing fetal development, perinatal problems, acquired childhood illnesses, and psychosocial factors. The majority of individuals with mental retardation will be in the mildly retarded range. These individuals may not stand out until a later age. Individuals with more severe retardation will present with difficulties earlier in childhood.

Mental retardation is more common in males than females. The male/female ratio is approximately 1.5 to 1. Mental retardation differs from the pervasive developmental disorders in that in the pervasive developmental disorders there is a *qualitative* impairment of normal development. The abnormalities of pervasive developmental disorders are not normal for any stage of development. In mental retardation, development is largely delayed, but with the development in these areas "normal" for the adjusted developmental age.

A. Emotional/Behavioral Problems in Mental Retardation: A number of emotional and behavioral symptoms are commonly associated with mental retardation including poor impulse control, aggressiveness, low self-esteem, self-injurious behavior, and sometimes passivity. The prevalence of other mental disorders is increased in patients with mental retardation, including pervasive development disorder, attention deficit hyperactivity disorder, and stereotypy/habit disorder. Patients with mental retardation may also develop other emotional/behavioral syndromes such as depression, mania, psychotic illnesses, etc. The diagnosis and treatment of these conditions may be difficult because of the difficulty assessing these patients, particularly those who are relatively nonverbal. Knowledge of baseline functioning and a good relationship with observant parents can be critical.

B. Treatment:

1. Rule out treatable causes.

2. Help the family grieve, accept the patient's limitations, and plan for the future.

3. Appropriate vision and hearing screening.

4. Be familiar with the patient's baseline functioning and work with parents to determine causes of deterioration. The parents' knowledge of the patient's cognitive baseline can help you interpret the mental status examination of the patient.

5. Advocate for resources.

6. There is a growing literature, which can be consulted, on the psychopharmacology of behavior problems in mental retardation. Many behavioral pediatricians and child psychiatrists have expertise in this area if behavioral problems become unmanageable.

Pervasive Developmental Disorders

Pervasive developmental disorders are characterized by (1) a qualitative impairment in reciprocal social interaction, (2) a qualitative impairment in verbal and nonverbal communication and in imaginative activity, and (3) a markedly restricted repertoire of activities and interests.

There are 2 pervasive developmental disorders: (1) autistic disorder, and (2) pervasive developmental disorder not otherwise specified. Patients with pervasive developmental disorders often also have mental retardation. These individuals may have abnormal movements (stereotypies) and may also show significant over or under response to particular sensory stimuli. These disorders may also involve abnormalities in eating, drinking, sleeping, and of mood. Self-injurious behavior such as head banging or finger/hand/wrist biting is common. Many parents report a very early awareness that something is "wrong."

Individuals do not generally "outgrow" these disorders although they may have symptom improvement over time. Seizure disorders are common, being present in approximately 25% or more cases of autism. The prevalence of pervasive developmental disorder including autistic and pervasive developmental disorder not otherwise specified has been estimated at 10 to 15 children in every 10,000. There is a male to female ratio estimated from 2:1 to 5:1. A number of conditions causing brain dysfunction are thought to predispose to the development of pervasive developmental disorders (eg, maternal rubella, tuberous scleroses, infantile spasms, and fragile X syndrome). The autistic disorder may be more common in siblings of children with the disorder.

A. Treatment:

1. Rule out physical causes or associated conditions and treat appropriately.

2. Develop a reciprocal treatment alliance. Parents have often been told that the child is normal or will outgrow the problems, leaving the parents with negative feelings about clinicians.

3. Help the family grieve, accept the patient's limitations, and plan appropriately for the future.

4. Advocate for resources.

5. Refer to a behavioral pediatrician or child psychiatrist for pharmacologic treatment of aggression, self abuse, or severe stereotypies.

Specific Developmental Disorders
(Learning Disabilities)

Learning disorders are disorders with specific deficits in academic, speech, language, and motor skills that are not secondary to a demonstratable physical disorder, pervasive developmental disorder, mental retardation, or inadequate schooling. It should be noted that the diagnosis is made if certain skill areas

---

Table 8–12. Side Effects of Methylphenidate and Dextroamphetamine.

Decreased growth has been reported though rebound growth that makes up most of the deficit often occurs when the medication is stopped

Poor sleep

Decreased appetite

Methylphenidate lowers seizure threshold (debatable clinical significance)

Increased pulse, blood pressure

Rebound restlessness/hyperactivity; remember the half life of these medications is relatively short such that patients is on AM and noon doses may show "rebound" symptoms during the evening hours requiring a dinner time dose

May precipitate tics; the literature on this is somewhat controversial but there appears to be an association between the onset or exacerbation of tics with the use of stimulants

Nervousness

Contraindicated in presence of glaucoma

are markedly below what is expected based on the patient's over-all cognitive functioning. Thus, a patient with mental retardation may, in addition, have an area where they are functioning much lower and therefore qualify for an additional diagnosis of a specific developmental disorder. A learning disorder diagnosis is based on standardized academic testing and should be suspected if performance in school lags in a particular area(s).

A. Treatment:

1. Look for this in patients with poor school performance, and refer for appropriate educational testing to make the appropriate diagnosis.

2. Rule out physical causes, especially hearing, visual, and neurologic conditions.

3. Refer for remedial academic intervention (usually available through school).

4. Screen for associated low self esteem or parent/child discord.

Disruptive Behavioral Disorders

These disorders are characterized by behavior that is socially disruptive. These disorders include attention deficit hyperactivity disorder, oppositional defiant disorder and conduct disorder. Symptoms of these disorders occur together frequently.

A. Attention Deficit Hyperactivity Disorder: These children have developmentally inappropriate levels of impulsivity, hyperactivity, and inattention. These may or may not be present across the child's environments. In some cases the disorder is only a problem in school. Children with attention deficit hyperactivity disorder may *not* show inattentiveness, impulsiveness, and hyperactivity in one-on-one situations, especially when the situations are novel. Therefore, these patients may not appear to have attention deficit hyperactivity disorder in your office. Standardized checklists such as the Connors scale may be useful in making the diagnosis and following medication response. Poor academic performance may be associated with attention deficit hyperactivity disorder. Early onset (not diagnosis) before age 4 is common. Approximately one-third of children with attention deficit hyperactivity disorder continue to have symptoms as adults. The disorder is common and may occur in as many as 3% of children, with a male-to-female ratio of between 6:1 to 9:1. This disorder is felt to run in families. Some patients do not have the impulsivety and hyperactivity and are given the diagnosis of undifferentiated attention deficit disorder.

1. Treatment:

a. Suspect this diagnosis when there is poor school performance or failure in usual limit setting.

b. Rule out potential physical causes (eg, hyperthyroidism and lead intoxication).

c. Educate the family regarding the nature of this disorder, especially the need for consistent limit setting and decreased stimulation, particularly in the classroom.

d. More involved psychological investigation and treatment is often indicated. Involvement of mental health professionals is often helpful.

e. It should also be noted that early onset of bipolar disorder may present similarly to attention deficit hyperactivity disorder. A strong family history of bipolar disorder should lead one to consider child psychiatric consultation.

f. Psychopharmacologic Management–Psychopharmacologic treatment is only indicated in the context of a complete treatment plan involving appropriate psychological, social, behavioral, and educational treatments. Stimulants are the first line drugs. These include methylphenidate (Ritalin), dextroamphetamine (Dexadrine), and pemoline (Cylert).

(1) Methylphenidate–Not approved for use under age 6. Over age 6 start with 5 mg in AM and at noon and increase by 5 mg per dose per week until desired effect is achieved. The usual optimal dose is between 0.3 and 0.7 mg/kg/dose. Maximum recommended daily dose is 60 mg. Many children also need a late afternoon dose. This is usually obvious to the parents as the patient's behavior falls off through the late afternoon and early evening. Remember that the half-life of this medication is short (approximately 4 hours), so rebound symptoms may occur. See Table 8–12 for common side effects. Patients need periodic monitoring of height, weight, pulse and blood pressure. Methylphenidate does come in a sustained-release form, but there are some questions about whether it has equal efficacy.

(2) Dextroamphetamine–Not approved for use under age 3. For children 3 to 5, begin with 2.5 mg daily, raised by 2.5-mg/24 hr increments weekly. For patients 6 years of age and older, begin with 5.0 mg and raise in 5.0-mg/24 hr increments weekly. The usual optimal daily dose normally falls between 0.15 and 0.5 mg/kg/dose administered one or two times a day. The usual maximum daily dose is less than 40 mg per day. Sustained-release forms are available. Regular monitoring of height, weight, pulse, and blood pressure are indicated.

(3) Pemoline–Not recommended under age 6. For patients 6 years of age and over, begin with 37.5 mg. This may be increased weekly by 18.75 mg. Maximal daily dose is 112.5 mg (usual range 56.25-75 mg/day). Pemoline has a relatively long half-life and is usually given once per day. It has fewer cardiovascular effects compared to the other stimulants. It appears to have a longer lag time before significant clinical benefit (perhaps 3 to 4 weeks). A significant number of patients develop increased liver function tests (felt to be reversible when medication stopped), and serious hepatotoxicity has been reported. Regular monitoring of liver functions is indicated. Regular monitoring of height and weight is also indicated.

(4) Tricyclic Antidepressants–These are usually the second-line medication for attention deficit hyperactivity disorder and are usually used by experienced clinicians (behavioral pediatricians, child neurologists, and child psychiatrists). A number of antidepressants have been used including imipramine, desipramine, and others. There are no official recommendations for dosing, though it appears that patients may respond to doses lower than that needed for depression. A recent very small series of sudden deaths in patients on desipramine (even in the recommended dosage ranges) has lead to recommendations of increased caution regarding potential cardiac toxicity, including the need for attention to patient and family histories of cardiac disease, syncope, or sudden death and EKG monitoring including at baseline, after dose increases and periodically at the final therapeutic dose. Look for conduction abnormalities including prolonged P-R interval, widened QRS, and prolonged Q-Tc interval. Although therapeutic drug ranges are available only for depression, drug levels can be used to avoid toxicity.

(5) Clonidine–This may also have a role in the treatment of attention deficit hyperactivity disorder. This medication is usually used by behavioral pediatricians and/or child psychiatrists familiar with the treatment of attention deficit hyperactivity disorder. See Table 8–13 for side effects.

B. Conduct Disorder: This disorder involves ongoing behaviors that violate the basic rights of others and major age-appropriate societal rules or norms. These behaviors may include physical aggression, destruction of property, stealing, and the use of tobacco, alcohol, or drugs at an age level before peers.

Table 8–13. Side effects of Clonidine.

Decreased blood pressure
Rebound hypertension if stopped abruptly
May have negative blood pressure effects if combined with a number of
  other medications
Sedation
Dizziness
Dry mouth
Constipation

Poor frustration tolerance, irritability, temper outbursts, and low
self-esteem are frequent characteristics. The age of onset is usually prepubertal. The course is variable with early onset associated with greater risk of continuation into adult life as antisocial
personality disorder. The disorder is common and affects as
many as 9% males and 2% of females under age 18.

   C. Oppositional Defiant Disorder: Oppositional defiant disorder is characterized by persistant, hostile, defiant, and oppositional behavior, without the more serious violation of basic rights
seen in conduct disorder. Symptoms are invariable present in
the home but *may not* be present in other settings. Impairment
is usually greatest within the home. These children commonly
develop conduct disorders. This disorder typically begins by 8
years of age. Before puberty, the disorder is more common in
males than females. After puberty, the sex ratio is probably
equal. Associated features may include low self-esteem, mood
lability, and psychoactive substance abuse.

   **D. Treatment of Conduct Disorder and Oppositional Defiant
Disorder:**

   1. Suspect these diagnoses in patients with significant antisocial activity or inability to follow limits.

   2. Psychoeducational approach with family about limit
setting.

   3. Refer for additional psychological evaluation if a psychoeducational approach fails or if there is a strong family history
of bipolar disorder.

Anxiety Disorders of Childhood or Adolescence

Anxiety, of course, is a "universal" symptom of people of all ages. The anxiety disorders of childhood or adolescence are characterized by persistent anxiety that is excessive for the child's developmental stage. There are 3 disorders included in this category:

A. Separation Anxiety Disorder: This disorder is characterized by at least 2 weeks of excessive anxiety concerning separation from attachment figures and may involve unrealistic fears of harm befalling the attachment figure or the child, reluctance to go to school, refusal to go to sleep, difficulties being alone, and complaints of physical symptoms. These children commonly have a depressed mood.

B. Avoidant Disorder of Childhood or Adolescence: This disorder involves avoidance of contact with unfamiliar people for a period of 6 months or longer along with generally satisfactory relationships with familiar people. The child must be at least 2½ years old as avoidance of unfamiliar people before this time can be developmentally appropriate. This is often associated with one of the other anxiety disorders.

C. Overanxious Disorder: This disorder involves excessive unrealistic anxiety for a period of 6 months or longer. This disorder is more general than the other 2 diagnoses and can involve worry about future events, concern about the appropriateness of past behavior, somatic complaints, self-consciousness, difficulty relaxing, etc.

D. General Information about Anxiety Disorders: Somatic complaints with multiple visits to the physician may be common in both separation anxiety and overanxious disorder. Complaints can include headaches, gastrointestinal problems, palpitations, dizziness, and others.

Anxiety disorders are relatively common. Many run in families and may have significant co-morbidity with other psychiatric conditions, especially depression. In addition, these disorders may have a relatively chronic course (perhaps even years).

E. Treatment:

1. Rule out physical causes (eg, hyperthyroidism or caffeinism).

2. Screen other family members for anxiety disorders.

3. Prevent unnecessary school avoidance by appropriate management.

4. Nonpsychopharmacologic treatment (behavioral/psychotherapeutic) is usually indicated.

5. Psychopharmacologic Management–Tricyclic antidepressants may have a role in the treatment of separation anxiety disorder; refer to a behavioral pediatrician or child psychiatrist for this. Use benzodiazepines with consultation.

Panic Disorder

Although this disorder is often thought of as occurring in adults, recent literature suggests that panic disorder with symptomatology similar to that in adults does occur in children and adolescents. In fact, isolated panic attacks may be relatively common. A panic attack involves physiologic symptoms of anxiety (eg, shortness of breath, dizziness, sweating, nausea, palpitations, trembling, paresthesia, hot flashes or chills, chest pain) along with a subjective sense of intense fear or discomfort. A fear of dying or going "crazy" may be associated. The symptoms often come on very quickly (within minutes). Panic disorder is diagnosed on how frequent and disabling panic attacks are.

A. Treatment:

1. Rule out medical causes (hyperthyroidism, caffeinism, amphetamines).

2. Refer to a child psychiatrist.

School Phobia

School phobia is defined here as the persistent avoidance of school because of anxiety regarding separation from a parent/caretaker *or* because of anxiety about what will happen at school to the child. Although not an official *DSM-III-R* diagnosis, this overlaps with the *DSM-III-R* diagnosis of separation anxiety disorder. The second form is more common in adolescence. This does not include truants who avoid school to do activities that they find pleasurable. Suspect this diagnosis whenever there are frequently missed school days because of somatic complaints with no identifiable etiology.

A. Treatment:

1. Appropriate ongoing medical evaluation to reassure the child and parent there is no serious physical cause and/or to rule out serious physical abnormalities.

2. Refer back to school once the diagnosis is made and provide reassurance to school, family, and parents as needed to accomplish this. This may be difficult, requiring a great deal of reassurance for parents.

3. Refer for evaluation by mental health professionals if the usual interventions don't work.

Simple Phobias

Simple phobias involve persistent fear of a circumscribed stimulus that is not a fear of having a panic attach (as in panic disorder) or public embarrassment as in social phobia. Animal phobia usually beings in childhood, and blood/injury phobias most frequently in adolescence or early adulthood. Most simple phobias that start in childhood disappear without treatment. For persistent phobias that interfere with daily living, behavioral techniques are usually most helpful.

Eating Disorders

See Chapter 9.

Mood Disorders

A. Major Depressive Disorder: Patients with major depressive disorder have had one or more occurrences of a major depressive episode without a history of manic or hypomanic (partial manic) episode(s). A major depressive episode involves at least 2 weeks of predominantly depressed mood (depressed or irritable in children or adolescents), or loss of interest or pleasure, which may or may not include each of a number of other specific features, including appetite and sleep disturbance, psychomotor agitation or retardation, loss of energy, feelings of worthlessness, excessive guilt, diminished concentration, recurrent thoughts of death, and suicidal ideation or plan *and* is not due to a known organic factor, normal grief, or part of a nonmood psychotic disorder. In most cases of major depression, these symptoms will be there much of the time. Psychotic symptoms may be present but prolonged psychotic symptomology in the absence of mood disturbance call the diagnosis into question. In prepubertal children there are some age-specific features; somatic complaints, psychomotor agitation, and mood congruent hallucinations (usually a single voice). Adolescents may show negative or antisocial behavior, drug and alcohol abuse, aggression, withdrawal, and hypersomnia.

1. Treatment:

a. Rule Out Medical Causes (eg, certain medications, hypothyroidism—*see* Tables 8–4 and 8–5)—A common screening laboratory evaluation given a normal physical would be: CBC with differential, electrolytes, glucose, calcium, phosphate, creatinine, BUN, liver function tests, thyroid function tests, and urine toxicology. If risk factors are present, serum syphilis and HIV should be added. If psychotics symptoms are present add work-up for psychoses (discussed in schizophrenia section).

b. Screen the patient for manic symptoms now or in the past.

c. Assess family history of depression and mania.

d. Screen for suicidal ideation and risk—even young children make suicide attempts.

e. Screen for psychotic thinking.

f. Psychopharmacologic Management—This is an evolving area. Some patients may respond to antidepressants. If psychosis is present, an antipsychotic medication is indicated. Patients with personal histories of mania or strong family history of bipolar illness will often be treated initially with lithium, as antidepressants may precipitate manic episodes.

g. Referral to child psychiatrist is indicated.

B. Dysthymia: Dysthymia is a more chronic (at least 1 year in children and adolescents), less pervasive depressive disorder with depressive symptoms that do not fully meet the criteria for a major depressive episode. The boundaries between major depressive disorder and dysthymia are somewhat unclear.

C. Biopolar Disorders: Refers to mood disorders that involve a manic episode(s), or hypomanic episode(s) (usually the hypomanic episodes also involve a history of major depressive epidsode[s]). Manic episodes are marked by persistently elevated, expansive, or irritable mood, which interferes with functioning in a major way and are not due to a known organic factor or superimposed on a non mood psychotic disorder. Mood lability, including some depressive symptoms, commonly occurs. These episodes often come on quickly over a few days. Although retrospective studies show mean age of onset to be in the twenties, onset can occur in both adolescence and childhood. Psychotic symptoms (hallucinations, delusions) can occur during these episodes. Persistent psychotic features in the absence of mood disturbance calls for diagnosis into question.

1. Treatment

a. General Considerations: Manic patients are notoriously resistant to treatment, as they often do not perceive any problems. Irritability and even aggression are common, especially when you need to insist on treatment. Bipolar disorder is relatively common (perhaps as many as 1% of adults). It is also more and more frequently diagnosed in adolescence and even in young children. This disorder runs in families. A strong family history of bipolar disorder should lead one to consider this diagnosis in patients who present with depression, presumed attention deficit hyperactivity disorder, or episodic aggression.

b. Rule out organic factors (eg, medications, illicit drugs, hyperthyroidism, etc. *See* Tables 8–6 and 8–7). A suggested screening laboratory evaluation would include a CBC with differential, urinalysis, electrolytes, glucose, liver function tests, thyroid function tests, creatinine, BUN, calcium, phosphorus, and urine toxicology. If risk factors are present, add serum syphilis tests and HIV. If psychotic symptoms are present, add work-up for psychosis (described in schizophrenic section).

c. Consultation with a child psychiatrist. When manic these patients usually need urgent hospitalization.

d. These patients (when manic) may need emergency containment (police, hospital security) and can be quite volatile.

e. Psychopharmacologic Management—Manic episodes usually respond to lithium. Antipsychotics may be used for short-term treatment because of the many-day latency of lithium's antimanic affect. Carbamazepine (Tegretol), and perhaps other anticonvulsants, may also be effective antimanic drugs.

f. Do not give these patients medications known to precipitate manic episodes, especially antidepressants (Table 8–6), without consultation.

D. Cyclothymia: Cyclothymia is a condition in which there are alternating episodes of hypo- (or partial) mania and depressive symptoms that do not meet the criteria for a major depressive episode.

Substance Abuse
    See Chapter 9.

Obsessive Compulsive Disorder

Obsessive compulsive disorder is defined as the presence of (1) obessions—these are recurrent thoughts experienced as intrusive by the person, which are egodystonic (that is, not something that the person would usually be thinking); and (2) compulsions—that is, behaviors that one feels one must do, usually in order to prevent a negative event. These patients often feel compelled to do things a certain number of times (eg, washing their hands or opening or closing a door) or do particular things (such as stepping on all sidewalk cracks or touching certain things). Patients with obsessive compulsive disorder are often embarrassed by it and will hide these symptoms unless specifically asked. Good screening questions would be: "Do you ever have thoughts that bother you or go through your mind over and over and you can't get rid of them? Do you ever feel like you have to do things a specific way or a certain number of times to prevent something bad from happening?" Demographic studies of children and adolescents show this disorder may be considerably more common than previously thought.

A. Treatment:

1. Screen for this disorder by asking direct questions.

2. Make appropriate referral as this disorder is highly treatable using a combination of behavioral and psychopharmacologic intervention.

Schizophrenia

Schizophrenia is a chronic illness involving a thought disorder and a marked impairment or fall-off in functioning. It involves both negative (eg, withdrawal and lack of reactivity to environment) and positive (eg, delusions, hallucinations) symptoms. Onset is common during adolescence. Schizophrenia may present in adolescence with such nonspecific findings as a fall-off in school performance, personality change, or withdrawal. The screening mental status examination will often uncover the presence of a thought disorder.

A. Treatment:

1. Undertake work-up in collaboration with a child psychiatrist. This will involve ruling out common organic causes of psychosis. A suggested work-up would include CBC with differential, urinalysis, electrolytes, glucose, creatinine, calcium, phosphorus, urine toxicology, BUN, liver function tests, thyroid function tests, vitamin B$_{12}$, folate, copper, ceruloplasmin, sedimentation rate, MRI or CT scan of the head, and EEG. If risk factors are present, add serum syphilis test and HIV. Other studies (eg, CSF analysis, organic acids ANA, etc.) can be added based on clinical suspicion. Neurologic consultation may also be helpful.

2. Provide well child and acute illness care, realizing that the presence of a thought disorder may interfere or complicate compliance with medical care.

Post-traumatic Stress Disorder

Post-traumatic stress disorder probably occurs relatively frequently in children and adolescents and may be a common sequelae of child abuse. Post-traumatic stress disorder involves exposure to a trauma outside of usual human experience and involves symptoms of numbing, re-experiencing of the trauma, and symptoms of increased arousal. These patients may show withdrawal, avoidance of situations that cause re-experiencing of the trauma, and hypersensitivity to experiences that resemble the trauma. These patients may also show inappropriate behavior related to the trauma. For example, young children with histories of sexual abuse often show an inappropriate interest in sexuality, including public masturbation or fondling of others.

A. Treatment: At this time psychologically based treatments appear to be the most efficacious in children and adolescents. Ask about the symptoms when a history of severe trauma is known and make appropriate referral.

Enuresis

Enuresis is the developmentally inappropriate wetting of the bed or clothing. To qualify for a diagnosis of enuresis, the patient must be at least 5 years of age and have a mental age of at least 4. This disorder is common—age 5: 7% males, 3% females; age 10: 3% males, 2% females; age 18: 1% males, almost nonexistent in females. The great majority of children with enuresis *do not* have a coexisting serious psychiatric problem. This disorder strongly runs in families.

A. Treatment:

1. Reassurance of parents regarding age-related norms.

2. Organic causes such as diabetes, seizure disorder, and urinary tract infections need to ruled out (Table 8–14). With a normal history and physical, urinalysis may be the only necessary laboratory work-up.

Table 8–14. Causes of enuresis.[1]

Nonpathologic causes (97%)
    Small functional bladder capacity
    Inability to delay micturition urge
    Nighttime polyuria because ADH levels fail to rise at night
    Nighttime polyuria because child drinks too much in the evening
    Child doesn't wake up when his bladder feels full
Disease States (3%)
Medically treatable
    UTI
    Diabetes insipidus
    Diabetes mellitus
    Fecal impaction or constipation
Surgically treatable
    Ectopic ureter
    Lower urinary tract obstruction
    Neurogenic bladder
    Bladder calculus or foreign body
    Sleep apnea secondary to large adenoids

[1] From Schmitt BD: Nocturnal enuresis: Finding the treatment that fits the child. *Contemp Pediatr* September, 1990, p 72.

3. Assess and deal with the family conflict that commonly arises around this disorder through a psychoeducational approach.

4. Be sensitive to the potential negative effects on self-esteem.

5. Be familiar with treatment:

a. Behavioral techniques are the most efficacious. They have the least side effects and the lowest recurrence rate. Simply helping the child go to bed expecting to get up to urinate during the night may be sufficient. It is helpful to be familiar with enuresis alarms in order to be able to teach parents and children how to use these.

b. Psychopharmacologic intervention is generally overused and should be reserved for situations in which behavioral treatment is not possible or hasn't worked. A typical situation may be one in which a child must obtain control quickly to avoid embarrassment, such as when going off to camp. Psychopharmacologic agents that may be useful include imipramine (in doses lower than that use for antidepressant effect) and DDAVP. Imipramine carries significant risks and may require EKG monitoring (Table 8–15 and page 211).

Encopresis

Encopresis is the age-inappropriate soiling of one's self. By definition the child must have a chronological and mental age of 4 years. Encopresis is estimated to be present in 1% of 5-year-olds. Encopresis is related to an organic cause in 5% or less of cases (Tables 8–16 and 8–17). Most encopresis is related to leakage from an impaction. In these cases soiling will occur frequently with multiple episodes each day involving some loose stools. Nonretentive soiling is less common and more clearly deliberate and involves formed, less-frequent stooling.

    A. Treatment:

    1. Rule out physical causes (Table 8–16 and 8–17).

    2. Educate the family about appropriate diet and bowel habits. This disorder commonly involves severe constipation with leaking from around an impaction. Reregulating the child is often the initial approach. Enemas can free the impaction; then stool softeners (mineral oil or milk of magnesia) and a nonconstipating diet should be instituted. Laxatives (dulcolax) may also be needed (after the impaction is freed). Avoid using oral laxatives or rectal suppositories to remove an impaction, or before the impaction is freed, because they can cause abdominal pain.

    3. Children with nonretentive encopresis may need additional behavioral and psychological intervention.

    4. Assess and deal with the familial conflict that arises around this disorder through a psychoeducational approach. Be sensitive to the potential negative effects on self-esteem. Mental health referral may be indicated in some cases.

Tic Disorders

A tic is a recurrent, nonrhythmic, rapid, involuntary, stereotyped, motor movement or vocalization. Although it is experienced as uncontrollable, it can sometimes be suppressed for short periods of time. Stress may make tics worse. Tics may be reduced during activities requiring attention or during sleep. Tic disorders are often complicated by self-consciousness, low self-esteem, and at times depression. They may have marked social consequences. Evidence suggests that stimulants may bring out or exacerbate tic disorders. The differential diagnosis of tic disorders includes other movement disturbances, including chorei-

Table 8–15. Treating enuresis with drugs.[1]

	Desmopressin (DDAVP)	**Imipramine**
How supplied	5-mL spray bottle (delivers 10 µg/spray)	25–mg tablets
Dosage	2 sprays hs Increase by 1 spray weekly to maximum of 4 sprays/night	8–12 yr: 25–50 mg hs >12 yr: 50–75 mg hs
Cautions	Avoid excessive fluids to prevent hyponatremia	Overdose can be lethal Keep out of reach of younger siblings
Tapering	By 1 spray q2wk	By 25 mg q2wk
Enuresis alarm	Use simultaneously	Use simultaneously

[1] From Schmitt BD: Nocturnal enuresis: Finding the treatment that fits the child. *Contemp Pediatr* September, 1990, p 88.

Table 8–16. Organic causes of constipation and retentive soiling.[1]

Entity	Diagnosis Criteria
Constipating medication	History positive
Chronic anal fissure	Examination positive
Hypothyroidism	Linear growth delayed
Anterior displacement of anus	Examination positive
Anal or rectal stenosis	Finger cannot enter rectum
Pelvic mass	Mass on rectal examination (usually posteriorly)
Hirschsprung's disease	Rectal ampulla repeatedly empty; rectum is tight
Postsurgical anal stricture	Examination positive

[1] With permission, from Schmitt BD: Symposium on Common Pediatric Problems—Encopresis; Primary Care—Volume 11, No. 3, September 1984, p 500.

Table 8–17. Nonretentive encopresis.[1]

Exclusion of Organic Causes: Nonretentive Encopresis

1. Severe ulcerative colitis can cause fecal incontinence during relapses, but the presence of bloody diarrhea should suggest the correct diagnosis. Disease processes that cause loose stools but do not involve the rectum do not lead to fecal incontinence.
2. Acquired spinal cord disease (for example, sacral lipoma, diastematomyelia, or spinal cord neoplasm) can be diagnosed by reduced anal wink reflex and anal sphincter tone. Bladder incontinence and gait problems are usually associated. Many types of neurogenic bowel dysfunction can be treated.
3. A rectoperineal fistula with an imperforate anus will cause leakage of stool through the ectopic anus. Because the internal anal sphincter is intact, these children can be trained at a later age to become continent.
4. Postsurgical damage to the anal sphincter can result in fecal incontinence.

[1] Adapted, with permission, from Schmitt BD: Symposium on Common Pediatric Problems—Encopresis; Primary Care—Volume 11, Number 3, September 1984, p 506.

form movements, dystonic movements, myoclonic movements, athetoid movements, etc.

A. Tourettes Disorders: Tourettes disorder involves multiple motor and one or more vocal tics. The vocal tics can include nonverbal sounds or words, even including socially unacceptable obscenities (coprolalia). The motor tics may be simple or involve more complex movements such as deep knee bends, squatting, etc. The median age of onset is 7 years of age. Most patients have an onset before age 14. The course is usually life-long with periods of exacerbation and remission. Life-long prevalence is estimated to at least be 0.5 per 1000. The male-to-female ratio is 3:1. It appears to be familial. A significant number of patients with Tourettes disorder will also have attention deficit hyperactivity disorder and obsessive compulsive disorder.

B. Chronic Motor or Vocal Tic Disorder: These are patients that have tics that are either motor or vocal but not both (as in Tourettes disorder).

C. Transient Tic Disorder: This disorder applies to single or multiple motor and/or vocal tics that occur for at least 2 weeks but no longer than 1 year. The age of onset is always during childhood or adolescence. The male-to-female ratio is 3:1. This disorder appears to run in families.

D. Treatment:

1. Rule out potential physical causes (eg, neurologic disorders, amphetamine intoxication).

2. Screen for concurrent attention deficit hyperactivity disorder and obsessive compulsive disorder.

3. Help ensure appropriate education of patient, family, and school personnel about these disorders.

4. Stop medications that may exacerbate tics if possible (eg, stimulants and caffeine).

5. Transient tics are relatively common and may require no intervention. Patients with chronic or troublesome tics should usually be referred to a neurologist or child psychiatrist. These disorders are often medication responsive, although each of the medications have significant side effects. Medications include haloperidol, pimozide, and clonidine.

Sleep Disorders

See Chapter 20.

Factitious Disorders

Factitious disorders involve the conscious production of symptoms for reasons that are not readily apparent. The production of symptoms for an obvious gain (eg, getting out of going to detention) would be labeled malingering. Factitious disorders with physical symptoms have also been called Munchausen syndrome. Though infrequent, Munchausen syndrome by proxy (eg, parents who create illnesses in their children) often is a very difficult diagnosis to make and can present a very complicated and interesting clinical picture.

Sexual Disorders

See Chapter 9.

Somatoform Disorders
(Also see Chapter 9).

The vast majority of children and adolescents presenting for evaluation of physical complaints for which no organic etiology can be uncovered do not have somatoform disorders. Most of these symptoms are helped with careful evaluation, availability of the clinician over time to reassess for organic pathology as needed, evaluation of current psychosocial stressors, reassurance, and time.

Some patients will have more pervasive symptoms that do not respond to the usual interventions and they may have somatoform disorders.

There are 3 essential features of these disorders:

1. Symptoms suggesting physical disorder.
2. No demonstrable organic findings or known pathophysiologic mechanism.
3. Positive evidence, or a strong presumption, that the symptoms are linked to psychological factors or conflicts.

Note that these are not disorders that can be diagnosed merely by ruling out a list of possible organic causes. Flexible thinking allowing one to reconsider organic factors is critical to good clinical care. Many patients with presumed somatoform disorders eventually have organic causes uncovered. In addition, patients with somatoform disorders also develop physical illnesses.

A. Treatment:

1. Rule out organic causes as appropriate. Ongoing care should be designed to provide appropriate reassurance, appropriate re-evaluation for physical causes as needed, and to minimize complications (unnecessary surgery, narcotic addiction, school avoidance).

2. Refer for mental health evaluation if the patient/family is interested or there is an emergency.

Trichotillomania

This disorder involves repeatedly acting on the recurrent impulse to pull out one's own hair. It may be associated with eating of the hair. These patients present with patchy areas of incomplete alopecia. Patients often try to hide this disorder. It usually begins in childhood. It is probably more common than known because of the tendency of patients to hide it. There is some recent promising data suggesting that serotonin reuptake blockers may be helpful in this disorder.

Child Abuse and Neglect

Child abuse and neglect is epidemic and cuts across all socioeconomic levels. Approximately 2 million reports of potential child abuse are filed in the USA each year. These include cases of physical abuse, sexual abuse, emotional abuse, and neglect.

Signs of physical abuse may include pathognemonic physical findings, for example, bruising of the frontal dental ridges in infants by forcable feeding or characteristic marks from cigarette burns. A skeletal survey may be useful in confirming a diagnosis by showing healing fractures of various ages. Signs of neglect include inadequate nutrition, poor hygiene, and failure to thrive. Inpatient treatment may be indicated in suspected cases of failure to thrive. These children may show dramatic improvement relatively quickly in the hospital.

Sexual abuse is quite common and most often involves a perpetrator known to the child. This complicates the psychological adaptation by the child, particularly in the area of basic trust. There may be physical signs (vaginal or anal lesions) but often the signs are purely emotional and may be nonspecific, such as depression, poor sleep, hypersexuality, runaway behavior, and vague somatic complaints.

Once abuse or neglect is identified it must be reported (see Emergency Assessment section). Individual psychotherapy or group psychotherapy may be very helpful. Family therapy may be indicated both in the case of a perpetrator who is a family member and one who is not, as the abuse often effects the entire family.

ISSUES REGARDING HOSPITALIZATION

Hospitalization is a potentially traumatic event for any child or adolescent for a number of reasons. First of all, it undoubtably involves some health threats and may also involve painful procedures. In addition, there may be uncertainty about future health. Finally, there may be significant concerns regarding separation from the family. A patient's primary concern may vary depending on developmental level. Younger children will be more focused on the separation aspects. Grade school children may have more prominent concerns about body mutilation. A number of factors can help alleviate the potentially traumatic experiences of hospitalization.

1. Frequent family contact with rooming-in (if available and appropriate depending on the child's age).
2. Adequate explanation of the illness and procedures at a level that is developmentally appropriate for the child.

Table 8–18. Diagnoses in childhood and adolescence for which pharmacotherapy may be therapeutically indicated.[1]

DSM-III-R Diagnosis	Medication
Mental retardation (with severe behavioral disorder and/or self-injurious behavior)	Thioridazine
	Chlorpromazine
	Haloperidol
	Lithium
	(?) Propranolol
	(?) Naltrexone
Pervasive developmental disorders	Haloperidol
	(?) Fluphenazine
	(?) Naltrexone
	(?) Fenfluramine
Attention deficit hyperactivity disorder	Stimulants
	Tricyclics
	Antipsychotics
	(?) Clonidine
	(?) Clomipramine
	(?) MAOIs
	(?) Bupropion
Conduct disorder (severe, aggressive)	Antipsychotics
	Haloperidol
	Lithium
	(?) Propranolol
	(?) Carbamazepine
Separation anxiety disorder	Imipramine
	(?) Chlordiazepoxide
Overanxious disorder	(?) Benzodiazepines
	Diphenhydramine
Tourettes's disorder	Haloperidol
	Pimozide
	Clonidine
Functional encopresis	(?) Lithium
Functional eneuresis	Imipramine
	(?) Benzodiazepines
	(?) Carbamazepine
	(?) Amphetamines
	(?) Clomipramine
Schizophrenia	Antipsychotics
Mania (acute and maintenance)	Lithium
	Antipsychotics
Major depression	Antidepressants
	(?) Lithium for prophylaxis
	(?) Fluoxetine
	(?) Clomipramine
Obsessive–compulsive disorder	Clomipramine
	(?) Fluoxetine
Posttraumatic stress disorder (acute)	(?) Propranolol

(continued)

Table 8–18. Diagnoses in childhood and adolescence for which pharmacotherapy may be therapeutically indicated.[1] *(continued)*

DSM-III-R Diagnosis	Medication
Sleep disorders	
Insomnia disorders	Benzodiazepines
	Diphenhydramine
	Hydroxyzine
Sleep-wake schedule disorder	Benzodiazepines
	Diphenhydramine
	Hydroxyzine
Sleep terror disorder	Benzodiazepines
	(?) Imipramine
	(?) Carbamazepine
Sleepwalking disorder	Benzodiazepines
	(?) Imipramine
Intermittent explosive disorder	(?) Propranolol

[1] Adapted with permission from Green WH: *Child and Adolescent Clinical Pschopharmacology.* Baltimore: Williams & Wilkins; 1991. (Tables on inside cover.)

3. Adequate attention to parental anxiety with explanations to the parents regarding the illness and procedures. Children are often cued from the parents on how anxious to be.
4. Availability of recreational activities if possible. This may be limited to in-the-room board games, television, etc. Child life or therapeutic recreation specialists can be quite helpful.
5. Realize that as the primary caretaker you may not be in the best position to adequately assess the level of trauma of a particular diagnosis, prognosis, or procedure because of the natural tendency to need to distance from the traumatic aspect of one's intervention.

Familiarity with available consultation resources can prove to be very helpful. Many hospitals have the easy availability of medical social work or consultation liaison child psychiatric services.

CHRONIC ILLNESS

More and more children and adolescents are living with serious chronic illnesses. Chronic illness is an ongoing stressor for

Table 8–19. Side effects of antidepressant medications: tricyclic and newer agents (does not include MAO inhibitors).

Tricyclics
1. Overdosing may easily be lethal
2. Tachycardia
3. Dizziness (may be secondary to orthostatic hypotension)
4. Cardiac toxicity. Abnormal EKG may occur. (Conduction problems, widening of P-R and QRS intervals, prolongation of QTc; *see* page 211 for further discussion).
5. Syncope (uncommon, some cases may be associated with prolonged QTc)
6. Anticholinergic effects (dry mouth, constipation, blurred vision, urinary retention, delirium)
7. Cholinergic rebound with flu like symptoms if stopped abruptly
8. May precipitate glaucoma
9. Sedation
10. Significantly decreased white blood cell count
11. Lowered seizure threshold
12. Precipitation of manic episodes
13. Sexual dysfunction

Newer Agents
Side effects overlap to some degree with the tricyclics but there are numerous differences.
Selected properties:

Buproprion: Less cardiac and anticholinergic effect. Perhaps greater lowering of seizure threshold. Should not be used in patients with bulimia or anorexia nervosa because of frequent reports of seizures.

Fluoxetine: Less cardiac and anticholinergic effect. May cause anxiety, appetite suppression and weight loss. The very long half life of fluoxetine and its metabolites complicates its usage particularly in the area of drug interactions as active compounds may be around long after the patient stops taking it. Fluoxetine has been associated with case reports of increased violence. Given the small number of cases it is hard to know what to make of this. However, patients and families have often read about this in the popular media.

Amoxapine: May cause both extrapyramidal side effects and neuroleptic malignant syndrome because of its dopaminergic properties.

Table 8–20. Side effects of antipsychotics.

1. Sedation.
2. Dizziness (may be secondary to orthostatic hypotension).
3. Anticholinergic effects (dry mouth, constipation, blurred vision, urinary retention, delirium).
4. May precipitate glaucoma.
5. Liver toxicity.
6. Weight gain.
7. Significantly decreased white blood cell count.
8. Lowered seizure threshold.
9. Increased sensitivity to sunburn.
10. Poor temperature regulation with increased propensity to heat stroke.
11. Sexual dysfunction.
12. Extrapyramidal reactions:
    a. Dystonia: This is a sustained contraction of a muscle group, often the neck and eyes (torticollis) but can be any muscle group. On *rare* occasions it can involve the vocal chords making this condition life threatening.
    b. Pseudoparkinsm: Masked faces, drooling, akinesia, cogwheel rigidity.
    c. Tardive dyskinesia: Often oral/facial/buccal dyskinesia. It can also be truncal. This is more common in patients with prolonged exposure to antipsychotics. However, it can happen with relatively brief exposure. Because this side effect may be irreversible it is important to discuss it in detail with the patient and family and watch for it carefully.
    d. Akathisia: Restlessness, often of the legs. This may also be associated with severe dysphoria.
13. Neuroleptic malignant syndrome: This is a relatively uncommon life threatening reaction to antipsychotic medication that may involve autonomic disregulation, altered level of consciousness, stiffness, and increased CPK. Early recognition and supportive care and treatment with Dantrolene (dantrolene sodium) and/or Bromocriptine (bromocriptine mesylate) have greatly reduced the mortality related to this illness. It often requires intensive care unit care.
14. Combined lithium/neuroleptic neurotoxicity: This has been most commonly reported with lithium and Haldol but has also been reported with other combinations as well.
15. *Special considerations:*
    a. *Clozaril* (clozapine) is a relatively new antipsychotic with significantly fewer extrapyramidal side effects than the other antipsychotics. It has proven to be an excellent agent in some relatively treatment resistant chronic psychosis. Unfortunately, a small but significant number of patients may develop life threatening lowered white blood cell count.
    b. *Moban* (molindone) may be the only antipsychotic not to cause weight gain.

Table 8-21. Side effects of lithium.

1. Concern for long term renal toxicity. More recent literature suggests this may be somewhat less of a problem than originally thought. However renal function should be assessed periodically.
2. Polyuria and sometimes even frank nephrogenic diabetes insipidus. Most patients adapt, in milder cases, largely by increasing fluid intake. Frank nephrogenic diabetes insipidus should be pursued in concert with a nephrologist. Thiazide type diuretics may help but renal consultation is indicated before using these with lithium.
3. Thyroid suppression. Check thyroid functions every six months. Add supplement if needed. This is not usually a reason to discontinue lithium. Endocrinology consultation is indicated.
4. EKG changes (often related to repolarization but not limited to this).
5. Potential cardiac toxicity such that screening EKG should be done. In adults in combination with anthracyclines (chemotherapy agent) reported to cause sudden death likely by arrhythmia.
6. Worsening of acne.
7. Fine tremor.
8. Gastrointestinal distress. This is common. It usually responds to taking the medication with meals and/or taking slow release preparations. Frank nausea, vomiting, or diarrhea may indicate toxicity.
9. Increased stool frequency.
10. Weight gain.
11. Combined neurotoxicity with lithium and an antipsychotic.
12. Many medications may affect lithium levels. (eg, nonsteroidal anti-inflammatories and most diuretics).
13. Lithium toxicity can occur whenever a patient becomes dehydrated for any reason. Lithium is a salt and when dehydration occurs, the kidneys hold onto it tightly. Patients should take care to maintain hydration and should also consult their physician before making significant changes in salt intake. Patients who have nausea, vomiting, diarrhea, or a great appetite diminishment should not take lithium until they recover and should contact their physician. In addition, patients who are sweating profusely should take care to replenish fluid and electrolytes on a regular basis. Lithium toxicity may first present with nausea and vomiting. Higher levels may produce neurotoxicity involving confusion, slurred speech, staggering gait, and a course tremor. Lithium is highly dialyzable and this can be life saving with highly toxic levels.

Table 8–22. Anticholinergics: Artane (trihexphenydyl hydrochloride) and Cogentin (benztropine mesylate).

1. Sedation
2. Dry mouth
3. Tachycardia
4. Constipation
5. Anticholinergic delirium
6. Urinary retention
7. Blurred vision
8. May precipitate glaucoma
9. *Special Considerations:* It should be noted that many of the psychoactive medications including many of the antidepressants, antipsychotics, and obviously the anticholinergics, have strong anticholinergic properties and thus the combined anticholinergic load on many patients is high.

both the child and family. The child and family often have the task of regrieving the illness with each developmental phase. As the child grows and is unable to do all the things that they want to do at each developmental phase this challenges their self esteem, sense of vitality, and overall sense of self. There is a similar stress on the family, who must grieve their image of an ideal child and childhood through each developmental stage. Grief is a process that involves considerable work and can be skewed by many processes including familial conflict, psychiatric disturbances in the child or family members, or significant external stressors. Because of this, incomplete grieving is common. This is often manifested by any or all of the following:

1. Unrealistic expectations on the part of the child and/or family
2. Overprotection and infantalization
3. Disruption in limit setting
4. Serious noncompliance

Mental Health consultation and/or treatment can be extremely valuable with any of these presentations.

PSYCHOPHARMACOLOGY

The clinical practice of psychopharmacology in children is still largely based on clinical experience as opposed to double-blind controlled studies. However, the *DSM* systems of classification have helped make research in this area easier to do and to evaluate. Older literature may be difficult to interpret at times, because it may be difficult to know exactly what patient populations are being studied, or how to compare patient populations across studies. There currently is a rapid growth of knowledge in child and adolescent psychopharmacology. Although many pediatricians develop comfort with and expertise in the pharmacologic treatment of some psychiatric disorders (most commonly attention deficit hyperactivity disorder and enuresis), it is probably not indicated for the pediatrician to be an expert in psychopharmacology. Appropriate referral to a behavioral pediatrician or a child psychiatrist is often helpful.

Table 8–18 lists disorders that may respond to medication, along with the range of medications that may be effective for the disorder. In addition to having a familiarly with the range of indications for the use of psychotropic medication, an awareness of common side effects is useful. Although most pediatricians may use psychotropics in their practices infrequently, they may follow many patients prescribed psychotropics by someone else. Tables 8–12, 8–13 and 8–19 through 8–22 outline some of the common/clinically relevant side effects. These tables are designed to help the pediatrician recognize some of the side effects of psychotropic medications. They are not complete lists of side effects or drug interactions nor intended as a guide for usage (in pregnancy, nursing, or general usage).

SUMMARY

Pediatricians are in a unique position to diagnose and treat emotional and behavioral problems of children and adolescents. The pediatrician is often intimately involved with a child and family from a very early age and thus can place difficulties in an individual and familial developmental context. The pediatrician's training including developmental, psychosocial and psychological backgrounds also provide the framework for holistic assessment. The vast majority of emotional and behavioral problems presenting to a pediatrician can be managed by careful evaluation, rule-out or -in of concurrent or causative medical problems, and a psycho-educational approach. A good working relationship with a mental health colleague can be valuable in more severe cases.

Adolescence | 9

David W. Kaplan, MD, MPH, &
Kathleen A. Mammel, MD

Adolescence is a unique period of rapid physical, emotional, cognitive, and social growth and development bridging childhood and adulthood. Generally, adolescence "begins" at age 11–12 years and ends between ages 18 and 21.

The developmental passage from childhood to adulthood encompasses:

(1) Completing puberty and somatic growth.

(2) Developing socially, emotionally, and cognitively—moving from concrete to abstract thinking.

(3) Establishing an independent identity and separating from the family.

(4) Preparing for a career or vocation.

DEMOGRAPHY

In the United States in 1990, 17.8 million adolescents were between the ages of 15 and 19 years and 19.0 million were 20–24 years of age. The adolescent/young adult population—15–24 years–comprises 15% of the US population.

MORTALITY

The 3 leading causes of mortality in the adolescent population ages 15–19 years in 1988 were unintentional injuries 53.1% (82% of all unintentional injuries were caused by motor vehicle crashes), suicides 12.8%, and homicides 13.3%. During the past 20 years, mortality due to motor vehicle crashes, suicide, and homicide have increased between 300 and 400%. The major threats of death for the adolescent population are due to societal and environmental, rather than organic, factors.

MORBIDITY

The major morbidity during adolescence is primarily psychosocial: unintended pregnancy, sexually transmitted disease, substance abuse, smoking, dropping out of school, depression, running away from home, physical violence, and juvenile delinquency. Early identification of the teenager at risk for these problems is important not only to prevent the immediate complications but also to prevent any future associated problems. High-risk behavior in one area is often associated with or may lead to problems in another area (Figure 9–1).

Some of the early indicators of an adolescent at high risk include:

(1) Decline in school performance.
(2) Excessive school absences or cutting class.
(3) Frequent or persistent psychosomatic complaints.

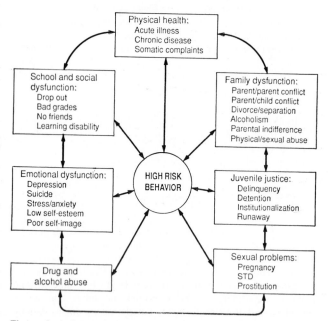

Figure 9–1. Interrelationship of high-risk adolescent behavior.

(4) Changes in sleeping or eating habits.

(5) Difficulty concentrating or persistent boredom.

(6) Signs or symptoms of depression, extreme stress, or anxiety.

(7) Withdrawal from friends or family, or change to a new group of friends.

(8) Unusually severe violent or rebellious behavior, and/or radical personality change.

(9) Parent–adolescent conflict.

(10) Sexual acting out.

(11) Conflict with the law.

(12) Expressing suicidal thoughts or preoccupation with themes of death.

(13) Drug and alcohol abuse.

(14) Running away from home.

DELIVERY OF HEALTH SERVICES

How, where, why, and when adolescents seek health care depends on a number of different factors: ability to pay for care, distance, transportation, accessibility of services, time out of school, and privacy. Teenagers having concerns about pregnancy or contraception, symptoms of a sexually transmitted disease or depression, or problems with substance abuse are often reluctant to confide in their parents for fear of disappointing them and being punished. For the physician, establishing a trusting and confidential relationship is basic to meeting an adolescent patient's health-care needs. If the patient senses the physician is going to tell parents about a confidential problem, the patient may lie or not disclose information essential for proper diagnosis and treatment.

RELATING TO THE ADOLESCENT PATIENT

The manner in which the physician initially approaches the adolescent may determine the success or failure of the visit. The physician should act in a simple and honest fashion, without an authoritarian or excessively "professional" aura. Because many young adolescents have a fragile self-esteem, the physician must be careful not to overpower and intimidate the patient. In communicating with an adolescent, the physician needs to be especially sensitive to developmental level, recognizing that physical appearance and chronological age may be misleading as a measure of cognitive development.

CONFIDENTIALITY

It is helpful at the beginning of the visit to talk with the adolescent and his or her parents as to what to expect. Confidentiality should be addressed, telling the parents you want to meet with the teenager alone, and then with them. Adequate time must be spent with both the patient and parent or important relevant information may be missed. At the beginning of the interview with the patient, it is useful to say something like "I am likely to ask you some personal questions. This is not because I am trying to snoop into your private life, but it may be important to your health. I want to assure you that what we talk about is confidential, just between the two of us. If there is something I feel we should discuss with your parents, I will ask your permission first, unless I feel it is life-threatening."

THE INTERVIEW

How the interview is conducted in the first few minutes of the visit may determine whether a trusting relationship can be established. Spending a few minutes getting to know the patient is time well spent.

The history should include an assessment of progress with psychodevelopmental tasks as well as those health behaviors that are potentially detrimental to the patient's health. The review of systems should include questions about:

(1) Nutrition: Number and balance of meals, calcium, iron, cholesterol intake.

(2) Sleep: Number of hours, problems with insomnia or frequent wakening.

(3) Seatbelt: Regularity of use.

(4) Self care: Knowledge of testicular or breast self examination, dental hygiene, and exercise.

(5) Family relationships: Parents, siblings, relatives.

(6) Peers: Best friend, involvement in group activities, boy/girl friend.

(7) School: Attendance, grades, activities.

(8) Educational and vocational interests: College, career, short- and long-term vocational plans.

(9) Tobacco: Use of cigarettes, snuff, chewing tobacco.

(10) Substance abuse: Frequency, extent and history of alcohol and drug use.

(11) Sexuality: Sexual activity, contraceptive use, pregnancies, history of sexually transmitted disease, number of sexual partners, risk for HIV.

(12) Emotional health: Signs of depression or excessive stress.

The physician's personal attention and interest is likely to be a new experience for the teenager who has probably only experienced medical care through his or her mother. The teenager should leave the visit with a sense of having his or her "own physician."

THE PHYSICAL EXAMINATION

During early adolescence many teenagers may be quite shy and modest, especially if examined by a physician of the opposite sex. The examiner should address this concern directly as it can usually be allayed by verbally acknowledging the uneasiness, explaining the purpose of the examination, and commenting on the findings during the examination. A pictorial chart of sexual development (Figure 9–2) is extremely useful to show the patient current development and the changes to expect in the future.

GROWTH AND DEVELOPMENT

PHYSICAL GROWTH

Pubertal growth and physical development are a result of activation in late childhood of the hypothalamic–pituitary–gonadal axis. Before the onset of puberty, pituitary and gonadal hormones remain at very low levels. With the onset of puberty, the inhibition of gonadotropin-releasing hormone (GnRH) in the hypothalamus is removed, thus allowing pulsatile production and release of the gonadotropins, luteinizing hormone (LH) and follicle-stimulating hormone (FSH). In early to middle adolescence,

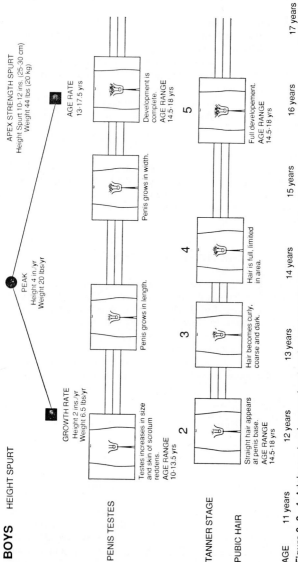

Figure 9–2. A. Adolescent male sexual maturation and growth. B. Adolescent female sexual maturation and growth. (Adapted from Tanner JM: *Growth at Adolescence.* Blackwell, 1962.)

BOYS HEIGHT SPURT

APEX STRENGTH SPURT
Height Spurt 10-12 ins. (25-30 cm)
Weight 44 lbs (20 kg)
AGE RATE
13-17.5 yrs

PEAK
Height 4 in./yr
Weight 20 lbs/yr

GROWTH RATE
Height 2 ins./yr
Weight 6.5 lbs/yr

PENIS TESTES

Testes increases in size and skin of scrotum reddens.
AGE RANGE
10-13.5 yrs

Penis grows in length.

Penis grows in width.

Development is complete.
AGE RANGE
14.5-18 yrs

TANNER STAGE   2   3   4   5

PUBIC HAIR

Straight hair appears at penis base.
AGE RANGE
14.5-18 yrs

Hair becomes curly, coarse and dark.

Hair is full, limited in area.

Full developement.
AGE RANGE
14.5-18 yrs

AGE   11 years   12 years   13 years   14 years   15 years   16 years   17 years

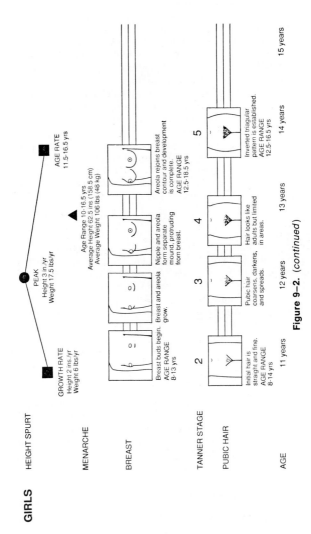

GIRLS

HEIGHT SPURT

PEAK
Height 3 in./yr.
Weight 17.5 lbs/yr

GROWTH RATE
Height 2 ins./yr
Weight 6 lbs/yr

AGE RATE
11.5-16.5 yrs

MENARCHE

Age Range 10-16.5 yrs
Average Height 62.5 ins (158.5 cm)
Average Weight 106 lbs (48 kg)

BREAST

Breast buds begin.
AGE RANGE
8-13 yrs

Breast and areola
grow.

Nipple and areola
form separate
mound, protruding
from breast.

Areola rejoins breast
contour and development
is complete.
AGE RANGE
12.5-18.5 yrs

TANNER STAGE

2   3   4   5

PUBIC HAIR

Initial hair is
straight and fine.
AGE RANGE
8-14 yrs

Pubic hair
coarsens, darkens,
and spreads.

Hair looks like
adults but limited
in areas.

Inverted triagular
pattern is established.
AGE RANGE
12.5-16.5 yrs

AGE

11 years   12 years   13 years   14 years   15 years

Figure 9–2. *(continued)*

there is an increase in pulse frequency and amplitude of LH and FSH secretion, which stimulates the gonads to produce sex steroids (estrogen or testosterone). In the female, FSH stimulates ovarian maturation, granulosa cell function, and estradiol secretion. LH is important in ovulation of the mature ovum and is also involved in corpus luteum formation and progesterone secretion. Initially, estradiol has an inhibitory effect on the release of LH and FSH. Eventually, estradiol becomes stimulatory and the secretions of LH and FSH become cyclic. There is a progressive increase in estradiol that results in maturation of the female genital tract and development of the breasts.

In the male, LH stimulates the interstitial cells of the testes, which produce testosterone. FSH stimulates the production of spermatocytes in the presence of testosterone. The testes also produce inhibin, which is a Sertoli-cell protein that inhibits the secretion of FSH. During puberty circulating testosterone increases more than 20-fold. Levels of testosterone correlate with the physical stages of puberty and the degree of skeletal maturation.

Tanner's scale of sexual maturation is useful clinically to categorize genital development. Tanner staging includes age ranges of normal development and specific descriptions for each stage of pubic hair growth, penis and testes development in boys, and breast maturation in girls. Figures 13–2 A and B graphically represent the chronologic development of this process with reference to each Tanner stage.

The pubertal growth spurt usually takes 2–4 years. It begins nearly 2 years earlier in girls than in boys, but lasts longer in boys. Girls reach their peak height velocity (PHV) between 11.5 and 12 years of age and boys at ages 13.5–14 years. Linear growth at peak velocity is 9.5 ± 1.5 cm per year for boys and 8.3 ± 1.2 cm per year for girls. During adolescence, a teenager's weight doubles, and height increases by 15–20%. In the US, the average age of menarche is $12\frac{3}{4}$ years. However, menarche may be delayed until age 16 or begin as early as age 10. The first conspicuous sign of puberty in girls is development of breast buds between the ages of 8 and 11 years. The first sign of puberty in the male, usually between the ages of 10 and 12, is thinning of the scrotum and testicular growth.

PSYCHOSOCIAL DEVELOPMENT

Adolescents are struggling to find out who they are, what they want to do in the future, and what their personal strengths and weaknesses are to accomplish that end. These questions arise primarily because teenagers are in the process of establishing their own identity. Adolescence is a period of progressive individuation and separation from the family. Because of the rapid physical, emotional, cognitive, and social growth that occur during adolescence, it is useful to divide the period into 3 sequential phases of development. Early adolescence occurs roughly between ages 10 and 13, middle adolescence between ages 14 and 16, and late adolescence at age 17 and older.

Early Adolescence

Early adolescence (ages 10–13) is characterized by rapid growth and development of secondary sex characteristics. Young adolescents are often preoccupied with the physical changes taking place in their bodies. Because of the rapid physical changes, body image, self-concept, and self-esteem fluctuate dramatically. Worries about how their growth and development deviates from their friends may be of great concern, especially issues of short stature in boys and delayed breast development or delayed menarche in girls. As the young teenager begins to become more independent, and family ties loosen, allegiance shifts from parents to peers, who become much more important. Young teenagers still think concretely and cannot easily conceptualize about the future. They may have vague and unrealistic professional goals such as becoming a lead singer in a rock group or a famous movie star.

Middle Adolescence

During middle adolescence (14–16 years), with the rapid pubertal growth of early adolescence decreasing, teenagers begin to adjust and become more comfortable with their "new" bodies. Intense emotions and wide mood swings are typical. Cognitively, as teenagers move from concrete thinking to formal operations, they develop the ability to think abstractly. With this new mental power comes a sense of omnipotence and a belief that the world can be changed merely by thinking about it. Sexually active teenagers may believe they don't need to worry about using contraception because they "can't get pregnant—it won't happen to me." In an effort to establish their own identity, relationships with other people, including peers, are primarily narcissistic, and experimenting with different images is quite common. Peers determine the standards for identification, behavior, activities, and fashion, and provide emotional support, intimacy, empathy, and the sharing of guilt and anxiety, during the struggle for autonomy.

Late Adolescence

Late adolescents (17 years and older) are less self-centered and begin caring much more about others. Social relationships shift from the peer group to the individual. Dating becomes much more intimate. The older adolescent becomes more independent from the family. The ability to think abstractly allows older adolescents to think more realistically in terms of future plans, actions, and careers. Morally, older adolescents have very rigid concepts of right and wrong. Late adolescence is a period of idealism.

BEHAVIORAL AND PSYCHOLOGIC HEALTH

Adolescents with emotional disorders often present with somatic symptoms that do not appear to have biologic cause, eg, abdominal pain, headaches, dizziness/syncope, fatigue, sleep problems, and chest pain. The emotional basis of such a complaint may be varied: somatoform disorder, depression, or stress and anxiety.

PSYCHOPHYSIOLOGIC SYMPTOMS
AND CONVERSION REACTIONS

The most common somatoform disorders during adolescence are conversion reactions. A **conversion reaction** is a psychophysiologic process in which unpleasant feelings, especially anxiety, depression and guilt, are communicated through the use of a physical symptom. The symptom may appear at times of stress such as parental conflict, serious illness in a parent or grandparent, or a change in school. Psychophysiologic symptoms result when anxiety activates the autonomic nervous system, resulting in tachycardia, hyperventilation, and vasoconstriction. The degree to which the conversion symptom lessens anxiety, depression, or the unpleasant feeling is referred to as "primary gain." Conversion symptoms not only diminish unpleasant feelings, but also benefit the adolescent by removing him or her from conflict or an uncomfortable situation. This is referred to as "secondary gain." Specific symptoms may be based on existing or previous illness such as pseudoseizures in adolescents with epilepsy. Adolescents with conversion symptoms tend to have overprotective parents and to become increasingly dependent on their parents as the symptoms becomes the major focus of both the parent's and adolescent's life.

Diagnosis and Treatment

In cases of suspected conversion reaction, history and physical findings are usually inconsistent with anatomic and physiologic concepts. It is critical that from the onset the physician emphasize to the patient and the family that both physical and emotional etiologies for the symptom need to be considered. The relationship between physical causes of emotional pain and emotional causes of physical pain needs to be described. The patient should be encouraged to understand that the symptom may persist, and that at least a short-term goal is to help the patient continue normal daily activities in school and with friends. Medication is rarely helpful in relieving or resolving the symptom. Discussion of the symptom itself should be minimized; however, the physician should be supportive and never suggest that the pain is not real. As the parents gain further insight into the etiology of the symptom, they will become less indulgent of the complaints, facilitating the resumption of normal activities. If management is successful, the adolescent will acquire increased coping skills and become more independent, with decreasing secondary gain.

If the symptom persists in interfering with daily activities, school attendance, participation in extracurricular activities, and involvement with peers, and the patient and parents feel that no progress is being made, psychologic referral is definitely indicated.

DEPRESSION

Presentation

Serious depression during adolescence may present in a variety of ways. It may be similar to the presentation in adults, with vegetative signs such as depressed mood nearly every day, crying spells or inability to cry, discouragement, irritability, sense of emptiness and meaninglessness, negative expectations of self and the environment, low self-esteem, isolation, helplessness, markedly diminished interest or pleasure in most activities, significant weight loss or weight gain, insomnia or hypersomnia, fatigue or loss of energy, and diminished ability to think or concentrate. However, it is not unusual for a serious depression to be ''masked'' because the teenager cannot tolerate the severe feelings of sadness. The teenager may present with recurrent or persistent psychosomatic complaints, such as abdominal pain, chest pain, headache, lethargy, weight loss, dizziness and syncope, or other nonspecific symptoms. Other behavioral manifestations of a masked depression may include school truancy, running away from home, defiance of authorities, self-destructive behavior, drug and alcohol abuse, sexual acting out, and delinquent acts.

Diagnosis

A complete history and physical examination should be performed, including a careful review of the patient's past medical and psychosocial history. The family history should be explored for psychiatric problems.

The teenager should be questioned directly about any specific symptoms of depression (as noted above), expression of suicidal thoughts, or preoccupation with themes of death. The history should include an assessment of the patient's school performance, change in work or other outside activities, changes in the family, or death of a close relative. The teenager may have withdrawn from friends or family, or changed to a new group of friends. Is there a history of drug and alcohol abuse, conflict with law, sexual acting out, running away from home, unusual severe violent or rebellious behavior, or radical personality change?

Because a number of physical disorders can mimic, cause, or exacerbate major depression, adolescents presenting with significant symptoms of depression deserve a thorough medical evaluation to rule out any contributing or underlying medical illness. Commonly prescribed medications in this age group, such as birth control pills and anticonvulsants, may be responsible for depressive symptoms, as may illicit drugs such as marijuana, phencyclidine, and amphetamine and cocaine.

The majority of physical disorders presenting with symptoms of depression are usually evident by history of present illness, past medical history, and physical examination. However, some routine laboratory studies are indicated, including CBC, sedimentation rate, urinalysis, electrolytes, BUN, calcium, T_4 and TSH, serology, and liver enzymes.

The risk of depression appears to be greatest in families with a history of depression of early onset and chronicity of depressive symptoms.

Treatment

The primary care physician may be able to counsel adolescents and parents if an underlying depression is mild or seems to be the result of an acute identifiable personal loss or frustration, and if the patient is not contemplating suicide or at risk for other life-threatening behaviors. If there is evidence of a longstanding depressive disorder, suicidal thoughts, or psychotic thinking, or if the physician does not feel competent or have the interest in counseling the patient, a psychologic referral should be made.

ADOLESCENT SUICIDE

In 1989 there were over 4870 suicides in persons aged 15 through 24. In the 15–19-year-old age group, males had a rate 400% higher than females, and white males had the highest rate. The estimated ratio of attempted suicides to actual suicides is estimated to be 50:1 to 100:1, and is 3 times higher in females than in males. Among actual suicides, deaths due to firearms are the number one cause for both males and females, accounting for over 60% of the suicide deaths.

Acute depressive reactions (transient grief responses) to the loss of a close family member or friend, due to death or separation, may result in depression lasting for weeks or even months. If an adolescent is unable to work through the grief and becomes increasingly depressed, is unable to function at school or socially, has sleep and appetite disturbances, and feelings of hopelessness and helplessness, the magnitude of the depression fulfills the criteria of a major depression and the teenager should be considered to be at increased risk for suicide. As discussed in the section on depression, symptoms of depression during adolescence may be "masked."

Another group of suicidal adolescents is composed of angry teenagers attempting to affect their environment. They may be only mildly depressed, and may not have a longstanding wish to die. Teenagers in this group—usually females—may "attempt'' or "gesture" suicide as a way of getting back at someone, or gaining attention by scaring another person.

The last group of adolescents at risk for suicide is made up of teenagers with a serious psychiatric problem such as acute schizophrenia or a true psychotic depressive disorder.

Diagnosis

The physician must determine the extent of the teenager's depression and the risk of the adolescent trying to self-inflict harm. The evaluation should include interviews with both the teenager and the family. The history should include the medical, social, emotional, and academic background, as described above. When seeing depressed patients, the physician should always inquire about thoughts of suicide: "Are things ever so bad that life doesn't seem worth living?" "Have you thought of taking your life?" If the patient has thoughts of suicide, the immediacy of risk can be assessed by determining if there is a concrete, feasible plan. Although the patients who are at greatest risk have a concrete plan that can be carried out in the near future, especially if they have rehearsed the plan, the physician should not dismiss the potential risk of suicide in the adolescent who does not describe a specific plan. The physician should pay attention to "gut feelings." There may be subtle nonverbal signs that the patient is at greater risk than is apparent on the surface.

Management

The primary care physician is often in a unique position to identify an adolescent at risk for suicide, because many teenagers who attempt suicide seek medical attention within weeks preceding the attempt. These visits are often for vague somatic complaints or subtle signs of depression. If there is evidence of depression, the physician must assess the severity of the depression and suicidal risk. The physician should always get emergency psychologic consultation for any teenager who is severely depressed, psychotic, or acutely suicidal. It is the psychologist's or psychiatrist's responsibility to assess the seriousness of suicidal ideation and decide whether hospitalization or outpatient treatment is most appropriate.

SUBSTANCE ABUSE

Substance abuse is a serious problem in our society of quick fixes for complex problems. In 1991, a national survey of high-school seniors reported that 54.0% had used alcohol and 13.8% smoked marijuana in the past 30 days; 7.8% reported they had tried cocaine.

Risk Factors

The causes of substance abuse are multifactorial, including personality characteristics, genetic influences, peer pressure, and parental and cultural influences.

Children whose parents give clear messages against drugs and provide consistent authoritative discipline involving warmth and discussion, those whose peers do not use drugs, those with knowledge of the consequences of substance abuse, and those possessing personal values placing importance on health and achievement tend to be protected from substance abuse.

Stages of Substance Abuse

Chemical dependency is the result of a gradual process. Donald Macdonald, MD, has suggested five stages of substance abuse, 0–4, which are outlined in Table 9–1. Progression through these stages may occur at a variable rate, and not every user will progress to stage 4. However, the younger the user, the greater the risk for development of chemical dependency.

Substances Abused

While tobacco and alcohol are considered "gateway" drugs, marijuana is also commonly used during adolescence. See Table 9–2 for a list of drugs commonly abused and their effects.

Diagnosis

History is the key to diagnosis of substance abuse, and a history obtained in a nonjudgmental manner may be highly enlightening. In later stages of involvement, however, denial may cause the adolescent to minimize use. Clues to diagnosis include episodes of acute drug abuse (such as overdose or suicide gestures), deteriorating school performance, personality changes (mood swings, lack of motivation), worsening family relationships, change of peer groups, trouble with the law, or persistent regular drug use despite parental or physician discussion with the teenager. When substance abuse is suspected or established in an adolescent, an assessment of the adolescent's involvement with the drug (age at onset, drugs used, duration of use, frequency of use, attitude toward use), involvement with a drug-using peer group, family relationship, and psychologic profile

Table 9–1. Stages of substance abuse.[1]

Stage	Drugs	Sources	Frequency	Feelings	Behavior	Treatment
Stage 0 Curiosity	None	Available— but not used	—	Curious	Risk-taking Desire for acceptance	Optimum time. Anticipatory guidance to develop good coping skills and strong self-esteem. Clear family guidelines on drug and alcohol use. Drug education.
Stage 1 Experimentation	Tobacco Alcohol Marijuana	House supply Friends Siblings	Weekend use for recreational purposes	Excitement Pleasure Few consequences Learns how easy it is to feel good	Lying Little change	Drug education. Attention to societal messages, reduce supply. Strict, loving rules at home. Drug-free alternative activities established.
Stage 2 Regular use	As above, plus hashish or hash oil, tranquilizers, sedatives, amphetamines	Buying	Progresses to mid-week use. Purpose is to get high.	Excitement followed by guilt	Mood swings Faltering school performance Truancy Changing peer groups Changing style of dress	Drug-free self-help groups (Alcoholics or Narcotics Anonymous). Family involvement. Psychiatric counseling unhelpful unless family therapy and after-care provided.

Stage 3 Psychologic or chemical dependency	As above, plus stimulants, hallucinogens	Selling to support their habit. Possibly stealing or prostitution in exchange for drugs.	Daily	Euphoric highs followed by depression, shame, guilt, and perhaps suicidal thoughts	Pathological lying School failure Family fights Involvement with the law over curfew, truancy, vandalism, shoplifting, or driving under the influence, breaking and entering, violence	Inpatient or foster-care programs that require family involvement and provide after-care.
Stage 4 Using drugs to feel "normal"	As above; any available drug, including opiates	Any way possible	All day	Euphoria rare and harder to achieve Chronic depression	Drifters with repeated failures and psychologic symptoms of paranoia and agression Overdosing, blackouts, amnesia occur regularly Chronic cough, fatigue, malnutrition	Inpatient or foster-care programs that require family involvement and provide after-care.

Table 9–2. Subjective, objective, and adverse effects of commonly abused drugs.

Drug	Street Name	Subjective Effects	Objective Effects	Adverse/Overdose Reactions
Cannabis Marijuana Hashish Hash oil THC	Pot Grass Weed Maryjane Hash Tea Reefer Joint	Sedation Tranquilization Mild hallucination or pleasurable change in perception	Tachycardia Conjunctival irritation Impaired abstract thinking, reading comprehension, verbal ability, short-term memory, counting, color discrimination Impaired driving ability	Acute anxiety Serious reaction uncommon unless adulterated with hallucinogens
Alcohol	Booze	Stimulation as blood level rises Subsequent sedation, release of inhibitions	Slurred speech Ataxia Impaired driving performance	Poor judgment Impaired cognitive and motor abilities Emotional changes Respiratory depression Decrease in temperature Coma, shock, death
CNS Stimulants Cocaine Amphetamines	Cocaine Coke Snow Dust Uppers Speed Meth Bennies Dexies	Euphoric effects: exhiliration, calmness, sense of power; omnipotence and unlimited energy in high doses Perception of decrease in appetite, thirst, fatigue Dysphoria or "wired" irritability after euphoric phase	Local anesthetic Sympathomimetic: mydriasis, hypertension, tachycardia, tachypnea, temperature elevation, tremor, agitation	Anxiety Elevated temperature Seizures Respiratory arrest Arrhythmia Death Hallucinations and paranoia
CNS Depressants Group I Sedatives Tranquilizers	Downers Quaaludes, Ludes Blues, Bluebirds Reds, Red devils Yellows, Yellow jackets	Relaxation Facilitation of social behavior With higher doses, loss of inhibitions, sedation, drowsiness	Nystagmus on lateral gaze Slurred speech, ataxia Impulsiveness	Coma Death

252

Drug	Street names	Effects	Signs	Adverse/severe reactions
CNS Depressants Group II Nitrous oxide Toluene Trichlorethylene Methanol Acetone Gasoline Fluorinated hydrocarbons		Sedation Heightened visual imagery Hallucination Euphoria	Drowsiness Rhinitis, bronchitis Odor of inhalant on breath Metabolic abnormalities	Coma is rare Idiosyncratic reaction to fluorinated hydrocarbons resulting in sudden death by cardiac arrhythmia
Nitrites Amyl nitrite Isobutyl nitrite	Rush Lockerroom Poppers Bolt	Sudden, transient, pleasurable tingling Headache Pounding heart	Tachycardia Hypotension	Exacerbation of preexisting cardiac disease, syncope Elevated intraocular pressure Coma, rarely sudden death Methemoglobinemia
Hallucinogens Group I Lysergic acid diethylamide Mescaline Psilocybin	Acid LSD Peyote Button Mesc Mushrooms	Vivid sensory stimulation and distortion Introspection Awareness of drug-induced state	Dizziness, nausea Paresthesias Sympathomimetic effects Varying mental status as changes from hallucinating to coherent recountings	Idiosyncratic "bad trips" or panic reactions with terrifying hallucinations that may last from hours to more than a day
Hallucinogens Group II Phencyclidine	PCP Angel dust	Low doses (1–5 mg) produce floating euphoria or numbness Doses of 5–15 mg cause confusion, agitation, impairment of communication, and distorted body perception Higher doses may cause psychotic reactions lasting from days to months	Sympathomimetic effects Drooling Rotatory nystagmus Decreased response to pain Combative and aggressive or silent and withdrawn	Muscle rigidity, opisthotonus, seizures, coma Toxic psychosis (rotatory nystagmus and fever may be the only signs to differentiate from nontoxic psychosis) Hypertensive crises with CNS hemorrhage and death
Opiates Heroin Morphine Meperidine Propoxyphene Methadone Codeine	Dope H Horse Smack Meth	With IV use a sudden "rush" and sensation similar to orgasm With other routes, euphoria, drowsiness, decreased appetite and libido Nausea, vomiting, and dizziness may occur in novices	Oriented but indifferent Slurred speech, unsteady gait Slowed heart and respiratory rates Pinpoint pupils Needle tracks in IV users	CNS and respiratory depression responsive to naloxone (Narcan) Pulmonary edema 24–36 hours after use, not responsive to naloxone Death

(any preexisting psychiatric, developmental, or educational difficulties) will assist in decisions on appropriate management. Information should also be obtained from the parents, who may suspect substance abuse or may be enabling the adolescent and therefore deny its significance.

Physical examination will provide few clues. Laboratory tests are generally helpful only with acute intoxication, when a blood alcohol and urine toxin screen should be obtained. When it is known that one chemical has been used at the time of acute intoxication, a drug screen should be obtained to look for other substances due to the possibility of multiple drug abuse or adulteration or misrepresentation of material. Drug testing outside of an episode of acute intoxication or a drug-free maintenance program is generally of little help and may endanger the patient-physician relationship.

Management

Prevention and early intervention during experimental use is most effective. Management will depend on the stage of involvement (Table 9–1).

EATING DISORDERS

It is estimated that 5–10% of adolescent girls and young women have an eating disorder. The typical patient is a middle or upper-middle class female, but this trend is changing. The causes of eating disorders remain unclear. There are contributing psychosocial and cultural factors, with the emphasis in today's society on thinness and the "superwoman" image.

Presentation and Diagnosis

Often the patient presents with abdominal pain, nausea, fainting spells, hair loss, or amenorrhea, and it is the clinician who discovers the true diagnosis. In some instances, a school nurse, coach, or parent may become suspicious after observing weight loss, overconcern with weight, or unusual eating and exercise behaviors. Bulimics, however, may present on their own and may feel relieved to share their burden with someone.

The diagnosis of anorexia nervosa or bulimia nervosa is largely based on history and meeting specific diagnostic criteria

Table 9–3. Diagnostic criteria for eating disorders.[1]

Anorexia Nervosa:
A. Weight loss or failure to gain weight during growth such that weight is 15% below that expected for age and height.
B. Fear of weight gain or fatness despite being underweight.
C. Distorted body image—feels all or part of the body is fat even when severely underweight.
D. Interruption of menstrual cycles for at least 3 months (secondary amenorrhea) or failure to menstruate when expected (primary amenorrhea).

Bulimia Nervosa
A. Repeated binge eating (large number of calories in short period of time) with a frequency of at least twice a week for 3 or more months.
B. Perception by patient that eating behavior is out of control.
C. Recurrent purging behavior to prevent weight gain—self-induced emesis; use of laxatives, diuretics, or emetics; excessive exercise; or severely restricted intake.
D. Overly focused on body image.

[1] Modified and reproduced, with permission, from *Diagnostic and Statistical Manual of Mental Disorders*. Third edition-Revised. American Psychiatric Association, 1987.

(Table 9–3). The history needs to include the presenting symptoms; weight history, including desired weight; dietary intake, unusual eating behaviors, or avoided foods; history of any purging behaviors such as vomiting, excessive exercise, or use of diet pills, diuretics, emetics, or laxatives; and menstrual history for irregular cycles, secondary amenorrhea, or delay in menarche. Social history may provide clues to a perfectionistic drive in anorexics or impulsiveness in bulimics (eg, substance abuse or sexual promiscuity), or family dysfunction. Review of systems should focus on symptoms of possible complications of the above behaviors and on symptoms of other diseases in the differential diagnosis.

Physical Findings

The physical examination is most often normal, but this does not rule out the diagnosis of an eating disorder. The anorexic's weight will quantitate the actual loss; however, bulimics are usually of normal weight or within 10 pounds (under or over) of normal weight. The vital signs of the anorexic may show hypothermia, bradycardia, or hypotension. Other findings in anorexia include dry skin, presence of fine, downy lanugo hair on the body or more pigmented body hair, limpness and loss of shine to the scalp hair, excoriation over the sacral spine from excessive situps, prominent ribs, atrophied breasts, scaphoid abdomen, palpable hard stool in the rectal vault, cold extremities, squaring off of the convergence of the thighs, or edema of the extremities. In patients with self-induced emesis there may be loss of tooth enamel, particularly on the posterior aspect of the front teeth, or callouses on the dorsum of the fingers.

Laboratory Findings

The goal of laboratory tests is to exclude other diagnoses and to assess the patient's status. Most laboratory studies will not change until late in the disease. A CBC is useful to assess nutritional status and a sedimentation rate to help exclude other disorders such as inflammatory bowel disease or collagen vascular disease. Electrolytes may detect the presence of hypochloremic alkalosis and hypokalemia from vomiting or the metabolic acidosis of laxative abuse. Serum total protein and albumin are usually normal until late; low serum phosphorus and magnesium levels are an ominous sign. Other laboratory studies, such as thyroid function tests, x-rays, upper gastrointestinal series, or CT scan of the head need only be done as indicated by the presentation.

Differential Diagnosis

The list of causes of weight loss is legend. Etiologies such as malignancy, collagen vascular disease, diabetes mellitus, hyperthyroidism, malabsorptive syndromes, inflammatory bowel disease, or chronic renal, pulmonary, or cardiac disease warrant consideration in the suspected anorexic. However, with these disorders there may be weight loss but there is no associated disturbance of body image or fear of obesity. One must also remember that a number of psychiatric disturbances, including depression, may be associated with loss of appetite and weight loss. Some unusual central nervous system disorders may present like bulimia, but again there is no distorted body image or overconcern with body shape or weight.

Complications

Eating disorders can result in severe consequences to nearly every system of the body including electrolyte and acid-base disturbances; depressed gonadotropins; altered thyroid tests; disturbed menstruation; dysrhythmias; congestive heart failure; osteoporosis; disturbed thermoregulation; constipation; gastric dilatation, delayed emptying, and rupture; and bone marrow suppression.

Management

The patient needs to know that the clinician appreciates her struggle, aims to restore her to health, won't let her become fat, and will help her to regain control. The parents need to understand that eating disorders are symptoms of underlying issues, often a family problem; that the family is very important to the solution; and that treatment requires the intervention of the mental health disciplines.

Restoration of the nutritional and physiologic state is an early goal. An individualized contract can be drawn up and signed by the patient that addresses such issues as long-term weight goal, rate of weight gain, amount of exercise, frequency of visits and of labwork, minimal weight signalling need for hospitalization, and consequences of failed weight goals.

Most often, the patient can eat adequately to replace nutrient deficits and to gain weight. In extremely malnourished and noncompliant hospitalized patients, nasogastric tube feedings or hyperalimentation may initially be necessary. Hospitalization may become necessary for medical or psychiatric reasons (Table 9–4).

Prognosis

It appears that 40–60% of significantly ill anorexics make a good physical and psychosocial recovery and that 75% improve

Table 9–4. Criteria for hospitalization of eating-disorder patients.

Medical
Weight loss greater than 30% of body weight over 3 months
Severe metabolic disturbance
   HR < 40
   T < 36°C
   SBP < 70
   Serum K^+ < 2.5 despite oral K^+ replacement
   Severe dehydration
Severe binging and purging

Psychiatric
Severe depression or risk of suicide
Psychosis
Family crisis
Failure to comply with a therapeutic contract, or inadequate response to
   outpatient treatment

weight. The mortality rate ranges from 0 to 19%, and is at least 5% in those receiving therapy. As few as 40–50% of treated bulimics are felt to be ''cured,'' and there is a greater likelihood of serious medical complications, risk of suicide, and death than for anorexics without bulimic behavior.

EXOGENOUS OBESITY

Background

If a child enters adolescence obese, the odds are 4:1 against later achievement of normal weight; but if a child leaves adolescence obese, the odds are 28:1 against later normal weight. The associated medical risks of obesity include pediatric and adult hypertension, elevated triglyceride levels, cerebrovascular accidents, diabetes mellitus, gallbladder disease, slipped capital-hard femoral epiphyses, degenerative arthritis, and pregnancy complications. The psychosocial hazards of obesity tend to be the greatest consequence for adolescents, who may experience alienation, distorted peer relations, poor self-esteem, guilt, depression, or distorted body image.

Diagnosis

History should include onset of obesity, eating and exercise habits, amount of time spent in sedentary activities such as television watching, problem foods, previous successful and unsuccessful attempts at weight loss, and family history of obesity. In addition, one needs to assess the patient's readiness to lose weight. A complete physical examination should be performed. Height, weight, and weight index should be plotted; an index greater than 1.2 is considered diagnostic of obesity. Triceps skinfold (TSF) thickness is the most practical way to measure obesity in children and teenagers, but reproducibility is inconsistent. A TSF more than one standard deviation above the mean (85th percentile) defines obesity; one at the 95th percentile indicates superobesity. Laboratory evaluation should include CBC, urinalysis, and cholesterol level. Endocrine causes such as hypothyroidism or Cushing's disease can generally be excluded on the basis of history and physical examination, but in individual cases exclusion of these may require additional studies.

Management

An age-appropriate behavior modification program incorporating good dietary counseling and exercise is optimal (Table 9–5).

Table 9–5. Program components for weight-control interventions.[1]

Component	Specific Aspects
Physical activity Cardiovascular fitness High calorie equivalent	a. Frequency: 3–4 ×/week b. Intensity: 50–60% maximal ability (55–65% max heart rate) c. Duration: 15 min at start, building to 30–40 min d. Mode: use of large muscle activity such as walk/jog, swim, or cycle e. Interest: encourage a wide variety of recreational activities f. Enjoyment: focus on the fun of movement and the enjoyment of being physically active
Nutrition education	a. Teach critical aspects of quality nutrition, ie, food groups, serving requirements, and variety b. Develop understanding for calorie balance: calories in vs calories out c. Alert children to pressures of media advertising d. Instruct on role of snacks and ideas for "good" snacking e. Assist children on balancing fast-food eating and calorie intake f. Teach children to reduce intake of high-calorie, low-nutrition treats
Behavior modification Change eating habits Increase habitual physical activity	a. Identify those cues that affect eating, eg, location of meals, size of plates, food in easy-to-see places b. Identify behavior that negatively affects weight control: speed of eating, chronic second portions, high calorie food choices, "pickiness" c. Contract for increased levels of activity using record cards or activity contracts d. Develop strategies for more functional activity, such as walking to school, taking stairs, sitting rather than lying e. Develop interest in a variety of recreational areas: tennis, dance, skating, etc f. Identify cues that lead to inactivity: frequent TV watching, lying down after school or meals, friends who do not like active play

[1] Reproduced with permission, from Ward DS, Bar-Or O: Role of the physician and physical education teacher in the treatment of obesity at school. *Pediatrician* 1986;**13**:44.

SCHOOL FAILURE

When children graduate from grade school to middle school or junior high school, the course work content, amount, and complexity increases significantly. Academic failure presenting at adolescence has a broad differential diagnosis: 1) limited intellectual abilities, 2) specific learning disability, 3) depression or emotional problems, 4) physical causes such as visual or hearing problems, 5) excessive school absenteeism secondary to chronic disease such as asthma or neurologic dysfunction, 6) lack of ability to concentrate, 7) attention deficit disorder, 8) lack of motivation, or 9) drug and alcohol problems. Each of these possible etiologies must be explored in depth.

Diagnosis

A thorough history, physical examination, appropriate laboratory studies, and educational and psychologic testing should be performed. A detailed medical history looking for the presence of chronic disease or any sensory deficits should be evaluated. The amount of school missed secondary to absences and the response of the parents, eg, "too sick to go to school," overlaps with school avoidance. A history of attention deficit disorder or stimulant medication use in the past may be an indication of ongoing problems with concentration. Educational records including previous educational and intelligence testing is important background information to obtain. The emotional history may reveal past episodes of counseling for depression or other significant psychiatric problems. The presence of conflict in the family, such as divorce or alcoholism, may have an important role, distracting the adolescent from academic responsibilities. There may be a family history of school problems in other siblings or family members.

Treatment

Management must be individualized to address specific needs, foster strengths, and implement a feasible program. With specific learning disabilities an individual prescription for regular and special educational courses, teachers, and extracurricular activities is important. Counseling is helpful to work on coping skills, self-esteem, and socialization. If there is a history of hyperactivity or attention deficit disorder, with poor concentrating ability, a trial of stimulant medication may be useful. If the teenager appears to be depressed, or other serious emotional problems are uncovered, further psychologic evaluation should be recommended.

BREAST DISORDERS

The breast examination should become part of the routine physical exam in females as soon as breast budding occurs. The breast examination begins with inspection of the breasts for symmetry and Tanner stage. Asymmetry is usually a normal variation but may be due to unilateral breast hypoplasia or amastia, absence of the pectoralis major muscle, or virginal hypertrophy.

BREAST MASSES

Most breast masses in adolescents are benign; however, approximately 150 cases of adenocarcinoma are reported each year in the US in women under 25 years of age. Fibroadenomas account for 90% of breast lumps in teenagers seen in referral clinics, with the remainder being cysts. In practice, cysts may account for as many as 50% of breast masses in adolescents, but they are readily diagnosed and many spontaneously resolve. Suspicious lesions should be immediately referred to a surgeon (Table 9–6).

GALACTORRHEA

In teenagers, **galactorrhea,** or inappropriate nipple discharge, is most often benign, although a careful history and work-up are necessary. Numerous prescribed and illicit drugs are associated with galactorrhea (Table 9–7), as are a number of CNS, endocrine, or chest-wall disorders (Table 9–8).

Evaluation
If there is no history of pregnancy or drug use, TSH and prolactin levels should be obtained. An elevated TSH confirms the diagnosis of hypothyroidism. An elevated prolactin and normal TSH, often accompanied by amenorrhea, suggests a hypothalamic or pituitary tumor, and CT scan is indicated. When the

Table 9-6. Breast lesions.

Type	Clinical Findings	Progression	Treatment
Fibroadenoma	Rubbery, well-demarcated, nontender mass, usually in upper outer quadrant. Most < 5 cm; 25% will be multiple or recurrent.	Slow growing, quiescent after teen years.	Follow for 2–3 menstrual cycles. If no change, ultrasound differentiates solid tumor from cyst. Solid tumors should be referred for excisional biopsy.
Cysts	Tender, spongy masses, often multiple. Increased symptoms premenstrually.	About half of cysts spontaneously regress over 2–3 menstrual cycles.	Persistent cysts may be drained by needle aspiration. Refer suspicious lesions to breast surgeon.
Fibrocystic breasts	Cyclical tenderness and nodularity bilaterally, most common in third and fourth decades, but seen in adolescence.	Increase and diminish under cyclical influence of estrogen–progesterone balance.	Reassurance. Oral contraceptives reduce the risk of fibrocystic breasts. Some women report decreased symptoms after methylxanthines are limited in the diet, vitamin E treatment or when methylxanthines are limited in the diet, but recent studies have not proven this.
Breast abscess	Unilateral breast pain with overlying inflammatory changes, breast mass palpable late in course. Often due to *Staphylococcus aureus*.	Infection may extend deeper than suspected on exam.	Surgical incision and drainage when fluctuant. Oral antibiotics (dicloxacillin or cephalosporin) for 2–4 weeks.
Adenocarcinoma	Hard, nonmobile, well-circumscribed, painless mass.	Generally indolent course.	Refer for surgical treatment.
Cystosarcoma phylloides	Firm, rubbery, tender, warm, cystic; associated with skin necrosis.	May suddenly enlarge. Most often benign; rarely metastasizes.	Surgical removal is indicated.
Giant juvenile fibroadenoma	Remarkably large fibroadenoma with overlying dilated superficial veins.	Benign.	Requires excision to prevent breast atrophy for cosmetic reasons.
Intraductal papilloma	Cylindrical tumor arising from epithelium of duct; often subareolar but may be in periphery in adolescents; associated nipple discharge.	Most are benign.	Requires excision for cytologic diagnosis.
Fat necrosis	Localized inflammatory process in one breast; follows trauma in half of cases.	Subsequent scarring may be confused with malignancy.	Biopsy if suspicious in scarring stage.
Virginal or juvenile hypertrophy	Massive enlargement of both, or less often one, breasts, attributed to end-organ hypersensitivity to normal hormones levels around menarche.	Benign. May cause embarrassment.	Cosmetic reduction may be done at a later date.

Table 9–7. Drugs associated with breast symptoms (galactorrhea, gynecomastia, pain, mass).[1]

Street drugs (illicit or abused)
  Marijuana
  Opiates
  Amphetamines
  Meprobamate

Hormones or related drugs
  Oral contraceptives
  Estrogens
  Tamoxifen
  Bromocriptine withdrawal
  Methyltestosterone
  Human chorionic gonadotropin

Chemotherapeutic agents
  Vincristine
  Busulfan

Prescription medications
  Antidepressants
  Benzodiazepines
  Butyrophenones
  Cimetidine
  Digoxin
  Isoniazid
  Methyldopa
  Phenothiazines & derivatives
  Reserpine
  Spironolactone

[1] Modified and reproduced, with permission, from Beach RK: Routine breast exams: A chance to reassure, guide, and protect. *Contemp Pediatr,* 1987;**Oct**:70.

prolactin level is normal, uncommon causes such as adrenal, renal, or ovarian tumors should be considered. For those with a negative work-up and persistent galactorrhea, careful follow-up is required. In many cases symptoms resolve spontaneously without a diagnosis.

Treatment

Treatment of galactorrhea depends upon the underlying cause. Prolactinomas may be surgically removed or suppressed with bromocriptine. Bromocriptine may also be beneficial to some amenorrheic females with normal prolactin levels.

Table 9–8. Causes of galactorrhea[1]

1. Hypothalamic disorders
    Functional
        Postpartum
        Without pregnancy
    Pathologic
        Infiltrative
            Sarcoid
            Histiocytosis X
            Hypothalamic tumors
        Section of pituitary stalk
2. Drug therapy
    Tranquilizers
    Tricyclic antidepressants
    Methyldopa
    Rauwolfia alkaloids
    Oral contraceptives
    Estrogens
3. Neoplasms
    Pituitary tumors
        Prolactin secretion only
        Prolatin and ACTH secretion (Cushing's disease)
        Growth hormone secretion with or without prolactin secretion
            (acromegaly)
    Ectopic prolactin-secreting tumors
4. Hypothyroidism
5. Neurogenic stimulation
    Breast stimulation
    Chest-wall lesions (herpes zoster, thoracotomy)

[1] Reproduced, with permission, from Fraser WM, Blackard WG: Medical conditions that affect the breast and lactation. *Clin Obstet Gynecol* 1975; **18**:51.

GYNECOMASTIA

Gynecomastia is a common concern of male adolescents, the majority of whom (60–70%) develop transient subareolar breast tissue during Tanner stage II–III development. Proposed etiologies include testosterone-estrogen imbalance, increased prolactin level, or abnormal serum binding protein levels.

Clinical Findings

In type I idiopathic gynecomastia the adolescent presents with a unilateral (20% bilateral), tender, firm mass beneath the areola. More generalized breast enlargement is classified as type

Table 9–9. Disorders associated with gynecomastia.[1]

Klinefelter's syndrome
Traumatic paraplegia
Male pseudohermphroditism
Testicular feminization syndrome
Reifenstein's syndrome
17-Ketosteroid reductase deficiency
Endocrine tumors (seminoma, Leydig cell tumor, teratoma, feminizing adrenal tumor, hepatoma, leukemia, hemophilia, bronchogenic carcinoma, leprosy, etc)
Hypothyroidism
Hyperthyroidism
Cirrhosis
Herpes zoster
Friedreich's ataxia

[1] Reproduced, with permission, from McAnarney ER, Greydanus DE: Adolescence. In: *Current Pediatric Diagnosis and Treatment*, 9th ed. Kempe CH, Silver HK, O'Brien D, Fulginiti VA (eds). Appleton and Lange, 1987.

II. Pseudogynecomastia refers to excessive fat tissue or prominent pectoralis muscles.

Differential Diagnosis

Gynecomastia may be drug-induced (Table 9–7) or related to any one of a host of disorders (Table 9–9).

Treatment

If gynecomastia is idiopathic, reassurance of the common and benign nature of the process should be given. Resolution may take several months to 2 years. Pharmacotherapeutic agents, such as dihydrotestosterone heptanoate, danazol, clomiphene, and tamoxifen, have been used with variable results. Surgery is reserved for adolescents with significant psychologic trauma or severe breast enlargement.

GYNECOLOGIC DISORDERS IN ADOLESCENCE

MENSTRUAL PHYSIOLOGY

The menstrual cycle is divided into 3 phases: follicular, ovulatory, and luteal. Hypothalamic, pituitary, and ovarian hor-

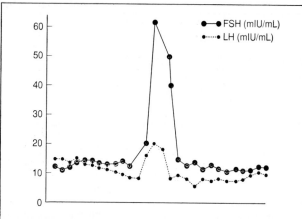

Gonadotropins

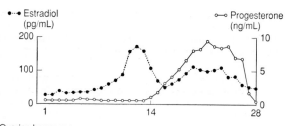

Ovarian hormones

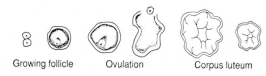

Ovarian follicle

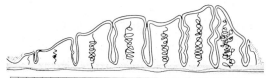

Endometrium

mones work in concert through a complex system of positive and negative feedback to bring about monthly ovulation (Figure 9–3) and, if fertilization does not occur, menstruation.

MENSTRUAL DISORDERS

Amenorrhea

Amenorrhea is the lack of menses when otherwise expected to occur. It may be the result of anatomic abnormalities, chromosomal deviations, or physiologic delay (Table 9–10).

Primary amenorrhea refers to delay in menarche such that there are no menstrual periods or secondary sex characteristics by 14 years of age, or no menses in the presence of secondary sex characteristics by 16 years of age. **Secondary amenorrhea** is defined as the absence of menses for at least 3 cycles after regular cycles have been established. In some instances evaluation should begin immediately, without waiting for the specified age or duration of lapsed periods, for example, in suspected pregnancy, short stature with the stigmata or Turner's syndrome, or an anatomic defect.

A. Evaluation for Primary Amenorrhea: The history should include whether puberty has commenced and the age at menarche for other female relatives. A careful physical examination should be performed, keeping in mind that estrogen is responsible for breast development; maturation of the external genitalia, vagina, and uterus; and menstruation. If pelvic examination reveals normal female external genitalia and pelvic organs, a vaginal smear for estrogen influence or a progesterone challenge may be done (Fig. 9–4).

If signs of virilization are present (Fig. 9–5), LH level should be obtained as the first step, to rule out polycystic ovaries. If the LH level is low in the face of virilization, an adrenal disorder is the most likely diagnosis.

If physical examination reveals the absence of a uterus (Fig 13–5), karyotyping should be performed to differentiate testicu-

←———————————————————————

Figure 9–3. Physiology of the normal ovulatory menstrual cycle: gonadotropin secretion, ovarian hormone production, follicular maturation, and endometrial changes during one cycle. FSH = follicle-stimulating hormone; LH = luteinizing hormone.

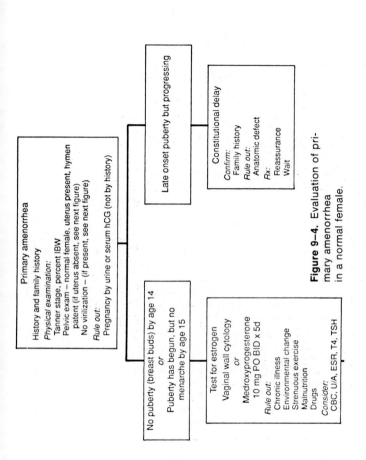

Figure 9–4. Evaluation of primary amenorrhea in a normal female.

Primary amenorrhea

History and family history

Physical examination:
Tanner stage, percent IBW
Pelvic exam – normal female, uterus present, hymen patent (if uterus absent, see next figure)
No virilization – (if present, see next figure)

Rule out:
Pregnancy by urine or serum hCG (not by history)

No puberty (breast buds) by age 14
or
Puberty has begun, but no menarche by age 15

Test for estrogen
Vaginal wall cytology
or
Medroxyprogesterone
10 mg PO BID x 5d

Rule out:
Chronic illness
Environmental change
Strenuous exercise
Malnutrition
Drugs

Consider:
CBC, U/A, ESR, T4, TSH

Late onset puberty but progressing

Constitutional delay

Confirm:
Family history
Rule out:
Anatomic defect
Rx:
Reassurance
Wait

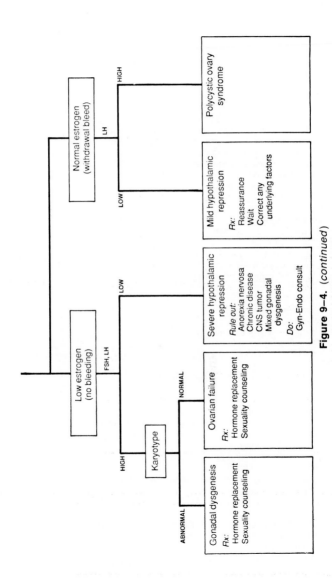

Figure 9–4. *(continued)*

Table 9–10. Causes of amenorrhea.

Hypothalamic–Pituitary Axis
Hypothalamic repression
  Emotional stress
  Depression
  Chronic disease
  Weight loss; severe dieting
  Obesity
  Strenuous athletics
  Drugs (post-BCP, phenothiazines)
CNS lesion
  Pituitary lesion—adenoma, prolatinoma
  Craniopharyngioma and other brainstem or parasellar tumors
  Head injury with hypothalamic contusion
  Infiltrative process (sarcoidosis)
  Vascular disease (hypothalamic vasculitis)
Congenital conditions[1]
  Kallman's syndrome

Ovaries
Gonadal dysgenesis[1]
  Turner's syndrome (XO)
  Mosaic (XX/XO)
Injury to ovary
  Autoimmune disease (may include thyroid, adrenal, islet cells)
  Infection (mumps, oophoritis)
  Toxins (alkylating chemotherapeutic agents)
  Irradiation
  Trauma, torsion (rare)
Polycystic ovary syndrome (Stein-Leventhal)
  (virilization may be present)
Ovarian failure
  Premature menopause—may result from causes of ovarian injury above
  Resistant ovary
  Variant of gonadal dysgenesis (mosaic)

Uterovaginal Outflow Tract
Müllerian dysgenesis[1]
  Congenital deformity or absence of uterus, fallopian tubes, or vagina
Imperforate hymen, transverse vaginal septum, vaginal agenesis, agenesis of the cervix[1]
Testicular feminization (absent uterus)[1]
Uterine lining defect
  Asherman's syndrome (intrauterine synechiae postcurettage or endometritis)
  TB, brucellosis

Defect in Hormone Synthesis/Action (virilization may be present)
Adrenal hyperplasia[1]
Cushing's syndrome
Adrenal tumor
Ovarian tumor (rare)
Drugs (steroids, ACTH)

[1] Indicates condition usually presenting as primary amenorrhea.

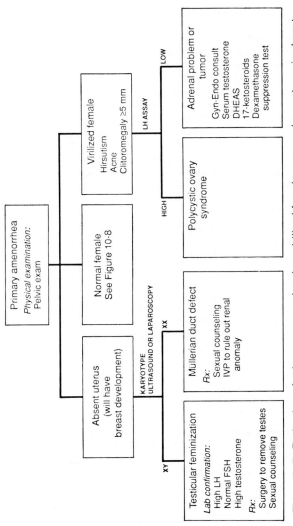

Figure 9–5. Evaluation of primary amenorrhea in a virilized female or one whose uterus is absent.

lar feminization from Müllerian duct defect, since the managements differ.

B. Evaluation and Management of Secondary Amenorrhea:
Secondary amenorrhea results when there is unopposed estrogen stimulation, maintaining the endometrium in the proliferative phase. The most common causes are pregnancy, stress, or Stein-Leventhal syndrome (polycystic ovaries) (Fig. 9–6 and Table 9–11). The history should focus on issues of stress, weight change, strenuous exercise, sexual activity, and contraceptive use. Review of systems should include questions about headaches, visual changes, and galactorrhea. Physical examination should be sure to include a careful funduscopic examination, visual fields, palpation of the thyroid, measurement of blood pressure and heart rate, compression of the areola to check for galactorrhea, and a search for signs of androgen excess such as hirsutism, clitoromegaly, severe acne, or ovarian enlargement.

The first laboratory study obtained is a pregnancy test, even if the patient denies sexual activity. If the test is negative, vaginal smear for estrogen or progesterone challenge should be done to determine whether the patient has an estrogen-primed uterus that will respond with withdrawal bleeding.

Dysmenorrhea

Dysmenorrhea is the most common gynecologic complaint of adolescent girls, with an incidence of about 60%. Dysmenorrhea can be divided into primary and secondary dysmenorrhea on the basis of whether there is any underlying pelvic pathology. **Primary spasmodic dysmenorrhea** accounts for 80% of adolescent dysmenorrhea and most often affects women under 25 years of age. **Secondary dysmenorrhea** is most often due to sexually transmitted infection, endometriosis, congenital anomalies, or a complication of pregnancy (Table 9–12).

Dysfunctional Uterine Bleeding

Dysfunctional uterine bleeding (DUB) may be referred to as hypermenorrhea or polymenorrhea. It results when an endometrium that has proliferated under unopposed estrogen stimulation finally begins to slough, but incompletely, causing irregular, painless bleeding. The unopposed estrogen stimulation occurs during anovulatory cycles, common in younger adolescents who have not been menstruating for long, but also seen in older adolescents during times of stress or illness.

Table 9-11. Management of secondary amenorrhea by cause.

	Cause	Lab	Management
A. Mild hypothalamic dysfunction	Recent pregnancy Physical illness Weight loss Obesity Emotional stress Environmental change Strenuous athletics Drugs (post birth control pills, phenothiazines)	CBC, urinalysis ESR T4, TSH, etc (as indicated)	Reassurance; assessment of birth control needs Repeat of progesterone test every 3 months (after ruling out pregnancy) LH, FSH, prolactin if no menses for 1 year
B. Androgen excess	Polycystic ovary syndrome (PCO) Cushing's syndrome Adrenal hyperplasia Adrenal tumor Ovarian tumor Drugs (steroids, ACTH)	LH, FSH (high LH suggests PCO); consultation with endocrinologists to help evaluate adrenals	If PCO, birth control pills (Demulen) to control hirsutism and menses Treatment of underlying problem
C. Asherman's syndrome	Uterine synechiae post TAb or D&C	No bleeding after 1 cycle of combination oral contraceptive (Ovulen)	Referral to gynecologist
D. Severe hypothalamic dysfunction	Anorexia nervosa Severe emotional stress Chronic systemic disease CNS tumor Pituitary infarction	Low estrogen Low LH Check T4, TSH, ESR, neurologic exam	Treatment of cause; slow hormone recovery expected
E. Ovarian failure	Variant of gonadal dysgenesis (mosaicism) XX/XO) Postirradiation Postchemotherapy Autoimmune oophoritis Resistant ovarian syndrome Premature menopause	Chromosomes Antiovarian antibodies Laparoscopy Ovarian biopsy	Referral to gynecologist; hormone replacement therapy

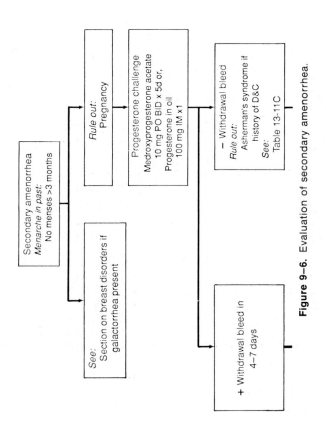

Figure 9-6. Evaluation of secondary amenorrhea.

274

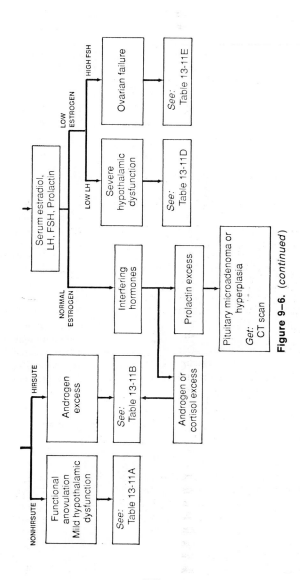

Figure 9-6. (continued)

Table 9-12. Dysmenorrhea in the adolescent.

Primary Dysmenorrhea—no pelvic pathology

	Etiology	Onset and Duration	Symptoms	Pelvic Exam	Treatment
Primary spasmodic	Excessive amount of prostaglandin F2α, which attaches to myometrium causing uterine contractions, hypoxia, and ischemia. Also, directly sensitizes pain receptors.	Begins with onset of flow or just prior and lasts 1–2 days. Does not start until 6–18 months after menarche, when cycles become ovulatory.	Lower abdominal cramps radiating to lower back and thighs. Associated nausea, vomiting, diarrhea, and urinary frequency also due to excess prostaglandins.	Normal. May wait to examine if never sexually active and history is consistent with primary spasmodic dysmenorrhea.	Mild—heating pad, warm baths, nonprescription analgesics. Moderate–severe: prostaglandin inhibitors at onset of flow or pain. Oral contraceptives for sexually active patients.
Psychogenic	May have history of sexual abuse or may have difficulty adjusting to womanhood. May have secondary gain from school or work avoidance.	Starts at menarche. Pain begins with anticipation of menses and lasts throughout flow.	Abdominal cramps.	Normal.	Educate regarding normal menstrual function. Reassure that pain does not indicate pathology. Relaxation techniques and biofeedback. Counseling to understand underlying issues.

Secondary Dysmenorrhea—underlying pathology present. (Always perform pelvic exam if secondary dysmenorrhea suspected or patient is sexually active. Gonorrhea culture, test for chlamydia, CBC, and ESR should be obtained.)

	Etiology	Onset and Duration	Symptoms	Pelvic Exam	Treatment
Infection	Most often due to a sexually transmitted disease such as chlamydia or gonorrhea.	Recent onset of pelvic cramps.	Pelvic cramps, excessive bleeding, intermenstrual spotting or vaginal discharge.	Mucopurulent or purulent discharge from cervical os, cervical friability, cervical motion tenderness, adnexal tenderness, positive culture for STD.	Appropriate antibiotics.

Endometriosis	Aberrant implants of endometrial tissue in pelvis or abdomen; may result from reflux.	Generally starts more than 2 years after menarche.	Pelvic pain, may occur intermenstrually.	Two thirds are tender on exam, expecially during late luteal phase.	Hormonal suppression by oral contraceptives or danazol. Surgery may be necessary for extensive disease.
Complication of pregnancy	Spontaneous abortion, ectopic pregnancy.	Acute onset.	Pelvic cramps associated with a delay in menses.	Positive hCG, enlarged uterus or adnexal mass.	Immediate gynecologic consult.
Congenital anomalies	Transverse vaginal septum, septate uterus, or cervical stenosis.	Onset at menarche.	Pelvic cramps.	Underlying congenital anomaly may be apparent. May require exam under anesthesia.	Gynecologic consult for ultrasound, hysteroscopy, or laparoscopy.
IUD	Increased uterine contractions, or increase risk for pelvic infection.	Onset after placement of IUD or acutely if due to infection.	Pelvic cramps, heavy menstrual bleeding, may have vaginal discharge.	Normal, or see infection above.	Prostaglandin inhibitors or mefenamic acid may be drug of choice because it also reduces flow. Appropriate antibiotics and consider removal of IUD if infection is present.
Pelvic adhesions	Previous abdominal surgery or pelvic inflammatory disease.	Delayed onset after surgery or PID.	Abdominal pain, may or may not be associated with menstrual cycles; possible alteration in bowel pattern.	Variable.	Surgery.

277

Table 9–13. Differential diagnosis of dysfunctional uterine bleeding in adolescents.

Pelvic inflammatory disease or cervicitis

Complication of pregnancy: ectopic pregnancy, threatened abortion, incomplete abortion, missed abortion

Breakthrough bleeding on oral contraceptives

Blood dyscrasias: iron deficiency, thrombocytopenia, coagulopathy, von Willebrand's disease, leukemia

Endocrine disorders: hypothyroidism, hyperthyroidism, diabetes mellitus, adrenal disease, hyperprolactinemia

Trauma

Foreign body

Uterine, vaginal, ovarian, abnormalities: carcinoma, fibroids, adenosis from DES, premature menopause

A. Findings: Typically, the adolescent will present with a history of several years of regular cycles; she then begins to have menses every 2 weeks, or complains of bleeding for 2–3 weeks after 2–3 months of amenorrhea. A past history of painless, irregular periods at intervals of less than 3 weeks may also be elicited. Bleeding for more than 10 days should be considered abnormal. Dysfunctional uterine bleeding must be considered a diagnosis of exclusion (Table 9–13).

B. Management: A pregnancy test and pelvic examination with appropriate cultures should be performed in sexually active patients. A CBC with platelets should also be obtained. Additional coagulation or hormonal studies can be based on the history and physical findings. Management depends on the severity of the problem (Table 9–14).

Severe dysfunctional bleeding requires hospitalization if the patient presents with a low hemoglobin and orthostatic symptoms in the face of heavy vaginal bleeding with disruption of menstrual cycles. Clotting studies should be obtained. Hemodynamic instability should be treated with fluids and blood transfusions as needed. Premarin, 25 mg intravenously, may be given for its hemostatic effect (Table 9–14). Gynecologic consult should be obtained.

Mittelschmerz

Mittelschmerz refers to the pain caused by spillage of fluid from the ruptured follicular cyst at the time of ovulation, irritating the peritoneum. The patient presents with a history of midcycle, unilateral dull or aching abdominal pain lasting a few min-

Table 9–14. Management of dysfunctional uterine bleeding (DUB).[1]

	Mild	Moderate	Severe
Characteristics	Hct >33% or Hgb >11 g/dL	Hct 27–33% or Hgb 9–11 g/dL	Hct <27% or Hgb <9 g/dL (or dropping)
Acute treatment	Menstrual calendar Iron supplementation Consider OCPs if patient is sexually active and desires contraception (standard once-daily dose)	*Begin:* OCPs (1/35) cycle 4 pills/day × 4 days 3 pills/day × 4 days 2 pills/day × 13–19 days withdrawal bleeding × 7 days	Blood transfusion, PRN *Consider:* Conjugated estrogens, 25 mg IV q 4–6 h × 24 h until bleeding stops; antiemetic *Begin:* OCPs (1/35) cycle 4 pills/day × 4 days 3 pills/day × 4 days 2 pills/day × 13–19 days withdrawal bleeding × 7 days
Long-term treatment	*Monitor:* Iron status (Hgb/Hct) *Follow-up* in 2 months	*Next:* OCPs(1/35)[2] cycle for 3 months. Begin OCPs the Sunday after withdrawal bleeding begins. Length of use dependent on resolution of anemia. Iron supplementation. *Monitor:* Iron status *Follow-up* within 2–3 weeks and every 3 months	*Next:* OCPs(1/50)[3] cycle for 3 months. Begin OCPs the Sunday after withdrawal bleeding begins. Length of use dependent on resolution of anemia. Iron supplementation. *Monitor:* Iron status *Follow-up* within 2–3 weeks and every 3 months

[1] DX = Prolonged painless menses (≥8 days); heavy flow (>6 tampons/pads per day); short cycles (≤21 days); no other etiology found.
[2] Triphasic OCP is acceptable.
[3] Use pill with 50 mcg of ethinyl estradiol for first 3 months, then 30–35 mcg monophasic or triphasic pill.

279

utes or as long as 8 hours. Rarely this pain mimics the acute abdominal findings of appendicitis, torsion or rupture of an ovarian cyst, or ectopic pregnancy, in which case a laparoscopy may be necessary. The patient should be reassured and treated symptomatically.

Ovarian Cysts

Functional cysts account for 20–50% of ovarian masses in adolescents and are a variation of the normal physiologic process. They may be asymptomatic, or may cause menstrual irregularity, constipation, or urinary frequency. Functional cysts, unless large, rarely cause abdominal pain. However, torsion or hemorrhage of an ovarian cyst may present as an acute or subacute abdomen. **Follicular cysts** account for the majority of ovarian cysts; they are usually less than or equal to 4 cm in diameter, and resolve spontaneously. **Lutein cysts** occur less commonly, and may be 5–10 cm in diameter. The patient should be referred to a gynecologist for laparoscopy if she is premenarchal, the cyst has a solid component or is larger than 5 cm by ultrasound, there are symptoms or signs suggestive of hemorrhage or torsion, or the cyst fails to regress after 2 to 3 menstrual cycles.

CONTRACEPTION

Sexually active adolescent females wait an average of 1 year before seeking contraception. However, one half of teen pregnancies in the United States occur in the first 6 months of initiating sexual intercourse. Sexuality, contraception, and pregnancy prevention are areas with which the pediatrician has become familiar out of necessity.

Counseling Teenagers About Contraception

Adolescents may have poorly formulated skills for making decisions of any kind, and often benefit from a decision-making framework that can be applied to a variety of situations, particularly those involving peer pressure. By talking with teenagers about their alternatives to sexual intercourse and the implications of coitus (unintended pregnancy; sexually transmitted diseases; possible emotional trauma; and effects on education, career, income, and responsibilities if a pregnancy occurs) the physician can help them to make better-informed decisions before they find themselves in a dilemma.

Abstinence is the most commonly used method of birth control. However, it is prudent to encourage the adolescent to use contraception at the time they do initiate sexual intercourse. Adolescents should understand the menstrual cycle and be taught either that there is no "safe" period or that ovulation occurs 2 weeks before the next menstrual period and may be difficult to predict. Since teenagers frequently have irregular cycles and sexual intercourse is often spontaneous and unplanned, the rhythm or calendar method is not effective for them. Adolescents also need to be educated that withdrawal is not a method of contraception (Table 9–15).

A. Beginning Birth Control Pills and Follow-up: Before beginning oral contraceptives, a careful menstrual history, medical history, and family medical history should be taken. In addition, baseline weight and blood pressure should be established, breast and pelvic examination should be performed, and specimens for urinalysis. Papanicolaou smear, gonorrhea culture, and chlamydia culture or antigen-detection test obtained.

If there are no contraindications (Table 9–16), the patient may begin her first pack of pills with her next menstrual period. A triphasic or a low-dose combined oral contraceptive is used for teenagers without contraindications to the use of estrogen. It is wise to always use 28-day packs with adolescents rather than 21-day packs to reduce the chance of missed pills. The patient should be instructed on the use of her type of pills, as well as possible risks and side effects and their warning signs. She should use a back-up method such as condoms and foam for the first 2 weeks to assure protection. A follow-up visit in 1 month and then every 2–3 months for the first year may improve compliance, as teenagers often discontinue birth control pills for nonmedical reasons or because of minor side effects.

B. Management of Side Effects: A different type of combined oral contraceptive should be tried if the patient has a persistent minor side effect for more than the first 2 or 3 months. Adjustments should be made on the basis of hormonal effects. Changes are most often made for persistent breakthrough bleeding not related to missed pills.

PREGNANCY

There are more than 1 million teen pregnancies in the US each year. Of these, about 40% result in abortion, 13% in miscar-

Table 9–15. Commonly used contraceptives in the United States.

Method	Action	Effectiveness (%)	Side Effects	Benefits	Comments
Condoms	Barrier, spermicidal action of nonoxynol-9 in some	88–98	None	Protect against STD	Require no medical visit or prescription
Spermicides	Spermicidal action	79–97	Local irritation	Non-oxynol 9 is bactericidal and viricidal	
Sponges	Barriers, spermicidal	72–95	Possible risk of toxic shock syndrome		Higher failure rates in parous than nulliparous women
Combined oral contraceptives	1) Suppress ovulation 2) Thicken cervical mucus and make sperm penetration difficult 3) Atrophy of endometrium diminishes chance of implantation	96–99	Risk of thromboembolism, MI, stroke, hypertension, hepatoma, death exist but rare in teenagers	Improve dysmenorrhea and acne Protect against PID, ovarian and endometrial cancer, benign breast masses. Decrease menstrual blood loss.	May be method of choice for adolescents who have unplanned intercourse. Serious risks increase after age 30, especially in smokers. See Table 13–14 for contraindications.
Mini pill	1) Thicken cervical mucus 2) Atrophy of endometrium 3) Ovulation suppressed in only 15–40% of cycles	97–98	Less predictable menstrual patterns		May be used in patients who should avoid exogenous estrogens

282

Method	Mechanism	%	Side effects/risks	Relationship to sexual activity	Comments
IUD	Prevent implantation through local inflammatory response and local production of prostaglandins	95–98	STDs, PID and its sequelae, heavy menstrual flow, dysmenorrhea	No temporal relationship to sexual activity	Not the most ideal method for teens who have multiple partners and their childbearing years ahead of them, given STD risk
Diaphragm	Barrier Spermicidal action of contraceptive gel used in conjunction	82–97	None		Must be comfortable inserting and checking fit
Subdermal progestin implant (Norplant)	1) Thicken cervical mucus 2) Atrophy of endometrium 3) Suppression of LH surge	>99	Irregular bleeding, mood changes, hair loss, pigmentation change at insertion site	No temporal relationship to sexual activity	Emphasize need for annual check-ups despite 5 year method. Contraindicated in those with active liver disease, acute thromboembolic disorder, undiagnosed genital bleeding, pregnancy

Table 9–16. Contraindications to combined birth control pills.[1]

Absolute contraindications

History of thrombophlebitis, thromboembolic disorder, cerebrovascular disorder, ischemic heart disease

Known or suspected cardinoma of the breast or estrogen-dependent neoplasia

Known or suspected pregnancy

History of benign or malignant liver tumor

Undiagnosed abnormal vaginal bleeding

Strong relative contraindications

Severe vascular or migraine headaches

Hypertension

Diabetes

Active gallbladder disease

Mononucleosis, acute phase

Sickle cell disease or sickle C disease

Upcoming major surgery

Long leg cast or major injury to lower leg

Known impaired liver function at present time

Completion of term pregnancy within past 10–14 days

[1] Modifiied and reproduced, with permission, from *Contraceptive Technology 1988–1989*, 14th revised ed. Breedlove B. Judy B, Martin N (eds). Irvington Publishers, Inc., 1988.

riage, and 47% in live births. About 45% of 15–19-year-old females are sexually active and more than one third of these become pregnant within 2 years of the onset of sexual intercourse. More than 80% of these pregnancies are unintended, and about 60% of pregnancies in women less than 20 years old occur out of wedlock.

Young maternal age and associated maternal risk factors have been linked to adverse neonatal outcome, including higher rates of low-birth-weight babies (<2500 g) and neonatal mortality. The psychosocial consequences for the teen mother and her infant are extensive.

Presentation

An adolescent may present with delayed or missed menses, or may even request a pregnancy test, but often they present with an unrelated concern (hidden agenda) or a vague somatic complaint. Clinicians need to have a low threshold for suspecting pregnancy. If there is *any* suspicion, a urine pregnancy test should be obtained.

Diagnosis

History, as above, and physical examination may assist in making the diagnosis of pregnancy. Bluish coloring and softening of the cervix may be noted on speculum examination. The uterine fundus may be palpable on abdominal examination if sufficient time has lapsed. If uterine size on bimanual examination does not correspond to dates, one must consider ectopic pregnancy, incomplete or missed abortion, twin gestation, or inaccurate dates. Laboratory tests for human chorionic gonadotropin (hCG) are simple to perform and usually make the diagnosis.

Special Issues in Management

When an adolescent presents for pregnancy testing, it is wise to find out before performing the test what she hopes the results will be and what she thinks she will do. If she wants to be pregnant and the test is negative, further counseling into the implications of teen pregnancy should be undertaken. For those who do not wish to be pregnant, this is a good time to begin contraception.

If the adolescent is pregnant, discuss her support systems and her options with her. Many teenagers need help in involving their parents. Since teenagers are often ambivalent about their plans and may have a high level of denial, it is prudent to follow-up with her in a week to be certain that a decision has been made and to assist her into prenatal care if she has chosen to maintain the pregnancy.

It has been shown that maternal age in and of itself is not responsible for low birth weight and poor fetal outcome, but that low maternal prepregnancy weight, poor weight gain, delay in prenatal care, low socioeconomic status, and black race are contributing factors. The poor nutritional status of some teenagers and their erratic diets, habits of smoking, drinking, or substance abuse, and high prevalence of sexually transmitted diseases also play a role. Teenagers are also at greater risk of toxemia of pregnancy, iron deficiency anemia, cephalopelvic disproportion, prolonged labor, premature labor, and maternal death. Early prenatal care and good nutrition can make a difference with a number of these potential complications.

Because of the high risk of a second unintended pregnancy within the next 2 years, postpartum contraceptive counseling and follow-up is imperative.

VULVOVAGINITIS

Vaginitis has two main causes: pathogens or indigenous flora after a change in milieu of the vagina. Monilia vulvovaginitis and bacterial vaginosis (formerly referred to as gardnerella, hemophilus, or nonspecific vaginitis) may be found in non-sexually active patients and are examples of indigenous flora that may cause infection. Bacterial vaginosis is more prevalent in those who are sexually active. In sexually active patients, trichomonas or cervicitis from sexually transmitted pathogens must be considered. (See section on STDs.) For this reason, sexually active patients or those suspected to be victims of sexual abuse should have appropriate specimens taken for STDs even if yeast or bacterial vaginosis is identified (Table 9–17).

SEXUALLY TRANSMITTED DISEASES AND PELVIC INFLAMMATORY DISEASE

The 15–25-year-old age group has the highest incidence of sexually transmitted diseases (STDs) because of multiple sexual partners, lack of use of barrier methods of contraception, and delay in seeking treatment.

Chlamydia trachomatis, an obligate intracellular body half the size of the gonococcus, is the most common cause of STD, with 2–3 million new cases per year in the US; peak incidence is in 15–20 year olds. One quarter to one half of those infected are asymptomatic, and one quarter to one half are coinfected with gonorrhea. Chlamydia accounts for 20–30% of the 170,000 cases of pelvic inflammatory disease (PID) per year and is responsible for more than 60% of PID cases in women under 20 years old (Table 13–16).

Neisseria gonorrhoea is the second most common cause of STD, with peak incidence in the 15–25-year-old age group. Five to 25% of cases are associated with another STD, and more than 50% of those infected are asymptomatic (Table 9–18).

In view of the prevalence of STD in the adolescent population and the reluctance of teenagers to talk about them, the clinician needs to routinely ask adolescents about sexual activity, number of partners, and symptoms of STD when they present for routine physical examinations or sexually related symptoms

Table 9–17. Vulvovaginitis.

	Cases	Description	Tests	Treatment
Physiologic leukorrhea	Physiologic	Clear, white, nonodorous discharge beginning around menarche	Wet prep may show few squamous epithelial cells and <5 PMN/hpf	Reassure patient that this is normal
Monilia vulvovaginitis	Candida (yeast)	Thick, white, adherent, cheesy discharge; erythematous mucosa; associated pruritus	Leukocytes on wet prep. Budding yeast or mycelia on KOH prep. Slides may be negative.	Treat on basis of exam if slides negative. Nystatin, clotrimazole, or terconazole vaginal creams or suppositories for 3–7 nightly doses.
Bacterial vaginosis	Indigenous vaginal floragardnerella, bacteroides, peptococcus, lactobacilli	Thin, homogenous, gray-white discharge adherent to vaginal wall; diffuse vaginal erythema; malodorous.	Whiff test (KOH drop added to smear of discharge) results in fishy odor. Abundance of clue cells (stippled vaginal epithelial cells) on wet prep.	Metronidazole 500 mg orally twice a day for 7 days. Ampicillin 500 mg orally four times daily for 7 days is alternative during pregnancy.
Sexually transmitted diseases (see next section)	See next section	Cervix may appear inflamed, friable, ulcerated, or normal.	Wet prep, gonorrhea culture, chlamydia culture or antigen detection should be performed.	See next section
Foreign body vaginitis	Retained tampons most common	Extremely malodorous purulent discharge.	Speculum exam to visualize.	Remove foreign body. Antibiotics are generally not necessary.
Allergic or contact vaginitis	Bubble baths, feminine hygiene sprays, vaginal contraceptives	Erythematous vaginal mucosa	Rule out sexually transmitted diseases	Discontinue use of offending agent

Table 9–18. Urethritis, cervicitis, and pelvic inflammatory disease.

	Agents	Symptoms	Physical Findings	Laboratory Findings	Complications
Urethritis	Chlamydia Gonorrhea *Ureaplasma* *Mycoplasma* Trichomonas	Dysuria Urethral discharge May be asymptomatic	Exam may be normal. Clear, white, or purulent penile discharge. (May occur in females, often in association with cervicitis.)	U/A: Moderate WBCs without bacteriuria Gramstain: PMNs, may show gram-negative intracellular diplococci if due to gonorrhea. Gonorrhea culture: may be positive. Chlamydia culture or antigen detection test: may be positive.	Nontender penile edema Prostatitis Epididymitis Orchitis
Cervicitis	Chlamydia Gonorrhea Herpes Trichomonas	Asymptomatic Possible vaginal discharge or dysuria	Cervix may appear normal, or may have erythema, petechiae, irregular raised surface, friability, or ulcerations. Mucopurulent or purulent cervical discharge.	Wet prep: >10 WBCs/hpf if due to gonorrhea or chlamydia. Gonorrhea culture: may be positive. Chlamydia culture or antigen detection test: may be positive	Pelvic inflammatory disease Infection of Bartholin glands
PID	Chlamydia Gonorrhea Normal vaginal aerobic and anaerobic flora may be secondary invaders	Abdominal pain may be minimal Vaginal discharge in 75% Excessive menstrual bleeding or intermenstrual spotting in 40% Fever in 40% Dysuria in 15%	Lower abdominal tenderness. Uterine, adnexal, or cervical motion tenderness. Abnormal cervical discharge in half.	May have elevated WBC, ESR, but may be normal. Cervical culture for gonorrhea or chlamydia may be positive.	Tuboovarian abscess Fitz-Hugh-Curtis syndrome Tubal occlusion Infertility Ectopic pregnancy Chronic abdominal pain

(dysuria, penile or vaginal discharge, genital lesion, or abdominal pain). As females are frequently asymptomatic, obtaining wet prep, gonorrhea culture, and test for chlamydia at the time of the annual Pap smear in sexually active females is advised. Although males are usually symptomatic, a significant number of those with chlamydia are asymptomatic, or symptoms of gonorrhea may resolve, and the adolescent fails to seek treatment.

When an STD is diagnosed, the adolescent and his or her partner(s) should be treated simultaneously with the appropriate antibiotic regimen (Tables 9–19, 9–20, 9–21, and 9–22). They should be followed closely because poor compliance with treatment is common in this age group. A test-of-cure culture for gonorrhea should be obtained no sooner than 4–5 days after completion of treatment to allow clearing of antibiotic from the blood. Serology will need to be followed in the case of syphilis. It is essential to emphasize abstinence until both partners complete treatment to avoid reinfection and/or spread, and to advise use of barrier methods of contraception to prevent future infections. Possible complications and the implications of recurrent infections with regard to fertility and ectopic pregnancy should also be discussed. Adolescents should also be made aware of the possibility of transmission of an STD to the fetus.

Table 9–19. Treatment of urethritis or cervicitis in adolescents[1]

	Drug of Choice	**Alternatives**
Gonorrhea	Ceftriaxone 125–250 mg IM once, followed by treatment for *Chlamydia*, below	Cefixime 400 mg orally once or ciprofloxacin[2] 500 mg orally once or ofloxacin[2] 400 mg orally once or spectinomycin 2 g IM once plus treatment for *Chlamydia*
Chlamydia trachomatis	Doxycycline[3] 100 mg orally bid for 7 days or tetracycline[3] 500 mg orally 4 times daily for 7 days	Erythromycin 500 mg orally 4 times daily for 7 days

[1] Modified and reproduced, with permission, from Treatment of sexually transmitted diseases. *Med Lett Drugs Ther* 1991;33:119.
[2] Quinolones, such as ciprofloxacin, are contraindicated during pregnancy and in children 16 years of age or younger.
[3] Contraindicated during pregnancy.

Table 9–20. Treatment of pelvic inflammatory disease.[1]

	Drug of Choice	Dosage	Alternatives
Hospitalized patients	Cefoxitin or	2 g IV every 6 hours	Clindamycin 900 mg IV every 8 hours plus gentamicin 2 mg/kg IV once followed by gentamicin 1.5 mg/kg IV every 8 hours until improved followed by doxycycline[2] 100 mg orally twice daily to complete 14 days
	cefotetan	2 g IV every 12 hours	
	either one plus doxycycline followed by	100 mg IV every 12 hours until improved	
	doxycycline[2]	100 mg orally twice daily to complete 10–14 days	
Outpatients	Cefoxitin plus probenecid or ceftriaxone either one followed by doxycycline[2]	2 g IM once 1 g orally once 250 mg IM once	
		100 mg orally twice daily for 14 days	

[1] Modified and reproduced, with permission, from Treatment of sexually transmitted diseases. *Med Lett Drugs Ther* 1991;33:119.
[2] Contraindicated during pregnancy.

PELVIC INFLAMMATORY DISEASE

Acute PID, or salpingitis, is the most common serious infection occurring in young women (Table 9–18). The adolescent age group has the highest rate of PID, with an annual rate of 1.5% of females 15–19 years old. Risk factors for PID include sexual activity, multiple partners (5 times greater risk than for one partner), age less than 25, presence of an IUD (2–4 times greater risk than for nonusers), nulliparous, prior history of PID (2 times greater risk), prior history of uncomplicated STD, and prior induced abortion.

The diagnosis of PID is not straightforward, hence, the following guidelines have been suggested. The 3 major criteria of

Table 9–21. Diagnosis and treatment of genital lesions.

Lesion	Agent	Clinical Findings	Treatment
Condyloma acuminata (genital warts)	Human papilloma virus	Verrucous skin lesion most often occurring on the glans penis or corona in males and posterior introitus in females.	Apply 20–25% Podophyllin in tincture of benzoin to wart after applying petroleum jelly to normal skin. Wash off in 4 hours. Do not use on vaginal or anal mucosa, nor during pregnancy. Refer for colposcopy if HPV effects are noted on Pap smear. (Additional treatments: liquid nitrogen, laser, 5-FU, surgical excision, trichloroacetic acid, interferon.)
Herpes	Herpes simplex virus (HSV-2 in 80–95% and HSV-1 in remainder)	Cluster of painful papules which progress to vesicles, pustules, ulcers, and crusts. Systemic symptoms with primary episode. Prodromal tingling with recurrences.	Acyclovir 400 mg orally 3 times a day for 7–10 days (primary) or 5 days (recurrence). May shorten duration of eruptions. Institute with prodromal symptoms.
Syphilis Primary	Treponema pallidum	Painless, clean ulcer with an erythematous, indurated border (chancre) which is positive on darkfield exam.	Penicillin G benzathine 2.4 million units IM once OR doxycycline 100 mg orally twice daily for 14 days OR ceftriaxone 250 mg IM once daily for 10 days OR Erythromycin 500 mg orally 4 times a day for 15 days.
Secondary		Broad-based, flat, mucoid lesions (condyloma lata) on the genitals.	

Table 9–22. Diagnosis and treatment of sexually transmitted parasites.

	Symptoms	Clinical Findings	Treatment
Trichomoniasis	Asymptomatic or pruritic vaginal discharge in females or clear penile discharge in males.	Copious frothy vaginal discharge. Motile flagellated trichomonad seen on wet prep of vaginal discharge or spun urinalysis	Metronidazole 2 g orally once or 500 mg orally 2 times a day for 7 days. During pregnancy, use clotrimazole 100 mg intravaginally at bedtime for 7 days instead.
Pediculosis pubis (crab lice)	Pruritic rash.	Lice and opalescent nits found anchored to pubic hairs.	Lindane or pyrethrins is applied to pubic hair and surrounding skin, lathering for 4–10 minutes, and rinsed off. Nits are combed. Fomites and linens need to be washed in hot water. Treat close contacts.
Scabies	Pruritic rash of groin, thighs, or abdomen.	Scabetic burrows and erythematous, maculopapular scaliness and tendency to impetignize.	Permethrin 5% (Elimite cream) is applied from head to soles, left on for 8–14 hours, then showered off. Fomites & close contacts must be treated.

lower abdominal pain and tenderness, cervical motion tenderness, and adnexal tenderness must be present. In addition one of the following minor criteria must be present: temperature greater than 38°C, leukocytosis above 10,500 WBC/mm^3, culdocentesis yielding peritoneal fluid containing WBCs and bacteria, inflammatory mass noted on pelvic examination or ultrasound, elevated ESR, cervical Gram stain suggestive of gonorrhea or positive chlamydia antigen detection test, or more than 5 WBCs per oil-immersion field on Gram stain of endocervical discharge.

The differential diagnosis of PID includes acute appendicitis, mesenteric lymphadenitis, cholecystitis, ectopic pregnancy, intrauterine pregnancy, ovarian cyst or tumor, endometriosis, urinary tract infection, and renal calculus.

If there is the slightest suspicion of PID the patient should be treated with appropriate antibiotics while cultures are pending (Table 9–20). The patient should be hospitalized if she exhibits significant fever or toxicity, is unable to tolerate oral medication and fluids, has not responded to outpatient therapy or is unlikely to comply with it, is a younger adolescent, or is seriously ill with an unclear diagnosis.

GENITAL LESIONS

Condyloma acuminata, or genital warts, are caused by human papilloma virus (HPV). Warts typically occur at the site of minute skin trauma on the external genitalia, but may be present on the cervix and indiscernible to the unaided eye. It is now accepted that HPV is the most important etiologic agent in the development of cervical intraepithelial neoplasia and invasive cervical cancers, and appears to be associated with penile cancer (Table 9–21).

Herpes Simplex Virus

The primary episode of genital herpes is generally more symptomatic and prolonged than recurrences, and is characterized by systemic symptoms such as fever, headache, malaise, myalgias, and a cluster of painful papules that progress to vesicles, pustules, ulcers, and finally crusts (Table 9–21). Fifty percent of new cases may be asymptomatic.

Syphilis

The primary stage of syphilis typically presents with a painless chancre. Diagnosis is by immediate darkfield examination of a microscope slide that has been pressed to the base of the lesion with a drop of saline added. VDRL can be done for further investigation, but may be negative early in the course of the disease. The chancre may be self-limited, and after a latency period of 4–6 weeks the disease may resurface in the secondary stage, characterized by a diffuse, nonpruritic, maculopapular rash that includes the palms and soles, mucous patches on the mucosal surfaces, generalized lymphadenopathy, constitutional symptoms, and the presence of condylomalata on the genitals. At this stage, diagnosis is by VDRL. The tertiary stage is divided into early latent and late benign, and may include the cardiovascular and central nervous system complications of dissection of the ascending aorta, seizures, stroke, optic atrophy and tabes dorsalis. All stages may be treated with penicillin. The VDRL should be repeated 3, 6, and 12 months after treatment.

PARASITES

See Table 9–22.

HUMAN IMMUNODEFICIENCY VIRUS (HIV)

AIDS results from infection with the human immunodeficiency virus (HIV), which is transmitted in blood and semen, and potentially other bodily fluids, through sexual and needle contact.

As of 1992 only 0.39% of AIDS cases in the U.S. occurred in 13–19 year olds. It is unknown what percentage of those who are HIV seropositive are teenagers. While 87% of AIDS cases are attributed to men having sex with men, injectable drug use, or both, in the 13–19 year old group only 41% are attributed to these causes. Fourteen percent of adolescent AIDS is due to heterosexual transmission compared to 6% of all cases. Adolescents are at significant potential risk due to their propensity for multiple sexual partners and their limited use of barrier contraceptives, as well as the use of drugs by some. A large number of infected young adults 20–29 years old acquired the infection as adolescents.

Preventive measures need to be taken to ensure that adolescents have the necessary knowledge to protect themselves from HIV in current and future relationships, and to eliminate AIDS hysteria. They need to be instructed in risk factors for HIV, modes of transmission, means of protection, and availability of confidential testing. The safer sex practices promoted as a result of AIDS can reduce the rate of all kinds of STD if heeded. Adolescence is an ideal time to promote these practices, as it is a time when intimate relationships are beginning and sexual decisions become important.

10 | Infectious Diseases: Viral & Rickettsial

Mark J. Abzug, MD

VIRAL DISEASES

ROSEOLA INFANTUM
(Exanthema Subitum)

Roseola infantum is an acute febrile disease of infants and young children characterized by fever followed by a faint rash. The incubation period is estimated to be 5–15 days. Human herpesvirus-6 has been implicated as the causative agent.

Clinical Findings (Table 10–1)

A. Symptoms and Signs: The onset is sudden, with sustained or spiking fever as high as 41.1°C (106°F). Fever persists for 1–5 days (average, 3 days), falls by crisis, and then may be subnormal for a few hours just before the rash appears. Rash appears when the temperature returns to normal. It is faintly erythematous, maculopapular, and principally confined to the trunk. Other physical findings may include mild pharyngitis, enlargement of the postoccipital nodes, and irritability.

B. Laboratory Findings: Findings include progressive leukopenia to 3000–5000 white cells, with a relative lymphocytosis as high as 90%.

Complications

Seizures are the principal complication (they may be the first sign of illness) and are related to the rapidly rising temperature. A parainfectious type of encephalitis has been reported (see Chapter 20).

Treatment

A. Specific Measures: None available.

B. General Measures: Antipyretics and tepid water sponge baths may be used to minimize discomfort and the risk of febrile seizures.

C. Treatment of Complications: Barbiturate anticonvulsants may prevent febrile seizures in children with convulsive tendencies.

Prognosis

The prognosis is excellent.

MEASLES
(Rubeola)

Measles is a highly communicable disease; the highest incidence is between the ages of 2 and 14 years. The incubation period is 8–14 days, with a majority of cases occurring 10 days after exposure.

Clinical Findings (Table 10–1)
  A. Symptoms and Signs:
  1. Prodrome–Fever is usually the first sign and persists throughout the prodrome. It ranges from 38.3 to 40°C (101 to 104°F), tends to be higher just before the appearance of the skin rash, and may be lower after eruption of the rash. Sore throat, nasal discharge, and dry, "barking" cough are common during the prodrome. Nonpurulent conjunctivitis appears toward the end of the prodrome and is accompanied by photophobia. Lymphadenopathy of the posterior cervical lymph nodes may occur. The causative virus is easily transmitted via nose and throat secretions during the prodromal period, which lasts 3–5 days.

Koplik's spots are fine white spots on a faint erythematous base that appear first on the buccal mucosa opposite the molar teeth and by about the third or fourth day of the prodrome may spread over the entire inside of the mouth. They usually disappear as the exanthem becomes well established.

  2. Rash–Rash appears on about the fifth day of disease. The pink, blotchy, irregular, macular erythema rapidly darkens and characteristically coalesces into larger red patches of varying size and shape. The rash first appears on the face and behind the ears; it then spreads to the chest and abdomen and, finally, to the extremities. It lasts 4–7 days and may be accompanied by mild itching. A fine brawny desquamation, especially of the face and trunk, may follow, lasting 2 or 3 days; light brown pigmentation may then appear.

  B. Laboratory Findings: Leukopenia is present during the prodrome and early stages of the rash. There is usually a sharp

Table 10–1. Diagnostic features of some acute exanthems.

Disease	Prodromal Signs and Symptoms	Nature of Eruption	Other Diagnostic Features	Laboratory Findings
Chickenpox (varicella)	0–1 d of fever, anorexia, headache.	Rapid evolution of macules to papules, vesicles, crusts; vesicles extremely fragile; all stages simultaneously present in successive outcroppings; lesions superficial; distribution centripetal.	Lesions on scalp and mucous membranes.	Specialized complement fixation and virus neutralization in tissue culture. Fluorescent antibody test of smear of lesions.
Drug eruption	Occasionally fever.	Maculopapular rash resembling rubella, rarely papulovesicular.		Eosinophilia.
Enterovirus infection	1–2 d of fever, malaise.	Maculopapular rash resembling rubella, rarely papulovesicular or petechial.	Aseptic meningitis.	Virus isolation from stool or cerebrospinal fluid; complement fixation titer rise.
Erythema infectiosum	No prodrome. Usually in epidemics.	Red, flushed checks; circumoral pallor, maculopapules on extremities.	"Slapped face" appearance.	White blood count normal.
Exanthema subitum	3–4 d of high fever.	As fever falls by crisis, pink maculopapules appear on chest and trunk; fade in 1–3 d.		White blood count low.
Infectious mononucleosis	Fever, adenopathy, sore throat.	Maculopapular rash resembling rubella, rarely papulovesicular; distribution scattered, asymmetrical.	Splenomegaly, tonsillar exudate.	Atypical lymphs in blood smears; heterophil agglutination. Slide agglutination test.

Meningococcemia	Hours of fever, vomiting.	Maculopapules, petechiae, purpura.	Meningeal signs, toxicity, shock.	White blood count high. Cultures of blood and cerebrospinal fluid.
Rocky Mountain spotted fever	3–4 d of fever, chills, severe headache.	Maculopapules, petechiae; distribution centrifugal.	History of tick bite.	Agglutination (O × 19, O × 2), complement fixation.
Rubella (German measles)	Little or no prodrome.	Maculopapular, pink; begins on head and neck, spreads downward, fades in 3 d. No desquamation.	Lymphadenopathy, postauricular or occipital.	White blood count normal or low. Serologic tests for immunity and definitive diagnosis (hemagglutination inhibition, complement fixation).
Rubeola (measles)	3–4 d of fever, coryza, conjunctivitis, cough.	Maculopapular, brick-red; begins on head and neck; spreads downward. In 5–6 d, rash is brownish, desquamating.	Koplik's spots on buccal mucosa.	White blood count low. Virus isolation in cell culture. Antibody tests by hemagglutination inhibition and complement fixation or neutralization.
Scarlet fever	½–2 d of malaise, sore throat, fever, vomiting.	Generalized, punctate, red; prominent on neck, in axilla, groin, skin folds; circumoral pallor; fine desquamation involves hands and feet.	Strawberry tongue, exudative tonsilitis.	Group A hemolytic streptococci cultures from throat; antistreptolysin O titer rise.

rise in the white cell count with the onset of any bacterial complication. In the absence of complications, the white cell count slowly rises to normal as the rash fades.

Complications

   A. Bacterial Infection:

   1. Otitis Media–This may appear toward the end of the prodrome or during the course of the rash (see Chapter 13).

   2. Tracheobronchitis–Besides the specific inflammation due to rubeola, there may be secondary bacterial involvement. This is usually accompanied by a more productive cough.

   3. Bronchopneumonia–While rubeola virus itself often causes a specific pneumonitis, secondary bacterial invasion is a relatively common complication.

   B. Encephalitis: Encephalitis (see Chapter 20) occurs in about 1 of 2000 cases (no relation to severity of measles). The first sign may be increasing lethargy or seizures. Lumbar puncture shows 0–200 cells, mostly lymphocytes. Subacute sclerosing panencephalitis (SSPE) is a late degenerative central nervous system complication that results from persistent infection.

   C. Hemorrhagic Measles: This rare form of the disease has a high mortality rate and is characterized by generalized bleeding and purpura.

   D. Tuberculosis: Active pulmonary tuberculosis may be aggravated by measles.

Treatment

   A. Specific Measures: None available.

   B. General Measures: Measures include isolation for 4 days from onset of rash, and supportive therapies: rest, antipyretics, mist, and antitussives.

   C. Treatment of Complications: Bacterial complications should be treated with appropriate antibacterials. For treatment of patients with encephalitis, see Chapter 20.

Prophylaxis

   Live measles virus vaccine should be given at 15 months of age—or at any age thereafter in susceptible persons (see Chapter 6). Recommendations call for a second vaccination, either at the time of school entry (ie, at approximately 5 years) or at the time of middle/junior high school entry (ie, at approximately seventh grade). Measles vaccine may be given between 6 and 12 months of age in high-risk areas. Measles vaccine is contraindicated in immunocompromised children, except for HIV-infected patients. Measles vaccine given within 72 hours of measles exposure may be effective as postexposure prophylaxis. Standard immune globulin can prevent the disease in exposed susceptible persons if it is administered within 6 days of exposure and at a dose of 0.25 mL/kg (0.5 mL/kg in immunocompromised children). One of these methods of postexposure prophylaxis is recommended for exposed infants < 12 months old.

Prognosis

In uncomplicated cases or those with bacterial complications, the prognosis is excellent. In patients with encephalitis, the prognosis is guarded; the incidence of permanent sequelae is high.

RUBELLA
(German Measles)

Rubella is a mild febrile virus infection that frequently occurs in epidemics. Transmission is probably by the droplet route. The incubation period is 12–21 days (average, 16 days).

Clinical Findings (Table 10–1)

 A. Symptoms and Signs:

 1. Typical Rubella–The prodrome, if present, lasts only a few days and is characterized by slight malaise, occasional tender postauricular and occipital lymph nodes, and no catarrhal symptoms. Rash may be the first sign of disease and consists of faint, fine, discrete, erythematous maculopapules, which may coalesce, appearing first on the face and spreading rapidly over the trunk and extremities. The rash generally disappears by the third day. The temperature rarely exceeds 38.3°C (101°F) and usually lasts less than 2 days.

 2. Rubella Without Rash–Rubella sine eruptions occurs as a febrile lymphadenopathy that may persist for a week or more. During epidemics, this syndrome may represent over 40% of cases with infection.

 3. Congenital Rubella–This is a syndrome generally involving infants born to mothers affected with rubella in the first trimester of pregnancy. The majority of infants show growth retardation and microcephaly, hepatosplenomegaly, and purpura, in addition to mental deficiency and congenital defects of the heart, eye, and ear. Marked thrombocytopenia and radiographic metaphysitis are common findings. Rubella virus is easily isolated from such patients, and they must be considered to be highly contagious. A late-onset congenital rubella syndrome, with minimal signs at birth and an acute onset of severe clinical disease after 3–6 months, has been reported.

B. Laboratory Findings: Transient leukopenia is generally noted.

Complications

If rubella occurs during the first month of pregnancy, there is a 50% change of fetal abnormality. By the third month of pregnancy, the risk of abnormalities decreases to less than 10%.

Encephalitis and thrombocytopenic purpura are rare. Polyarthritis occurs in 25% of cases in persons over 16 years of age.

Treatment

A. Specific Measures: None available.

B. General Measures: Isolation is required for 7 days after the onset of rash. Infants with congenital rubella may be contagious for more than 1 year. Symptomatic measures are rarely necessary.

C. Treatment of Complications: For treatment of encephalitis and purpura, see Chapters 19 and 20, respectively.

Prophylaxis

Live rubella vaccine is normally administered in combination with measles and mumps vaccine at 15 months of age and is advised to be given along with the second recommended dose of measle vaccine (see Chapter 6). Live rubella vaccine can be administered at any age after 12 months in susceptible persons; adolescents and young adults with no history of vaccine should be identified and vaccinated. A history of disease is unreliable and should not be used to determine the need for vaccine. Females of childbearing age should avoid pregnancy for 3 months after vaccination, although surveillance data suggest that no cases of congenital rubella syndrome have occurred in the offspring of women inadvertently given live rubella vaccine shortly before or within 3 months of conception. Rubella vaccine is contraindicated in immunocompromised patients, except those with HIV infection.

Standard immune globulin is not reliable in preventing infection in pregnant women exposed to rubella virus infection and is therefore not routinely recommended. Rubella serology should be measured immediately after exposure and then, if negative (susceptible), again at 3 and 6 weeks, to document whether maternal infection has occurred. All pregnant women—regardless of their immune status—should be cautioned against exposure to any person with an illness suggestive of rubella.

Prognosis

The prognosis in patients with acquired infection is excellent. In patient with congenital disease, the prognosis is universally poor. A progressive, degenerative panencephalitis has been reported. Late manifestations of brain damage such as behavior problems, increasing mental retardation, and minimal brain dysfunction (see Chapter 8) may occur.

ERYTHEMA INFECTIOSUM
(Fifth Disease & Parvoviruses)

Erythema infectiosum is a mild, minimally febrile contagious disease usually occurring in family or institutional epidemics. The incubation period is estimated to be 4–14 days. Human parvovirus B19 has been demonstrated to be the causative agent.

Clinical Findings (Table 10–1)

A. Symptoms and Signs: There is usually no prodrome. The first symptom is rash, which appears first on the cheeks and ears as red coalescent macules that are warm and slightly raised. Circumoral pallor is marked, leading to a "slapped cheek" appearance. This eruption fades within 4 days, followed 1 day later by a lacy, reticulated maculopapular erythematous rash that appears on the extensor surfaces of the extremities and spreads, over 2–3 days, to the flexor surfaces and trunk. The rash lasts 3–7 days but may recur over 1–3 weeks in response to environmental changes. Pruritus, headache, and arthralgia are occasional additional symptoms.

B. Laboratory Findings: The white blood cell count is normal.

Complications

Human parvovirus has been implicated in arthritis syndromes, particularly in adults, and is the cause of aplastic crises in patients with chronic hemolytic disorders. Intrauterine parvovirus infection may produce fetal hydrops and fetal death. Infection in immunocompromised patients may lead to chronic infection and chronic anemia.

Treatment

Treatment in uncomplicated cases is not indicated. Patients with hemolytic conditions may require transfusions. Intrauterine transfusion has been suggested for fetal infections. Intravenous immune globulin may be effective in immune deficient patients with chronic infection.

Prophylaxis

Pregnant women can be advised to avoid exposure to a known outbreak of erythema infectiosum. Should exposure occur, acute serology (IgG and IgM) can be measured; if negative (susceptible), repeat IgG and IgM titers can then be checked in 3 or more weeks to document whether maternal infection has occurred. Pregnant women with known infection may be followed with serum alpha-fetoprotein levels and frequent ultrasound examinations for the earliest detection of fetal hydrops.

Prognosis

Prognosis of uncomplicated erythema infectiosum and aplastic crises, if adequately supported by transfusion therapy, is excellent. It appears that most intrauterine infections that produce hydrops will result in fetal loss unless transfusion therapy can be implemented.

VARICELLA
(Chickenpox)
& HERPES ZOSTER
(Shingles)

Varicella is an acute, extremely communicable disease caused by the varicella zoster virus. It is spread from person to person by droplets from a respiratory source or by direct contact with freshly infected vesicles. Varicella is communicable from 1 to 2 days before until 6 days after appearance of the rash. The incubation period is 10–21 days (average, 15 days).

With rare exceptions, immunity to varicella after attack is probably lifelong, although the individual with a history of varicella may later develop herpes zoster.

Clinical Findings (Table 10–1)

A. Symptoms and Signs:

1. Prodrome–The prodrome is usually not apparent; there may be slight malaise and fever for 24 hours.

2. Rash–Usually, the first sign is rash. Lesions tend to appear in crops (2–4 crops in 2–6 days), and all stages and sizes may be present at the same time and in the same vicinity. Lesions occur first on the scalp and mucous surfaces and then on the body. They are numerous over the chest, back, and shoulders; less numerous on the extremities; and seldom seen on the palms and soles. Successive stages include macules, papules, vesicles on erythematous bases, and pustules or scabs.

3. Pruritus–Pruritus is minimal at first but may become severe in the pustular stage.

4. Fever–Fever may occur during the first few days of rash, but systemic symptoms are usually minimal.

5. Herpes Zoster–Herpes zoster (shingles) occurs in individuals who have had varicella and is rarely seen in very young children. There may be pain in the area of the rash before the vesicles erupt. Lesions resemble those of varicella but are confined to dermatomal distributions. The most common site is the chest, but lesions may also follow the distribution of the trigeminal nerve root. The vesicles have usually dried and are healing by the fourth or fifth day.

B. Laboratory Findings: Leukopenia occurs early. The white blood cell count may rise with extensive secondary infection of vesicles.

Complications

Secondary infection of vesicles is a common complication. Encephalitis, nephritis, hepatitis, arthritis, glomerulonephritis, thrombocytopenia, and Reye's syndrome occur rarely. Severe disease with visceral involvement (including pneumonia) occurs in some immunocompromised individuals and in some normal adults and newborns. Congenital infection, with cicatricial skin lesions and neurologic and eye abnormalities, occasionally results from infection during the first or early second trimester of pregnancy.

Treatment

A. Specific Measures: Intravenous acyclovir or vidarabine is generally reserved for complicated cases, eg, immunocompromised patients or those with disseminated, visceral involvement.

Oral acyclovir, which reduces the duration and extent of skin lesions and fever, may be beneficial in children with underlying diseases or at otherwise increased risk of severe disease.

B. General Measures: Pruritus may be relieved by local application of calamine lotion or mild local anesthetic ointments, or by administration of systemic antihistamines.

C. Treatment of Complications: Treat secondary infection with antibiotics directed toward group A streptococcus and *Staphylococcus aureus*. For general measures of treatment in patients with encephalitis, see Chapter 20.

Prophylaxis

Varicella zoster immune globulin (VZIG) may modify the course of progressive disease or prevent it in susceptible immunodeficient individuals exposed to the virus. For maximal benefit, it should be administered within 96 hours of exposure. Protection with VZIG is also recommended for susceptible, exposed pregnant women, adolescents, and adults, for neonates whose mothers develop chickenpox between 5 days before and 2 days after delivery, and for premature neonates exposed postnatally.

Prognosis

In uncomplicated disease, the prognosis is excellent. Scarring is not uncommon. Encephalitis may lead to significant neurologic sequelae in some patients. Severe illness and death may occur in immunodeficient patients or neonates with disseminated disease. Congenital disease may result in long-term extremity, neurologic, or ocular abnormalities. In patients with herpes zoster, pain along the nerve root may persist for several months.

MUMPS
(Epidemic Parotitis)

Mumps is an acute viral disease that commonly affects the salivary glands, chiefly the parotid gland (about 60% of cases), and frequently the central nervous system. It is uncommon before 3 and after 40 years of age. Mumps is spread directly from person to person by a respiratory route. It is communicable from 2 days before the appearance of symptoms to the disappearance of salivary gland swelling. The incubation period is usually 12–24 days (average, 16–18 days).

Clinical Findings (Table 10–1)

A. Symptoms and Signs:

1. Gland Involvement–A prodrome of 1 or 2 days may precede the salivary gland involvement and is characterized by fever, malaise, and pain in or behind the ear on chewing or swallowing. Tender swelling and brawny edema of the parotid gland is common (submaxillary and sublingual glands may be involved also or in the absence of parotid gland involvement). Pain is referred to the ear and is aggravated by chewing, swallowing, opening the mouth, and sometimes by ingestion of sour substances. Tenderness persists for 1–3 days and swelling is present for 7–10 days. Skin over the gland is normal. Openings of ducts of the involved gland and especially the papilla of Stensen's duct (opposite the upper second molar) may be puffy and red. Fever may be absent or as high as 40°C (104°F). Malaise, anorexia, and headache may be present.

2. "Inapparent" Mumps Infection–This infection has a short course, with fever lasting 1–5 days and without apparent salivary gland involvement.

3. Central Nervous System Involvement–Mumps encephalitis may precede, accompany, or follow inflammation of the salivary glands but may occur without such involvement. Mumps meningitis is heralded by the sudden onset of meningeal irritation. Headache, vomiting, stiff neck and back, and lethargy are characteristic. Fever recurs or increases, up to 41.1°C (106°F). Symptoms seldom last more than 5 days. Transient paresis may suggest poliomyelitis. Asymptomatic central nervous system inflammation with pleocytosis may be found in over half of cases of mumps.

4. Other Organ Involvement–Mastitis, arthritis, and thyroiditis may occur. Other organs may be involved, including the following:

a. Testicles and Ovaries–Involvement is usually during or after adolescence, but orchitis can occur in childhood. This may occur in the absence of distinctive salivary gland involvement.

b. Pancreas–There is a sudden onset of pain in the mid or upper abdomen, with vomiting, prostration, and usually, fever.

c. Kidney–Nephritis is rare and mild, with complete recovery in most cases.

d. Ear–Deafness occasionally occurs and may be permanent.

B. Laboratory Findings: The white blood cell count usually shows leukopenia and relative lymphocytosis. Serologic tests will confirm the diagnosis. Skin testing is unreliable as an indication of immunity in exposed persons.

Complications

Paresis of the facial nerve has been reported. Serious sequelae of central nervous system involvement are rare. Testicular involvement (usually unilateral) may produce atrophy, but sterility is rare.

Treatment

A. Specific Measures: None available.

B. General Measures: Measures include bed rest, isolation of the patient until the salivary swelling is gone, local warm or cold applications to areas of salivary gland swelling, analgesics, mouth wash with fat-free broth or slightly saline solution, and avoidance of highly flavored or acidic foods and drinks.

C. Treatment of Complications:

1. Central Nervous System Involvement–Treatment is symptomatic for mild encephalitis. Lumbar puncture may be useful in reducing headache.

2. Orchitis–Suspension of the scrotum in a sling or suspensory, application of ice packs, and use of analgesics may be indicated. Infiltration around the spermatic cord at the external inguinal ring with 10–20 mL of 1% procaine solution may produce dramatic relief.

3. Pancreatitis and Oophoritis–Treatment is symptomatic only.

Prophylaxis

Live mumps virus vaccine is usually given in combination with measles and rubella vaccine at 15 months of age. It may be administered to any preadolescent or adolescent with a negative history for vaccine (see Chapter 6). A second dose of vaccine is recommended (with measles and rubella vaccine) at school entry or at entry into middle school/junior high school. There is no effective passive protection for mumps exposure.

Prognosis

The prognosis is excellent even with extensive organ system involvement. Sterility very rarely results from orchitis in the postadolescent male. Death may occasionally result from encephalitis.

ENTEROVIRUS INFECTION
(Coxsackieviruses, Echoviruses, & Other Nonpolio Enteroviruses)

Enteroviruses are responsible for a large variety of illnesses, chiefly occurring during epidemics in the summer and fall months. They are spread by the enteric–oral route and perhaps by the respiratory route; incubation periods are usually 3–6 days.

Clinical Findings (Table 10–1)

A. "Summer Grippe": An acute, brief febrile illness lasting 1–4 days without other specific signs or symptoms.

B. Exanthematous Disease: A febrile illness associated with a macular or maculopapular or petechial rash on the face, trunk, and extremities. The illness may be accompanied by pharyngitis or gastrointestinal symptoms. Frequently caused by echovirus strains.

C. Herpangina: A febrile illness lasting 1–4 days associated with pharyngitis, including hyperemia of the anterior tonsillar pillars and vesicles in the posterior oropharynx. Usually associated with Coxsackie A viruses.

D. Hand-Foot-Mouth Syndrome: Also caused by Coxsackie A viruses; a papulovesicular eruption is present on the oropharynx, hand or foot, and, often, on the buttocks.

E. Aseptic Meningitis: Caused by both Coxsackie viruses and echoviruses, this self-limited febrile illness is accompanied by headache, nausea, vomiting, meningismus, and, sometimes, rash. Spinal fluid generally shows a pleocytosis, usually less than 500/mL, and usually mononuclear cells, although these findings are variable. Paralytic disease occasionally occurs with some viral strains. Chronic meningoencephalitis may occur in patients with humoral immunodeficiency.

F. Pleurodynia (Bornholm Disease): Fever is accompanied by dyspnea and pleuritic chest pain, and, often, abdominal pain. Usually pleurodynia is caused by Coxsackie B viruses, and tends to occur in older children and adults.

G. Myocarditis and Pericarditis: Enteroviruses, especially Coxsackie B viruses, are a major cause of viral myocarditis. They may occasionally lead to sudden cardiac death or chronic heart failure.

H. Neonatal Infection: Infected neonates may have variable combinations of sepsis, meningoencephalitis, myocarditis (especially Coxsackie B viruses), hepatitis (especially echoviruses), and pneumonia. Epidemics in newborn nurseries have been reported.

I. Conjunctivitis: Specific serotypes have been implicated in acute (epidemic) hemorrhagic conjunctivitis.

J. Upper Respiratory Tract Infection

K. Gastroenteritis: Particularly seen in young infants.

Treatment

No specific therapies are available. Immune globulin may be beneficial for infections in immunodeficient hosts and, perhaps, in some neonatal infections.

Prophylaxis

Good hand washing can minimize spread of infection.

Prognosis

Prognosis is generally excellent. Paresis, when present, is usually transient. Myocarditis occasionally will lead to chronic heart failure or death. Severe neonatal disease has a high mortality.

VIRAL HEPATITIS

Viral hepatitis is an acute contagious disease involving inflammation of the liver, and often accompanied by jaundice. Several viral etiologies are presently recognized, with distinct morphologic and antigenic characteristics.

Hepatitis A virus is transmitted by the fecal–oral route and by contaminated food or water. Daycare centers have been identified as an important site of hepatitis A virus spread. The incubation period is 15–50 days (average, 25–30 days).

Hepatitis B virus is transmitted via blood, mucous membrane secretions, and open wounds. Transmission may occur either from acutely infected patients or from chronically infected carriers. Perinatal transmission can occur prior to or, more commonly, at the time of birth, from a mother who is hepatitis B surface antigen (HBsAg) positive (especially if she is also hepatitis B e antigen positive). The incubation period of hepatitis B is 50–180 days (average, 120 days).

Hepatitis delta virus is a helper virus that, only in the presence of coinfection with hepatitis B virus, leads to accelerated acute or chronic hepatitis. It is transmitted via the same routes as hepatitis B virus, although perinatal transmission is unusual. The incubation period is approximately 28–56 days.

Hepatitis C is the major etiologic agent of parenterally-acquired non-A, non-B hepatitis. It is transmitted by blood and is probably also sexually transmitted and can be perinatally acquired. A significant number of infected individuals have no identified risk factor. The incubation period is 14–84 days (average, 49–63 days).

Hepatitis E is an enterically transmitted agent of hepatitis that has been evident in Asia, Africa, and Central America. It has an incubation period of 15–60 days (average, 40 days).

Clinical Findings

A. Symptoms and Signs:

1. Hepatitis A–This is most often asymptomatic or mild and nonspecific in infants and young children. It may produce acute clinical hepatitis with fever, jaundice, anorexia, nausea and vomiting, abdominal pain, and hepatomegaly; generally resolves within 2–4 weeks. Fulminant hepatitis rarely occurs. Chronic infection does not occur.

2. Hepatitis B–This may also produce asymptomatic or mild anicteric illness in children. Hepatitis tends to be subacute; fever, jaundice, anorexia, nausea, malaise, and tender liver enlargement may be accompanied by rash or arthralgias/arthritis. Fulminant hepatitis, chronic hepatitis, or chronic asymptomatic viral carriage may occur.

3. Hepatitis Delta–Can accelerate acute or chronic disease in patients with hepatitis B infection.

4. Hepatitis C–This virus may produce asymptomatic infection or an insidious, mild illness with jaundice and malaise. Symptoms and transaminase values may fluctuate. Chronic infection and chronic hepatitis may occur. Fulminant hepatitis may also occur.

5. Hepatitis E–Produces an acute illness consisting of jaundice, malaise, fever, abdominal pain, and arthralgia. Chronic infection is not described. Fulminant infection may occur, particularly in pregnant women.

B. Laboratory Findings:

Elevations in hepatic transaminases associated with elevated bilirubin levels are frequent. Specific serologic markers are available to diagnose infections by hepatitis A, hepatitis B, hepatitis delta, and hepatitis C viruses.

Complications

Complications of acute severe hepatitis include hemorrhage, encephalopathy, ascites, renal failure, and hepatic necrosis. Chronic and/or recurring hepatitis, which may proceed to cirrhosis, can occur after acute infection with hepatitis B, delta, or hepatitis C virus. Infection with hepatitis B virus (especially perinatal infection), or hepatitis C virus may lead to chronic viral carriage, which is associated with an increased risk of cirrhosis and hepatocellular carcinoma.

Treatment

A. Specific Measures: Interferon may be useful for some cases of chronic hepatitis caused by hepatitis B or C viruses.

B. General Measures: Rest as dictated by degree of illness and attention to dietary needs (including vitamins).

Prophylaxis

Standard immune globulin can prevent overt disease from hepatitis A infection but may not prevent infection. A dose of 0.02 mL/kg given within 2 weeks of exposure is recommended for household, sexual, and daycare contacts. Travelers to endemic regions should receive 0.02 mL/kg for stays up to 3 months; 0.06 mL/kg every 5 months is recommended for longer stays. Vaccines for hepatitis A virus are currently under investigation.

Hepatitis B immune globulin (HBIG) is effective in preventing hepatitis B infection in exposed susceptible individuals, eg, those who have had contact with the blood of an infected person via a needle prick or a splash onto a mucosal surface or those with sexual exposure of some household exposures. HBIG is given in a dose of 0.06 mL/kg as soon as possible after exposure (but within 7 days); the hepatitis B vaccine series should also be initiated. Perinatal exposure requires administration of 0.5 mL of HBIG as soon after birth as possible, preferably in the delivery room but within 12–48 hours, and initiation of hepatitis B vaccine (see below).

Inactivated hepatitis B vaccine, either plasma-derived or recombinant, is effective in the prevention of hepatitis B. The vaccine regimen consists of 3 doses administered intramuscularly. The first dose is followed in 1 month by the second and in 6 months by the third. Alternative regimens are available. In addition to use following blood exposure and use following perinatal exposure, vaccination (and HBIG) is recommended for some household and sexual contacts of persons with hepatitis B and for other high-risk groups. In addition, vaccination is now recommended universally for all newborns and, when feasible, for unimmunized adolescents. Following the neonatal vaccine series (when given for perinatal exposure), serum anti-HBs antibody and hepatitis B surface antigen should be measured at 9 months of age. If the antibody titer and surface antigen are negative, give another dose of vaccine and retest antibody 1 month later; if surface antigen is positive, perform followup testing to determine whether chronic carriage has occurred. Prophylaxis for exposure to blood from a patient with hepatitis C infection may be attempted with immune globulin (0.06 mL/kg), but efficacy is unclear.

Prognosis

Hepatitis A is usually a self-limited disease. In the absence of acute hepatic failure, the prognosis is good. Severe acute hepatitis or chronic progressive or recurrent liver disease may result from hepatitis B and hepatitis C infections and may lead to cirrhosis. Hepatitis E may occasionally produce fatal disease, particularly in pregnant women.

HERPES SIMPLEX INFECTIONS

Herpes simplex virus typically produces a subclinical or clinical primary infection, followed by latent persistence of the virus in a sensory ganglion. Recurrences are triggered by fever, trauma, stress, etc. Herpes simplex virus type 1 (HSV-1) occurs principally around the mouth and produces lesions on the face and upper part of the body; it is transmitted commonly by saliva or respiratory droplets. Herpes simplex virus type 2 (HSV-2) occurs principally on the genitals and the lower parts of the body and is often a sexually transmitted disease. It is the virus type more commonly implicated in neonatal herpes infection. The incubation period of genital HSV-2 infection is approximately 2–14 days.

Clinical Findings

A. Symptoms and Signs:

1. Acute Herpetic Gingivostomatitis–This is a typical primary infection of young children, with extensive vesicles and ulcers on the gums, palate, and buccal mucous membranes; pain, bleeding, and fever are common. It is self-limited and heals in 1–2 weeks. Primary oral infection is often subclinical.

2. Recurrent "Cold Sores"–These are most common at the mucocutaneous junctions of the lips or nose. They recur at the same site in a given person, with the virus latent in the trigeminal ganglion between recurrences. Individual vesicles develop 36–60 hours after a "trigger" (eg, sunburn), persist for 2–4 days, and then rupture, leaving an ulcer that crusts and heals without scarring.

3. Whitlow–This is a vesicular paronychia caused by primary or secondary infection of a finger with HSV.

4. Genital Herpes–This is seen as vesicles and ulceration on the genitalia, with much surrounding inflammation. Recurrent lesions occur at the same site (penis, vulva, cervix), liberating virus and serving as a source of infection for sexual contact.

Primary episodes may be severe, while recurrent lesions may be associated with minimal inflammation and symptoms.

5. Keratoconjunctivitis–This may be a primary or recurrent infection, usually with HSV-1. Recurrent lesions often take the form of dendritic lesions or ulcers of the corneal epithelium. Sometimes the corneal stroma may be involved, leading to opacity and impairment of vision or to blindness.

6. Eczema Herpeticum–Vesicular lesions concentrate in areas of eczematous dermatitis. Unless the child is immunodeficient, these widespread lesions usually heal.

7. Encephalitis–This may be a primary or a recurrent infection; it begins with headache, fever, impairment of the sensorium, seizures, or signs pointing to a lesion of the temporal lobe (aphasia, behavioral disorders, psychomotor convulsions). This necrotizing encephalitis is often fatal in untreated patients. Brain biopsy permits virus isolation; cerebrospinal fluid findings are often negative, but may have viral DNA detectable by polymerase chain reaction. HSV-1 may also be responsible for 2–5% of cases of viral aseptic meningitis, with an almost universally favorable outcome.

8. Neonatal Herpes–This is a primary infection transmitted from asymptomatically shed virus or lesions on the mother's genitalia to the child during or shortly before birth. Manifestations include cutaneous and oral vesicles; keratoconjunctivitis and chorioretinitis; meningoencephalitis; and/or multisystem disease affecting the liver, lungs, and other organs; disease usually occurs in the first month of life. Congenital disease apparent at birth also occurs.

9. Infection in Immunocompromised Hosts–Herpes simplex may produce disseminated mucocutaneous and/or visceral disease. Pneumonia, hepatitis, or encephalitis may occur.

B. Laboratory Findings: Scrapings from ulcerations on the base of vesicles show multinucleated giant cells in Giemsa-stained smears or positive antigen testing. Swabs or aspirates from early lesions (first to fourth days) inoculated into cell cultures permit growth of the virus in 1–3 days.

Treatment

Several drugs can inhibit herpes simplex virus replication. Idoxuridine, vidarabine, and trifluridine ophthalmic preparations, applied topically for herpetic keratitis, and local debridement will greatly accelerate corneal healing but will not affect the rate of recurrence. In the case of a neonate, intravenous acyclovir must be used in addition to topical treatment of herpes keratitis.

Intravenous acyclovir is indicated for the treatment of neonatal HSV infection, HSV disease in immunocompromised hosts, HSV encephalitis, severe eczema herpeticum, and severe primary genital herpes infection.

Oral acyclovir may be used for treatment or prophylaxis of genital herpes and for treatment or prophylaxis of HSV infections in immunocompromised patients.

Prophylaxis

Susceptible individuals should avoid contact with open lesions. Transmission of genital herpes may be minimized by the use of condoms. Cesarean section may prevent some neonatal infections when active genital lesions are present in the mother at the time of delivery. Cultures obtained from at-risk mothers and babies at the time of delivery, or after 24–48 hours, may be useful in guiding management.

Prognosis

In most cases of mucocutaneous disease, the prognosis is excellent. In patients with central nervous system involvement and in newborns or other compromised hosts with systemic disease, the prognosis is guarded.

INFECTIOUS MONONUCLEOSIS

Infectious mononucleosis is the prototype disease caused by Epstein-Barr (EB) virus, although EB virus produces a range of illnesses, from asymptomatic infection to severe, progressive disease. Infectious mononucleosis may occur at any age up to 30 years; it is rare in infancy and most common in the later years of childhood and early adult years. Intimate person to person contact is required for transmission. The incubation period ranges from approximately 30 to 50 days.

Clinical Findings

A. Symptoms and Signs: There is usually a gradual onset of malaise and fever to 38.9°C (102°F). A sore throat becomes apparent and sometimes becomes severe, with swelling of the neck and a membrane on the tonsils and pharynx. There is generalized lymphadenopathy, especially of the cervical nodes. The liver and spleen are characteristically enlarged, usually after the first week of symptoms. A morbilliform, scarlatiniform, or petechial rash may appear.

B. Laboratory Findings: A leukocytosis develops very early, with a predominant lymphocytosis, including large immature vacuolated lymphocytes. A rising titer of heterophil agglutinins usually appears in the serum by the second week; a slide agglutination test demonstrates the same antibody and can be used for diagnostic purposes. In uncertain cases, an EB virus serology panel can determine the timing of EB virus infection.

Complications

A secondary infection in the throat with group A streptococcus is the most common complication. Myocarditis, encephalitis, meningitis, Guillain–Barré syndrome, thrombocytopenia, hemolytic anemia, and agranulocytosis have been reported. Rupture of the spleen may occur from trauma to the abdomen. EB virus infection in immunodeficient patients, including transplant recipients, may produce disseminated infection and/or B-cell lymphomas. EB virus also causes African Burkitt lymphoma and nasopharyngeal carcinoma.

Treatment

A. Specific Measures: None available.

B. General Measures: Pharyngitis complicated by group A streptococci should be treated with penicillin (see Chapter 11). Steroids may be useful for severe tonsillar swelling that threatens airway patency. Contact sports and trauma should be avoided during the acute illness and convalescence.

Prognosis

Infectious mononucleosis usually runs its course in 10–20 days. The prognosis is excellent in most cases. Rupture of the spleen is a serious complication requiring surgical intervention.

CYTOMEGALOVIRUS DISEASE

Cytomegalovirus is the cause of severe congenital infection as well as generally milder acquired infections. Routes of viral acquisition include transplacental, from cervical secretions during birth, from breast milk, via contact with saliva or urine, and by blood transfusion or tissue transplantation. While most infections are asymptomatic, certain clinical entities may result.

Clinical Findings

A. Symptoms and Signs:

1. Congenital Cytomegalic Inclusion Disease–A minority of congenitally infected infants show evidence of this severe illness. Most infants with severe disease were infected as a result of a primary maternal infection during pregnancy. In such babies there is onset of jaundice shortly after birth, with hepatosplenomegaly, purpura, pneumonitis, and signs of encephalitis. Laboratory findings include thrombocytopenia, erythroblastosis, hyperbilirubinemia, and marked lymphocytosis. Sequelae include intracranial calcifications, microcephaly, mental retardation, and chorioretinitis. The prognosis is poor. Fortunately, the majority of congenital infections cause only mild symptoms (hearing loss, mild developmental delay) or are asymptomatic.

2. Acute Acquired Disease–This resembles the syndrome of infectious mononucleosis (see above). There is a sudden onset of fever, malaise, joint pain, and myalgia. Pharyngitis is minimal, and respiratory symptoms are absent. Lymphadenopathy is generalized. The liver shows enlargement and often slight tenderness. Laboratory findings include the hematologic picture of mononucleosis as well as hyperbilirubinemia. Heterophil antibody does not appear.

3. Generalized Systemic Disease–This occurs in immunosuppressed individuals, especially following organ transplant procedures, and in patients with acquired immunodeficiency syndrome (AIDS). Manifestations include pneumonitis, hepatitis, colitis, chorioretinitis, and leukopenia, often with a lymphocytosis. Generalized disease is occasionally fatal. Transplant patients without serologic evidence of previous infection are at especially high risk of serious disease.

B. Laboratory Findings: Infection may be diagnosed by virus culture of urine, saliva, leukocytes, or other secretions and tissues. Serologic tests are also available.

Treatment

Ganciclovir and Foscarnet are available for the treatment of severe CMV-associated disease. CMV immune globulin may be synergistic with ganciclovir in bone marrow transplant patients with CMV pneumonia.

Prophylaxis

Good hand washing is the most effective way of preventing infection. Attempts should be made to avoid CMV-contaminated transfusions to high-risk groups (eg, premature newborns or immunosuppressed patients) by freezing blood in glycerol, by filtering out white blood cells, or by using blood from seronegative donors. Infection or illness with CMV in immune compromised patients may be reduced with prophylactic regimens consisting of acyclovir, ganciclovir, and/or (CMV) immune globulin. CMV vaccines are being developed.

Prognosis

Ninety percent of survivors of the congenital cytomegalic inclusion disease are neurologically impaired, with microcephaly, mental retardation, and hearing loss. Up to 10–15% of asymptomatic congenitally infected neonates will go on to have hearing loss and/or mild developmental delay. Acquired infection may be severe in immunocompromised hosts.

INFLUENZA

Influenza is an acute systemic viral disease that usually occurs in epidemics. It is caused by a distinct class of virus divided into 3 main serotypes (A, B, and C) based on ribonucleoproteins. Further classification of each type is based on the surface proteins hemagglutinin and neuraminidase. The incubation period is 1–3 days.

Clinical Findings

Onset is abrupt, with sudden fever to 39.4–40°C (103–104°F), extreme malaise, myalgia, headache, a dry, nonproductive cough, and nasal congestion. Small infants may exhibit only fever, cough, and marked irritability. Physical findings are minimal; they may include nasal congestion, pharyngitis, and myositis.

Complications

Primary complications are rare but may include pneumonia, croup, myocarditis, and toxic encephalopathy. Secondary complications due to bacterial agents include pneumonia and otitis media. The bacterial agent most often responsible is *Staphylococcus aureus*. Reye's syndrome is a rare complication of influenza B infection.

Treatment

Amantadine reduces symptoms of influenza A if begun early in the illness. Treatment for 2–5 days is recommended for children with severe disease and in those with underlying conditions that place them at high risk for severe infection.

Acetaminophen should be used for antipyresis; salicylates are to be avoided for fear of Reye's syndrome.

Prophylaxis

Immunization against influenza is recommended annually for high-risk children (and their close contacts), including those with chronic cardiopulmonary disease, immunocompromised patients, children with hemoglobinopathies, those with chronic metabolic or renal diseases, and children on chronic aspirin therapy.

Chemoprophylaxis with amantadine (against influenza A) is an alternative during an identified community outbreak. Rimantadine is a related drug that is being evaluated for prophylaxis (and treatment) against influenza A.

Prognosis

The prognosis of influenza is good in normal hosts. The course of illness may be severe in those with underlying diseases, especially those with preexistent cardiopulmonary disease and in those who develop primary complications such as myocarditis or secondary bacterial superinfections, eg, pneumonia.

KAWASAKI DISEASE
(Mucocutaneous Lymph Node Symdrome)

Kawasaki disease is a vasculitic illness of unknown etiology. It occurs primarily in children under 8 years of age.

Clinical Findings

A. Symptoms and Signs: The onset is abrupt, with fever as high as 40°C (104°F) and a diffuse rash over the body. The lips are very red, and the tongue has a bright "strawberry" appearance. The conjunctivae and the palms and soles are red and swollen. The lymph nodes in the neck are often enlarged. Fever usually subsides in 1–3 weeks, and there is a characteristic peeling of the skin, beginning around the fingertips and toenails. Associated symptoms or findings may include carditis, arthralgia, pyuria, gallbladder hydrops, and aseptic meningitis. Young infants may not show the full range of clinical findings.

B. Laboratory Findings: Leukocytosis, elevated sedimentation rate, and sterile pyuria are common, and the platelet count generally rises as the illness progresses.

Echocardiographic and electrocardiographic evaluations are critical both at the time of diagnosis and during follow-up.

Complications

Complications include carditis; arthritis; dilatation or aneurysms or coronary arteries; and aneurysms in other large arteries.

Treatment

Intravenous gamma globulin reduces the acute inflammatory signs of Kawasaki disease and also appears to reduce the frequency of coronary artery dilatation and aneurysm. Aspirin is generally used at high, anti-inflammatory doses during the acute phase of illness, followed by low-dose antiplatelet doses during the subacute and convalescent phases.

Prognosis

Patients with coronary artery involvement are at risk of coronary thrombosis, myocardial infarction, and/or sudden death. Mild coronary vessel dilatation often regresses over weeks or months.

ACQUIRED IMMUNODEFICIENCY SYNDROME (AIDS)

AIDS is caused by human immunodeficiency virus (HIV), a human retrovirus that infects the helper-inducer subset of T cells as well as other cells and tissues.

Adults and older children at risk include intravenous drug

abusers, recipients of infected blood or blood products, and individuals with infected sex partners (homosexual or heterosexual). New pediatric infections with HIV most commonly (>80%) occur in offspring of parents infected with HIV, whether or not either of the parents is symptomatic. Approximately 30% of infants of HIV antibody–positive mothers will be infected. The relative importance of transplacental infection versus intrapartum infection is not known.

Clinical Findings

A. Symptoms and Signs: Common findings in pediatric AIDS include failure to thrive, lymphadenopathy, hepatosplenomegaly, persistent thrush, recurrent bacterial infections, diarrhea, parotitis, and lymphoid interstitial pneumonitis. Opportunistic infections occur, including *Pneumocystis carinii* pneumonia, cryptosporidiosis, cytomegalovirus infection, cryptococcal meningitis, tuberculosis, and *Mycobacterium avium-intracellulare* infection. Cardiomyopathy, hepatitis, retinitis, or nephropathy may develop. Developmental delay and encephalopathy are frequent.

B. Laboratory Findings: Frequent features include hypergammaglobulinemia, thrombocytopenia, lymphopenia, and decreased T4 (helper) lymphocytes. Diagnosis is generally made via serum ELISA and Western blot assays for IgG antibody; other modalities include viral culture, antigen detection, nucleic acid detection (polymerase chain reaction), and anti-HIV IgA detection. Diagnosis is difficult in the first 15 months of life because of the presence of passively acquired maternal antibodies.

Complications

Many infants with HIV infection have a rapidly progressive illness in the first 2 years of life, with *Pneumocystis carinii* pneumonia, encephalopathy, recurrent bacterial infections, failure to thrive, and, frequently, death. Other children have more benign illness, with minimal symptoms during early childhood.

Treatment

AZT, DDI, and DDC are antiviral agents that have in vitro activity against HIV and are effective in treating symptomatic patients. Studies currently in progress are addressing the utility of early treatment of mildly symptomatic children. Intravenous immune globulin may benefit patients with recurrent bacterial infections; study of this therapeutic modality is continuing.

Treatment of typical bacterial and opportunistic infections is important in the total care of AIDS patients.

Prophylaxis (usually with trimethoprim-sulfamethoxazole) against *Pneumocystis carinii* pneumonia is instituted according to age-dependent thresholds in the T_4 lymphocyte count and may be given to all HIV-infected infants < 1 year. Immunizations for the HIV-infected child should include DPT, inactivated poliovirus, *Haemophilus influenza* B, measles/mumps/rubella, and, when > 2 years, pneumococcal vaccine. Annual influenza vaccine is also recommended, particularly in symptomatic children.

Prognosis

Children infected with HIV have displayed a spectrum of prognoses ranging from rapid death to survival for many years from the time of diagnosis. While most HIV infections are presumed to eventually produce progressive, symptomatic illness, the potential for prolonged asymptomatic infection and/or prolonged survival is still to be determined. Poor prognostic factors include symptoms in the first year, pneumocystis pneumonia, encephalopathy, and severe wasting.

POLIOMYELITIS

Poliomyelitis is an acute viral infection of the spinal cord and brainstem. In its severe form, it leads to neuron destruction and irreversible muscular paralysis and, in 10% of the paralytic forms, to death. In countries where immunization is widely used, this disease is very rare.

The disease is caused by poliovirus serotypes 1, 2, and 3, which are enteroviruses. They are transmitted by the fecal–oral route and possibly by the respiratory route. The incubation period is 3–6 days for abortive poliomyelitis and 7–21 days for paralytic disease.

Clinical Findings

A. Symptoms and Signs: Poliovirus infection may be asymptomatic or produce a nonspecific febrile illness (abortive poliomyelitis). Other forms of infection include:

1. Nonparalytic Poliomyelitis–Symptoms and signs are those of a febrile aseptic meningitis. Diagnosis can rarely be established except by inference in epidemics.

2. Paralytic Poliomyelitis (Spinal Type)–Paralysis may occur without obvious antecedent illness, especially in infants. Paralysis usually begins and progresses during the febrile stage of the illness. Tremor upon sustained effort may be the first clue to diagnosis and may be present before weakness occurs. Muscle tightness and pain on stretching may cause malfunction and simulate paralysis. The cerebrospinal fluid white cell count may be normal in 10–15% of cases.

3. Bulbar Polioencephalitis–This is paralytic poliomyelitis that includes involvement of the cranial nerves and brainstem. Significant lower spinal involvement may be absent. Any cranial nerve may be affected, but swallowing difficulties, predominate. This form of poliomyelitis is more likely to occur in patients whose tonsils have been removed. Polioencephalitis is the term applied when there is impairment of cerebral function. It follows a fulminant course.

4. Respiratory Difficulty in Poliomyelitis–Respiratory difficulty may occur with paralysis of intercostal muscles, manifested by anxiety, increased respiratory rate, and reluctance to vocalize. The upper arm and shoulder muscles are often involved. Paralyses of the diaphragm, which are easily overlooked, are usually associated with intercostal paralysis. Weakness of the intercostal muscles and diaphragm is demonstrated by diminished chest expansion and decreased vital capacity. Damage to the medullary respiratory center may also occur, sometimes with severe symptoms of irregular, shallow, spasmodic breathing. Obstruction of the pharynx or trachea, due to aspiration of saliva secondary to pharyngeal or palatal paralysis (or both), may occur.

B. Laboratory Findings: Poliovirus can be grown from stool and throat specimens; it is rarely recovered from the cerebrospinal fluid. Serology can demonstrate seroconversion.

Treatment

A. Specific Measures: None available.

B. General Measures: Many patients with mild forms of poliomyelitis can be cared for at home. The need for isolation in special hospitals is questionable, since in epidemic conditions the virus is universally distributed. Special facilities and trained professional personnel are required for the more severely ill patient.

Bed rest is indicated, with careful observation for further paralysis during the first week of disease. Hot packs, hot soaks, bed boards, foot boards, and splints may be used. Physiotherapy is the most important single factor in recovery. During the acute stage passive motion is begun, to the point of pain only. All extremities must be exercised to prevent joint immobilization. Active motion is begun when pain subsides. Uncoordinated or unnatural function must be avoided as long as possible. Resistance-type exercises should be postponed until all tightness has subsided. Braces and surgery are indicated only after physiotherapy has been attempted.

C. Treatment of Respiratory Difficulties: Intercostal or diaphragm paralysis requires artificial ventilation before cyanosis appears. A tank respirator, operated by experienced personnel, may be used. The chest respirator (cuirass) is about 60% as efficient as the tank. It is useful in rehabilitation and simplifies the problem of nursing care. A positive-pressure ventilator may also be considered. Tracheostomy may be required in patients with paralysis of muscles of swallowing, weakness of muscles of respiration, or bulbar poliomyelitis.

Prophylaxis

The paralytic consequences of infection with poliomyelitis virus can be avoided by prophylactic use of live oral (or inactive/intramuscular) vaccine (see Chapter 6). The vaccine should be administered to infants and children according to the routine schedule.

The oral, live attenuated vaccine has a very small risk of causing paralytic poliomyelitis; this risk is increased in immunocompromised hosts. Therefore, inactivated, intramuscular vaccine should be used for people with immune deficiency and for people who are in close contact with immunocompromised hosts. The inactivated vaccine is also the preferred vaccine for adults, as they have a slightly higher risk of developing vaccine-associated paralytic poliomyelitis than do children. Adults who are at increased risk for exposure to poliovirus, eg, those traveling to or residing in areas with endemic or epidemic disease, are candidates for immunization.

Prognosis

The prognosis with paralytic polio is guarded, although muscle function may improve within the first 2 years after infection. In the bulbar form, prognosis is good if complications are overcome. Patients with polioencephalitis usually have a poor prognosis for survival. If the respiratory center is severely involved, the prognosis is poor.

RESPIRATORY SYNCYTIAL VIRUS

Respiratory syncytial virus (RSV) is the most frequent cause of viral lower respiratory tract infection in infants. The incubation period ranges between 2 and 8 days. Annual epidemics in winter and early spring typically occur in temperate climates.

Clinical Findings

A. Symptoms and Signs: RSV typically causes upper respiratory infection, bronchiolitis or pneumonia. Symptoms include fever, anorexia, lethargy, tachypnea, cough, and respiratory distress. Patients may have nasal flaring, retractions, rales, rhonchi, or wheezes. Apnea may be a presenting manifestation.

B. Laboratory Findings: Chest radiographs may show hyperexpansion, atelectasis, and/or scattered infiltrates. Blood gas or oximetry may reveal hypoxemia. Diagnosis can be made by viral isolation from nasopharyngeal secretions or rapid antigen detection (ELISA, immunofluorescence).

Complications

RSV infections in young infants may produce severe apnea and/or progressive pulmonary infection. Children at particular risk include premature babies, infants with congenital heart disease or chronic pulmonary disease (including bronchopulmonary dysplasia), and patients who are immunodeficient.

Treatment

Most infants require only supportive care. Oxygen is used for hypoxemia; mechanical ventilation may be required for significant apnea or pulmonary involvement. Ribavirin is an antiviral that may be delivered via aerosol to infants with RSV disease; it is generally reserved for those with severe disease or for those in high-risk groups. Studies of new methods of passive and active immunization are currently in progress.

Prognosis

The prognosis varies with the degree of illness and the presence of underlying risk factors. The majority of patients recover fully, although some may exhibit reactive airway diseases in the future.

PARAINFLUENZA VIRUS

Parainfluenza viruses are RNA viruses with 4 subtypes that are frequent causes of pediatric respiratory infections. They are the most frequent cause of croup. Transmitted by direct person–person contact and by nasopharyngeal secretions, the incubation period is 2–6 days.

Clinical Findings:

A. Symptoms and Signs: Parainfluenza viruses may cause croup, upper respiratory tract infections and lower respiratory tract disease.

1. Croup–Parainfluenza 1 is responsible for most croup in autumn; parainfluenza 2 is sometimes implicated. Parainfluenza 3 tends to predominate in spring and summer. Affected toddlers and young children develop stridor, barky cough, and respiratory distress, usually with upper-respiratory symptoms and low-grade fever.

2. Lower Respiratory Infections–Parainfluenza viruses may cause pneumonia and bronchiolitis in infants and young children. Severe and persistent infection can occur in immunocompromised children.

B. Laboratory Findings: Diagnosis may be made by viral isolation from or detection of viral antigen in respiratory secretions or, less commonly, by acute and convalescent serologic evaluation.

Treatment

Treatment is generally supportive, including mist, oxygen, and a non-invasive environment (particularly for croup). Patients with croup may have clinical improvement with aerosolized epinephrine (short-lived) and with dexamethasone. Severe croup or lower respiratory disease occasionally requires intubation and mechanical ventilation. Ribavirin aerosol has been used for some immune deficient patients with progressive or chronic pneumonia.

Prognosis

Prognosis is good for those with mild to moderate illness. Patients with severe disease and those with immune compromise may have long-term morbidity.

ROTAVIRUS

Rotaviruses are RNA viruses whose major clinical association is diarrheal illness. They are the most frequent cause of gastroenteritis worldwide.

Table 10-2. Rickettsial diseases.

Disease	Agent	Natural Host	Vector	Geographic Prevalence
Epidemic typhus	Rickettsia prowazekii	Man	Body louse	Asia, Africa, Europe, Central & S. America
Endemic typhus	R typhi	Rat	Rat flea	Worldwide, including Southeast US
Rocky Mtn. spotted fever	R rickettsii	Tick, small animals, dogs	Tick	Americas, including southern & eastern US & upper Rocky Mtn. states
Q Fever	Coxiella burnetii	Farm & wild animals (including sheep, goats, cows)	—	Australia, Africa, Canada, Europe, Western US
Rickettsial pox	R akari	House mouse	Mouse mite	US, Asia, Africa

Disease	Clinical Findings	Complications	Treatment	Prophylaxia
Epidemic typhus	Nausea, vomiting fever, headache, maculopapular-hemorrhagic rash	Encephalopathy, myocarditis, renal failure, bacterial pneumonia	Tetracycline; chloramphenicol; pediculocides	Epidemic typhus vaccine (not available in US); delousing
Endemic typhus	Fever, headache, myalgia, macular rash	Unusual	Tetracycline, chloramphenicol	Insecticides; rat control
Rocky Mtn. spotted fever	Fever, maculopapular-hemorrhagic rash, headache, myalgia, nausea, vomiting, conjunctivitis	Shock, disseminated intravascular coagulation, multisystem failure	Chloramphenicol; tetracycline; supportive care	Minimize tick exposure
Q fever	Fever, malaise, headache, cough, weakness, hepatosplenomegaly	Pneumonia, endocarditis, hepatitis	Tetracycline; chloramphenicol	Reduce animal exposure, pasteurize milk
Rickettsial pox	Papulovesicular rash, fever, headache, myalgia, photophobia. Eschar & lymphadenopathy at site of mite bite	Rare	Tetracycline; chloramphenicol	Insecticides & rodent control
Ehrlichiosis	Fever, chills, myalgia, headache, arthralgia, vomiting, ± rash	Pneumonitis, renal failure	Tetracycline; chloramphenicol	Minimize tick exposure

Clinical Findings

A. Symptoms and Signs: Vomiting, watery diarrhea, and mild fever are frequent. Cough and rhinorrhea may also be present. Severe infection, particularly in infants, may induce dehydration and acidosis.

B. Laboratory Findings: Serum electrolytes may reflect dehydration and/or acidosis. Diagnosis may be made by detection of viral antigens in stool via ELISA or latex agglutination, or by visualization of virus in stool with electron microscopy.

Treatment

A. Specific Measures: None available. Oral immune globulin may be helpful for prolonged infection in immune compromised patients.

B. General Measures: Fluid therapy, oral or parenteral, is essential to prevent and treat dehydration.

Prophylaxis

Hand washing and good hygiene are the major preventive measures. Live attenuated oral vaccines are being developed.

Prognosis

Prognosis is good if hydration is maintained. Some patients with severe diarrhea may malabsorb for a period after the acute enteritis subsides. Deaths are usually due to severe dehydration and/or electrolyte imbalance.

RICKETTSIAL DISEASES

The rickettsiae are very small intracellular organisms that irregularly stain gram negative. They are divided immunologically into distinct groups and subgroups. While most groups stimulate the production in humans of agglutinins against strains of *Proteus vulgaris*, the determination of complement-fixing antibodies is a more accurate and acceptable serologic testing method (Table 10–2).

Infectious Diseases: Bacterial, Spirochetal, Protozoal, Metazoal, & Mycotic | 11

Mark J. Abzug, MD

BACTERIAL DISEASES

STREPTOCOCCAL DISEASES

A variety of disease states directly or indirectly ascribed to streptococci are very important in the pediatric age groups. These are spread from person to person by droplets.

Etiology

Streptococci are gram-positive and characteristically appear in chains. They may be classified as follows:

A. β-Hemolytic Streptocci: These exhibit beta hemolysis on blood agar culture and are divided into a number of groups, of which A, B, and D are the principal pathogens. Group A infections most commonly occur in children and adults, and group B may cause severe disease in infants, pregnant women, and the elderly.

B. Non-β-Hemolytic Streptococci: These commonly exhibit alpha hemolysis or no hemolysis on blood agar culture. Viridans streptococci and some group D streptococci are included in this category.

C. Peptostreptococci: These are anaerobic, produce variable hemolysis, are found in the pharynx and intestinal tract, and are sometimes pathogenic.

Clinical Findings

A. Symptoms and Signs: Streptococci produce a great variety of clinical diseases. Certain entities show a definite concentration in specific age groups.

1. Infection in Neonates–Neonatal infections are principally caused by group B streptococci, especially type III. There are 2 clinical syndromes—early onset and late onset. In the early onset syndrome (at less than 5 days of age), infection is acquired from the maternal vagina. Early onset disease frequently includes apnea, shock, pneumonia, sepsis, and meningitis. There is a high mortality rate. In the late-onset syndrome (between 1 week and 4 months), which may result from person-to-person transmission, meningitis, cellulitis, and osteomyelitis are common manifestations.

2. Infection in Young Children (< 3 Years Old)–In the early childhood type (group A) infection, the onset is insidious, with mild constitutional symptoms, mucopurulent nasal discharge, and suppurative complications (otitis media, lymphadenitis). Exudative tonsillitis is uncommon, and sore throat is apparently absent. Rheumatic fever, nephritis, and scarlet fever rarely occur in association with this form of the disease.

3. Infection in Older Children–In the middle childhood type (group A) infection, the onset is usually sudden, with temperature over 39°C (102.2°F). The throat is moderately sore and beefy red, with edema of anterior pillars and palatal petechiae. Exudative tonsillitis, with a white-yellow membrane, is relatively frequent. Anterior cervical lymph nodes are large and tender. Scarlet fever, which occurs in association with this form of disease, consists of streptococcal pharyngitis plus a rash due to host susceptibility to erythrogenic toxin. The rash appears 12–48 hours after the onset of fever; it begins in the areas of warmth and pressure, spreads rapidly to involve the entire body below the chin line, and reaches its maximum in 1 or 2 days (see Table 11–1). It is characterized by a diffuse erythema of the skin, with prominence of the bases of the hair follicles. It fades on pressure and does not involve the circumoral region. Transverse lines that do not fade on pressure are found at the elbow (Pastia's sign). The exanthem usually is followed by desquamation beginning in the second week, with peeling of the fingertips. The tongue may be coated but then desquamates and becomes beefy red.

4. Skin Infection–In streptococcal disease of the skin (see Impetigo, Chapter 12), streptococci may enter the skin and subcutaneous tissues through abrasions or wounds and may produce impetigo; erysipelas, a superficially spreading infection with edema and erythema; or cellulitis. Wound infection with streptococci may result in "surgical scarlet fever" when the organism produces the erythrogenic toxin in a patient lacking antibody to toxin.

B. Laboratory Findings: The white blood cell count is usually elevated in patients with uncomplicated group A streptococcal upper respiratory tract infection; it may go to 20,000/μL or higher in patients with suppurative complications. An anti–group A streptococcal antibody screen (Streptozyme) will generally become positive, and antistreptolysin titers will rise above 150 units in the course of Group A streptococcal infection. A documented rise (or fall) in titer is a more reliable measure of recent streptococcal infection. Throat culture is generally positive for group A streptococci and is the diagnostic method of choice. Positive rapid agglutination tests correlate well with culture results. Negative test results should be confirmed by culture, since rapid agglutination may fail to detect small numbers of streptococci.

Neonatal group B streptococcal infection may be identified by positive culture of blood, cerebrospinal fluid, or other involved body site or by positive latex agglutination of urine, serum, or cerebrospinal fluid for group B streptococcal antigen.

Complications

A wide variety of clinical conditions may result from the presence of streptococci in the upper respiratory tract, skin, or blood of the patient.

A. Otitis Media: This is commonly caused by streptococci as a complication of upper respiratory tract infection.

B. Adenitis: Streptococci are a common cause of adenitis (which is usually cervical) in children.

C. Septicemia: Septicemia occurs, especially in compromised hosts or the very young. A toxic-shock-like syndrome may also occur.

D. Pneumonia: Group A streptococcus is occasionally the cause of pneumonia, which may be severe and is frequently complicated by empyema.

E. "Metastatic Foci": These include meningitis, septic arthritis, osteomyelitis, and omphalitis (neonates).

F. Vaginitis and Perianal Cellulitis: Streptococci may cause vaginitis and perianal cellulitis.

G. Nonsuppurative Complications: These include rheumatic fever (see Chapter 16) and acute glomerulonephritis (see Chapter 18).

Table 11–1. Gastrointestinal bacterial & protozoal pathogens.

Organism	Organism Description	Epidemiology	Disease Manifestations	Laboratory Findings	Treatment	Prophylaxis
Salmonella typhi cholerasuis enteriditis	Gram-negative bacillus	Fecal–oral transmission and acquisition from contaminated foods, poultry, eggs, and pet turtles.	Gastroenteritis, bacteremia, localized infections (osteomyelitis, meningitis, pneumonia, peritonitis), enteric fever. Complications: dehydration, hemorrhage, perforation.	Leukopenia (enteric fever); leukocytosis (gastoenteritis). Stool WBCs; positive cultures from stool, blood, bone marrow, involved site.	Ampicillin, amoxicillin, chloramphenicol, trimethoprim–sulfamethoxazole, ceftriaxone, or cefotaxime (depending on susceptibilities) for enteric fever, bacteremia, invasive disease, or gastroenteritis in patients at high risk for invasive disease (<3 months of age, immune compromised, hemoglobinopathy, severe colitis). Antibiotic treatment may promote prolonged carriage and is not used for uncomplicated illness. Corticosteroids for severe enteric fever.	Sanitation. Typhoid vaccine for travelers to endemic regions.
Shigella sonnei flexneri dysenteriae boydii	Gram-negative bacillus	Fecal–oral transmission and acquisition from contaminated water and foods. Flies may serve as vectors.	Gastroenteritis, bacillary dysentery, encephalopathy. Complications: dehydration, seizures, hemolytic-uremic syndrome. Reiter's syndrome.	Leukocytosis; stool WBCs; positive culture from stool, rarely blood.	Trimethoprim–sulfamethoxazole, ampicillin, tetracycline, chloramphenicol (depending on susceptibilities); hydration.	Sanitation and hygiene.

Campylobacter jejuni fetus	Comma-shaped, gram-negative rods	Fecal–oral transmission; acquisition from infected poultry, pets, farm animals, contaminated foods.	Jejuni: Gastroenteritis, colitis, reactive arthritis, seizures, abdominal pain. Fetus: neonatal sepsis; sepsis in compromised hosts.	Motile rods in stool wet-mount; positive culture of stool (jejuni) or blood (fetus).	Erythromycin shortens excretion of *C. jejuni*	Hygiene, proper cooking of meat and pasteurization of milk.
Cholera *Vibrio cholerae*	Gram-negative, curved, flagellated rod.	Transmission via contaminated food, water, or shellfish.	Profuse watery diarrhea, vomiting, shock.	Darkfield microscopy of stools; positive culture of stool; positive serology	Trimethoprim–sulfamethoxazole, furazolidone, tetracycline Rehydration	Hygiene and adequate cooking of foods and boiling of water; antibiotic treatment for contacts; vaccine has limited efficacy
Escherichia coli enteropathogenic (EPEC) enterotoxigenic (ETEC) enteroinvasive (EIEC) enterohemorrhagic (EHEC; 0157:H7)	Gram-negative bacillus	Fecal–oral transmission and acquisition from contaminated food, milk, or water.	EPEC: diarrhea, dehydration, failure to thrive ETEC: diarrhea, including traveler's diarrhea EIEC: dysentery EHEC: diarrhea, hemorrhagic colitis, hemolytic-uremic syndrome	Positive stool culture with serotyping and/or in vitro analysis. Lack of sorbitol fermentation for EHEC strains.	Hydration; EPEC: non-absorbable antibiotic, trimethoprim–sulfamethoxazole, ampicillin ETEC: trimethoprim–sulfamethoxazole EIEC: ampicillin, trimethoprim–sulfamethoxazole EHEC: role of antibiotic treatment unclear	Hygiene, prophylactic neomycin or colistin during EPEC nursery outbreak; food and water precautions during foreign travel and empiric antibiotic treatment for traveler's diarrhea

(continued)

333

Table 11-1. Gastrointestinal bacterial & protozoal pathogens *(continued)*.

Organism	Organism Description	Epidemiology	Disease Manifestations	Laboratory Findings	Treatment	Prophylaxis
Amebiasis *Entamoeba histolytica*	Protozoan transmitted as cysts which produces invasive trophozoites	Fecal-oral transmission and acquisition from contaminated food or drink.	Gastroenteritis, dysentery, abdominal pain, liver abscess, metastatic abscesses	Trophozoites and/or cysts in stool or rectal biopsy; serology for invasive disease	Asymptomatic or mild: lumenal amebocide (iodoquinol, diloxanide furoate, paromomycin); Severe: tissue amebocide (metronidazole, emetine) and lumenal amebocide	Hygiene, sanitation
Giardiasis *giardia lamblia*	Flagellated protozoan, transmitted as cysts	Fecal-oral transmission and acquisition via contaminated food or water.	Chronic diarrhea, cramping, flatulence, steatorrhea, failure to thrive, malabsorption.	Trophozoites and/or cysts in stool, duodenal aspiration, or biopsy.	Furazolidone, metronidazole, quinacrine, paromomycin. Rehydration and nutritional support.	Hygiene and sanitation; boil water from streams; filter municipal water.
Cryptosporidiosis *Cryptosporidium*	Coccidian protozoan	Fecal-oral transmission and acquisition via contaminated water.	Watery diarrhea, abdominal pain, anorexia. Chronic in immunocompromised; occasional dissemination in immunocompromised.	Oocytes in stool or intestinal biopsy.	Hydration and nourishment in normal hosts; treatment regimens in immunocompromised under investigation.	Hygiene and sanitation.

Treatment

A. Specific Measures:

1. Group B Streptococcal Infections–Parenteral penicillin or ampicillin is the therapy of choice. Combination therapy with an aminoglycoside is recommended until clinical stabilization and improvement have been observed. Treatment is ordinarily administered for 10–14 days.

2. Group A Streptococcal Infections–Oral penicillin V for 10 days or intramuscular benzathine penicillin are recommended for uncomplicated group A streptococcal infections. Alternatives for penicillin-allergic patients include erythromycin, cephalosporins, and clindamycin. Some also advise use of these antibiotics in cases of failure of penicillin therapy. Severe infections should be treated with parenteral antibiotics. Prompt therapy for group A streptococcal infections will prevent acute rheumatic fever in the majority of cases.

3. Group A Streptococcal Carriers–These usually do not require antibiotic therapy unless there is a personal or family history of acute rheumatic fever. However, illnesses accompanied by a positive throat culture require a course of antibiotic treatment.

Prophylaxis

Antibiotic prophylaxis against group A streptococcal infection with penicillin or sulfadiazine is indicated for persons with a history of rheumatic fever, in order to prevent recurrent disease.

Prenatal identification and antibiotic treatment of mothers or neonates carrying group B streptococci may be effective in preventing infection of high-risk newborns. A vaccine for pregnant carriers is being investigated.

Prognosis

The prognosis for patients with early childhood and adult types of group A streptococcal infection is excellent with penicillin treatment. Uncomplicated cases of older childhood–type infection subside in 4–5 days with or without specific treatment, but treatment is recommended for all children to prevent nonsuppurative complications. Cases of group A streptococcal sepsis, visceral infection, and/or toxic-shock-like illness may have considerable morbidity and some prove fatal. The prognosis for neonates with group B streptococcal infection varies with the severity of infection. The prognosis for patients with severe sepsis, pneumonia, or meningitis is guarded.

PNEUMOCOCCAL DISEASES

Streptococcus pneumoniae produces a number of disease entities principally in the respiratory tract. The organisms are gram-positive diplococci, and are divided into more than 83 types on the basis of specific capsular polysaccharides. Types 6, 14, 18, 19, and 23 are more likely to cause disease in children than in adults. The disease is spread from person to person by respiratory droplets.

Clinical Findings

A. Symptoms and Signs:

1. Upper Respiratory Tract Infection–This occurs commonly as a consequence of primary viral infections; otitis media and sinusitis are the most frequent manifestations.

2. Bacteremia–*S pneumoniae* is a frequent cause of bacteremia, with fever and leukocytosis occurring in children over 1 month of age. (A presumptive diagnosis can be made when a characteristic gingival cystic swelling is found on the posterior buccal surface of the alveolar ridge.) However, fever without any localizing signs may be the only presenting finding of "occult" bacteremia.

3. Pneumonia–Pneumonia is usually peribronchial in the child under 6 years of age. Typical lobar pneumonia occurs more commonly in older children.

4. Meningitis–Meningitis occurs usually as a result of pneumonococcal bacteremia.

5. Peritonitis–Peritonitis may occur, especially in patients with chronic glomerulonephritis and nephrosis.

B. Laboratory Findings: Leukocytosis is the rule in pneumococcal infection. Blood cultures should be done when pneumonia, meningitis, or peritonitis is suspected; Gram's stain and culture of material from the site of infection should be obtained where possible. Rapid tests such as latex agglutination or counterimmunoelectrophoresis may also be helpful.

Complications

Localized pneumococcal infection may result from bacteremia or respiratory spread; infected sites may include joints, pericardium, pleural space, and bone.

Treatment

Penicillin is the drug of choice for susceptible isolates. In cases of penicillin allergy, patients may be treated with oral erythromycin, trimethoprimsulfamethoxazole, clindamycin, or cephalexin. Severe infections should be treated parenterally; if partial or full penicillin resistance is observed, an alternative antibiotic, such as vancomycin, chloramphenicol, or cefotaxime may be preferable (particularly for meningitis).

Prophylaxis

Polyvalent polysaccharide vaccine is available and contains antigens of 23 different types of pneumococci, which account for more than 90% of strains producing bacteremic disease in adults and children. Experience in children is limited, but the vaccine is ineffective under 2 years of age. It is recommended for children over 2 years old who are in the following high-risk categories: children with functional (sickle cell disease), congenital, or surgical asplenia; nephrotic syndrome or chronic renal failure; antibody-deficient states (response is not ensured in this group, but some children may respond); Hodgkin's disease and other immune deficiency states; and human immunodeficiency virus infection. Revaccination after 3–5 years should be considered for children in high risk groups.

Antibiotic prophylaxis is recommended by many to prevent pneumococcal infections in patients with anatomic or functional asplenia (including sickle cell disease). Parents and patients should be advised that vaccine and antibiotics may not prevent all infections and that they should report for medical care immediately if there is any febrile illness. Physicians seeing such children should treat them for potential bacteremia.

STAPHYLOCOCCAL DISEASES

The staphylococci are gram-positive organisms and are divided into several types. *Staphylococcus aureus*, which are coagulase-producing, are the most common pathogens. Coagulase-negative staphylococci, including *S epidermidis*, occasionally also cause invasive disease, particularly in compromised hosts and in patients with foreign bodies.

Staphylococci are common in the environment and are normally found in the nose and on the skin.

Clinical Findings

    A. Symptoms and Signs:

    1. *Staphylococcus Aureus*–

    a. Superficial Infection–Pyoderma/impetigo is the most common type of infection with this organism. Furuncles, folliculitis, carbuncles, and impetigo are discussed in Chapter 12.

b. Deep Infection–Osteomyelitis or septic arthritis can occur following bloodstream spread from a local inoculation or a superficial infection. Pneumonia may occur, especially after a viral infection, eg, influenza; it tends to be severe and is usually associated with an empyema. Septicemia, with focal abscesses in the chest, abdomen, and brain, may be present. Enterocolitis in the small infant is often the result of intestinal flora being modified through use of broad-spectrum antibiotics.

c. Toxin Disease–Food poisoning (see Table 11–1) may be the result of production of enterotoxin in contaminated foods, usually gravies or custards. The onset is abrupt, with vomiting, prostration, and diarrhea within 4 hours of ingestion. Staphylococcal scalded skin syndrome is an exfoliative skin disease caused by an exotoxin that occurs in infants colonized by staphylococcus aureus. Toxic shock syndrome, also caused by an exotoxin, may result from staphylococcal infection in surgical wounds, in the vagina during menstruation and with the use of tampons, in localized abscesses, and in fulminant staphylococcal sepsis. The onset is sudden with fever, vomiting, diarrhea, and hypotension, followed by a generalized erythroderma that desquamates.

2. Coagulase-Negative Staphylococci–

a. Bacteremia–Bacteremia with coagulase-negative staphylococci occurs in compromised patients, including premature infants and immunosuppressed patients. Bacteremia with these organisms frequently occurs as a consequence of indwelling vascular catheters.

b. Other Foreign Body Infections–Coagulase-negative staphylococci are frequently the causative organisms of infections affecting ventriculoperitoneal shunts, peritoneal dialysis catheters, and other indwelling foreign bodies.

c. Urinary Tract Infections–*S saprophyticus* is a cause of urinary tract infections, mostly in adolescents and adults.

B. Laboratory Findings: Leukocytosis occurs in patients with deep infection. Culture of the blood yields positive results in many cases of deep infection. A Gram's stain and culture of pus from the local infection or a rectal smear in enterocolitis easily demonstrates the organism.

Treatment

Most *S aureus* are resistant to penicillin and require treatment with penicillinase-resistant penicillins, eg, nafcillin or oxacillin. Alternative agents include first-generation cephalosporins, clindamycin, or vancomycin. Vancomycin is the drug of choice for methicillin-resistant *S aureus* (infrequent) and methicillin-resistant coagulase-negative staphylococci (frequent). Deep infections may require several weeks of antibiotic therapy. Abscesses generally need to be drained and foreign bodies may need to be removed.

Prophylaxis

For prophylaxis of recurrent furunculosis, see Chapter 12. Prevent food poisoning by adequate refrigeration and sanitation. Cleanliness and antiseptic measures can control excessive spread from draining lesions. Hand washing by attendants and other personnel is an important control measure.

Prognosis

In the typical case of local infection with adequate local treatment, the prognosis is excellent. In deep infections with sepsis, pneumonia, brain abscess, or other localization, the prognosis is guarded. Patients with osteomyelitis have an excellent prognosis if they are promptly treated.

HAEMOPHILUS INFLUENZAE B DISEASES

Haemophilus influenzae B is an important bacterial pathogen found in infants and young children and was the cause of the majority of bacterial meningitis in pediatrics. The organism is an encapsulated gram-negative pleomorphic rod. It generally infects children under the age of 6 years. Its incidence is decreasing as a result of immunization.

Clinical Findings

A. Symptoms and Signs: *H influenzae B* causes a wide spectrum of disease, including meningitis, pneumonia, empyema, bacteremia, epiglottitis, cellulitis (buccal, periorbital, or other), septic arthritis, osteomyelitis, pericarditis, and uvulitis. More than one of these processes may coexist. Patients usually present with fever and irritability and then develop specific localizing findings depending on the site of infection.

B. Laboratory Findings: Leukocytosis with a shift to the left is frequently present. Gram's stain of fluid obtained from the site of infection is frequently positive; latex agglutination or counterimmunoelectrophoresis of such fluid or urine is frequently positive. The organism can be cultured on chocolate agar from the blood or from fluid or swabs obtained from the site of localization.

Treatment

A. Specific Measures: Useful parenteral antibiotics for *H influenzae B* include ampicillin, chloramphenicol, cefotaxime, ceftriaxone, and cefuroxime. Antibiotic susceptibility testing will guide the choice of antibiotic; ampicillin resistance is common (up to 40%) and chloramphenicol resistance is occasional. Parenteral therapy is usually administered initially; oral agents that may be used to complete a course of therapy for non-meningitic disease include amoxicillin, cefaclor, trimethoprim-sulfamethoxazole, amoxicillin-clavulanic acid, erythromycin-sulfisoxazole, cefuroxime axetil, and cefixime.

B. General Measures: Intensive support may be needed for severely ill patients, including those with meningitis, sepsis, pneumonia, pericarditis, and epiglottitis. Patients with epiglottitis require emergent tracheal intubation to assure an adequate airway. Patients with pericarditis, empyema, and arthritis generally benefit from aspiration or drainage of infected fluid.

Prophylaxis

Rifampin (20 mg/kg/d once daily for 4 days; adult dose 600 mg daily) is recommended for children who develop *H influenzae B* disease and for their household contacts. In addition, many experts recommend similar prophylaxis of daycare and nursery school contacts of index patients, particularly if there are attendees under 2 years of age. (Prophylaxis is indicated both for children vaccinated and unvaccinated against *H influenzae B*.) Children exposed to *H influenzae B* who develop a febrile illness should receive medical attention.

Immunization against *H influenzae B* disease is currently recommended for children beginning in infancy with a vaccine that conjugates *H influenzae B* capsular polysaccharide to a protein carrier. All children younger than 60 months should receive the vaccine series and children older than 60 months of age who are in high-risk groups, eg, those with asplenia, sickle cell disease, or malignancy, should receive a conjugate vaccine. Children who have had invasive *H influenzae B* disease prior to the age of 24 months should be vaccinated with a conjugate vaccine; those with invasive disease after 24 months do not need to be vaccinated.

Prognosis

Patients with mild to moderate disease who receive prompt therapy usually have a good prognosis. Patients with severe infections, including sepsis, pericarditis, meningitis, and epiglottitis, have a more guarded outlook, particularly if there is a delay in therapy.

MENINGOCOCCAL DISEASES

Neisseria meningitidis is a gram-negative diplococcus that is a common pathogen of children as well as adults.

Clinical Findings

A. Symptoms and Signs: Septicemia, or meningococcemia, presents with fever, irritability, lethargy, and, often, a maculopapular or petechial rash. In severe cases, hypotension, disseminated intravascular coagulation, and coma may occur (Waterhouse-Friderichsen syndrome). Meningococcal meningitis may also occur, with or without the signs of meningococcemia. Other meninococcal infections include bacteremia, pericarditis, arthritis, and pneumonia, alone or in combination. Chronic meningococcemia is a form of bacteremia that persists for more than 1 week and is associated with fever, rash, and arthralgias.

B. Laboratory Findings: Leukocytosis with a leftward shift is common; thrombocytopenia is present in severe meningococcemia.

The diagnosis may be made by Gram's stain identification in a culture of blood, cerebrospinal fluid, joint fluid, or petechiae. Latex agglutination or counterimmunoelectrophoresis of urine, serum, or cerebrospinal fluid may be positive, although sensitivity is lacking.

Treatment

A. Specific Measures: The antibiotic of choice is penicillin G or ampicillin (except where resistance is reported). Alternatives include chloramphenicol, cefotaxime, ceftriaxone, and cefuroxime.

B. General Measures: Intensive supportive care may be required for patients with meningococcemia or meningitis, particularly if shock and coagulopathy are present.

Prophylaxis

Prophylaxis is recommended for contacts of a patient with meningococcal disease, eg, household, daycare, and nursery contacts as well as any other people who have had contact with oral secretions of the index patient. Medical personnel involved with resuscitation or airway care should receive prophylaxis. The drug of choice for prophylaxis is rifampin (10 mg/kg every 12 hours for 2 days; adult dose 600 mg every 12 hours); sulfisoxazole is an alternative. Contacts who develop a febrile illness should receive medical attention.

Meningococcal vaccine is a quadrivalent polysaccharide vaccine. It is recommended for children 2 years of age and older who are in a high-risk group for meningococcal disease, eg, asplenic children or those with a deficiency of terminal complement. In addition, it is administered to people traveling to regions with hyperendemic or epidemic disease and to aid in interrupting outbreaks.

Prognosis

Patients with isolated focal disease who receive prompt therapy have a good prognosis. Patients with overwhelming meningococcemia have a guarded prognosis; features suggestive of a poor prognosis include hypotension, leukopenia, purpura, and absence of meningitis.

PERTUSSIS
(Whooping Cough)

Bordetella pertussis is a gram-negative bacillus. Transmission is by droplets during the catarrhal and paroxysmal stages of whooping cough. Pertussis is communicable from 1 week before to 3 weeks after onset of paroxysms. The incubation period is 7–10 days. A pertussis-like syndrome may be caused by *B parapertussis, Chlamydia trachomatis,* or several respiratory tract viruses.

Clinical Findings

A. Symptoms and Signs: Insidious onset of symptoms of a mild upper respiratory tract infection occurs, with rhinitis, sneezing, lacrimation, slight fever, and irritating cough (catarrhal stage). Within 2 weeks, the cough becomes paroxysmal; a repeated series of many coughs during one expiration is followed by a sudden deep inspiration with a characteristic crowing sound, or "whoop." Eating often precipitates paroxysms, which may also cause vomiting. Tenacious mucus may be coughed and vomited. The paroxysmal stage lasts 2–6 weeks, but a habit pattern of coughing may continue for many weeks (convalescent stage). Typical paroxysms and "whoops" may not be present in young infants or older children and adults.

B. Laboratory Findings: The white blood cell count may be very high, with predominant lymphocytosis. Cultures are best obtained by nasopharyngeal swab or washings. The nasopharyngeal culture on Bordet-Gengou medium yields positive results. Results are generally positive during the catarrhal stage and the first week or two of the paroxysmal stage. The fluorescent antibody test may give a rapid diagnosis but has variable sensitivity and specificity.

Complications

Pneumonia accounts for most of the deaths due to pertussis. Atelectasis, emphysema, and bronchiectasis are other pulmonary complications. Neurologic complications include seizures, apnea, and encephalopathy.

Treatment

A. Specific Measures: Erythromycin will quickly eradicate organisms and reduce the possibility of spread of infection. It will not influence the course of the clinical disease unless begun during the catarrhal stage. Corticosteroids and albuterol may have benefit in reducing coughing paroxysms.

B. General Measures:

1. Respiration–Because of anoxic periods during paroxysms, infants may require constant attendance and such measures as insertion of an airway, artificial respiration, and suction of oropharynx. Oxygen should be administered to infants who have significant desaturation during coughing paroxysms. Bacterial superinfections of the respiratory tract require specific antimicrobial treatment.

2. Parenteral Fluids–Severe paroxysms may prevent adequate intake of fluids and necessitate parenteral therapy.

3. Feedings–Frequent small feedings are less likely to cause vomiting than the usual 3-meals-a-day schedule. Thick feedings are often retained better than more fluid ones. If vomiting occurs during or immediately after a feeding, the child should be fed again. Paroxysms are less likely to occur at this time.

Prophylaxis

For active immunization in early infancy, see Table 6–3. Exposed household, daycare, and other close contacts of a patient with pertussis should receive a 14-day course of erythromycin.

Prognosis

Disease in infants under 1 year of age may be severe and is sometimes accompanied by a poor prognosis (especially if complications have occurred). The prognosis is good in patients over 1 year of age and in those with uncomplicated infection.

DIPHTHERIA

Diphtheria is an acute febrile infection, usually of the throat, and is most common in the winter months in temperate zones. With active immunization in early childhood, the disease has become rare in the USA.

Diphtheria is caused by a gram-positive, pleomorphic rod, *Corynebacterium diphtheriae*. The disease is transmitted by droplets from the respiratory tract of a carrier or patient. The incubation period is 1–7 days (average, 3 days).

Clinical Findings

A. Symptoms and Signs:

1. Pharyngeal–Findings include mild sore throat, moderate fever to 38.5°C (101.2–102.2°F), rapid pulse, severe prostration, and exudate. A membrane forms in the throat and spreads from the tonsils to the anterior pillars and uvula. It is typically dirty gray or gray-green when fully developed but may be white early in the course. The edges of the membrane are slightly elevated, and bleeding results if it is scraped off. (This procedure is contraindicated as it will hasten absorption of toxin.)

2. Nasal–Nasal discharge is a potent source of spread of infection to others, and serosanguineous nasal discharge may excoriate the patient's upper lip. A membrane may be visible on turbinates; constitutional manifestations are slight.

3. Laryngeal–Findings of laryngeal involvement are the most serious and include hoarseness or aphonia, croupy cough, fever up to 39.5–40.0°C (103–104°F), marked prostration, cyanosis, difficulty in breathing, and, eventually, respiratory obstruction. Brawny edema of the neck may occur, and membrane formation may be visible in the pharynx.

4. Cutaneous, Vaginal, and Wound–Findings include ulcerative lesions with membrane formation. The lesions are persistent and often anesthetic.

B. Laboratory Findings: The white blood cell count is normal, or there may be a slight leukocytosis. A smear of exudate stained with methylene blue shows rods with mid polar bars. Cultures on Loffler's medium yield positive results.

Complications

A. Myocarditis: Myocarditis is a direct result of toxin. Clinical diagnosis is discussed in Chapter 16. The ECG shows T-wave changes and partial or complete atrioventricular block.

B. Neuritis: Neuritis is usually a late development. Both sensory loss and motor paralyses develop rapidly once neuritis becomes apparent. Complete recovery is usual.

1. Pharyngeal and Palatal Muscles–These are the earliest muscles to become involved. Manifestations include nasal voice, dysphagia, and nasal regurgitation of fluids. Vocal cord paralysis may occur.

2. Extrinsic Eye Muscles–Diplopia and strabismus are manifestations.

3. Skeletal Muscles–Involvement of the legs and arms may end in quadriplegia.

C. Bronchopneumonia:

D. Proteinuria: Proteinuria usually clears as the temperature returns to normal, but nephritis may occur.

E. Thrombocytopenia

Treatment

A. Specific Measures: The following measures are for the treatment of all types of diphtheria.

1. Antitoxin–Diphtheria antitoxin in sufficient dosage must be given promptly. The longer the time between onset of disease and administration of antitoxin, the higher the mortality. Give antitoxin if disease is considered possible from clinical manifestations; do not wait for reports of cultures. The dosage is 20,000–100,000 units for patients of any age, depending on the site, severity, and duration of the disease. Always test for horse serum sensitivity before administration (see Administration of Animal Sera, Chapter 6); the preferred route is intravenous.

2. Antibiotics–Erythromycin (best) or penicillin G for 14 days should be used in treatment and to shorten the carrier state. The administration of these antibiotics before specimens for culture are collected may prevent diagnosis of diphtheria by inhibiting growth of the organisms.

3. Toxoid–Diphtheria may not confer immunity. Patients recovered from diphtheria should receive a full primary course of immunization (see Chapter 6).

B. General Measures: Parenteral fluids, bed rest, and monitoring of the adequacy of the patient's airway are important elements of supportive care. Special measures for the treatment of patients with the laryngeal form of diphtheria include avoidance of sedation, suction of the larynx as necessary, tracheal intubation or tracheostomy for respiratory obstruction, and use of an atmosphere with high humidity.

C. Treatment of Complications:

1. Myocarditis–Treat with oxygen, antiarrhythmics, and blood pressure support as indicated.

2. Neuritis–Dysphagia may necessitate the use of an indwelling nasogastric tube. Intercostal paralysis may necessitate the use of a mechanical respirator.

Prophylaxis

Prophylactic measures include active immunization in early childhood (see Table 6–3), culture of close contacts and antibiotic treatment of identified culture-positive individuals, and booster immunization of contacts.

Prognosis

The prognosis is always guarded, varying with the day of disease on which antitoxin treatment is given. After 6 days without treatment, mortality is almost 50%. Myocarditis within the first 10 days is an ominous sign.

TETANUS

Tetanus is an acute disease characterized by painful muscular contractions. The causative organism of tetanus, *Clostridium tetani,* is an anaerobic, spore-forming, gram-positive organism that produces a very powerful neurotoxin. Bacilli and spores are widely distributed in soil and dust and are present in the feces of animals and humans. Inoculation of a wound with dirt or dust is most likely to occur with puncture wounds. In many cases, the original wound may have been very minor or overlooked entirely. In the newborn, transmission may occur by contamination of the umbilical cord, which, as it becomes necrotic, permits growth of the organism. The exotoxin acts upon the motor nerve endplates and anterior horn cells of the spinal cord and brainstem.

Clinical Findings

A. Symptoms and Signs: The incubation period varies from 3 days to 3 weeks, depending upon the size of the inoculum and the rapidity of its growth. The onset may be with spasm and cramplike pain in the muscles of the back and abdomen or about the site of inoculation, together with restlessness, irritability, difficulty in swallowing, and (sometimes) convulsions. A gradual increase in muscular tension occurs in the following 48 hours, with stiff neck, positive Kernig sign, tightness of masseters, anxious expression of the face, and stiffness of the arms and legs. Facial expression is modified by inability to open the mouth (trismus). Swallowing is difficult. Recurring tetanic spasms occur and last 5–10 seconds; they are characterized by agonizing pain, stiffening of the body, retraction of the head, opisthotonos, clenching of the jaws, and clenching of the hands. Fever is usually low-grade but may rarely be as high as 40°C (104°F). Auditory or tactile stimuli may initiate convulsions. Severe spasms may occur for ≥ 1 week and then gradually subside. Local tetanus, with muscle spasms only near the initial wound, may also occur.

B. Laboratory Findings: Cerebrospinal fluid shows a slight increase in pressure, with a normal cell count. Anaerobic culture of excised necrotic tissue may yield positive results; however, the diagnosis is usually made on clinical presentation.

Treatment

A. Specific Measures:

1. Tetanus immune globulin (TIG) is preferred in a single dose of 3000–6000 units, part delivered intramuscularly and part infiltrated locally around the wound (Table 11–2). If human TIG is not available, give tetanus antitoxin (equine), 50,000–100,000 units intravenously, after testing for horse serum sensitivity. The value of antitoxin treatment is questionable in mild cases and when treatment is delayed for several days after the appearance of symptoms.

2. Surgical exploration of the wound, with excision of necrotic tissue and cleaning and drainage, is indicated to eliminate a local source of infection.

3. Give parenteral penicillin or tetracycline for 10–14 days.

Table 11–2. Guide to tetanus prophylaxis in wound management.[1]

History of Tetanus Immunization	Clean, Minor Wounds		All Other Wounds	
	Td[3]	TIG[3]	Td[2]	TIG[3]
Uncertain, or <3 doses	Yes	No	Yes	Yes
≥3 doses	No[4]	No	No[5]	No

[1] Modified and reproduced, with permission, from *Report of the Committee on Infectious Diseases*, 21st ed. American Academy of Pediatrics, 1988, p 412.

[2] Td = tetanus toxoid and diphtheria toxoid, adult form. Use this preparation (Td adult) only in children over 7 years of age. Use DT or DTP in children <7 years of age.

[3] TIG = tetanus immune globulin.

[4] Yes, if more than 10 years since last dose.

[5] Yes, if more than 5 years since last dose.

B. General Measures:

1. Keep the patient in a quiet, dark room. Minimize handling.

2. Give sedation as indicated; benzodiazopines and barbiturates are useful.

3. Gentle aspiration of secretions in the nasopharynx should be done as required.

4. Oxygen and intravenous fluids are given as required.

5. Airway maintenance may necessitate tracheal intubation or tracheostomy.

Prophylaxis

Active immunization with a booster every 10 years will prevent tetanus in children and adults.

Adequate debridements of wounds is one of the most important preventive measures. In addition, administration of tetanus toxoid and/or tetanus immune globulin may be indicated depending on the type of wound and the immunization status (see Table 11–1).

Prognosis

The mortality rate in infants is 70%; in other age groups, mortality rates range from 10 to 60%.

BOTULISM

Classification

Three clinical syndromes due to the neuromuscular paralytic effects of the neurotoxins produced by *Clostridiumbotulinum* are recognized:

A. Endogenous Toxin Syndrome: Infant botulism is the result of colonization of the infant's intestinal tract with *C botulinum*, probably from food sources other than milk. Contaminated honey and corn syrups have been implicated in some cases. Toxin is produced in the infant bowel and absorbed to produce symptoms.

B. Exogenous Toxin Syndrome: Poisoning from contaminated food, in which the organism has grown and produced toxin, may occur especially if the food is improperly processed or canned.

C. Wound Infection: Botulism may result from growth of *C botulinum* and toxin production in a colonized wound.

Clinical Findings

A. Symptoms and Signs:

1. Endogenous Toxin Syndrome–Onset of infant botulism occurs within the first 6 months of life. Manifestations include apathy, weakness, constipation, floppiness, sudden apnea (occasionally), and ocular palsies.

2. Exogenous Toxin Syndrome–Sudden onset of food poisoning occurs 12–36 hours after ingestion of contaminated food. Double vision, nystagmus, dry mouth, and dysphagia may occur. There may be progressive descending motor paralysis with no sensory impairment or meningeal signs.

3. Wound Infection–Onset is 4–14 days after injury. Symptoms are similar to those found in patients with exogenous toxin syndrome.

B. Laboratory Findings: All possible food sources should be sampled for culture when exogenous botulism is suspected. Exogenous toxin can be demonstrated in the wound, vomitus, serum, stool, and/or implicated food. In infant disease, endogenous toxin may be found in the stool or serum. The organism can sometimes be cultured from the feces of the infant. Other laboratory findings are usually normal. Cerebrospinal fluid findings are normal. Electromyography shows responses characteristic of neuromuscular block.

Treatment

   A. Specific Measures: Equine antitoxin should be given for food-borne and wound botulism after testing for hypersensitivity. Endogenous disease in the infant does not require antitoxin. Antibiotic therapy (penicillin) is recommended only for wound botulism.

   B. General Measures: Respiratory paralysis requires mechanical aids. Tracheal intubation or tracheostomy may be necessary to remove pooled secretions. Tube feeding may be necessary with prolonged paralysis. In infant disease, the possibility of sudden death due to respiratory arrest dictates constant and careful observation. The use of aminoglycoside antibiotics may exacerbate symptoms.

Prophylaxis

   The best prophylaxis for exogenous disease is to assure proper food preservation, eg, use of a pressure cooker to kill *C botulinum* spores in home canned foodstuffs. Honey should not be given to small infants.

Prognosis

   The mortality rate in exogenous disease is 20–50%. In endogenous disease, most infants recover after an illness that may last several weeks to months.

TUBERCULOSIS

   Tuberculosis, caused by the acid-fast bacillus *Mycobacterium tuberculosis,* is a cause of significant morbidity and mortality world-wide. High risk groups include people living in developing regions, and, in the U.S., minority groups (especially in urban areas) and homeless or institutionalized people. Tuberculosis is currently linked to the AIDS epidemic, as individuals with impaired cellular immunity are at risk of severe disease.

   Transmission occurs via droplets from the respiratory tract of patients with active pulmonary tuberculosis. Transplacental infection or acquisition from infected amniotic fluid occasionally occurs. The incubation period to skin test reactivity is 2–10 weeks, although disease may not result for many years or may never follow. The risk of disease is greatest in the 2 years following infection.

Clinical Findings

A. Symptoms and Signs:

1. Primary Infection–Initial pulmonary infection may be asymptomatic or may produce symptomatic pulmonary disease, lymphadenopathy, and/or metastatic disease (eg, meningitis, mastoiditis, osteomyelitis, arthritis, cutaneous infection, renal disease, or miliary tuberculosis). Meningeal, bony, and miliary disease are relatively more common in children.

2. Reactivation–Latent infection may reactivate years after the primary infection, generally in the lung, but also in the kidney and other organs.

B. Laboratory Findings: The diagnosis is based on clinical findings and typical radiographic findings in combination with identification and isolation of *M tuberculosis* in body fluids or tissues. Skin testing by the Mantoux (intradermal) technique often provides supportive evidence of the diagnosis when isolation of the causative organism is not possible. Skin testing may be negative in the presence of infection in immunocompromised patients, in patients in the early phase of infection, and in infants < 6 months of age.

Complications

The most dreaded complication is tuberculous meningitis, which may be progressive, causing increased intracranial pressure, severe neurologic sequelae, and/or death.

Other complications include central nervous system tuberculoma, pericarditis, ocular tuberculosis, and gastrointestinal infection.

Treatment

A. Specific Measures: Tuberculous therapy utilizes prolonged, multiple drug protocols to eradicate the slow-growing organisms and limit the emergence of resistant organisms. Currently recommended regimens use 6–12 month treatment courses of 2–4 drugs, depending on the extent of disease. Uncomplicated pulmonary infection may be treated with a 6 month regimen utilizing isoniazid, rifampin, and pyrazinamide (the latter for the first 2 months). Severe extrapulmonary disease such as bone/joint, meningeal, and miliary infection is treated for up to 12 months, with 4 drugs used during the first couple of months (eg, isoniazid, rifampin, pyrazinamide, and streptomycin), followed by administration of isoniazid and rifampin.

Treatment of tuberculosis must be guided by in vitro susceptibility testing. Drug-resistant tuberculosis usually is treated with more than 2 drugs (at least initially), for prolonged courses.

Immunocompromised patients such as those with HIV infection are generally treated with more than 2 drugs (at least initially) for prolonged courses. Congenital disease is generally treated with more than 2 drugs for 9–12 months.

B. General Measures: Corticosteroids are considered as adjunctive treatment with antituberculous medication for tuberculous meningitis, pleural effusions, pericarditis, miliary disease, and obstructive endobronchial disease.

Prophylaxis

Regular (annual) tuberculin test screening is recommended in high risk populations, eg, minority groups, underpriviledged populations, families with members who have immigrated from high-risk countries, communities with high rates of tuberculosis, and individuals in contact with a known case of tuberculosis. Periodic screening is appropriate in low-risk groups.

Isoniazid prophylaxis (''preventive therapy'') is indicated for all individuals < 35 years old with a positive skin test and no evidence of disease; a 9-month course is recommended for normal children.

Isoniazid is also given to contacts of a patient with active tuberculosis. If a skin test 2–3 months later is negative, prophylaxis is discontinued; if it is positive, prophylaxis is continued for a total of 9 months. If contact is with a patient with Isoniazid-resistant tuberculosis, rifampin may be substituted.

Bacillus Calmette-Guérin (BCG) vaccine, consisting of live attenuated strains of Mycobacterium bovis, is used widely worldwide. It is indicated in the U.S. in situations where repeated exposure to tuberculosis is anticipated and is not otherwise able to be prevented. The vaccine is contraindicated in immunodeficient individuals.

GONORRHEA

Neisseria gonorrhoeae is a gram-negative, coffee bean–shaped diplococcus usually found both intracellularly and extracellularly in purulent exudate. The neonatal infection may be acquired during delivery by direct contact with infected material in the mother's vagina. In childhood, infection may be acquired by contact with infected vaginal or urethral discharge or, perhaps, very rarely, from household exposure.

Clinical Findings

  A. Symptoms and Signs: For gonococcal conjunctivitis of the newborn, see Chapter 14. Urethritis with purulent discharge may occur in males, and gonorrheal vulvovaginitis may occur in prepubertal females. While the vaginal mucosa in adults is resistant to gonococcal infection, both the vagina and the vulva are readily infected before puberty, most commonly from birth to 5 years of age. The infection can be spread by contact with contaminated articles or infected children or adults and is manifested by itching and burning of the vulva and vagina. The mucous membranes of the vulva and vagina are red and edematous, and there is a profuse yellow purulent discharge. Vulvovaginitis due to gonococci must be differentiated from nonspecific vulvovaginitis due to improper hygiene. Acute salpingitis (pelvic inflammatory disease) may develop suddenly after several weeks or months of inapparent infection; however, this is more common in postpubertal females. Nongonococcal salpingitis may have an indentical clinical picture. Perihepatitis in conjunction with salpingitis is characterized by right upper abdominal tenderness and, occasionally, abnormal results of liver function tests. Pharyngitis and proctitis are occasional manifestations of gonococcal disease.

  B. Laboratory Findings: A smear of purulent exudate may show intracellular organisms. Cultures on Thayer-Martin medium or other suitable media should be carried out for any suspected case. All isolates from children should be confirmed by a reference laboratory because of their medicolegal implications.

Complications

  Complications of conjunctivitis include corneal ulceration and opacity. Vaginitis may spread to regional organs or (through the bloodstream) to joints. Bacteremia with purulent arthritis and distinctive skin lesions can occur. The skin lesions have an erythematous base, with central hemorrhage. They later become necrotic and vesicular. Nonpurulent polyarthritis also may occur, with low-grade fever, pain and swelling of joints, and redness and tenderness of areas over the wrist, ankle, knee, finger, foot, and other joints of the extremities. Tenosynovitis is also common.

Treatment

A. Specific Measures: The drugs useful for treating gonococcal infections include penicillin G and amoxicillin (often in combination with probenecid), tetracycline and doxycycline, spectinomycin, and ceftriaxone, and cefotaxime, and cefixime. Local resistance patterns as well as susceptibilities of individual isolates should be used to guide therapy. The dosage and duration of therapy vary with the site of infection.

B. General Measures:

1. Neonates with gonococcal infection should be hospitalized. In addition to parenteral antibiotics, frequent irrigation of the eyes is crucial.

2. Expectant therapy of potential copathogens, eg, *Chlamydia trachomatis,* is important for any patient with gonorrhea. In addition, serologic testing for syphilis should be performed.

3. Children who have gonococcal infections should be evaluated for the possibility of sexual abuse.

4. Children and adolescents with gonococcal infections should be considered for screening for human immunodeficiency virus and for hepatitis B immunization.

Prophylaxis

For prophylaxis of conjunctivitis, see Chapter 14. Pregnant women should undergo routine screening for gonorrhea. In addition, pregnant women with vaginitis should be examined and cultured prior to delivery with appropriate treatment of the neonate if maternal cultures are positive. Examination, culturing, and treatment of sexual partners of any person with gonorrhea must be carried out. (Asymptomatic vaginal or urethral infection is common.)

Prognosis

The prognosis is excellent with prompt treatment. Untreated conjunctivitis may result in corneal scarring. Salpingitis as a result of spread from the vagina may be asymptomatic and chronic and may lead to sterility.

TULAREMIA

The causative agent of tularemia is *Francisella tularensis,* a gram-negative coccobacillus. The infection is transmitted through direct contact with the blood of an infected rabbit, ground squirrel, or (more rarely) any one of many species of wild or domestic mammals; through bites of infected ticks or mosquitoes; or through ingestion of improperly cooked meat from wild mammals, usually rabbits, or of contaminated water. The incubation period is 1–21 days (average, 3–5 days).

Clinical Findings

A. Symptoms and Signs: Onset is sudden, with fever to 40–40.5°C (104–105°F), vomiting, chills in older children, and seizures in the rarely infected infant. Cutaneous eruptions of various types occur in about 10% of children. The clinical picture depends upon the portal of entry.

1. Ulceroglandular Type–The lesion on the extremity where the bacteria enter the skin is at first papular but rapidly breaks down and becomes a punched-out ulcer. It is accompanied by enlargement and tenderness of regional lymph nodes and sometimes by nodules along the course of the lymphatics. Without therapy, suppuration of the lymph nodes frequently occurs. In some cases, there is lymphadenopathy but no primary lesion can be detected (glandular type).

2. Oropharyngeal Type–Ulceration and formation of a membrane on the pharynx and tonsils are accompanied by enlargement of the cervical lymph nodes.

3. Oculoglandular Type–Infection is acquired when material is rubbed into the eye. Findings include acute conjunctivitis with edema; photophobia; itching and pain in the eye; swelling of the upper lid, which may show scattered small yellow nodules; and enlargement of lymph glands of the neck, axilla, and scalp.

4. Typhoidal Type–The point of entry of the organisms cannot be recognized, and the symptoms are systemic.

5. Pneumonia

B. Laboratory Findings: The white blood cell count may be normal, or there may be a slight leukocytosis. The serologic agglutinin test shows a positive rising titer, beginning around 7 days from onset. Culture of blood and material from other sites of infection may be positive (on special media); an indirect fluorescent antibody stain can also be done on potentially infected tissues or exudates.

Treatment

Give streptomycin or gentamicin for 7–10 days. Tetracyclines or chloramphenicol may be used as alternatives; they are associated with a greater chance of relapse.

Prophylaxis

Prophylactic measures include proper handling and cooking of meat from wild mammals, wearing rubber gloves in handling potentially infected animals, using extreme care in handling laboratory materials, and minimizing the chances of tick and mosquito bites. A live attenuated vaccine is recommended for persons with repeated exposures.

Prognosis

The mortality rate in patients with untreated ulceroglandular tularemia is 5%, and that in patients with the pneumonic type is 30%. Early chemotherapy eliminates fatalities. Skin tests and agglutinin tests suggest that subclinical infection is common in endemic areas.

PLAGUE

Plague is a disease primarily of rats and other small rodents. It is transmitted to humans by a variety of rodent fleas, as well as by direct contact with infected rodents, rabbits, and domestic animals. The pneumonic form of the disease may be transmitted from person to person by the inhalation of infected droplets.

The causative agent is *Yersinia pestis*, a gram-negative, bipolar-staining, pleomorphic bacillus.

Clinical Findings

A. Symptoms and Signs: The incubation period is 2–6 days, and there are 3 clinical syndromes of the disease:

1. Bubonic Plague–Onset is sudden, with chills, fever to 40°C (104°F), vomiting, and lethargy. There is tender, firm enlargement of the inguinal, axillary, and cervical lymph nodes (buboes) by the third day. Meningismus, seizures, and delirium may occur.

2. Pneumonic Plague–Findings are as above but with the absence of buboes and onset of cough on the first day. Mucoid or thin, blood-tinged or bright-red sputum may be brought up. Clinical signs of pneumonia may be absent at first.

3. Fulminant (Septicemic) Plague–Onset is as above but with overwhelming bloodstream invasion before enlargement of nodes or pneumonia.

B. Laboratory Findings: Leukocytosis appears early, with counts as high as 50,000/μL (mostly polymorphonuclear leukocytes). Early blood cultures show positive results. Organisms can be cultured from lymph node contents, sputum, and sometimes from cerebrospinal fluid. The organism may also be identified in stains of blood smears, lymph node aspirates, cerebrospinal fluid, or sputum. Serologic testing may also indicate the occurrence of recent infection.

Treatment

A. Specific Measures: Streptomycin is the drug of choice. A tetracycline (for older children) or chloramphenicol may be used as an alternative. Chloramphenicol should be included in the therapy of meningitis.

B. General Measures: Strict isolation of patients with pneumonic plague and disinfection of all secretions are mandatory.

Prophylaxis

Periodic surveys of rodents and their ectoparasites in endemic areas will provide guidelines for extensive rodent and flea control measures. Total eradication of plague from wild rodents in an endemic area is rarely possible. Active immunization in endemic areas and for those with occupational exposure may be indicated (see Chapter 6). Antibiotic prophylaxis with tetracycline or a sulfonamide may provide temporary protection for those exposed to plague infection, especially by the respiratory route.

Prognosis

If treatment can be started early enough in the disease, the prognosis is excellent. Delay in treatment may result in death from the fulminant form of disease. Without treatment, the prognosis is poor.

BRUCELLOSIS
(Undulant Fever, Malta Fever)

Brucellosis is caused by one of the 4 strains of gram-negative brucellae (*Brucella abortus, B melitensis, B canis,* and *B suis*). Although these varieties are most commonly found in cattle, goats, dogs, and hogs respectively, they have also been isolated in other species of animals. The incubation period ranges from a few days to greater than 1 month.

Transmission is by direct contact with diseased animals,

their tissues, or unpasteurized milk or cheese from diseased cows and goats.

Clinical Findings

A. Symptoms and Signs: In the acute disease, the onset is gradual and insidious, with fever and loss of weight. Fever may at first be low-grade and present in the evening only, but in the course of days or weeks it may reach 40°C (104°F) and present a wavelike character over a period of 2–4 days. The chronic disease is manifested by low-grade fever, sweats, malaise, arthralgia, depression, hepatomegaly and splenomegaly, and leukopenia.

B. Laboratory Findings: The white blood cell count is usually normal to low, with a relative or absolute lymphocytosis. The organism can be recovered from the blood, bone marrow, urine, and local abscesses, usually with difficulty and requiring long incubation in a special medium. An agglutination titer greater than 1:160 or a rising titer will support the diagnosis. A prozone phenomenon in which the agglutination occurs in high dilutions but not in low ones is common. Skin tests are of no value. Serologic tests may give a cross-reaction with tularemia, yersinia, and cholera.

Complications

Complications can include endocarditis, pneumonia, meningoencephalitis, and osteomyelitis.

Treatment

Tetracyclines are the drugs of choice. Rifampin may be added in refractory cases. Continue treatment for a minimum of 3 weeks. In severe illness, add streptomycin. Trimethoprim-sulfamethoxazole may be used in lieu of tetracycline in young children.

Prophylaxis

Milk and milk products should be pasteurized.

Prognosis

In patients with the acute form of infection, the prognosis is good with adequate treatment. In patients with the chronic form, response to treatment may be poor, although the disease generally is not fatal.

NOCARDIOSIS

Nocardia asteroides is a gram-positive filamentous aerobic bacterium causing chronic pulmonary and systemic disease or local infection of the skin. The organism exists in soil; infection is acquired via airborne particles, usually via the respiratory tract or by skin inoculation. Infection usually occurs in immunocompromised hosts.

Clinical Findings

A. Symptoms and Signs: The lungs are the most common site of initial infection, with systemic spread resulting in a chronic febrile illness, especially in immunologically deficient children. Local skin infection or mycetoma (Madura foot) occurs by inoculation through an abrasion. Systemic disease includes multiple abscesses in the lungs, liver, brain, and lymph nodes.

B. Laboratory Findings: Partially acid-fast, branching gram-positive rods may be visible in smears of sputum, cerebrospinal fluid, pus, or tissue biopsies. The organism can also be cultured from these specimens.

Treatment

Trimethoprim-sulfamethoxazole or sulfadiazine are the drugs of choice; prolonged therapy is indicated. In case of poor response streptomycin, amikacin, or tetracycline may be added. In addition, surgical incision and drainage of abscesses may be useful.

Prognosis

Infections can usually be treated and controlled effectively, although this ability is influenced by the underlying immunodeficiency.

ACTINOMYCOSIS

Actinomyces israelii is a branching, anaerobic, filamentous bacterium that is found in the normal flora of the human tonsils and oropharynx.

Clinical Findings

A. Symptoms and Signs: After local trauma, organisms may invade tissues to form cervicofacial abscesses and draining sinuses. If organisms are aspirated, lesions may develop in the lung; after intestinal operations, abdominal lesions may occur. The lesions tend to be hard and painless, draining pus through sinuses. Fever and anemia are the systemic manifestations of infection.

B. Laboratory Findings: The diagnosis rests on either microscopic observation of beaded gram-positive rods and masses of filaments (''sulfur granules'') in pus or growth of the organism in anaerobic culture.

Treatment

Administration of penicillin for prolonged periods (months) tends to be curative, but surgical drainage and/or excision may also be required.

MYCOPLASMA PNEUMONIAE INFECTIONS

Mycoplasmas are free-living organisms without cell walls. The common clinical diseases caused by *Mycoplasma pneumoniae* are pneumonia and tracheobronchitis, which are most frequent in persons 5–18 years of age and especially in young adults. The incubation period is 2–3 weeks.

Clinical Findings

A. Symptoms and Signs: There is a gradual onset of moderate fever, with malaise and sore throat. Nonproductive cough occurs after 3–5 days. The cough becomes persistent and sometimes paroxysmal, resembling pertussis. Other findings include abdominal pain, vomiting, nausea, and dry rales occasionally accompanied by friction rub.

B. Laboratory Findings: The white blood cell count is normal early in the disease but later may show leukocytosis. Autohemagglutinins for type O human erythrocytes (cold agglutinins) appear usually after the first 10 days of disease. Complement fixation and other antibody tests are all useful, particularly when a 4-fold rise in titer is demonstrated. The organism may be grown on special media and will indicate either current or recent infection.

C. Imaging: The x-ray findings are those of pneumonitis, with infiltrates developing around the hilum and gradually spreading. Pleural effusion may be apparent.

Complications

Otitis media or bullous myringitis is common in younger individuals. Central nervous system disease, hemolytic anemia, exanthems, Stevens-Johnson syndrome, and arthritis have all been reported. Severe respiratory disease may be seen in immunocompromised hosts and in children with sickle cell disease.

Treatment

Erythromycin in young children or tetracycline in those over 9 years of age is the drug of choice (see Chapter 31).

Prognosis

With adequate treatment, the prognosis is excellent.

CHLAMYDIAL INFECTIONS

The species of the genus *Chlamydia* are obligate intracellular bacteria and are classified as *C trachomatis*, *C psittaci*, and *C pneumoniae* (TWAR agent). These agents cause several disease entities.

Clinical Findings

A. Symptoms and Signs:

1. Inclusion Conjunctivitis and Trachoma–Neonatal inclusion conjunctivitis (inclusion blennorrhea) and trachoma are caused by *C trachomatis*. The neonatal infection is acquired during passage through the cervix and causes a purulent conjunctivitis within the first few weeks after birth which usually heals without scarring. Trachoma is a chronic keratoconjunctivitis which may cause scarring and blindness. (see Conjunctivitis, Chapter 25).

2. Pneumonitis–Neonatal pneumonitis, also a result of *C trachomitis* infection acquired during birth, is characterized by onset during early infancy, with progressive tachypnea, staccato cough, cyanosis, and vomiting. It is an afebrile illness. Chest x-ray shows bilateral infiltrates.

3. Lymphogranuloma Venereum–Infection is caused by particular strains of *C trachomatis*. There is inguinal and pelvic lymph node involvement after sexual contact with penile, vaginal, or rectal surfaces. The inguinal nodes in the male and the perirectal nodes in the female become infected, enlarge, and suppurate. This process is apparent as buboes in the male and proctitis in the female or in the homosexual male.

4. Urethritis and Cervicitis–Infection is caused by *C trachomatis*. It is clinically similar to disease produced by gonococci and may be mistaken for resistant gonococcal infection. Infection may be asymptomatic and it may be persistent.

5. Psittacosis–Psittacosis (ornithosis) is caused by *C psittaci* and is acquired by contact with parrots, parakeets, pigeons, chickens, ducks, and other wild birds. There is a sudden onset of fever, chills, and nonproductive cough, with clinical signs of pneumonia or bronchiolitis (see Chapter 15). Multisystem involvement rarely occurs.

6. Chlamydia Pneumoniae–A febrile respiratory illness consisting of pharyngitis, fever, cough, cervical adenopathy, and pneumonia has been described caused by this chlamydial agent, which is antigenically distinct from *C trachomatis* and *C psittaci*.

B. Laboratory Findings: Chlamydiae can be cultured, with difficulty, on special media. This test is available for *C trachomatis*, *C pneumoniae*, and *C psittaci*. Characteristic inclusion bodies are found on Glemsa-stained smears of discharge in neonatal conjunctivitis and trachoma. Fluorescent antibody staining and enzyme-linked immunoassay tests are widely available for diagnosing *C trachomatis* infections. Complement fixation tests are diagnostic in lymphogranuloma venereum, psittacosis, and in *C pneumoniae* agent infection.

Complications

Neonatal inclusion conjunctivitis (rarely) and trachoma (relatively commonly) may produce corneal scarring and vision problems if untreated. Untreated lymphogranuloma venerum in boys may produce extensive scarring around draining inguinal nodes; in girls, perirectal scarring may cause rectal stricture. Untreated urethritis in boys may cause chronic discharge and dysuria persisting for many weeks. Untreated cervicitis in girls may spread to cause salpingitis with resultant scarring and sterility. Untreated neonatal chlamydial pneumonia may produce chronic illness.

Treatment

A. Specific Measures:

1. Inclusion Conjunctivitis–Therapy with oral erythromycin continued for 14 days (see Chapter 14) is the recommended treatment. Sulfonamides are an acceptable alternative. Topical therapy does not eradicate nasopharyngeal carriage.

2. Trachoma–Give oral tetracyclines (doxycycline) or erythromycin in addition to local antibiotic treatment. Therapy may have to be continued for as long as 40 days.

3. Pneumonitis–Treat with oral erythromycin or sulfisoxazole for 14 days.

4. Lymphogranuloma Venereum–Give tetracycline or sulfonamides orally for several weeks to months (see Chapter 31).

5. Urethritis and Cervicitis–Oral tetracyclines or erythromycin may reduce symptoms but will not always eradicate the organisms.

6. Psittacocis–Give tetracyclines or erythromycin orally (see Chapter 31).

7. *C pneumoniae*–Erythromycin and tetracycline are the drugs of choice.

Prophylaxis

Topical erythromycin, tetracycline, or silver nitrate will not prevent all neonatal chlamydial conjunctivitis. In addition, identification and treatment of pregnant women who are infected may prevent neonatal conjunctivitis and pneumonia. Sexual partners of patients with identified or probable chlamydial infections should be treated.

Prognosis

With early diagnosis and treatment of chlamydia infections, complications are minimal and the prognosis excellent.

CAT-SCRATCH FEVER
(Benign Lymphoreticulosis)

Cat-scratch fever is an acute illness due to a tiny pleomorphic gram-negative bacillus, *Afipia felis*.

Clinical Findings

A. Symptoms and Signs: Cat-scratch fever is characterized by low-grade fever, malaise, an erythematous papular or pustular cutaneous lesion at the site of contact, and regional lymphadenopathy occurring about 2–4 weeks later. The lymph nodes are usually not very painful, but they may become warm, fixed to surrounding tissue, and suppurative; the enlargement may persist for 1 week to several months. A history of cat scratch, cat bite, or contact with healthy cats before onset is characteristic.

B. Laboratory Findings: Heat-inactivated purulent material from enlarged and fluctuant lymph nodes has served as a skin test antigen under research conditions and produces a tuberculin-like reaction in convalescent cases. Warthin-Starry silver stain of lymph node tissue may reveal gram-negative bacilli.

Culture is not widely available.

Complications

An encephalopathy associated with cat-scratch fever has been reported, and a conjunctivitis associated with inoculation on the face has also been described. Other complications include osteomyelitis, hepatitis, thrombocytopenia, erythema multiforme and systemic disease.

Treatment

No specific therapy is known; the illness is generally self-limited. Surgical removal or needle evacuation of the affected node will usually be followed by marked improvement.

Gentamicin or trimethoprim-sulfamethoxazole may be effective in patients with systemic disease.

Prognosis

Complete recovery usually occurs within a few months.

BACTERIAL INFECTIONS OF THE CENTRAL NERVOUS SYSTEM

GENERAL CONSIDERATIONS IN MENINGITIS

The most important step in diagnosis of infection of the central nervous system is to suspect that it may be present.

The most frequent etiologic agents are group B streptococcus and gram-negative enterics in neonates and *Haemophilus influenza B, Streptococcus pneumoniae,* and *Neisseria meningitidis* in infants and children (Table 11–3).

Symptoms and Signs

A. "Meningeal" Signs: Signs include stiffness of the neck (inability to touch the chin to the chest), stiffness of the back (inability to sit up normally), a positive Kernig sign (inability to extend the knee when the leg is flexed anteriorly at the hip), and a positive Brudzinski sign (bending the head forward produces flexure movements of the lower extremity).

B. Increased Intracranial Pressure: Findings include bulging fontanelles in small infants, irritability, headache (may be intermittent), projectile vomiting (or vomiting may be absent), diplopia, "choking" of the optic disks, "cracked pot" percussion note over the skull (sometimes found in normal children also), slowing of the pulse, irregular respirations, and increase in blood pressure.

C. Change in Sensorium: Changes range from mild lethargy to coma.

D. Seizures: Seizures usually are generalized and are more common in infants.

E. Fever: Onset of high or low-grade fever may be sudden or insidious, or there may be a marked change in pattern during a minor illness.

F. Shock: Shock may appear in the course of many types of infection of the central nervous system.

G. Other: In the child under 2 years of age, irritability, persistent crying, poor feeding, diarrhea, or vomiting may be the *only* symptoms. Fever may be absent or low-grade, and meningeal signs as above may not be found. Therefore, the index of suspicion must be higher for infants.

Examination of Cerebrospinal Fluid

When infection of the central nervous system is suspected, lumbar puncture and examination of the cerebrospinal fluid must be performed to establish the diagnosis. The gross examination, cell count, chemistries, and microscopic examination for bacteria may all be performed immediately after lumbar puncture. Latex agglutination and counterimmunoelectrophoresis are rapid diagnostic tests that may be used to identify capsular antigens of meningococci, pneumococci, *Haemophilus influenzae,* or Group B Streptococcus in cerebrospinal fluid. Cerebrospinal fluid must be cultured both aerobically and anaerobically.

Differential Diagnosis

Bacterial meningitis must be differentiated from other types of central nervous system infection and disease (eg, granulomatous meningitis due to tuberculosis, coccidiomycosis, cryptococcosis, histoplasmosis, and syphilis) and from aseptic meningitis and viral encephalitis.

Table 11–3. Bacterial meningitis: specific agents.

Organism	Epidemiology	Clinical Findings	Laboratory Findings	Complications	Treatment	Prophylaxis
Haemophilus influenzae B	Previously most frequent cause of pediatric meningitis (now decreasing due to immunization); most frequent under 5 yrs, especially <2 yrs.	May be of rapid or insidious onset, frequently follows URI. May have associated foci of infection, eg, arthritis, cellulitis.	Gram stain of CSF may show gram-negative pleomorphic rods (coccobacilli). CSF culture and, often, blood culture positive. Latex agglutination or counterimmunoelectrophoresis (CIE) may be positive in CSF, serum, or urine.	Persistent or recurrent fevers; secondary sites of infection (athritis, pericarditis; subdural effusions or empyemas). Long-term morbidity, especially hearing loss, may ensue.	Ampicillin, cefotaxime, ceftriaxone, chloramphicol depending on susceptibilities. Ampicillin resistance ranges from 25–50%.	Rifampin prophylaxis of contacts; *Haemophilus influenzae B* vaccine.
Neisseria meningitidis	Most frequent in infants & young children. Increased risk in patients with terminal complement deficiency.	Morbilliform, petechial, or purpuric rash frequent. May present with shock.	Gram stain of CSF may show gram-positive diplocci. Organism may be grown from CSF, blood & petechial lesions. Latex agglutination or CIE may be helpful, though lack sensitivity	Secondary sites of infection may occur. DIC, myocarditis, pericarditis. Waterhouse-Friderichson syndrome, shock.	Penicillin G, ampicillin, chloramphenicol, cefotaxime, ceftriaxone. Rarely penicillin-resistant.	
Streptococcus pneumoniae	Increased risk in children with deficiencies of humoral immunity or splenic function; common cause of posttraumatic meningitis.	Frequently follows URI or other infection (otitis, sinusitis, pneumonia).	Gram stain of CSF may show gram-positive diplococci. Organism often isolated from CSF and or blood. Latex agglutination or CIE may be positive in CSF, serum, or urine.	Secondary sites of infection may occur. Long-term morbidity common, including hearing loss, seizures, motor deficits, & intellectual impairment.	Penicillin G or ampicillin. If strain is not fully susceptible to penicillin, alternatives include vancomycin, chloramphenicol, & cefotaxime.	Antibiotic prophylaxis for asplenic and sickle cell patients; pneumococcal vaccine.
Group B streptococcus	Neonates; increased risk with prematur-	May present as early onset or late onset	Gram stain of CSF may show gram-posi-	Long-term sequelae may include intellec-	Penicillin G or ampicillin; an aminoglyco-	Antibiotic prophylaxis of pregnant

		disease. Findings may be nonspecific.	tive cocci in chains; CSF & blood cultures usually positive. Latex agglutination or CIE frequently positive (urine, CSF, serum).	tual impairment, motor deficits, hearing loss, seizures.	side may be added for possible synergy.	women or neonates carrying group B streptococcus may be considered.
	ity, prolonged rupture of membranes, maternal infection.					
Gram-negative Enterics (Escherichia coli, Klebsiella pneumoniae, Pseudomonas aeruginosa, Citrobacter diversus, Enterobacter species)	Increased risk in premature neonates or other compromised hosts; may be associated with UTI, foreign body, other focus of infection. break in skin or mucosal integrity.	Usually acute onset, with systemic illness.	Gram stain of CSF may reveal gram-negative rods. Cultures of CSF, often blood, positive.	Tends to have severe course, with resultant morbidity. Brain abscess may occur.	Cefotaxime, ceftazidime, or an aminoglycoside, depending on susceptibilities.	—
Listeria monocytogenes	Neonates; patients with defective cell-mediated immunity.	May present as early onset or late onset disease in neonates. May be associated with maternal illness.	Gram stain of CSF shows gram-positive rods. Cultures of CSF & blood usually positive.	May have long-term morbidity if severe and/or treatment delayed.	Ampicillin, plus an aminoglycoside initially.	Maternal avoidance of foods implicated in listeriosis outbreak; treat maternal infections when identified.
Mycobacterium tuberculosis	Infected contact can usually be identified; patient often in high-risk geographic or ethnic group.	Onset may be gradual; encephalopathic symptoms may predominate. Tuberculous pneumonia often present.	Positive tuberculin skin test; moderate CSF pleocytosis with very low CSF glucose. Acid-fast bacilli may be identified in or grown from CSF or detected with DNA probes.	Long-term sequelae may develop as for other bacterial meningitis.	Prolonged antituberculous therapy with isoniazid, rifampin and, initially, usually a third and fourth drug (pyrazinamide, streptomycin, or ethambutol) depending on susceptibilities. Corticosteroids for increased intracranial pressure	Prophylactic administration of isoniazid to contacts with active tuberculosis & to PPD converters. Use of BCG in rare circumstances in USA.

Partially treated bacterial meningitis may present with the same course and same laboratory findings as aseptic meningitis following inadequate antimicrobial therapy.

The "neighborhood reaction" (ie, a response to a purulent infectious process in close proximity to the central nervous system) introduces elements of the inflammatory process—white cells or protein—into the cerebrospinal fluid. Such a parameningeal infection might be brain abscess, osteomyelitis of the skull or vertebrae, epidural abscess, or mastoiditis.

Meningismus may occur in such infections as pneumonia, shigellosis, salmonellosis, otitis media, and meningeal invasion by neoplastic cells. In the latter instance, there may be not only increased numbers of cells in the spinal fluid but also a lowered glucose level.

Complications

Central nervous system infection may produce fatality rates of up to 20% and long-term sequelae in up to 30% of survivors. Complications include hydrocephalus, especially in infants (uncommon since the advent of specific therapy); subdural accumulation of fluid, especially in a patient under 2 years of age; deafness; paresis; mental retardation; focal epilepsy; or psychologic residua. Persistent fever may be due to brain abscess, lateral sinus thrombosis, mastoiditis, drug reaction, continued sepsis, or simply to persistent inflammation.

Treatment

A. Emergency Measures: Treat shock (see Chapter 6). Avoid overhydration and aggravation of brain edema.

B. Specific Measures:

1. Infection with Known Organism–Treat with antibiotics appropriate for organism.

2. Suspected Infection with Undetermined Bacterial Organism–Obtain all possible diagnostic material before instituting antimicrobial therapy. Meningitis of unknown cause in premature infants and infants under 1 month of age should be treated with ampicillin plus cefotaxime or ampicillin plus gentamicin. Children over 1 month of age should be given cefotaxime, ceftriaxone, or chloramphenicol, in combination with ampicillin for infants in the first few months of age. After 3 months of age, empiric treatment with cefotaxime or ceftriaxone is suitable; a second drug, eg, vancomycin, should be added if *Streptococcus pneumoniae* is suspected.

3. Increased Intracranial Pressure–Increased pressure may cause death before antimicrobial treatment takes effect. Treat as for encephalitis (see Chapter 20).

4. Corticosteroids–Dexamethasone has been shown in some studies to reduce hearing loss and some neurologic sequelae of bacterial meningitis (particularly when caused by *Haemophilus influenzae B*). When given, it should be started with (or before) the administration of antibiotics. Studies in neonates have not yet been performed.

BRAIN ABSCESS

Brain abscess is usually caused by one of the common pyogenic bacteria: streptococci, oral anaerobes, pneumococci, staphylococci, or gram negatives. The source of infection is usually a septic focus elsewhere in the body (eg, oropharyngeal infection, sinusitis, otitis media, pneumonia, osteomyelitis, subacute infective endocarditis, furuncles). After skull fracture organisms may enter through the sinuses or middle ear.

Clinical Findings

A. Symptoms and Signs: Findings may be few and diagnosis difficult. Onset is gradual, with fever, vomiting, lethargy, and coma. Increased intracranial pressure may be present, manifested by bulging fontanelles (infants) or papilledema (older children). Neurologic signs related to special areas of the brain may be present, and focal seizures may occur (see Convulsive Disorders, Chapter 27). A history of infection elsewhere in the body should be sought.

B. Laboratory Findings: Leukocytosis, elevated sedimentation rate, and cerebrospinal fluid changes may occur.

C. Imaging: Cranial sutures may be widened. CT scan, magnetic resonance imaging, radionuclide brain scan, and arteriography may give specific diagnosis and location.

Treatment

A. Specific Measures: Surgical aspiration and drainage, for diagnosis and therapy, are usually indicated. Identification of the pathogens will allow specific antibiotic therapy. Until this can be performed, broad-spectrum antimicrobial therapy should be initiated (eg, combinations of penicillin, nafcillin, chloramphenicol, cefotaxime, or metronidazole, as dictated by particular circumstances).

B. General Measures: Give anticonvulsants for seizures.

Prognosis

When the organism is known and is susceptible to antibiotics, and when treatment is initiated early, the prognosis is good. For extensive disease or delayed therapy, the prognosis is guarded. Brain damage may occur, with resultant cortical deficits.

SPIROCHETAL DISEASES

SYPHILIS

Syphilis is caused by *Treponema pallidum*. It occurs in congenital and acquired forms. Congenital syphilis is transmitted transplacentally, particularly from mother to infant during the latter half of pregnancy. Infection may also be transmitted at the time of delivery. If infection of the mother has occurred recently, the infant is almost always affected. The longer the interval between infection of the mother and conception, the greater the likelihood that the infant will be free of the disease. Intrauterine infection may produce intrauterine fetal death or congenital syphilis.

Syphilis may be acquired in childhood by contact of an abrasion or laceration with infectious secretions, by contact with infected nipples, through kissing of infectious lesions, or by sexual contact.

Clinical Findings

A. Symptoms and Signs: Childhood syphilis may occur in early or late congenital forms or may occur in the same way as adult disease.

1. Early Congenital Syphilis–Signs generally appear before the sixth week of life. The more severe the infection, the earlier the onset. Rhinitis or "snuffles"—a profuse, persistent, mucopurulent nasal discharge—is usually the first symptom. The discharge may be blood-tinged. Skin rash follows onset of rhinitis and appears as a maculopapular or morbilliform eruption, heaviest on the back, buttocks, and backs of thighs. Bullous lesions on the hands and feet are suggestive. Other findings include bleeding ulcerations and fissures of mucous membranes of the mouth, anus, and contiguous areas; anemia, with erythroblasts often present in large numbers; osteochondritis or periostitis (or both), with pseudoparalysis, pathologic fractures, and a characteristic x-ray appearance of increased density, widening of the epiphyseal line, and scattered areas of decreased density; hepatomegaly and splenomegaly (jaundice may be prominent); pneumonia; and chorioretinitis, with eventual atrophy.

2. Late Congenital Syphilis–Symptoms do not usually occur until after the second year of life. There may be maldevelopment of bones of the nose (saddle nose) and legs (saber shins). Neurosyphilis may occur, with clinical evidence of meningitis, paresis, tabes, or a slowly developing hydrocephalus. Deciduous teeth are normal. Permanent dentition may show Hutchinson's teeth, in which upper central incisors have a characteristic V-shaped notch in a peg-shaped tooth. The first permanent molars may have multiple cusps ("mulberry molar"). Other findings include rhagades, or scars around the mouth and nose; interstitial keratitis, usually occurring in children between 6 and 12 years of age; and early conjunctivitis, which gradually infiltrates deeply into the cornea and produces opacity.

3. Acquired Syphilis–Symptoms in children are similar to those in adults, with 3 stages: mucocutaneous ulcerative lesions, rash, and tertiary syphilis with its cardiovascular or neurologic changes.

B. Laboratory Findings: Darkfield microscopic examination of scrapings from mucocutaneous lesions and nasal discharge may show treponemal spirochetes.

Serologic tests for syphilis include nontreponemal tests (VDRL, RPR, ART) and treponemal tests (FTA-ABS, MHA-TP, TPI). The nontreponemal tests are useful for screening; positive tests need to be confirmed with the specific treponemal tests. The nontreponemal tests should be followed after therapy; a declining titer correlates with successful treatment while a persistent elevated titer suggests persistent infection. The nontreponemal tests generally become nonreactive within 1–2 years after adequate therapy, while the treponemal tests remain positive indefinitely. IgM tests are under investigation.

The diagnosis of congenital syphilis is based on clinical findings as well as serologic tests. Positive nontreponemal and treponemal tests on neonatal serum may reflect neonatal infection or maternal infection (even a satisfactorily treated maternal infection). In some cases, the only way to define a neonatal infection is to follow the neonate's nontreponemal titer; a rising titer over the first few months suggests an active infection.

Children with suspected congenital syphilis or acquired syphilis of more than 1 year's duration should have their cerebrospinal fluid analyzed. Increases in protein or cell count, or a positive nontreponemal test (VDRL) on cerebrospinal fluid, suggest neurologic involvement by infection.

C. Imaging: Findings are characteristic in congenital syphilis. All of the long bones may be affected. Changes are apparent early in the disease. The epiphyseal line shows increased density, with decreased density proximal to it. In severe cases, destructive lesions occur near the ends of the long bones. Periostitis appears as a widening of the shaft of the long bones, with eventual calcification and distortion of the normal curvature.

Treatment

A. Specific Measures:

1. Congenital Syphilis–Give aqueous penicillin G, 100,000 units/kg/d intramuscularly or intravenously in 2 divided doses in the first week of life, for 10–14 days (150,000 units/kg/d divided every 8 hours between 8–28 days of life), or procaine penicillin G, 50,000 units/kg/d intramuscularly in 1 dose for 10 days.

Therapy should be provided for neonates with clinical syphilis and for newborns born to mothers who had syphilis during pregnancy but were untreated, had inadequate treatment, had unknown treatment, had nonpenicillin treatment, or had treatment during the last 4 weeks of pregnancy.

Infants who are asymptomatic and are born to mothers who received appropriate treatment for syphilis during pregnancy do not need therapy; their nontreponemal test titer should be followed monthly until negative. Treatment should be provided if the titer is not negative by 6 months or if follow-up cannot be assured.

2. Acquired Syphilis–Give benzathine penicillin G, 50,000 units/kg up to 2.4 million units in intramuscular injections of 1.2 million units each, for disease of less than 1 year's duration. Infection of more than 1 year's duration should be treated with the same dosage given once a week for 3 weeks.

3. Penicillin Sensitivity–In individuals sensitive to penicillin, give tetracycline or erythromycin for 14 days. Penicillin should be used whenever safely possible during pregnancy.

B. Complications of Specific Therapy: The Jarisch-Herxheimer reaction, with fever due to the sudden destruction of spirochetes by drugs, occurs within the first 24 hours and subsides within the next 24 hours. Treatment should not be discontinued unless aggravation of laryngitis, if present, obstructs the airway.

C. Follow-up Treatment: Nontreponemal serologic tests should be done at intervals of 3 months for at least 1 year. Retreatment should be considered if titers do not fall to the negative range. For those with initially abnormal cerebrospinal fluid, cerebrospinal fluid examinations need to be performed at 6-month intervals for at least 3 years or until normal.

Prophylaxis

All pregnant women should be screened for syphilis at least once, early in pregnancy, and again late in pregnancy in high-risk patients. If syphilis is diagnosed early in pregnancy, treatment may be completed before delivery. The chances of preventing the disease in the newborn are excellent even if the mother is not treated until the seventh or eighth month of pregnancy.

Sexual contacts of patients identified as having syphilis should be tested and treated.

Prognosis

Rapid treatment of infants with early congenital syphilis or of older patients with early acquired disease will usually result in a cure and normal growth and development. In children with late congenital syphilis, the prognosis for cure of the spirochetal infection is good, but pathologic changes in the bones, nervous system, and eyes will remain throughout life.

LEPTOSPIROSIS

Leptospirosis is an acute febrile disease caused by *Leptospira* serovariants of *L interrogans*. The most common species (or serovariants) implicated are *L canicola*, *L icterohaemorrhagiae*, and *L pomona*. The infection is transmitted through the ingestion of food or water contaminated with the urine of the reservoir animal (dogs, rats, cattle, and swine). Ingestion may occur while bathing in contaminated water. Rat bites are also a source. The incubation period is 6–12 days.

Clinical Findings

A. Symptoms and Signs: Onset is abrupt, with fever to 39.5–40.5°C (103–105°F). Pharyngitis, cervical lymphadenopathy, and conjunctivitis accompany the first phase of the disease, which lasts 3–5 days and is followed by subsidence of fever and symptoms. The second phase of the disease appears after 2 or 3 days, with recurrence of fever and the onset of joint pain, vomiting, headache, and often a rash, which is morbilliform and sometimes purpuric. Meningitis and (more rarely) uveitis may develop at this phase of the disease.

B. Laboratory Findings: The white blood cell count usually is markedly elevated (as high as 50,000 μL), sometimes with immature forms. Cerebrospinal fluid may show 100–200 cells/μL. Leptospirae may occasionally be seen on darkfield examination, silver stain, or fluorescent antibody stain of blood, urine, or cerebrospinal fluid. The organism can be cultured (on special media) from these body fluids. Serum bilirubin levels may be elevated, and the AST (SGOT) level may be abnormal. The diagnosis is most often made serologically; antibody is detectable after the first 7 days of disease.

Complications

Renal involvement, with hematuria, proteinuria, and oliguria, occurs in about 50% of cases. Jaundice, with an enlarged and tender liver, is also common. Symptomatic meningitis may become apparent in the second phase of the disease. Myocarditis may infrequently occur.

Treatment

A. Specific Measures: Give procaine penicillin G intravenously for 7 days. In patients with penicillin sensitivity, give doxycycline.

B. Complications of Specific Therapy: The Jarisch–Herxheimer reaction may occur, as in the treatment of syphilis (see above).

Prophylaxis

Methods used to prevent leptospirosis include rodent control, protective clothing in occupational exposures, and prophylactic doxycycline.

Prognosis

In the absence of renal or hepatic involvement, recovery is complete after 10–21 days. With severe kidney and liver involvement, the mortality rate may be as high as 30%.

RELAPSING FEVER

Relapsing fever is endemic in many parts of the world, especially in mountainous areas. The causative organisms are *Borrelia recurrentis* and related borrelia species, and the reservoir is rodents, other small mammals, or human beings with relapsing fever. Transmission to humans occurs by lice or ticks and occasionally by contact with the blood of infected rodents.

Clinical Findings
   A. Symptoms and Signs: After an incubation period of 2–14 days, the onset of disease is abrupt, with fever, chills, tachycardia, nausea, vomiting, headache, hepatosplenomegaly, arthralgia, and cough. A macular or morbilliform rash appears usually within the first 2 days over the trunk and extremities. Petechiae may also occur. Without treatment, the fever falls by crisis in 3–10 days. Relapse then characteristically occurs at intervals of 1–2 weeks, with relapses becoming progressively shorter and milder. As many as 10 such episodes may occur in the absence of treatment.
   B. Laboratory Findings: Diagnosis depends upon the clinical course and the observation of spirochetes in the peripheral blood by darkfield examination or by use of Wright's stain, Giemsa stain, or acridine orange stain on thick smears or buffy coat smears. Aids to diagnosis include inoculation of blood in mice and proteus OX-K agglutinin serology.

Complications
   Complications include meningitis, iridocyclitis, epistaxis, myocarditis, and intrauterine infection, which can lead to abortion or neonatal disease.

Treatment
   Treatment with erythromycin, penicillin, tetracyclines, or chloramphenicol is successful. As with syphilis and leptospirosis, the Jarisch–Herxheimer reaction may occur in the first 24 hours of treatment.

Prophylaxis
   Limiting contact with lice and ticks by good hygiene, appropriate clothing, and insect repellants is appropriate.

Prognosis

Prognosis is good except in debilitated patients.

LYME DISEASE

Lyme disease, caused by the spirochete *Borrelia burgdorferi*, is a multisystem disorder that is prevalent in the USA (upper Atlantic coast, Midwest, and West coast), Europe, and Australia. The major vectors are ticks, particularly *Ixodes* ticks.

Clinical Findings

A. Symptoms and Signs: The majority of patients develop an annular erythematous skin lesion—erythema chronicum migrans—at the site of a tick bite; the incubation period is 3–32 days. More extensive rashes, conjunctivitis, fever, malaise, arthralgia, or meningitis may also develop. Weeks to months later, involvement of several organ systems may occur: neurologic (Bell's palsy, cranial or peripheral neuritis, meningitis), cardiac (conduction block, myocarditis), or joints (chronic arthritis). These later findings may develop without the prior appearance of erythema chronicum migrans. Anecdotes of apparent intrauterine infection with adverse pregnancy outcome have been reported.

B. Laboratory Findings: The most widely available diagnostic test is the ELISA serology. Antibody may not be detectable for several weeks following onset of infection, and sensitivity and specificity may be lacking. Western blot testing may improve sensitivity and specificity. Antibodies may not develop in patients treated early in the disease. Culture is not routinely available and lacks sensitivity.

Treatment

A. Specific Measures: Oral tetracycline, penicillin V, or amoxicillin, or erythromycin for 14–30 days is recommended for early disease (erythema chronicum migrans). High-dose intravenous ceftriaxone or penicillin G for 14–21 days is recommended once the later stages of disease have developed.

B. General Measures: Nonsteroidal anti-inflammatory agents may be useful for patients with arthritis.

Prophylaxis

The major preventive measure is to avoid tick exposure, eg, by wearing protective clothing in endemic areas, and to remove ticks promptly.

Prognosis

Patients treated early in the infection generally have a favorable course; patients with delayed therapy have more chronic courses.

PROTOZOAL DISEASES

MALARIA

Malaria is an acute or chronic febrile disease caused by one of 4 types of plasmodia: *Plasmodium vivax, P malariae, P falciparum,* or *P ovale.* Transmission occurs through the bite of the female *Anopheles* mosquito, in which the sexual cycle of the parasite occurs. Transmission via transfusion and congenital infection are less common. The asexual cycle occurs in humans. Infection is widespread in the tropics and subtropics. The incubation period ranges from 6–30 days; relapses may occur with *P vivax, P ovale,* and *P malariae* infection.

Clinical Findings

In children, malaria does not always present the classic clinical picture seen in adults.

A. Symptoms and Signs: Sudden onset of paroxysms of fever to 39.5–40.5°C (103–105°F) may be accompanied by seizures in the very young. Chills are sometimes present, last at least 2–4 hours, and are followed by sweating. In young children, paroxysms may be continuous or very irregularly recurrent. In older children, recurrence of paroxysms varies with type of infection: 48 hours for *P vivax, P falciparum,* and *P ovale* infections and 72 hours for *P malariae* infection. Diarrhea and vomiting are frequent and splenomegaly is usually present. Hemolysis may lead to clinical jaundice and pallor. The child may be asymptomatic or have mild manifestations of illness between paroxysms. Infection in infants may cause lethargy, irritability, anorexia, and other findings suggestive of sepsis.

B. Laboratory Findings: There is rapid onset of anemia, and serum bilirubin levels are increased. Thin and thick blood smears and bone marrow smears show parasites.

Complications

''Blackwater fever'' is rare in childhood. It is usually associated with *P falciparum* infection and is characterized by hemoglobinuria and shocklike state. Coagulopathy, encephalopathy, and multiorgan failure may also result from *P falciparum* infection. Nephrosis may complicate chronic *P malariae* infection.

Treatment

A. Specific Measures: Treatment is dictated in part by the malarial species involved and the region in which infection was contracted.

1. Chloroquine–Chloroquine phosphate (Aralen), given once daily orally for 3 days, is the drug of choice for *P vivax*, *P ovale*, *P malariae*, and nonresistant *P falciparum* infections.

If oral therapy is not possible, give intravenous quinine dihydrochloride or quinidine gluconate, and begin oral chloroquine as soon as possible.

2. Quinine, Pyrimethamine, and Sulfadiazine–Oral quinine sulfate (3–7 days) and pyrimethamine-sulfadoxine (Fansidar) (1 dose). Alternatives are mefloquine hydrochloride or tetracycline.

Intravenous quinine dihydrochloride or quinidine gluconate is used for patients who cannot tolerate oral medication. Oral therapy should be initiated once it becomes possible.

3. Primaquine Phosphate–Use with chloroquine to prevent relapses in patients with *P vivax* and *P ovale* infections. Give orally once daily for 14 days. Patients should be screened for glucose-6-phosphate dehydrogenase (G6PD) deficiency before primaquine is begun.

B. General Measures: Fluid therapy is most important. Urge oral intake and, if not satisfactory, give parenteral fluids. Control high fever. Treat anemia with iron.

Prophylaxis

Pregnant women from nonendemic areas should be discouraged from traveling to malarial areas. Although chloroquine can be given safely in standard prophylactic doses during pregnancy, other antimicrobials may be fetotoxic.

Since true prophylaxis (prevention of infection by the destruction of sporozoites) is unavailable for travelers to endemic areas, a drug is given that suppresses schizogony and clinical symptoms. The most commonly used suppressive drug is chloroquine, given orally each week, beginning 1 week before travel to an endemic area and continued for 4 weeks after return from the endemic region. Travelers to areas where *P ovale* and *P vivax* are endemic may also generally be given primaquine phosphate for 14 days after departure from the endemic region, to prevent relapses (rule out G6PD deficiency before beginning primaquine).

Falciparum malaria resistant to chloroquine is widespread in Southeast Asia, Indonesia, some islands of the South Pacific (including the Philippines and Papua New Guinea), and South America and has been documented in the Indian subcontinent, East Africa, and parts of Panama. Chemoprophylaxis with chloroquine is not always effective in these areas. Chemoprophylaxis of travelers to areas with chloroquine-resistance is recommended with weekly mefloquine beginning 1 week before travel through 4 weeks after return. Alternatives when mefloquine is contraindicated include chloroquine prophylaxis with pyrimethamine-sulfadoxine (Fansidar) use for presumptive treatment of a febrile illness (while medical care is sought) and prophylaxis with doxycycline.

Caution: Pyrimethamine-sulfadoxine is contraindicated in patients with a history of sulfonamide or pyrimethamine intolerance, in pregnant women (at term), and in infants under 2 months of age. Severe, sometimes fatal, cutaneous reactions (such as Stevens-Johnson syndrome) have occurred; if any mucocutaneous signs or symptoms develop, the drug should be stopped immediately.

Mefloquine is not recommended in pregnant women (1st trimester), in patients with epilepsy or psychiatric disorders, in patients taking beta blockers, or in young children.

Since most malarial vectors are night biters, mosquito nets to sleep in and mosquito repellants are important preventive measures. While chemoprophylaxis and environmental engineering or chemical control of mosquito populations currently represent the most feasible mass preventive measures, biologic control of mosquitoes and malarial vaccines are under study for future use.

People who have traveled to areas endemic for malaria should seek medical care if they develop fever after return from their travel—even if they have taken prophylactic medication.

Prognosis

In the majority of cases, the prognosis is excellent with proper therapy. In small infants, in the presence of malnutrition or chronic debilitating disease, or with severe *P falciparum* disease the prognosis is more guarded.

TRICHOMONIASIS

Trichomoniasis is caused by *Trichomonas vaginalis*, a flagellate protozoon. Infection is usually spread by sexual intercourse, often with an asymptomatic male carrier.

Clinical Findings
A. Symptoms and Signs: The symptoms are vaginitis and cervicitis with itching and a frothy discharge that is usually yellow-green with a characteristic "fishy" odor. Other symptoms may include abdominal pain and dysuria. Males may have urethritis or prostatitis. Trichomoniasis is very uncommon in patients before menarche. Infection is often asymptomatic.

B. Laboratory Findings: The diagnosis is usually made by visualization of the organism in a wet mount of vaginal secretions.

Treatment
Treatment with oral metronidazole is most effective. The sexual partner should be treated concomitantly. Metronidazole should not be used in the first trimester of pregnancy; instead, clotrimazole may be used to reduce symptoms.

Prognosis
The prognosis for patients with vaginal trichomoniasis is excellent although reinfection or relapse may occur.

TOXOPLASMOSIS

Toxoplasma gondii, an obligate intracellular parasite, is found worldwide in humans and in many species of animals and birds. The parasite is a coccidian of cats, the definitive host. Human infection occurs by ingestion of oocysts from cat feces, by ingestion of cysts in raw of undercooked meat, by transplacental transmission, or, rarely, by direct inoculation of trophozoites, as in blood transfusion.

Clinical Findings
A. Symptoms and Signs:
1. Congenital Toxoplasmosis–Congenital transmission occurs only as a result of acute infection *during* pregnancy and may occur in any trimester. Infection has been detected in up

to 1% of women during pregnancy; about 45% of women who acquire the primary infection during pregnancy and who are not treated will give birth to congenitally infected infants. Signs of congenital toxoplasmosis are present at birth in 10% of infected infants. The others may develop symptoms in the first months of life. Symptoms and signs of congenital toxoplasmosis include microcephaly, hydrocephalus, seizures, mental retardation, hepatosplenomegaly, jaundice, thrombocytopenia, pneumonitis, rash, fever, chorioretinitis, and cerebral calcification. Chorioretinitis is usually a late sequela of congenital infection, with symptoms being first noted in the second or third decade of life.

2. Toxoplasmosis in the Immunocompromised Host–Toxoplasmosis may present as a disseminated disease, particularly in patients given immunosuppressive drugs or patients with acquired immunodeficiency syndrome or lymphoreticular, hematologic, or other malignant diseases. Encephalitis and focal brain abscesses are the most common manifestations; pneumonitis and myocarditis may also occur.

3. Acquired Toxoplasmosis–

a. There may be febrile lymphadenopathy resembling infectious mononucleosis but with a more prolonged course (sometimes 2–6 months) and with intermittent exacerbations.

b. There may be febrile disease without symptoms or signs of specific organ system involvement. Transient morbilliform rash may appear. A prolonged and recurrent course is not uncommon.

c. Chorioretinitis, with acute onset in children or young adults, may be recurrent and prolonged (almost pathognomonic of toxoplasmosis).

B. Laboratory Findings: The white blood cell count and differential count may resemble infectious mononucleosis (see Chapter 10) or may be entirely normal. The heterophil antibody titer is rarely elevated. The Sabin–Feldman dye test results become positive after initial infection and are positive in the mother of the child with congenital infection. Complement fixation, indirect hemagglutination, immunofluorescent antibody (IFA), and IgM-IFA tests are also available. A seroconversion or 4-fold rise in IgG titer, a very high single IgG titer, or a positive IgM tests will confirm the clinical diagnosis. To diagnose congenital infection, maternal and neonatal sera should be analyzed simultaneously for IgG and IgM. A positive neonatal IgM or a very high or rising IgG level suggests the diagnosis of congenital toxoplasmosis. Toxoplasmosis can be diagnosed occasionally by histologic examination of tissue or by isolation of the parasite in bone marrow aspirates, cerebrospinal fluid sediment, sputum, blood, and other tissue and body fluids. Only isolation from body fluids confirms acute infection; isolation from tissue could represent chronic infection.

Skull x-rays or head CT scans show intracranial calcifications in recovered congenital infection.

Treatment

Treatment is indicated in immunocompromised patients, in pregnant women with acute infection, in congenitally infected infants with or without symptoms, and in patients with acquired disease whose symptoms persist for more than 2 weeks or who have active chorioretinitis.

A. Specific Measures:

1. Pyrimethamine, Folinic Acid, and Sulfadiazine or Trisulfapyrimidines–Treatment is with a combination of pyrimethamine (Daraprim), folinic acid (calcium leucovorin), and either sulfadiazine or trisulfapyrimidines (Terfonyl). The duration of therapy is determined by the severity of illness; treatment is usually administered for 1 to several months. Pyrimethamine should not be used during the first trimester of pregnancy as it is teratogenic in animals. Alternatives include spiramycin and clindamycin.

2. Prednisone–For patients with chorioretinitis, prednisone may be used if disease is progressive and threatening the macula.

Prophylaxis in Pregnant Women

Women with negative IgG titers and pregnant women who do not know their toxoplasmosis status should take measures to prevent infection: (1) Avoid contact with or wear gloves when handling materials that are potentially contaminated (eg, cat litter boxes) or when gardening. (2) Avoid eating raw or undercooked meat. (3) Wash hands thoroughly after handling raw meat. (4) Wash fruits and vegetables before consumption. These same suggestions apply to the nonpregnant population, especially those who are immunosuppressed.

Prognosis

Nearly all children with congenital toxoplasmosis who are asymptomatic or have only mild abnormalities in the first year of life will subsequently develop untoward sequelae such as ophthalmologic and neurologic handicaps.

PNEUMOCYSTIS PNEUMONIA

Pneumocystis is an interstitial pneumonitis occurring in immunocompromised infants and children (eg, when receiving corticosteroids or cytotoxic drugs for neoplasms or transplants, from inborn or acquired immunodeficiency, or related to malnutrition and/or prematurity). It has emerged as a major problem in patients with acquired immunodeficiency syndrome (AIDS). The causative organism, *P carinii*, has not been classified definitively, although it is most commonly believed to be either a fungus related to the yeasts or a sporozoon. The organism occurs in many animal species. The roles of human–human and animal–human transmission are unknown.

Clinical Findings

X-rays show an interstitial pneumonitis, and physical signs may include tachypnea, dyspnea, cough, and fever. Onset may be acute and fulminant or subacute and gradual. Hypoxemia is characteristically present. The diagnosis may be established by lung puncture biopsy or open lung biopsy, or by staining of bronchoscopic brush biopsy specimens or washes or of induced sputum specimens. Elevated serum lactate dehydrogenase is frequently seen in HIV-infected patients with *P carinii* pneumonia.

Treatment

A. Specific Measures: Trimethoprim-sulfamethoxazole is the treatment of choice, given intravenously or orally. Pentamidine isethionate, given by the intravenous or intramuscular routes, is also an effective therapy, but can have significant toxicities. New therapeutic regimens involving aerosolized pentamidine, trimetrexate, dapsone, trimethoprim, pyrimethamine–sulfadoxine, difluoromethylornithine, and other drugs are being studied. Corticosteroids appear to be an efficacious adjunctive therapy in HIV-infected patients with *P carinii* pneumonia.

B. General Measures: Oxygen, and, if needed, mechanical ventilation are important supportive measures. The cause of impaired immunity should be eliminated if known and possible.

Prophylaxis

Use of trimethoprim combined with sulfamethoxazole in subtherapeutic doses prevents infection in patients at risk if administered throughout the period of increased susceptibility.

Other potentially useful prophylactic regimens include aerosol-ized pentamidine, intravenous pentamidine, oral pyrimeth-amine–sulfadoxine (Fansidar), dapsone, and dapsone–trimeth-orpim.

Prophylaxis is provided to HIV-infected patients at high risk for *P carinii* pneumonia, including those with a prior episode, those with low T_4 cell count ($< 200/mm^3$ or $< 20\%$ of lympho-cytes in adolescents and adults and according to age-specific criteria in children), and, according to some experts, to all HIV-infected children < 1 year of age.

METAZOAL DISEASES

Metazoal diseases are outlined in Table 11–4.

MYCOTIC INFECTIONS

Many of the systemic mycoses share a number of character-istics. Infection of humans occurs through inhalation of free-living infectious spores of the fungus, which are present in the dust in endemic areas. Primary pulmonary infections are usually mild or asymptomatic, and most infections have a tendency to heal, mainly through cellular immune mechanisms. Specific skin tests become positive after primary infection and remain positive throughout life. In a few specifically predisposed persons, the disease progresses after primary infection (immediately or after a latent period), becomes disseminated and involves many organs, and may be fatal. Dissemination may occur years after primary infection if the person is subsequently immunosuppressed by disease (eg, lymphoma) or drugs.

SYSTEMIC MYCOSES

Systemic mycoses are outlined in Table 11–5.

CANDIDIASIS

Candida albicans and other *Candida* species are found in the normal flora of human mucous membranes, especially in the

Table 11-4. Diseases caused by helminths.

Agent	Geographic Prevalence	Definitive Host (Mature Worms)	Intermediate Host (Larval Stages)	Route of Human Infection	Directly Communicable Human to Human	Eggs in Human Feces	Stage of Parasite Causing Disease	Pathology	Diagnostic Tests	Specific Treatment (Drugs Listed in Order of Preference)
Ancylostoma braziliense, A caninum (cat and dog hookworm)	Southern USA	Cats, dogs	Humans	Invasion of larvae in soil through skin	No	No	Larva	Cutaneous larva migrans, with serpiginous skin eruption at site of entry.	Clinical diagnosis	Self-limited; freezing, thiabendazole
Ancylostoma duodenale, Necator americanus (hookworm)	Tropics and subtropics. Europe, Asia	Humans	—	Larvae in soil enter through skin	Yes	Yes	Larva in skin and lungs; adult in bowel	Dermatitis and pneumonitis in larval stage; anemia, melena, anorexia from adult worm in bowel.	Detection of ova in stool	Mebendazole, pyrantel pamoate
Ascaris lumbricoides (roundworm)	Tropics and areas with poor sanitation	Humans	—	Ingestional of eggs in soil	Yes (via soil)	Yes	Larva in lungs; adult in bowel	Pneumonitis in larval stage; adult worm may cause intestinal obstruction, abdominal pain, peritonitis.	Detection of ova or adult worms in stool	Pyrantel pamoate, mebendazole, albendazole
Diphyllobothrium latum (fish tapeworm)	Worldwide	Humans, other mammals	Copepods, fish	Ingestion of fish containing larval worms	No	Yes	Adult	Vitamin B12 deficiency; intestinal irritation; anemia.	Identification of ova or proglottids in stool	Niclosamide, praziquantel

(continued)

Table 11-4. Diseases caused by helminths (continued).

Agent	Geographic Prevalence	Definitive Host (Mature Worms)	Intermediate Host (Larval Stages)	Route of Human Infection	Directly Communicable Human to Human	Eggs in Human Feces	Stage of Parasite Causing Disease	Pathology	Diagnostic Tests	Specific Treatment (Drugs Listed in Order of Preference)
Dipylidium caninum (dog tapeworm)	Worldwide	Dogs, cats, humans	Fleas	Ingestion of fleas containing larval worms	No	Yes	Adult	Intestinal irritation.	Identification of ova in stool	Niclosamide, praziquantel
Echinococcus granulosus (unilocular hydatid cyst)	Scattered foci worldwide	Dogs, wolves	Domestic and wild herbivores, (including sheep), humans	Ingestion of worm eggs from canine feces	No	No	Larva (hydatid)	Circumscribed unilocular cysts in lung, liver, other viscera.	History, radiographs, serology, biopsies	Surgical removal, mebendazole, albendazole
Echinococcus multilocularis (alveolar hydatid cyst)	Northern hemisphere	Foxes, dogs	Field rodents, humans	Ingestion of worm eggs from canine feces	No	No	Larva (hydatid)	Invasive multilocular cysts in liver.	History, radiographs, biopsies, serology	Surgical removal; mebendazole
Enterobius vermicularis (pinworm)	Worldwide	Humans	—	Ingestion of eggs on clothing, on food, in dust, etc	Yes	Yes	Adult female	Anal irritation and itching; vaginal inflammation; abdominal pain.	Scotch tape exam under microscope	Pyrantel pamoate, mebendazole
Hymenolepis nana (dwarf tapeworm)	Worldwide in warm climates	Humans, rodents	Humans, rodents	Ingestion of worm eggs from human feces or infected insects	Yes	Yes	Adult	Intestinal irritation.	Detection of ova in stool	Niclosamide, praziquantel

Organism	Distribution	Definitive host	Intermediate host	Mode of infection				Disease	Diagnosis	Treatment
Schistosoma mansoni, S japonicum, S haematobium (blood flukes)	S mansoni— tropics; S japonicum—Far East, SE Asia; S haematobium— Africa, Asia	Humans	Snails	Invasion of skin by cercariae in bodies of fresh water	No	Yes (S mansoni and S japonicum) (S haematobium in urine)	Adult	Maturation in veins draining intestines (S mansoni, S japonicum) or bladder (S haematobium), producing enteritis, hepatomegaly, portal hypertension, or hematuria and urinary symptoms.	Demonstration of eggs in stool or urine, tissue biopsies, serology	Praziquantel, oxamniquine (S mansoni), metrifonate (S haematobium), surgical removal
Strongyloides stercoralis (threadworm)	Tropics and subtropics	Humans, dogs, cats	—	Larvae enter through skin	Yes	Rare	Larva and adult	Pneumonitis and intestinal irritation, disseminated disease in immunocompromised host	Identification of larvae in stool or duodenal aspirate, serology	Thiabendazole, Ivermectin
Taenia saginata (beef tapeworm)	Africa, Central and South America, Europe, Asia	Humans	Cattle	Ingestion of beef containing larval worms	No	Yes	Adult	Intestinal irritation with nausea, diarrhea.	Identification of ova or proglottids in stool, serology	Niclosamide, praziquantel

387

(continued)

Table 11-4. Diseases caused by helminths (continued).

Agent	Geographic Prevalence	Definitive Host (Mature Worms)	Intermediate Host (Larval Stages)	Route of Human Infection	Directly Communicable Human to Human	Eggs in Human Feces	Stage of Parasite Causing Disease	Pathology	Diagnostic Tests	Specific Treatment (Drugs Listed in Order of Preference)
Taenia solium (pork tapeworm)	Africa, Asia, Central and South America, Europe	Humans	Hogs	Ingestion of pork containing larval worms	Yes	Yes	Adult	Intestinal irritation with nausea, diarrhea.	Identification of ova or proglottids in stool, serology	Niclosamide, praziquantel
			Humans	Ingestion of worm eggs from human feces	No	No	Larva (cysticercus)	Cysticercosis with lesions in muscles, brain, viscera, eyes. Seizures common.	Muscle or brain biopsy; CT scan (head); serology	Surgical removal, praziquantel, albendazole, corticosteroids
Toxocara canis, T. cati (dog and cat roundworm)	North America, Europe	Dogs, cats	Humans	Ingestion of worm eggs in soil	No	No	Larva	Visceral larva migrans with fever, systemic symptoms, and infection of eyes, lung, heart, brain, liver.	Eosinophilia, organ biopsy, serology	Thiabendazole, diethylcarbamazine, corticosteroids
Trichinella spiralis (trichina worm)	Worldwide	Hogs, bears, rats, humans	Hogs, bears, rats, humans	Ingestion of larvae in meat	no	No	Larva in muscle, heart, and brain	Encystment of larvae in tissue (especially muscle) causes necrosis and inflam-	Eosinophilia, serology, muscle biopsy, exam of suspect meat	Mebendazole, thiabendazole, corticosteroids

	Geographic distribution	Reservoir		Transmission			Stage	Pathology/Symptoms	Diagnosis	Treatment
Trichuris trichiura (whipworm)	Worldwide	Humans	—	Ingestion of eggs in soil	Yes (via soil)	Yes	Adult	mation. Symptoms produced include diarrhea, myalgia, fever, periorbital edema, urticaria, headache, myocardial failure. Adult worm in mucosa of colon usually produces no reactions or symptoms. Abdominal pain, colitis, and rectal prolapse may occur in severe infections.	Identification of ova in stool	Mebendazole
Wuchereria bancrofti, Brugia malayi, B timori (filaria)	Tropics, subtropics	Humans	Humans, mosquitoes	Bite by infected mosquito	No	No	Adult	Inflammation or obstruction of lymphatics, producing lymphadenopathy, lymphangitis, edema of extremities and genitalia.	Demonstration of microfilariae in blood, tissue biopsies, serology	Diethylcarbamazine citrate, Ivermectin, corticosteroids, surgical removal, treatment of superinfections

Table 11-5. Systemic mycoses.

Disease	Organism	Geographic Prevalence/ Environmental Source	Primary Infection	Disseminated Disease	Laboratory Findings	Treatment
Coccidioidomy- cosis	*Coccidioidesim- mitis*	S.W. USA, Mexico, Central and South America/Soil	Asymptomatic or fever, headache, myal- gias, arthralgias, rash, URI, bronchitis, ± pulmonary cavity.	Pneumonia, empy- ema, osteomyelitis, soft tissue infection, abdominal visceral in- volvement, meningitis	Elevated ESR, white blood cell count. CXR densities and enlarged nodes. Positive anti- body, smears and cul- tures.	Primary infec- tion—therapy gener- ally not required. Dis- seminated disease—Amphoteri- cin B; ketoconazole; fluconazole; itraco- nazole? Surgical exci- sion; CSF shunting.
Histoplasmosis	*Histoplasma cap- sulatum*	Central and South- ern USA/Dust, silos, bird and bat feces	Asymptomatic or in- fluenza-like. Also, pneumonitis, fever, cough, chest pain, and enlarged nodes, liver, spleen.	Fever, anemia, ade- nopathy, hepatomeg- aly, splenomegaly, pneumonitis, bone le- sions, cutaneous granulomas. Chronic pulmonary histoplas- mosis may occur.	Leukopenia, anemia, elevated ESR. Positive smears (bone marrow & other tissues), cul- tures, and antibody. CXR consolidations ± calcifications.	Primary infec- tion—generally not required. Dissemi- nated disease—am- photericin B; ketoco- nazole; itraconazole? Surgical excision.
Blastomycosis (North American)	*Blastomyces der- matitidis*	Central and South- eastern USA, Cen- tral and South Amer- ica/Soil	Cutaneous ulcerating papule and ab- scesses. Pulmonary densities, empyema, and lymph node en- largement.	Cough, fever, cuta- neous lesions; brain abscesses; abdomi- nal viscera, bone, muscle involvement.	Positive smears, cul- tures, and antibody.	Amphotericin B; keto- conazole

Paracoccidioidomycosis (South American Blastomycosis)	*Paracoccidioides brasiliensis*	Central and South America/Soil	Skin and mucous membrane granulomatous lesions.	Spread to lymph nodes, gut, lung, other viscera.	Positive smears, cultures, and antibody.	Ketoconazole; miconazole; amphotericin B
Cryptococcosis	*Cryptococcus neoformans*	Worldwide/Soil, bird feces	Asymptomatic or influenza-like. Pulmonary consolidation.	Meningitis, bone or skin lesions. lymphadenopathy	CSF inflammation, positive CSF antigen, India ink smear, culture.	Primary infection—generally does not require treatment. Disseminated disease—Amphotericin B, with flucytosine; fluconazole. Surgical excision.
Sporotrichosis	*Sporothrix schenkii*	Worldwide/Plant matter	Subcutaneous nodules and ulcers, with spread along lymphatics.	Spread to bones, joints, lung, brain uncommon	Positive smears and cultures from lesions (drainage or biopsy)	Potassium iodide; amphotericin B; itraconazole?
Aspergillosis	*Aspergillus fumigatus, Flavus niger*	Worldwide/Soil, vegetable matter	Allergic bronchopulmonary disease: episodic fever, wheezing, fleeting infiltrates. Fungus balls in prior pulmonary cavities.	Sinusitis; pulmonary infection; bone, abdominal viscera, CNS involvement	Positive smears and cultures. Allergic bronchopulmonary aspergillosis: elevated IgE and eosinophils, positive precipitins to Aspergillus, airway colonization	Amphotericin B ± flucytosine or rifampin; itraconazole. Surgical excision. Corticosteroids for allergic broncho-pulmonary disease.

respiratory, gastrointestinal, and female genital tracts. In these locations, *Candida* may proliferate and produce local lesions, and from these locations, may disseminate.

Clinical Findings

   A. Symptoms and Signs: Moist, warm, eroded skin in intertriginous areas, the diaper area, or nails are subject to chronic surface infection. Mucous membranes of the mouth (thrush) and vagina (vaginitis) are made more susceptible to overgrowth of *Candida* by use of antimicrobial agents that suppress normal flora or by use of corticosteroids. Rarely, *Candida* invades tissues or the bloodstream, as in patients with indwelling catheters, immunodeficiency, leukemia, parenteral drug abuse, or prematurity, and may then cause progressive systemic lesions, pneumonia, endocarditis, and involvement of other organs.

   B. Laboratory Findings: Diagnosis is based on visualization of yeast and pseudohyphae in material from lesions or infected tissues or on culture of *Candida* from blood, cerebrospinal fluid, urine, or involved organs.

Treatment

   Treatment consists of keeping local lesions dry and applying topical nystatin, clotrimazole, gentian violet, miconazole, amphotericin B, or other antifungals. Ketoconazole has proved effective in many cases of esophageal candidiasis and chronic mucocutaneous disease. Treatment with amphotericin B intravenously is the approach of choice for systemic infections. Oral flucytosine is added for synergy in severe infections. Therapy is usually prolonged (weeks to months). Fluconazole is useful for esophagitis, refractory thrush, candidemia, and some cases of disseminated disease.

Prognosis

   The prognosis is good for patients with local lesions but guarded for those with systemic dissemination.

Skin | 12

Joseph G. Morelli, MD, &
William L. Weston, MD

Terminology

A. Primary Lesions (The First to Appear):

1. Macule–Any circumscribed color change in the skin that is flat. Examples: White (vitiligo), brown (café au lait spot), purple (petechia).

2. Papule–A solid, elevated lesion smaller than 1 cm in diameter whose top may be pointed, rounded, or flat. Examples: Acne, warts, small lesion of psoriasis.

3. Plaque–A solid, circumscribed area greater than 1 cm in diameter, usually flat-topped. Example: Psoriasis.

4. Vesicle–A circumscribed, elevated lesion less than 1 cm in diameter and containing clear serous fluid. Example: Blisters of herpes simplex.

5. Bulla–A circumscribed, elevated lesion greater than 1 cm in diameter and containing clear serous fluid. Example: Bullous erythema multiforme.

6. Nodule–A deep-seated mass with indistinct borders that elevates the overlying epidermis. Examples: Tumors, granuloma annulare. If it moves with the skin on palpation, it is intradermal; if the skin moves over the nodule, it is subcutaneous.

7. Wheal–A circumscribed, flat-topped, firm elevation of skin resulting from tense edema of the papillary dermis. Example: Urticaria.

B. Secondary Changes:

1. Pustule–A vesicle containing a purulent exudate. Examples: Acne, folliculitis.

2. Scales–Dry, thin plates of keratinized epidermal cells (stratum corneum). Examples: Psoriasis, ichthyosis.

3. Lichenification–Dry, leathery thickening of the skin with deep and exaggerated skin lines and a shiny surface resulting from chronic rubbing of the skin. Example: Atopic dermatitis.

4. Erosion and Oozing–A moist, circumscribed, slightly depressed area representing a blister base with the roof of the blister removed. Examples: Burns, impetigo. Most oral blisters present as erosions.

5. Crust–Dried exudate of plasma on the surface of the skin following acute dermatitis.

6. Fissure–A linear split in the skin extending through the epidermis into the dermis. Example: Angular cheilitis.

7. Scar–A flat, raised, or depressed area of fibrotic replacement of dermis or subcutaneous tissue. Examples: Acne, scar, burn scar.

8. Atrophy–Depression of the skin surface due to thinning of one or more layers of skin.

C. Color: The lesion should be described as red, yellow, brown, tan, or blue. Particular attention should be given to the blanching of red or brown lesions, eg, petechiae.

D. Configuration: Clues to diagnosis may be obtained from the characteristic morphologic arrangement of primary or secondary lesions.

1. Annular (circular)–Annular nodules represent granuloma annular; annular papules are more apt to be due to dermatophyte infections.

2. Linear (straight line)–Linear papules represent lichen striatus; linear vesicles, incontinentia pigmenti; linear papules with burrow, scabies.

3. Grouped–Grouped vesicles occur in herpes simplex or zoster.

E. Distribution: It is useful to note whether the eruption is generalized, acral (hands, feet, buttocks, or face), or localized to a specific skin region.

F. Description of Skin Lesions: Skin lesions are described in reverse order from that of their identification. One begins with distribution, followed by configuration, color, secondary changes, and then primary lesion; eg, guttate psoriasis could be described as generalized discrete, red, scaly papules.

GENERAL PRINCIPLES OF TREATMENT
OF SKIN DISORDERS

Percutaneous Absorption & the Role of Water

Treatment should be simple and aimed at preserving or restoring the physiologic state of skin. It is essential to keep in mind that one is treating the child and not the anxious parent or grandparent. Topical therapy is often preferred because medica-

Table 12–1. Bases used for topical preparations.

Base	Combined With	Uses
Liquids		Wet dressings: relieve pruritus, vasoconstrict.
	Powder	Shake lotions, drying pastes: relieve pruritus, vasoconstrict.
	Grease and emulsifier; oil in water	Vanishing cream: penetrates quickly (10–15 minutes) and thus allows evaporation.
	Excess grease and emulsifier; water in oil	Emollient cream: penetrates more slowly and thus retains moisture on skin.
Grease		Ointments: occlusive (hold material on skin for prolonged time) and prevent evaporation of water.
Powder		Enhances evaporation.

(1) Most greases are triglycerides (eg, Aquaphor, petrolatum, Eucerin).
(2) Oils are fluid fats (eg, Alpha Keri, olive oil, mineral oil).
(3) True fats (eg, lard, animal fats) contain free fatty acids that increase in amount upon standing and cause irritation.
(4) Ointments (eg, Aquaphor, petrolatum) should not be used in intertriginous areas such as the axillas, between the toes, and in the perineum, because they increase maceration. Lotions or creams are preferred in these areas.
(5) Oils and ointments hold medication on the skin for long periods of time and are therefore ideal for barriers or prophylaxis and for dried areas of skin. Medication gets into the skin more slowly from ointments.
(6) Creams carry medication into skin and are preferable for intertriginous dermatitis.
(7) Solutions, gels, or lotions should be used for scalp treatment.

tion can be delivered in optimal concentrations at the exact site where it is needed.

Water is an important therapeutic agent that is often forgotten (it is the active ingredient in Burrow's solution, calamine lotion, potassium permanganate, and tannic acid soaks). When the skin is optimally hydrated, it is soft and smooth (Table 12–1). This occurs at approximately 60% environmental humidity. Since water evaporates readily from the cutaneous surface, the skin (stratum corneum of the epidermis) is dependent on the water concentration in the air, and sweating contributes little. However, if sweat is prevented from evaporating (eg, in the axilla or groin), the environmental humidity is increased and so is the hydration of the skin. As environmental humidity falls below

15–20%, the stratum corneum shrinks and cracks; the epidermal barrier is lost and allows irritants to enter the skin and induce an inflammatory response. Replacement of water will correct this if the water is not allowed to evaporate. Therefore, in treating dry and scaly skin, one would soak the skin in water for 5 minutes and then add a barrier to prevent evaporation. Oils and ointments prevent evaporation for 8–12 hours. Thus, oils and ointments must be applied once or twice a day. In areas already occluded (axilla, diaper area), ointments or oils will merely increase retention of water and should not be used.

Overhydration (maceration) can also occur. As environmental humidity increases to 90–100%, the number of water molecules absorbed by the stratum corneum increases and the tight lipid junctions between the cells of the stratum corneum are gradually replaced by weak hydrogen bonds (water); the cells eventually become widely separated, and the epidermal barrier falls apart. This occurs in immersion foot, diaper areas, axillas, and other areas of the body exposed to excessive hydration. It is desirable to enhance evaporation of water in these areas. Exposure to less humidity and the use of powders (talcum) that take up extra water are indicated in maceration.

Evaporation of water is also cooling, vasoconstrictive ("gets the red out"), and antipruritic—all desirable objectives in the management of itchy, red skin. Water applied frequently to the skin and allowed to dry will result in drying of the skin surface.

Wet Dressing

By placing the skin in an environment where the humidity is 100% and allowing the moisture to evaporate to 60%, pruritus is relieved. Evaporation of water stimulates cold-dependent nerve fibers in the skin—thereby, theoretically, tying up the circuits so that the itching sensation coming through the pain fibers will not reach the central nervous system. Water also is vasoconstrictive, which helps reduce the erythema and decrease the inflammatory cellular response.

Gauze of 20/12 mesh is commonly used for wet dressings. Parke-Davis 4-in gauze comes in 100-yard rolls, and 5 yards is usually sufficient for application to the extremities. Curity 18-in gauze can be used for application to the trunk. An alternative is to use the "2 longjohns" technique, in which a pair of wet cotton long-sleeved and long-legged underwear is covered by a dry pair.

Warm but not hot water is used, and the gauze or longjohns

are soaked in the water and then wrung out until no more drops come out. The dressings are then wrapped around the extremities and fastened with a safety pin. The wet dressing is then covered with dry flannel or dry longjohns, which will slow down the evaporation process but not completely retard it, so the wet dressings need only be changed every 3 or 4 hours.

Topical Glucocorticosteroids

Topical glucocorticosteroids (Table 12–2) can be used under wet dressings. Fluocinolone acetonide cream (Fluonid, Synalar 0.01%) is made specifically for this purpose. If these steroids are to be used, the wet dressings are removed completely and the medications replaced every 4–6 hours; this is usually sufficient to completely clear a severe generalized dermatitis. Prolonged use of this treatment will result in significant systemic absorption of steroids. Establishing a higher concentration of corticosteroid drugs in the skin by topical rather than systemic therapy will result in marked clearing. Because of the high concentration of steroids remaining in the skin, the mainstay of treatment of chronic forms of atopic dermatitis is application of topical glucocorticosteroid preparations twice daily (Table 12–2).

Table 12–2. Topical glucocorticosteroids.

	Concentrations (Percent)
Low potency = 1	
Hydrocortisone	1.0
Desonide	0.05
Moderate potency = 5–10	
Triamcinolone acetonide	0.025 and 0.1
Fluocinoline acetonide	0.01 and 0.025
Hydrocortisone valerate	0.2
Flurandrenolide	0.025
Flumethasone pivalate	0.03
Betamethasone valerate	0.1
Betamethasone acetate	0.2
Betamethasone dipropionate	0.05
Methylprednisolone acetate	0.25
Betamethasone benzoate	0.025
Desoximetasone	0.25
Diflorasone diacetate	0.05
High potency = 10–100	
Fluocinonide	0.05
Halcinonide	0.025 and 0.1

DISORDERS OF THE SKIN IN NEWBORNS

Transient Diseases in the Newborn

No treatment is required for any of these disorders, although treatment may be given as noted below.

Milia

Multiple white papules 1 mm in diameter scattered over the forehead, nose, and cheeks are present in up to 40% of newborn infants. Histologically, they represent superficial epidermal cysts filled with keratinous material associated with the developing pilosebaceous follicle. Their intraoral counterparts are called Epstein's pearls and are even more common than facial milia. All these cystic structures spontaneously rupture and exfoliate their contents.

Sebaceous Gland Hyperplasia

Prominent yellow macules at the opening of each pilosebaceous follicle, predominantly over the nose, represent overgrowth of sebaceous glands in response to the same androgenic stimulation that occurs in adolescence.

Acne Neonatorum

Open and closed comedones, erythematous papules, and pustules identical in appearance to adolescent acne may occur in infants over the forehead, cheeks, and chin. The lesions may be present at birth but usually do not appear until 3–4 weeks of age. Spontaneous resolution occurs over a period of 6 months to a year. Rarely, neonatal acne may be a manifestation of a virilizing syndrome.

Harlequin Color Change

A cutaneous vascular phenomenon unique to neonates occurs when the infant (particularly one of low birth weight) is placed on one side. The dependent half develops an erythematous flush with a sharp demarcation at the midline, and the upper half of the body becomes pale. The color changes usually subside within a few seconds after the infant is placed supine but may persist for as long as 20 minutes.

Mottling

A lacelike pattern of dilated cutaneous vessels appears over the extremities and often on the trunk of neonates exposed to lowered room temperature. This feature is transient and usually disappears completely upon rewarming.

Erythema Toxicum

Up to 50% of term infants develop erythema toxicum. Usually at 24–48 hours of age, blotchy erythematous macules 2–3 cm in diameter appear, most prominently on the chest but also on the back, face, and extremities. These are occasionally present at birth, and rarely have their onset after 4–5 days of life. The lesions vary in number from 2 to 3, up to as many as 100. Incidence is much higher in term infants than in premature ones. The macular erythema may fade within 24–48 hours or may progress to develop urticarial wheals in the center of the macules or, in 10% of cases, pustules. Examination of a Wright-stained smear of the lesion will reveal numerous eosinophils. This may be accompanied by peripheral blood eosinophilia of up to 20%. All the lesions fade and disappear by 5–7 days. A similar eruption in black newborns has a neutrophilic predominance and leaves hyperpigmentation.

Sucking Blisters

Bullae, either intact or in the form of an erosion representing a blister base without inflammatory borders, may occur over the forearms, wrists, thumbs, or upper lip. These presumably result from vigorous sucking in utero. They resolve without complications.

Miliaria

Obstruction of the eccrine sweat ducts occurs often in neonates and produces one of 2 clinical pictures depending upon the level of obstruction. **Miliaria crystallina** is characterized by tiny (1–2 mm) superficial grouped vesicles without erythema over intertriginous areas and adjacent skin (eg, neck and upper chest). Obstruction occurs in the stratum corneum portion of the eccrine duct. More commonly, obstruction of the eccrine duct deeper in the epidermis results in erythematous grouped papules in the same areas and is called **miliaria rubra.** Rarely, these may progress to pustules. Heat and high humidity predispose to eccrine duct port closure. Removal to a cooler environment is the treatment of choice.

Subcutaneous Fat Necrosis

Reddish or purple, sharply circumscribed, firm nodules occurring over the cheeks, buttocks, arms, and thighs and occurring between day 1 and day 7 in infants represent subcutaneous fat necrosis. Cold injury is thought to play an important role. These lesions resolve spontaneously over a period of weeks, although like all instances of fat necrosis they may calcify.

Sclerema

Premature newborns, especially those who suffer metabolic alterations (eg, metabolic acidosis, hypoglycemia, hypothermia) are susceptible to a diffused hardening of the skin that makes the skin look shiny and feel tight. Severe cold injury in under-nourished infants is assumed to be the cause.

Treatment consists of protecting the infant from undue exposure to cold and repairing metabolic and nutritional deficiencies.

BIRTHMARKS

Birthmarks may involve an overgrowth of one or more of any of the normal components of skin: pigment cells, blood vessels, lymph vessels, etc. A nervus is a hamartoma of highly differentiated cells that retain their normal function.

1. PIGMENT CELL BIRTHMARKS

Mongolian Spot

A blue-black macule found over the lumbosacral area in 90% of American Indian, black, and Oriental infants is called a mongolian spot. These spots are occasionally noted over the shoulders and back and may extend over the buttocks. Histologically, they consist of spindle-shaped pigment cells located deep in the dermis. The lesions fade somewhat with time, but some traces may persist into adult life.

Café au Lait Spot

A café au lait spot is a light brown, oval macule (dark brown on black skin) that may be found anywhere on the body. Ten percent of white and 22% of black children have café au lait spots greater than 1.5 cm in their longest diameter. These lesions persist throughout life and may increase in number with age. The presence of 6 or more café au lait macules greater than 1.5

cm in their longest diameter may represent a clue to neurofibromatosis. Patients with Albright's syndrome also have increased numbers of café au lait macules.

Junctional Nevus & Compound Nevus

Dark brown or black macules, usually few in number at birth but becoming more numerous with age, represent junctional nevi. Histologically, these lesions are large clones of melanocytes at the junction of the epidermis and dermis. With aging, they may become raised (papules) and contain intradermal melanocytes, creating a compound nevus. Often the surface becomes irregular and roughened.

Intradermal Nevus & Blue Nevus

Brown to blue solitary papules with smooth surfaces represent intradermal nevi. When pigmentation is present deeper in the dermis, the lesions appear blue or blue-black and are called blue nevi.

Spindle & Epitheloid Cell Nevus

A reddish-brown solitary nodule appearing on the face or upper arm of a child represents a spindle and epitheloid cell nevus. Histologically, it consists of pigment-producing cells of bizarre shape with numerous mitoses. Clinically, it is always a benign lesion.

Giant Pigmented Nevus (Bathing Trunk Nevus)

An irregular dark brown to black plaque over 10 cm in diameter represents a giant pigmented nevus. Often the lesions are of such size as to cover the entire trunk (bathing trunk nevi). Histologically, they are compound nevi. Transformation to malignant melanoma has been reported in as many as 10% of cases in some series, although the true incidence is probably somewhat less. Malignant change may rarely occur at birth or at any time thereafter.

2. VASCULAR BIRTHMARKS

Flat Hemangioma

Flat vascular birthmarks can be divided into 2 types: those that are orange or light red (salmon patch) and those that are dark red or bluish red (port wine stain).

A. Salmon Patch: The salmon patch is a light red macule found over the nape of the neck, upper eyelids, and glabella. Fifty percent of infants have such lesions over their necks. Eyelid lesions fade completely within 3–6 months and most glabella lesions by age 5 to 6; those on the nape of the neck fade somewhat but may persist into adult life.

B. Port Wine Stain: Port wine stains are dark red or purple maculas appearing anywhere on the body. A port wine stain covering a large portion of the face, including the first and second branches of the trigeminal nerve, may be a clue to **Sturge-Weber syndrome,** which is characterized by seizures, mental retardation, glaucoma, and hemiplegia. Most infants with unilateral port wine stains do not have Sturge–Weber syndrome.

Similarly, a port wine hemangioma over an extremity may be associated with hypertrophy of the soft tissue and bone of that extremity **(Kippel–Trenaunay syndrome).**

The newest treatment consists of a pulse dye laser. Infants as young as 2 weeks of age have been successfully treated.

Hemangioma

A red, rubbery nodule with a roughened surface is a hemangioma. The lesion is often not present at birth but is represented by a permanent blanched area on the skin that is supplanted at 2–4 weeks of age by red nodules. Histologically, these are benign tumors of endothelial cells. Fifty percent resolve spontaneously by age 5; 70% by age 7; 90% by age 9; and the rest do not resolve.

Hemangiomas resolve, leaving redundant skin, hyperpigmentation, telangiectasia, and fibrofatty deposits. The most common complication is ulceration and secondary bacterial infection. Treatment of noninfected ulceration is with the pulsed dye laser. Infected lesions require oral antibiotics.

Major complications are (1) thrombocytopenia due to platelet trapping within the lesion **(Kasabach–Merritt syndrome);** (2) airway obstruction (hemangiomas of the head and neck are often associated with subglottic hemangiomas); (3) visual obstruction (with resulting amblyopia); and (4) cardiac decompensation (high output failure). In these instances, the treatment of choice is prednisone, 1–2 mg/kg orally daily or every other day for 4–6 weeks. Recently, interferon α has been used to treat hemangiomas unresponsive to prednisone.

Lymphangioma

Deep lymphangiomas are rubbery, skin-colored nodules commonly occurring in the parotid area (**cystic hygroma**). Superficial lymphangiomas are clear. They often result in grotesque enlargement of soft tissue.

Surgical excision is the only treatment available, although the results are not satisfactory.

3. EPIDERMAL BIRTHMARKS

Nevus Unius Lateris & Ichthyosis Hystrix

Linear or groups of linear, warty, papular, unilateral lesions represent overgrowth of epidermis. These areas may range from dirty yellow to brown or may be darkly pigmented. The histologic features of the lesions include thickening of the epidermis and elongation of the rete ridges and hyperkeratosis. Clinically, the lesions are rarely associated with focal motor seizures, mental subnormality, and skeletal anomalies.

Treatment once or twice daily with topical tretinoin 0.05% (retinoic acid [Retin-A]) may keep the lesions flat.

Nevus Comedonicus

The lesion known as nevus comedonicus consists of linear groups of widely dilated follicular openings plugged with keratin, giving the appearance of localized noninflammatory acne. The treatment of choice is surgical removal. If this is not feasible, topical retinoic acid is helpful.

Nevus Sebaceous

The nevus sebaceous of Jadassohn is a hamartoma of sebaceous glands and underlying apocrine glands that is diagnosed by the appearance at birth of a yellowish, hairless, smooth, plaque in the scalp or on the face.

Histologically, nevus sebaceous represents an overabundance of sebaceous glands without hair follicles. At puberty, with androgenic stimulation, the sebaceous cells in the nevus divide, expanding their cellular volume, and synthesize sebum, resulting in a warty mass.

Because 15% of these lesions become basal cell carcinomas after puberty, excision before puberty is recommended.

4. CONNECTIVE TISSUE BIRTHMARKS

Connective tissue nevi are smooth, skin-colored papules 1–10 mm in diameter that are grouped on the trunk. A solitary, larger (5–10 cm) nodule is called a **shagreen patch** and is histologically indistinguishable from other connective tissue nevi that show thickened, abundant collagen bundles with or without associated increases of elastic tissue. Although the shagreen patch is a cutaneous clue to tuberous sclerosis, the other connective tissue nevi occur as isolated events.

These nevi remain throughout life, and no treatment is necessary.

HEREDITARY SKIN DISORDERS

The Ichthyoses

Ichthyosis is a term applied to several heritable diseases characterized by the presence of excessive scales on the skin. The nomenclature of this group of diseases is confusing. Major categories are listed in Table 12–3. X-linked ichthyosis is related to cholesterol sulfatase deficiency.

Control scaling with hydroxy acids, eg, 5% pyruvic, citric, lactic, or salicylic acid in petrolatum applied once or twice daily. Restoring water to the skin is also very helpful.

Epidermolysis Bullosa

The diagnostic feature of this group of diseases is the formation of hemorrhagic blisters in response to slight trauma. They can be divided into scarring and nonscarring types (Table 12–4).

Treatment usually consists of systemic antibiotics for infection, protective dressings of petrolatum or zinc oxide, and cooling the skin.

Incontinentia Pigmenti

Linear blisters in the newborn represent incontinentia pigmenti. These are replaced by hypertrophic, linear, warty bands within several months, followed by swirling brown hyperpigmentation. Most cases are thought to be X-linked dominant, lethal to the male. Mental retardation and seizures were reported in as many as 30% of cases in one series, but the true incidence is probably much less.

Table 12–3. Four major types of ichthyosis.[1]

Name	Age at Onset	Clinical Features	Histology	Inheritance
Ichthyosis with normal epidermal turnover				
Ichthyosis vulgaris	Childhood	Fine scales, deep palmar and plantar markings	Decreased to absent granular layer, hyperkeratosis	Autosomal dominant
X-linked ichthyosis	Birth	Palms and soles spared; thick scales that darken with age; corneal opacities in patients and carrier mothers	Hyperkeratosis	X-linked
Ichthyosis with increased epidermal turnover				
Epidermolytic hyperkeratosis	Birth	Verrucous, yellow scales in flexural areas and palms and soles	Hyperkeratosis, vacuolated reticular spaces in epidermis	Autosomal dominant
Lamellar ichthyosis	Birth; collodion baby	Erythroderma, ectropion, large coarse scales; thickened palms and soles	Hyperkeratosis, many mitotic figures	Autosomal recessive

[1] Reproduced, with permission, from Frost P, Weinstein GD: Ichthyosiform dermatoses. In: *Dermatology in General Medicine.* Fitzpatrick TB (editor). McGraw-Hill, 1971.

405

Table 12-4. Types of epidermolysis bullosa.

Name	Age at Onset	Clinical Features	Histology	Inheritance
Nonscarring types				
Epidermolysis bullosa simplex	Birth	Hemorrhagic blisters over the lower legs; cooling prevents blisters	Disintegration of basal cells	Autosomal dominant
Recurrent bullous eruption of the hands and feet (Weber-Cockayne syndrome)	First few years of life	Blisters brought out by walking	Cytolysis of suprabasal cells; keratotic cells	Autosomal dominant
Junctional bullous epimatosis (Herlitz disease)	Birth	Erosions on legs, oral mucosa; severe perioral involvement	Separation between plasma membrane of basal cells and PAS-positive basal lamina	Autosomal recessive
Scarring types				
Epidermolysis bullosa dystrophica, dominant	Infancy	Numerous blisters on hands and feet; milia formation	Separation of PAS-positive basal lamina; anchoring fibrils lost	Autosomal dominant
Epidermolysis bullosa dystrophica, recessive	Birth	Repeated episodes of blistering, secondary infection and scarring—"mitten hands and feet"	Separation below PAS-positive basal lamina; anchoring fibrils lost	Autosomal recessive

406

COMMON SKIN DISEASES IN INFANTS, CHILDREN, & ADOLESCENTS

ACNE

Clinical Findings

The common forms of acne in pediatric patients occur at 2 ages: in the newborn period and in adolescence. Neonatal acne is a response to maternal androgen, first appearing at 4–6 weeks of age and lasting until 4–6 months of age. It is characterized by inflammatory papules with all lesions in the same stage at the same time. The lesions are seen primarily on the face, upper chest, and back, in a distribution similar to that seen in adolescent acne. It has been hypothesized but not proved that infants who have severe neonatal acne will develop severe adolescent acne.

The onset of adolescent acne is between ages 8 and 10 in 40% of children. The early lesions are usually limited to the face and are primarily closed comedones (whiteheads; see below). Eventually, 85% of adolescents will develop some form of acne.

Acne occurs in sebaceous follicles, which, unlike hair follicles, have large, abundant sebaceous glands and usually lack hair. They are located primarily on the face, upper chest, back, and penis. Obstruction of the sebaceous follicle opening produces the clinical lesion of acne. If the obstruction occurs at the follicular mouth, the clinical lesion is characterized by a wide, patulous opening filled with a plug of stratum corneum cells. This is the open comedo, or blackhead. Open comedones are the predominant clinical lesion seen in early adolescent acne. The black color is due not to dirt but to oxidized material within the stratum corneum cellular plug. Open comedones do not often progress to inflammatory lesions. Closed comedones, or whiteheads, are caused by obstruction just beneath the follicular opening in the neck of the sebaceous follicle, which produces a cystic swelling of the follicular duct directly beneath the epidermis. The stratum corneum produced accumulates continuously within the cystic cavity. The resultant lesion is an enlarging sphere just beneath the skin surface. Most authorities believe that closed comedones are precursors of inflammatory acne. If open or closed comedones are the predominant lesions on the skin in adolescent acne, it is called **comedonal acne.**

In typical adolescent acne, several different types of lesions are present simultaneously, eg, open and closed comedones and inflammatory lesions such as papules, pustules, and cysts. Inflammatory lesions may also rarely occur as interconnecting, draining sinus tracts. Adolescents with cystic acne require prompt medical attention, since ruptured cysts and sinus tracts result in severe scar formation. New acne scars are highly vascular and have a reddish or purplish hue. Such scars return to normal skin color after several years. Acne scars may be depressed beneath the skin level, raised, or flat to the skin. In adolescents with a tendency toward keloid formation, keloidal scars can occur following acne lesions, particularly over the sternal area.

Treatment

A. Topical Keratolytic Agents: Two classes of potent keratolytic agents are available: retinoic acid and benzoyl peroxide gel. These have been found to be the most efficacious agents in the treatment of acne. Either agent may be used once daily, or the combination of retinoic acid cream applied to acne-bearing areas of the skin once daily in the evening and a benzoyl peroxide gel applied once daily in the morning may be used. This regime will control 80–85% of cases of adolescent acne.

B. Topical Antibiotics: Topical antibiotics are less effective than systemic antibiotics and at best are equivalent in potency to 250 mg of tetracycline orally once a day. One percent clindamycin phosphate solution is the most efficacious of all topical antibiotics; 1.5% and 2% topical erythromycin solutions are effective; while 1% topical tetracycline solution is minimally effective.

C. Systemic Antibiotics: Antibiotics that are concentrated in sebum, such as tetracycline and erythromycin, are very effective in inflammatory acne. The usual dose is 0.5–1 g taken once or twice daily on an empty stomach (nothing to eat 1 hour before or after the medication). Tetracycline or erythromycin should be continued for 2–3 months until the acne lesions are suppressed.

D. Oral Retinoids: An oral retinoid, 13-cis-retinoic acid (isotretinoin; Accutane), offers the most efficacious treatment of severe cystic acne. The precise mechanism of its action is unknown, but decreased sebum production, decreased follicular obstruction, decreased skin bacteria, and general antiinflammatory activities have been described. The initial dosage is 40 mg once or twice daily. This drug is not effective in comedonal acne or other mild forms of acne. Side effects include dryness and scaliness of the skin, dry lips, and, occasionally, dry eyes and dry nose. Up to 10% of patients experience mild, reversible hair loss. Elevated liver enzymes and blood lipids have been described. Isotretinoin is teratogenic. Use in young women of childbearing age is not recommended.

E. Other Acne Treatments: There is no convincing evidence that dietary management, mild drying agents, abrasive scrubs, oral vitamin A, ultraviolet light, cryotherapy, or incision and drainage have any beneficial effects in the management of acne.

F. Avoidance of Cosmetics and Hair Spray: Acne can be aggravated by a variety of external factors that result in further obstruction of partially occluded sebaceous follicles. Discontinuing the use of oil-base cosmetics, face creams, and hair sprays may alleviate the comedonal component of acne within 4–6 weeks.

Patient Education & Follow-up Visits

It is important to explain the mechanism of acne and the treatment plan to adolescent patients. Time should be set aside at the first visit to answer the patient's questions. Explain that there will not be much improvement for 4–8 weeks. Establish guidelines for ideal control, and explain that the best the patient might achieve is one or two new pimples a month. A written education sheet is most useful.

BACTERIAL INFECTIONS OF THE SKIN

Impetigo

Erosions covered by honey-colored crusts are diagnostic of impetigo. Staphylococci and group A streptococci are important pathogens in this disease, which histologically consists of superficial invasion of bacteria into the upper epidermis, forming a subcorneal pustule.

Although topical antibiotics may effect a clinical cure, parenteral penicillin or oral penicillin for 10 days is necessary to eradicate streptococci. The risk of nephritogenic strains varies considerably from area to area, but active treatment of patients and contacts with systemic penicillin will significantly reduce the incidence of acute glomerulonephritis in endemic areas. Dicloxacillin or other antistaphylococcal antibiotics are used when staphylococcal infection is suspected.

Ecthyma

Ecthyma is a firm, dry crust, surrounded by erythema, that exudes purulent material. It represents deep invasion by the streptococcus through the epidermis to the superficial dermis.

Cellulitis

Cellulitis is characterized by erythematous, hot, tender, ill-defined plaques accompanied by regional lymphadenopathy. Histologically, this disorder represents invasion of microorganisms into the lower dermis and sometimes beyond, with obstruction of local lymphatics. *Haemophilus influenza, Streptococcus pneumoniae,* and *S pyogenes* are the most common offending organisms.

Septicemia is common, and treatment with the appropriate systemic antibiotic is indicated.

Folliculitis

A pustule at the follicular opening represents folliculitis. If the pustule occurs at eccrine sweat orifices, it is correctly called **poritis.** Staphylococci and streptococci are the most frequent pathogens.

Treatment consists of measures to remove follicular obstruction—either cool wet compresses for 24 hours or keratolytics such as are used for acne as well as systemic antibiotics.

Abscess

An abscess occurs deep in the skin, at the bottom of a follicle or an apocrine gland, and is diagnosed as an erythematous, firm, acutely tender nodule with ill-defined borders. Staphylococci are the most common organisms.

Treatment consists of incision and drainage and systemic antibiotics.

Scalded Skin Syndrome

This entity consists of the sudden onset of bright red, acutely painful skin, most obvious periorally, periorbitally, and in the flexural areas of the neck, the axillas, the popliteal and antecubital areas, and groin. The slightest pressure on the skin results in severe pain and separation of the epidermis, leaving a glistening layer (the stratum granulosum of the epidermis) beneath. The disease is due to a circulating toxin (exfoliation) elaborated by group II staphylococci.

In all the forms of this entity, the causative staphylococci may not be isolated from the skin but rather from the nasopharynx, an abscess, blood culture, etc.

Treatment consists of systemic administration of antistaphylococcal drugs, eg, dicloxacillin, 25–50 mg/kg/d orally, or methicillin, 200–300 mg/kg/d intravenously. No topical therapy is necessary or warranted except in the newborn, where silver sulfadiazine or other burn therapy is used.

Bullous Impetigo

All impetigo is bullous, with the blister forming just beneath the stratum corneum, but in ''bullous impetigo'' there is, in addition to the usual erosion covered by a honey-colored crust, a border filled with clear fluid. Staphylococci may be isolated from the lesions, and systemic signs of circulating exfoliation are absent. ''Bullous varicella'' is a disorder that represents bullous impetigo in varicella lesions.

Treatment with dicloxacillin, 25–50 mg/kg/d orally for 5–6 days, is effective. Application of cool compresses to debride crusts is a helpful symptomatic measure.

FUNGAL INFECTIONS OF THE SKIN

1. DERMATOPHYTE INFECTIONS

Essentials of Diagnosis

- Red, scaly, round lesions.
- Hair loss with or without scaling in tinea capitis.

General Considerations

Dermatophytes become attached to the superficial layer of the epidermis, nails, and hair, where they proliferate. They grow mainly within the stratum corneum and do not invade the lower epidermis or dermis. Release of toxins from dermatophytes, especially those whose natural host is animals or soil, eg, *Microsporum canis* and *Trichophyton verrucosum,* results in dermatitis. Fungal infection should be suspected with any red and scaly lesion.

Diagnosis

A. Tinea Capitis: Thickened, broken-off hairs with erythema and scaling of underlying scalp are distinguishing features

Table 12–5. Clinical features of tinea capitis.

Most Common Organisms	Clinical Appearance	Microscopic Appearance in KOH
Trichophyton tonsurans (60%)	Hairs broken off 2–3 mm from follicle; "black dot"; no fluorescence	Hyphae and spores within hair
Microsporum canis (39%)	Thickened broken-off hairs that fluoresce yellow-green with Wood's lamp[1]	Small spores outside of hair; hyphae within hair
Microsporum audouini (1%)	Thickened broken-off, hairs that fluoresce yellow-green with Wood's lamp[1]	Small spores outside of hair; hyphae within hair

[1] Select fluorescent hairs for examination in KOH and culture.

(Table 12–5). Pustule formation and a boggy fluctuant mass on the scalp occur in *M canis* and *T tonsurans* infections. The mass, called a **kerion,** represents an exaggerated host response to the organism. Fungal culture should be performed in all cases of suspected tinea capitis.

B. Tinea Corporis: Tinea corporis presents either as annular marginated papules with a thin scale and clear center or as an annular confluent dermatitis. The most common organisms are *T mentagrophytes* and *M canis*. The diagnosis is made by scraping thin scales from the border of the lesion, dissolving them in 20% KOH, and examining for hyphae.

C. Tinea Cruris: Symmetric, sharply marginated lesions in inguinal areas are seen with tinea cruris. The most common organisms are *T rubrun, T mentagrophytes,* and *Epidermophyton floccosum.* Scrapings taken from the border should be examined under the microscope with 20% KOH for dermatophytes.

D. Tinea Pedis: The diagnosis of tinea pedis in a prepubertal child must always be regarded with skepticism; atopic feet or contact dermatitis is a more likely diagnosis in this age group. Tinea pedis is seen most commonly in postpubertal males with blisters on the instep of the foot. Fissuring between the toes is occasionally seen. Microscopic examination of thin scales or the undersurface of the blister roof confirms the diagnosis.

E. Tinea Unguium (Onychomycosis): Loosening of the nail plate from the nail bed (onycholysis), giving a yellow discoloration, is the first sign of fungal invasion of the nails. Thickening of the distal nail plate then occurs, followed by scaling and a crumbly appearance of the entire nail plate surface. *T rubrum* and *T mentagrophytes* are the most common causes. The diagnosis is confirmed by KOH examination. Usually one or 2 nails are involved. If every nail is involved, psoriasis or lichen planus is a more likely diagnosis than fungal infection.

Treatment

The treatment of dermatophytosis is quite simple: If hair or nails are involved, griseofulvin is the treatment of choice. Topical antifungal agents do not enter hair or nails in sufficient concentrations to clear the infection. The absorption of griseofulvin from the gastrointestinal tract is enhanced by a fatty meal; thus, whole milk or ice cream taken with the medication increases absorption. The dosage of griseofulvin is 20 mg/kg/d. With hair infections, it should be continued for a minimum of 6 weeks; in nail infections, for a minimum of 3 months. It is supplied in capsules containing 250 mg or as a suspension containing 125 mg/5 mL. The side effects are few, and the drug has even been used successfully in the newborn period.

The treatment of kerion includes suppression of the exaggerated inflammatory response with corticosteroids. Prednisone, 1.5 mg/kg/d orally for 7–10 days, is recommended for prevention of scarring and alopecia.

Tinea corporis, tinea pedis, and tinea cruris can be treated effectively with topical medication after careful inspection to make certain that the hair and nails are not involved. Treatment with clotrimazole (Lotrimin), miconazole (Micatin), econazole (Spectazol) or haloprogin (Halotex), applied twice daily for 3–4 weeks, is recommended.

2. TINEA VERSICOLOR

Tinea versicolor is a superficial infection caused by *Pityrosporon orbiculare* (also called *Malassezia furfur*), a yeastlike fungus. It characteristically causes polycyclic connected hypopigmented macules and very fine scales in areas of sun-induced pigmentation. In winter, the polycyclic maculas appear reddish-brown.

Treatment consists of application of selenium sulfide (Selsun), full-strength suspension. Selenium sulfide should be applied to the whole body and left on overnight. Treatment can be repeated again in a week and then monthly thereafter. It tends to be somewhat irritating, and the patient should be warned about this difficulty.

3. *CANDIDA ALBICANS* INFECTIONS

In addition to being a frequent invader in diaper dermatitis, *Candida albicans* also infects the oral mucosa, where it appears as thick white patches with an erythematous base **(thrush);** the angles of the mouth, where it causes fissures and white exudate **(perleche);** and the cuticular region of the fingers, where thickening of the cuticle, dull red erythema, and distortion of growth of the nail plate suggest the diagnosis of candida paronychia. *C albicans* is able to penetrate the stratum corneum layer and locally activate the complement system.

Nystatin (Mycostatin) is the drug of first choice for *C albicans* infections. It is supplied as an ointment or a cream, as an oral suspension, and as vaginal tablets. In diaper dermatitis, the cream form can be applied every 3–4 hours. In oral thrush, the suspension should be applied directly to the mucosa with the finger or a cotton-tipped applicator, since it is not absorbed and acts topically. In candida paronychia, nystatin is applied over the area, covered with an occlusive plastic wrapping, and left on overnight after the application is made airtight.

Haloprogin, miconazole, econazole nitrate, or clotrimazole is an effective alternative.

VIRAL INFECTIONS OF THE SKIN

Herpes Simplex

Grouped vesicles or grouped erosions suggest herpes simplex. The microscopic findings of epidermal giant cells after scraping the vesicle base with a No. 15 blade, smearing on a slide, and staining with Wright's stain (Tzank smear) suggests herpes simplex or varicella zoster. In infants, lesions due to herpes simplex type 1 are seen on the gingiva and lips, periorbitally, or on the thumb in thumb suckers. Recurrent erosions in the mouth are usually aphthous stomatitis rather than recurrent herpes simplex. Herpes simplex type 2 is seen on the genitalia and in the mouth in adolescents. Cutaneous dissemination of herpes simplex occurs in patients with atopic dermatitis **(eczema herpeticum, Kaposi's varicelliform eruption).**

In severe disseminated infection, oral acyclovir may be helpful.

Varicella Zoster

Grouped vesicles in a dermatome on the trunk or face suggest herpes zoster. Zoster in children is not painful and usually has a mild course. In patients with compromised host resistance, the appearance of an erythematous border around the vesicles is a good prognostic sign. Conversely, large bullae without a tendency to crusting imply a poor host response to a virus.

Varicella appears in crops, and many different stages of lesions are present at the same time. Itching is usually the symptom, and cool baths as frequently as necessary or drying lotions such as calamine lotion are sufficient to relieve symptoms. In immunosuppressed children, intravenous or oral acyclovir should be considered.

Varicella, zoster, and herpes simplex lesions undergo the same series of changes: papule, vesicle, pustule, crust, slightly depressed scar.

Virus-Induced Tumors

A. Molluscum Contagiosum: Molluscum contagiosum consists of umbilicated white or whitish-yellow papules found in groups on the genitalia or trunk. They are common in sexually active adolescents as well as in infants and preschool children. Crushing a lesion between glass slides followed by microscopic examination after staining with Wright's stain will demonstrate epidermal cells with inclusions. Molluscum contagiosum is a poxvirus that induces the epidermis to proliferate, forming a pale papule.

Removal of the lesion with a sharp curet or knife is curative. Other therapies include topical salicylic acid, podophyllin, or cantharone.

B. Warts: Warts are skin-colored papules with irregular, rough (verrucous) surfaces. They are intraepidermal tumors caused by infection with human papilloma virus. This DNA virus induces the epidermal cells to proliferate, thus resulting in the warty growth. The different forms of warts are caused by separate papilloma viruses.

No therapy for warts is ideal, and some types of therapy should be avoided because the recurrence rate of warts is high. Flat warts generally require no treatment. A good response to

0.05% tretinoin (Retin-A) cream, applied once daily for 3–4 weeks, has been reported.

The best treatment for the solitary **common ("vulgaris") wart** is to freeze it with liquid nitrogen. The liquid nitrogen should be allowed to drip from the cotton-tipped applicator onto the wart without pressure. Pressure amplifies the cold injury by causing vasoconstriction and may produce a deep ulcer and scar. Liquid nitrogen is applied by drip until the wart turns completely white and stays white for 20–25 seconds. Small plantar warts usually need not be treated. Large and painful ones are treated most effectively by applying 40% salicylic acid paste cut with a scissors to fit the lesion. The sticky brown side of the plaster is placed against the lesion, taped on securely with adhesive tape, and left on for 5 days. The plaster is then removed, and the white necrotic warty tissue can be gently rubbed off with the finger and a new salicylic acid plaster applied. This procedure is repeated every 5 days, and the patient is seen every 2 weeks. Most plantar warts resolve in 2–4 weeks when treated in this way.

Sharp scalpel excision, electrosurgery, and radiotherapy should be avoided, since the resulting scar often becomes a more difficult problem than the wart itself and there may be recurrence of the wart in the area of the scar.

Condyloma acuminatum is best treated with 25% podophyllum resin (podophyllin) in alcohol. This should be painted on the lesions and then washed off after 4 hours. Retreatment in 7–10 days may be necessary. A condyloma not on the vulvar mucous membrane but on the adjacent skin should be treated as a common wart and frozen.

For isolated warts and periungual warts, cantharidin (Cantharone) is effective and painless in children. It causes a blister and sometimes is difficult to control. An undesirable complication is the appearance of warts along the margins of the cantharidin blister. Cantharidin is applied to the skin, allowed to dry, and covered with occlusive tape such as Blenderm for 24 hours.

No wart therapy is immediate and definitive, and recurrences are reported in 20–30% of cases even with the best care.

HIV INFECTIONS

The onset of skin lesions in perinatally acquired AIDS is 4 months; it is 11 months in transfusion acquired AIDS. Persistent oral candidiasis and recalcitrant candida diaper rash are the most frequent cutaneous manifestations of infantile HIV infection. Severe herpetic gingivostomatitis, herpes zoster, and molluscum contagiosum are seen. Recurrent staphylococcal pyodermas, tinea of the face, and onychomycosis are also observed. A generalized dermatitis with features of seborrhea is extremely common. In general, persistent, recurrent or extensive skin infections should make one suspicious of AIDS.

INSECT INFESTATIONS
(Zoonoses)

Essentials of Diagnosis

- Discrete red papules, nodules, and S-shaped burrow on skin.
- Hand and foot involvement common.

Scabies

Scabies is suggested by the appearance of linear burrows about the wrists, ankles, finger webs, areolas, anterior axillary folds, genitalia, or face (in infants). Often, there are excoriations, honey-colored crusts, and pustules from secondary infection. Identification of the female mite or her eggs and feces is necessary to confirm the diagnosis. Slice off an unscratched papule or burrow with a No. 15 blade and examine it microscopically in either immersion oil or 10% KOH to confirm the diagnosis. In a child who is often scratching, scrape under the fingernails. Examine the parent for unscratched burrows.

Lindane (gamma benzene hexachloride 1%; Kwell) is an excellent scabicide. However, since lindane is concentrated in the central nervous system, and central nervous system toxicity from systemic absorption in infants has been reported, the following restricted use of this agent is recommended: (1) For adults and older children, one treatment of lindane lotion or cream applied to the entire body and left on for 4 hours, followed by a shower, is sufficient. (2) Infants tend to have more organisms and many more lesions and may have to be retreated in 7–10 days. All family members should be treated simultaneously. Elimite may be substituted for lindane in infants.

Pediculoses
(Louse Infestations)

Excoriated papules and pustules with a history of severe itching at night suggest infestation with the human body louse.

This louse may be discovered in the seams of underwear but not on the body. In the scalp hair, the gelatinous nits of the body louse adhere tightly to the hair shaft. The pubic louse may be found crawling among pubic hairs, or blue-black macules may be found dispersed through the pubic region (maculae ceruleae). The pubic louse is often seen in the eyelashes of newborns.

Lindane (gamma benzene hexachloride; Kwell) has been the treatment of choice. Since this agent is concentrated in the central nervous system and central nervous system toxicity from systemic absorption in infants has been reported, the following modification in its use is recommended: For head lice, a shampoo preparation is left on the scalp for 5 minutes and rinsed out thoroughly. The hair is then combed with a fine-tooth comb to remove nits. This may be repeated in 7 days. Lindane cream or lotion applied to the body for 4 hours may be necessary for body lice, but washing the clothing in boiling water followed by ironing the seams with a hot iron usually eliminates the organisms. Permethrin 1% cream rinse is also efficacious for lice.

Lindane cream or lotion applied to the pubic area for 24 hours is sufficient to treat pediculosis pubis. It may be repeated in 4–5 days.

Papular Urticaria

Papular urticaria is characterized by grouped erythematous papules surrounded by an urticarial flare and distributed over the shoulder, upper arms, and buttocks in infants. These lesions represent delayed hypersensitivity reactions to stinging or biting insects and can be reproduced by patch testing with the offending insect. Dog and cat fleas are the usual offenders. Less commonly, mosquitoes, lice, scabies, and bird and grass mites are involved. The sensitivity is transient, lasting 4–6 months.

The logical therapy is to remove the offending insect. Topical corticosteroids and oral antihistamines will control symptoms.

DERMATITIS
(Eczema)

Essentials of Diagnosis

- Red skin with disruption of skin surface.
- Vesicles, crusting, or lichenification may be present.

Atopic Dermatitis

Atopic dermatitis is not a clearly defined clinical entity but rather a general term for chronic superficial inflammation of the skin that can be applied to a heterogeneous group of patients. Many (not all) patients go through 3 clinical phases. In the first, infantile eczema, the dermatitis begins on the cheeks and scalp and frequently expresses itself as oval patches on the trunk, later involving the extensor surfaces of the extremities. The usual age at onset is 2–3 months, and this phase ends at age 18 months to 2 years. Only one-third of all infants with atopic eczema progress to phase 2—childhood or flexural eczema—in which the predominant involvement is in the antecubital and popliteal fossae, the neck, the wrist, and sometimes the hands or feet. This phase lasts from age 2 years to adolescence. Some children will have involvement of the soles of their feet only, with cracking, redness, and pain—the so-called atopic feet. Only a third of children with typical flexural eczema will progress to adolescent eczema, which is usually manifested by hand dermatitis only. Atopic dermatitis is quite unusual after age 30.

Atopic dermatitis has no known cause, and despite the high incidence of asthma and hay fever in these patients (39%) and their families (70%), evidence for allergy beyond this hereditary association is limited to testimonials. The evidence for food and inhalant allergens as causes of atopic dermatitis is not specific.

A few patients with atopic dermatitis have immunodeficiency with recurrent pyodermas, unusual susceptibility to herpes simplex and vaccinia virus, hyperimmunoglobulinemia E, defective neutrophil and monocyte chemotaxis, and impaired T lymphocyte function.

A faulty epidermal barrier may predispose the patient with atopic dermatitis to itchy skin. Inability to hold water within the stratum corneum results in rapid evaporation of water, shrinking of the stratum corneum, and "cracks" in the epidermal barrier. Such skin forms an ineffective barrier to the entry of various irritants—and, indeed, it may be clinically useful to regard atopic dermatitis as a primary irritant contact dermatitis and simply tell the patient, "You have sensitive skin." Chronic atopic dermatitis is frequently secondarily infected with *Staphylococcus aureus* or *Streptococcus pyogenes*.

A. Treatment of Acute Stages: Application of wet dressings and topical corticosteroids is the treatment of choice for acute, weeping atopic eczema. Topical steroid is applied 4 times daily and covered with wet dressings as outlined at the beginning of this chapter. Systemic antibiotics chosen on the basis of appropriate skin cultures may be necessary, since lesions in the acute stages are often secondarily infected with *S aureus* or streptococci.

B. Treatment of Chronic Stages: Treatment is aimed at avoiding irritants and restoring water to the skin. No soaps or harsh shampoos should be used, and the patient should avoid woolen clothing or any rough clothing. Restoring water to the skin is important in atopic dermatitis. This can be accomplished by 2 "drip-dry" baths daily, less than 5 minutes each, after which lubricating oils or ointments are applied. Moisturel is a useful lubricant. Plain petrolatum and lards are often too greasy and may cause considerable sweat retention. Liberal use of Cetaphil lotion as a soap substitute 3 or 5 times a day is also satisfactory as a means of lubrication. A bedroom humidifier is often helpful. Topical corticosteroids should be limited to the less potent ones. Hydrocortisone ointment, 1% twice daily, is often sufficient. There is never any reason to use high-potency corticosteroids in atopic dermatitis. In superinfected atopic dermatitis, systemic antibiotics for 10–14 days (erythromycin, 40 mg/kg/d; dicloxacillin, 50 mg/kg/d) are necessary.

Treatment failures in chronic atopic dermatitis are most often due to patient noncompliance. This is a frustrating disease for parent and child.

Nummular Eczema

Nummular eczema is characterized by numerous symmetrically distributed coin-shaped ("nummular") patches of dermatitis, principally on the extremities. These may be acute, oozing, and crusted or dry and scaling. The disease lasts 9 months to 2 years. The differential diagnosis should include tinea corporis and atopic dermatitis.

The same topical measures should be used as for atopic dermatitis, though treatment is often more difficult.

Primary Irritant Contact Dermatitis (Diaper Dermatitis)

Contact dermatitis is of 2 types: primary irritant and allergic eczematous. Primary irritant dermatitis develops within a few hours, reaches peak severity at 24 hours, and then disappears. Allergic eczematous contact dermatitis (see below) has a delayed onset of 18 hours, peaks at 48–72 hours, and often lasts as long as 2 or 3 weeks, even if exposure to the offending antigen is discontinued.

Diaper dermatitis, the most common form of primary irritant contact dermatitis seen in pediatric practice, is due to prolonged contact of the skin with urine and feces, which contain irritating chemicals such as urea and intestinal enzymes. The diagnosis of diaper dermatitis is based on the picture of erythema and thickening of the skin in the perineal area and the history of skin contact with urine or feces. In 80% of cases of diaper dermatitis lasting more than 4 days, the affected area is colonized with *Candida albicans* even before the classic signs of a beefy red, sharply marginated dermatitis with satellite lesions appear.

Treatment consists of changing diapers frequently. Because rubber or plastic pants serve as occlusive dressings and prevent the evaporation of the contactant and enhance its penetration into the skin, they should be avoided as much as possible. Air drying is useful. Streptococcal infection should be included in the differential diagnosis.

Treatment of long-standing diaper dermatitis should include application of nystatin (Mycostatin) cream with each diaper change.

Lichen Simplex Chronicus (Localized Neurodermatitis)

Lichen simplex chronicus is a sharply circumscribed single patch of lichenification. The patients produce the morphologic skin changes by chronic rubbing and scratching.

Treatment of the thickened lesions is with topical corticosteroids. Because the epidermal barrier has thickened, penetration of topical corticosteroids is poor. Penetration can be enhanced in several ways. Airtight occlusion with plastic dressings (eg, Saran Wrap) overnight over topical corticosteroids is useful, or flurandrenolide (Cordran) tape impregnated with corticosteroids will penetrate the lesion. Covering the lesion will also prevent scratching the area.

Allergic Eczematous Contact Dermatitis (Poison Ivy Dermatitis)

Children often present with acute dermatitis with blister formation, oozing, and crusting. Blisters are often linear and of acute onset. Plants such as poison ivy, poison sumac, and poison oak cause most cases of allergic contact dermatitis in children. Allergic contact dermatitis has all the features of delayed type

(T lymphocyte–mediated) hypersensitivity. Although many substances may cause such a reaction, nickel sulfate (metals), potassium dichromate, and neomycin are the most common causes. The true incidence of allergic contact dermatitis in children is not known.

Treatment of contact dermatitis in localized areas is with topical corticosteroids. In severe generalized involvement, prednisone, 1–2 mg/kg/d orally for 14–21 days, can be used.

Dry Skin
(Asteatotic Eczema, Xerosis)
Newborns and older children who live in arid climates are susceptible to dry skin, characterized by large cracked scales with erythematous borders. The stratum corneum is dependent upon environmental humidity for its water, and below 30% environmental humidity the stratum corneum loses water, shrinks, and cracks. These cracks in the epidermal barrier allow irritating substances to enter the skin, predisposing to dermatitis.

Treatment consists of increasing the water content of the skin's immediate external environment. House humidifiers are very useful. Two 5-minute baths a day with immediate application of oil; or ointments (petrolatum, Aquaphor) after the bath will allow the skin to retain water. Frequent soaping of the skin impairs its water-holding capacity and serves as an irritating alkali, and all soaps should therefore be avoided. Frequent use of emollients (eg, Moisturel, Cetaphil, Eucerin, Lubriderm) should be a major part of therapy.

Keratosis Pilaris
Follicular papules containing a white inspissated scale characterize keratosis pilaris. Individual lesions are discrete and may be red. They are prominent on the extensor surfaces of the upper arms and thighs and on the buttocks and cheeks. In severe cases, the lesions may be generalized. Such lesions are seen frequently in children with dry skin and have also been associated with atopic dermatitis and ichthyosis vulgaris.

Treatment is with keratolytics such as topical lactic acid or retinoic acid cream followed by skin hydration.

Pityriasis Alba
White, scaly macular areas with indistinct borders are seen over extensor surfaces of extremities and on the cheeks in children. Suntanning exaggerates these lesions. Histologic examina-

tion reveals a mild dermatitis. These lesions may be confused with tinea versicolor.

There is no satisfactory treatment.

Polymorphous Light Eruption

The appearance of vesicular, eczematous, or urticarial lesions in sun-exposed areas (cheeks, nose, chin, dorsum of the hands and arms) in the springtime should suggest a diagnosis of polymorphous light eruption: Confirmation can be made by skin biopsy demonstrating dense lymphocytic infiltrates in the dermis or by reproducing the lesion by daily exposure to artificial ultraviolet light. In American Indians, it is inherited as an autosomal dominant trait. Onset is usually at age 5 or 6, and spontaneous improvement occurs at puberty. The first rays of sunlight of sufficient energy reaching the earth's surface in early spring induce the disease. As summer progresses, the skin thickens in response to sunlight. Less ultraviolet energy enters the skin, and the disease subsides. The differential diagnosis includes erythropoietic protoporphyrin, in which patients experience severe pain and itching after 5 or 10 minutes of exposure to the sun but do not develop significant skin lesions except for small papules over the dorsum of the hand; and photodermatitis from plants (psoralens) or drugs, eg, thiazide diuretics, antihistamines, phenothiazine tranquilizers, tetracyclines, and sulfonamides.

Treatment of the dermatitis with topical corticosteroids, eg, 1% hydrocortisone cream to the face 3 times daily, and daily use of a sunscreen are sufficient.

COMMON SKIN TUMORS

If the skin moves with the nodule on lateral palpation, the tumor is located within the dermis; if the skin moves over the nodule, it is subcutaneous. Table 12–6 lists the tumors according to these categories.

Granuloma Annulare

Circles or semicircles of nontender interdermal nodules found over the lower legs and ankles, the dorsum of the hands and wrists, and the trunk, in that order, suggest granuloma annular. Histologically, the disease appears as a central area of tissue death (necrobiosis) surrounded by macrophages and lymphocytes.

Table 12–6. Common skin tumors.

Intradermal	Intradermal (cont'd)
Granuloma annulare	Lymphangioma
Dermatofibroma	Hemangioma
Epidermal inclusion cyst	Hair and sweat gland hamartomas
Neurofibroma	**Subcutaneous**
Neuroma	Lipoma
Leiomyoma	Rheumatoid nodule
Pylomatrixoma	Osteoma
Melanocytic nevus	
Pyogenic granuloma	

No treatment is necessary. Lesions resolve spontaneously within 1 or 2 years.

Pyogenic Granuloma

Rapid growth of a dark red papule with an ulcerated and crusted surface 1–2 weeks following skin trauma suggests pyogenic granuloma. Histologically, this represents excessive new vessel formation with or without inflammation (granulation tissue). It is neither pyogenic nor granulomatous but should be regarded as an abnormal healing response.

Excision with electrocautery is the treatment of choice.

Epidermal Inclusion Cysts

Epidermal inclusion cysts are smooth, dome-shaped nodules in the skin that may grow to 2 cm in diameter. In infants they may be found about the eyes and in older children and adolescents on the chest, back, and scalp. They are the most common superficial lumps in children.

Treatment, if desired, is surgical excision.

Keloids

Keloids are scars raised above the skin surface with many radial projections of scar tissue. They continue to enlarge over several years. They are often found on the face, earlobes, neck, chest, and back. Keloids show no racial predilection. Treatment includes intralesional injection with triamcinolone acetonide, 20 mg/mL, or excision and injection with glucocorticosteroids.

PAPULOSQUAMOUS ERUPTIONS
(See Table 12–7)

Pityriasis Rosea

Erythematous papules that coalesce to form oval plaques preceded by a large oval plaque with central clearing and a scaly border (the herald patch) establish the diagnosis of pityriasis rosea. The herald patch has the appearance of ringworm and is often treated as such. It appears 1–30 days before the onset of the generalized papular eruption. The oval plaques are parallel in their long axis and follow Langer's lines of skin cleavage. In whites, the lesions are primarily on the trunk. In blacks, lesions are primarily on the extremities. This disease is common in school-age children and adolescents and is presumed to be viral in origin. It lasts 6 weeks and may be pruritic for the first 7–10 days. The major differential diagnosis is secondary syphilis, and a VDRL test should be done if syphilis is suspected. A chronic variant of this disease may last 2 or 3 years and is called **chronic parapsoriasis** or **pityriasis lichenoides chronicus.**

Exposing the skin to sunlight until a mild sunburn occurs (slight redness) will hasten the disappearance of lesions. Ordinarily, no treatment is necessary.

Psoriasis

Psoriasis is characterized by erythematous papules covered by thick white scales. Guttate (droplike) psoriasis is a common form in children that often follows an episode of streptococcal pharyngitis by 2–3 weeks. The sudden onset of small (3–8 mm) papules, which are seen predominantly over the trunk and quickly become covered with thick white scales, is characteristic of guttate psoriasis. Chronic psoriasis is marked by thick, large (5–10 cm), scaly plaques over the elbows, knees, scalp, and other sites of trauma. Pinpoint pits in the nail plate are seen as well as yellow discoloration of the nail plate resulting from onycholysis.

Table 12–7. Papulosquamous eruptions in children.

Psoriasis	Pityriasis rubra pilaris
Pityriasis rosea	Tinea corporis
Secondary syphilis	Dermatomyositis
Lichen planus	Lupus erythematosus
Chronic papapsoriasis	

Thickening of all 20 fingernails and toenails is an uncommon feature. The sacral and seborrheic areas are commonly involved. Psoriasis has no known cause and demonstrates active proliferation of epidermal cells with a turnover time of 3–4 days, versus 28 days for normal skin. These rapidly proliferating epidermal cells produce excessive stratum corneum, giving rise to thick opaque scales. Papulosquamous eruptions that present problems of differential diagnosis are listed in Table 12–7.

All therapy is aimed at diminishing epidermal turnover time. Sunlight or artificial ultraviolet light (UVL) alone will produce some improvement. Coal tar enhances the effect of UVL and hastens the disappearance of psoriatic lesions. Bathing with a bath product containing tar (eg, Balnetar) at night, followed by UVL the next day, may be sufficient in mild cases. In more severe psoriasis, 2% crude coal tar in petrolatum should be applied after the bath. The newer tar gels (Estar gel, psoriGel) do not cause staining and are most effacious. They are applied twice daily for 6–8 weeks.

Crude coal tar therapy is messy and stains bed clothes, and patients may prefer to use topical corticosteroids. Penetration of topical corticosteroids through the enlarged epidermal barrier in psoriasis requires that more potent preparations be used, eg, fluocinonide (Lidex) 0.05%, or triamcinolone (Aristocort, Kenalog), 0.05%, 4 times daily. A successful alternative is to add a keratolytic agent to the topical corticosteroid to help remove scales and enhance penetration of the steroid. A cream consisting of salicylic acid, 2%, in fluocinonide, 0.05%, 4 times daily, is effective.

Anthralin therapy is also useful. Anthralin is applied to the skin for a short contact time (eg, 20 minutes once daily) and is then washed off with a neutral soap (eg, Dove). A 6-week course of treatment is recommended.

Scalp care using a tar shampoo (Polytar, Zetar, many others) requires leaving the shampoo on for 5 minutes, washing it off, and then shampooing with commercial shampoo to remove scales. It may be necessary to shampoo daily until scaling is reduced.

More severe cases of psoriasis are best treated by a dermatologist.

Lichen Planus

Lichen planus consists of pruritic, light-purple, flat-topped, many sided papules, predominantly on the lower legs, penis, wrist, and arms. A white lacy pattern in the buccal mucosa is often seen. Pruritis may be severe.

If pruritus is mild, no treatment is necessary, and the disease will disappear in 6–12 months. With severe pruritus, a trial of antihistamines, eg, diphenhydramine, 5 mg/kg/d, or hydroxyzine, 2 mg/kg/d orally, is warranted. Rapid relief of pruritus and disappearance of the lesions can be achieved by administering prednisone, 1 mg/kg/d orally for 3–4 weeks.

HAIR LOSS
(Alopecia)

Hair loss in children (Table 12–8) imposes great emotional stress on the parent and doctor—often more so than on the child. A 60% hair loss in a single area is necessary before hair loss can be detected clinically. Examination should begin with the scalp to determine if there are color changes or infiltrative changes. Hairs should be examined microscopically for breaking and structural defects and to see if growing or resting hairs are being shed. Placing removed hairs in mounting fluid (Permount) makes them easy to examine. Three diseases account for most cases

Table 12–8. Causes of hair loss in children.[1]

Hair loss with scalp changes
  Nodules and tumors
    Nevus sebaceus
    Epidermal nevus
  Thickening
    Linear scleroderma (morphea) (en coup de sabre)
    Burn
  Atrophy
    Lupus erythematosus
    Lichen planus
Hair loss with hair shaft defects (hair fails to grow out enough to require haircuts)
  Monilethrix—alternating bands of thin and thick areas
  Trichorrhexis nodosa—nodules with fragmented hair
  Trichorrhexis invaginata (bamboo hair)—intussusception of one hair into another
  Pili torti—hair twisted 180 degrees, brittle
  Pili annulati—alternating bands of light and dark pigmentation

[1] Price VH: Office diagnosis of hair shaft defects. *Cutis* 1975;**15**:231.

of hair loss in children: alopecia areata, tinea capitis, and trichotillomania.

REACTIVE ERYTHEMAS

Erythema Multiforme

Erythema multiforme begins with fixed papules for 7–10 days that later develop a dark center and then evolve into lesions with central blisters and the characteristic target lesions (iris lesions) with 3 concentric circles of color change. Primary injury is to endothelial cells, with later destruction of epidermal basal cells and blister formation. Erythema multiforme has sometimes been diagnosed in severe mucous membrane involvement, but **Stevens–Johnson syndrome** is the usual term for severe involvement of conjunctiva, oral cavity, and genital mucosa.

Many causes are suspected, particularly herpes simplex virus, drugs, and mycoplasma infections. Recurrent erythema multiforme is usually associated with reactivation of herpes simplex virus. Stevens–Johnson syndrome is more likely to be associated with a drug, especially nonsteroidals, anticonvulsants, and sulfonamides. In the mild form, spontaneous healing occurs in 10–14 days, but Stevens–Johnson syndrome may last 6–8 weeks if untreated.

Treatment is symptomatic in uncomplicated erythema multiforme. Removal of offending drugs is an obvious necessary measure. Oral antihistamines such as hydroxyzine, 2 mg/kg/d orally, are useful. Cool compresses and wet dressings will relieve pruritus.

Erythema Nodosum

Erythema nodosum consists of painful erythematous nodules on the anterior lower legs. In streptococcal infections, coccidioidomycosis, histoplasmosis, and tuberculosis, the onset of erythema nodosum parallels the appearance of cell-mediated immunity. Streptococcal infections and birth control pills are the most common causes of this panniculitis in the USA.

Treatment consists of removal of the offending drug or eradication of infection. Topical corticosteroids afford some relief, but prednisone, 1–2 mg/kg/d orally, may be necessary for 2–3 weeks.

Drug Eruptions

Drugs may produce urticarial, morbilliform, scarlatiniform, or bullous skin eruptions. Urticaria may appear within minutes after drug administration, but most reactions begin 7–14 days after the drug is first administered. Drugs commonly implicated in skin reactions are listed in Table 12–9.

NAIL DISORDERS

Nail biting and candida paronychia are the two most common nail disorders. Onychomycosis is uncommon. Nail pitting is seen in psoriasis and alopecia areata.

MISCELLANEOUS SKIN DISORDERS ENCOUNTERED IN PEDIATRIC PRACTICE

Aphthous Stomatitis

Recurrent erosions on the gums, lips, tongue, palate, and buccal mucosa are often confused with herpes simplex. A smear of the base of such a lesion stained with Wright's stain will aid in ruling out herpes simplex by the absence of epithelial giant cells. A culture for herpes simplex is also useful in this difficult differential diagnosis problem. It has been shown that recurrence of aphthous stomatitis correlates positively with lymphocyte-mediated cytotoxicity.

There is no specific therapy for this condition. Rinsing the mouth with liquid antacids will provide relief in most patients. Topical corticosteroids in a gel base that adheres to mucous membrane (eg, Lidex gel) may provide some relief. In severe cases that interfere with eating, prednisone, 1 mg/kg/d orally for 3–5 days, will suffice to abort an episode.

Morphea
(Linear Scleroderma)

Morphea is characterized by the appearance, anywhere on the body, of well-circumscribed, shiny, white, firmly adherent skin. It is particularly cosmetically deforming on the face. A light purple border is indicative of an early lesion or continuing activity. Skin biopsy reveals replacement of subcutaneous fat with thickened collagen fibers. The lesions tend to burn themselves out in 3–5 years. It may be difficult to differentiate mor-

Table 12–9. Common skin reactions associated with frequently used drugs.

Drug	Common Reactions
Aspirin	Urticaria rarely; purpuric eruptions.
Anti-infective agents Erythromycin	Urticaria.
Griseofulvin	Exanthematous eruptions; rarely, cold urticaria or photodermatitis.
Penicillin and synthetic penicillins	Serum sickness, urticaria, exanthematous eruptions, anaphylactic shock. Ampicillin causes a high incidence of exanthematous eruption in patients with infectious mononucleosis.
Streptomycin	Exanthematous eruptions, urticaria, stomatitis.
Sulfonamides	Urticaria, erythema multiforme, exanthematous eruptions, Stevens-Johnson syndrome, photodermatitis.
Tetracycline	Exanthematous eruptions, urticaria; rarely, bullous eruptions. Demeclocycline (Declomycin) can cause phototoxic reactions.
Antihistamines	Exanthematous eruptions, urticaria, photodermatitis.
Barbiturates	Maculopapular eruptions, urticaria, erythema multiforme, Stevens-Johnson syndrome, bullous eruptions.
Chlorothiazides	Exanthematous eruptions, urticaria, photodermatitis, hemosiderosis of the lower extremities, leading to development of petechiae with resultant pigmentation (Schamberg's phenomenon).
Cortisone and derivatives	Acneiform drug reactions on trunk—pustular, purpuric eruptions.
Insulin	Urticaria, erythema at injection site.
Iodides (cough syrups, antiasthma preparations)	Acneiform pustules over trunk, granulomatous reaction.
Phenytoin	Exanthematous eruptions usually in first 3 weeks of treatment; gingival hyperplasia, hypertrichosis; pseudolymphoma syndrome.

phea from lichen sclerosis et atrophicus, which has similar white patches that occur primarily on the upper back and genitalia. Histopathologic differentiation is often necessary and may be difficult. It has been noted that linear scleroderma in children may progress to severe systemic lupus erythematosus after several years. Borrelia infections have recently been implicated in morphea.

Lesions that are not consmetically disturbing should not be treated. Lesions on the face may be cleared by injections of repository corticosteroids, eg, triamcinolone acetonide diluted 1:4 with saline to make 2.5 mg/mL and injected through a 30-gauge needle. Less than 1 mL should be injected. Complications of local corticosteroid injection include atrophy, depigmentation, ulceration, and infection; therefore, this therapy should be reserved for unusual circumstances.

CUTANEOUS SIGNS OF SYSTEMIC DISEASE

Cutaneous signs of systemic disease in infants and children are outlined in Table 12–10.

Table 12–10. Cutaneous signs of systemic disease in infants and children.

Sign	Disease
Acnelike erythematous papules in mid face and white ash-leaf macules on trunk, shiny thickened patch on back, subungual fibromas	Tuberous sclerosis
Pruritic blisters on buttocks, elbows, knees, and scapula	Dermatitis herpetiformis (celiac disease)
Café au lait macules	Neurofibromatosis, Albright's disease
"Chicken skin"—yellow rows of soft papules with wrinkled valleys in between in neck, axillas, groin	Pseudoxanthoma elasticum
"Dirty" neck and axillas (hyperpigmented, velvety flexural papules)	Acanthosis nigricans and obesity (endocrinopathies)
Eczematous erosions around the mouth, eyes, perineum, fingers, and toes; alopecia and diarrhea	Acrodermatitis enteropathica (zinc deficiency)
Erythematous isolated papules on elbows, knees, buttocks, face	Papular acrodermatitis (viral infection, rarely Hepatitis B)
Erythematous truncal macules with central pallor	Juvenile rheumatoid arthritis
Erythematous flat-topped papules over knuckles	Dermatomyositis
Hemorrhagic (1–2 mm) macules on lips, tongue, palms (epistaxis, gastrointestinal bleeding)	Hereditary hemorrhagic telangiectasia (Osler–Weber–Rendu syndrome)

432

Hyperpigmentation in palmar creases, knuckles, scars, buccal mucosa, linea alba, scrotum	Addison's disease
Linear or oval vesicles on hands or feet, erosions on soft palate, tonsillar pillars	Hand, foot, and mouth syndrome (Coxsackie A16 and others)
Palpable purpura	Vasculitis
Pigmented macules on oral mucosa	Peutz–Jeghers disease (benign small intestinal polyps)
Purpuric lakes	Purpura fulminans—disseminated intravascular coagulation
Purpuric pustules on hands and feet	Gonococcemia
Purpuric (petechiae) seborrheic dermatitis	Histiocytosis X
Epidermal inclusion cysts (multiple) on face and trunk	Gardner's syndrome (premalignant polyps of colon and rectum)
Stretchy skin; healing with large purple scars	Ehlers–Danlos syndrome
Tight, hard skin, telangiectases, hypo- and hyperpigmentation	Scleroderma
Ulcers with undermined, liquifying borders	Pyoderma gangrenosum (ulcerative colitis, regional enteritis, rheumatoid arthritis)
Vitiligo (completely depigmented macules with hyperpigmented borders)	Pernicious anemia, Hashimoto's thyroiditis, Addison's disease, diabetes mellitus
Yellow papules (lower eyelids, joints, palms)	Xanthomas, hyperlipidemias

13 | Ear, Nose, & Throat

Stephen Berman, MD

DISEASES OF THE EAR

OTITIS MEDIA

Otitis media, defined as an inflammation of the middle ear, is usually associated with an effusion or collection of fluid in the middle ear space. Otitis media is classified by its onset, response to therapy, duration and complications as acute, residual, unresponsive, persistent, or chronic. **Acute** otitis media means onset of a new infection. **Residual** otitis media occurs when a middle ear effusion is present without tympanic membrane inflammation or symptoms 3–6 weeks following the initiation of antibiotic therapy for acute otitis media. **Unresponsive** otitis media occurs with continued tympanic membrane inflammation and/or symptoms despite initial antibiotic therapy. **Persistent** otitis media occurs with continued presence of a middle ear effusion 6–12 weeks despite initial antibiotic therapy. **Chronic** otitis media occurs when a middle ear effusion persists longer than 12 weeks despite therapy or there is irreversible damage to middle ear structures. At the 3 week post therapy visit for acute otitis media, resolution will be documented in approximately 50% of cases; 40% will have residual otitis media and 10% will have unresponsive otitis media. Approximately 75% of cases of residual otitis media resolve spontaneously during the subsequent 4 to 6 weeks. Classification based on the type of effusion (purulent, serous, or mucoid) has little clinical relevance since it is often difficult to distinguish the type of effusion with otoscopy and bacterial pathogens are frequently isolated from all 3 types of effusion.

In clinical practice, about one-third of the pediatrician's time is spent in the diagnosis and management of otitis media. By the time children reach 3 years of age, more than two-thirds of them have experienced one episode of otitis media, and one-third have had 3 or more episodes. More children present with otitis media in the winter months, when respiratory syncytial virus and other viruses are present in the community. These upper respiratory tract infections adversely affect eustachian tube function and predispose the child to middle ear inflammation. Since young children have shorter, more compliant and more horizontally placed eustachian tubes than older children and adults, colds in young patients will produce more severe eustachian tube dysfunction. This dysfunction promotes the accumulation of middle ear secretions and results in negative pressure in the middle ear space. Negative pressure predisposes the patient to periodic aspiration of contaminated nasopharyngeal secretions, which cause bacterial infection.

Specific conditions that cause eustachian tube dysfunction and predispose children to recurrent and/or chronic otitis media include frequent viral upper respiratory tract infections, allergic and vasomotor rhinitis, trisomy 21, cystic fibrosis, hypothyroidism, and anatomic abnormalities such as cleft palate, obstructing adenoids, and nasopharyngeal tumors. Bottle propping, passive exposure to smoking and day care outside the home also predispose children to recurrent or chronic otitis media.

Infants who experience their initial episode of otitis media in the first 2 or 3 months of life are more likely to have recurrent or chronic otitis media during their first year. Recurrence or persistence of disease places infants and children at risk for permanent ear damage and fluctuating or persistent hearing loss. Studies have shown that the amount of time the effusion is present during the first 6–12 months of life has the strongest correlation with delays in language development at 3 years of age. Therefore, early identification of otitis prone infants and children is essential for prevention of adverse sequelae.

The diagnosis of otitis media is based on specific otoscopic findings, which include the appearance of the tympanic membrane and an assessment of its mobility. In recent years, tympanometry has also become a useful technique in documenting middle ear effusions in children and infants older than 7 months. Unfortunately, it does not differentiate acute from residual otitis media. In pediatric practice, tympanometry is useful for screening patients uncooperative to examination, clarifying questionable otoscopic findings, and providing an objective measurement to follow the course of persistent effusions.

1. ACUTE OTITIS MEDIA

General Considerations

Bacteriologic findings in middle ear aspirates from Denver, Colorado can be summarized as follows: *Streptococcus pneumoniae*, 42% of isolations; *Haemophilus influenzae*, 41%; *Morexella catarrhalis*, 9%; *Streptococcus pyogenes*, 2%; *Staphylococcus aureus*, 4% and others (including enteric gram-negative organisms and anaerobic organisms), 2%. In 20% of cases, aspirates are sterile or grow presumed nonpathogens such as *Staphylococcus epidermidis* and diphtheroids. In about 11% of cases, multiple pathogens are isolated from a single middle ear aspirate. In children with bilateral acute otitis media, different pathogens can be recovered from each ear in 5–10% of cases. *S pneumoniae* is uniformly the most common pathogen throughout the country. *M catarrhalis* has become more frequently recognized as a causative agent of acute otitis media. *H influenzae* remains an important pathogen in cases throughout childhood and into early adulthood. In many areas, the prevalence of B-lactamase producing isolates for *H influenzae* is greater than 30%; that for *M catarrhalis* and *S aureus* are 80% or higher.

The microbiologic causes of acute otitis media in early infancy differ from those in later life. The risk of gram-negative enteric infection is especially high in infants who are under 6 weeks of age and have been or are hospitalized in a neonatal intensive care nursery. In infants seen during the first 3 months of life who were not hospitalized, acute otitis media is caused by *S aureus* and *Chlamydia trachomatis*, as well as *S pneumoniae*, *H influenzae*, and *M catarrhalis*.

Studies using antigen detection and/or culture of middle ear aspirates in cases of acute otitis media identify a virus in 16% of cases; 10% have mixed viral and bacterial isolation and 6% viral isolation alone. It remains unclear whether viruses are a primary cause of acute otitis media or whether they promote bacterial superinfection by impairing eustachian tube function and other host immune and non-immune defenses. The presence of virus in the middle ear space may compromise eradication of bacterial pathogens by antibiotics and predispose to unresponsive otitis media.

Clinical Findings

A. Symptoms and Signs: Acute otitis media often presents with pain in association with symptoms of upper respiratory tract infection (eg, rhinorrhea, stuffy nose, and cough) or purulent conjunctivitis. While older children may complain of earache, young children demonstrate pain by crying, increased irritability, and difficulty in sleeping or feeding. Irritability may be related to hearing loss as well as pain. Tugging at the ears, is often falsely positive, especially in infants with recurrent infections. Fever is present in less than half of cases. Facial palsy or ataxia occurs rarely.

The tympanic membrane appears either red or yellow, depending on the degree of inflammation and the amount of purulent material in the middle ear space. White exudate may be visible on the membrane. In early cases, bulging may be limited to the pars flaccida. Later, the entire eardrum bulges outward, giving a doughnutlike appearance. Tympanic membrane mobility is absent or markedly diminished. If the eardrum has spontaneously ruptured, cloudy to purulent discharge will be present in the ear canal, making examination of the tympanic membrane difficult. Cerumen that has melted with high fever or tears and is present in the ear canal can cause confusion with middle ear discharge. Occasionally, bullae form between the outer and middle layers of the tympanic membrane and produce acute bullous myringitis. This entity should be considered a form of acute otitis media and is described in detail in the next section.

B. Laboratory Findings: Nasopharyngeal and throat cultures are not useful because *S pneumoniae* and nontypeable *H influenzae* are often present in well children and thus of no significance. If perforation has occurred, it may be useful to culture the discharge, using a nasopharyngeal culture swab. If the discharge has been present for over 2 weeks despite therapy, pseudomonas is often isolated.

Beyond the neonatal period, acute otitis media infrequently presents with signs of systemic toxicity; therefore, blood cultures, urine culture, and lumbar puncture are indicated in the child with acute otitis media who also appears toxic or has signs of meningeal irritation.

Differential Diagnosis

Not all earaches are caused by acute otitis media. Mumps, toothaches, otitis externa, a foreign body in the ear canal, and ear canal furuncle, ear canal trauma, hard cerumen, and temporomandibular joint dysfunction can all present with a chief complaint of earache. Injected vessels at the drum periphery and along the malleus are frequently overdiagnosed as "early otitis media." An injected tympanic membrane as well as a flushed face can occur with fever or crying. Cleaning wax from the ear canal can cause reactive hyperemia of the same vessels. Such an eardrum may be red, but it will be mobile and not require treatment. Because acute otitis media is the most common complication of a cold, an infant with a cold and fever should never be sent home without examination of the eardrums. Cerumen removal (see below) will often be necessary.

Complications

The most common complication associated with acute otitis media is a hearing loss of 20–35 dB, which may persist for several months. The tympanic membrane may rupture spontaneously because of pressure necrosis and produce a sizable perforation. Acute otitis media may also cause labyrinthitis with ataxia, facial paralysis, cholesteatoma, mastoiditis, ossicular necrosis, pseudotumor cerebri (otitic hydrocephalus), or cerebral thrombophlebitis.

Treatment

An algorithm for the management of acute otitis media is shown in Fig. 13–1.

A. Specific Measures (Table 13–1):

1. Systemic Antibiotics–In areas where Beta-lactamase producing pathogens are common, the initial treatment for otitis media should be 10 days of trimethoprim, 10 mg/kg/d with sulfamethoxazole, in 2 divided doses. Otherwise, the drug of choice for acute otitis media in children of all ages is amoxicillin, 50 mg/kg/d in 3 divided doses, continued for 10 days. If symptoms persist beyond 48 hours of therapy, the patient should be reevaluated for an associated infection versus an unresponsive otitis media.

Clinical trials comparing commonly prescribed antibiotics have documented similar cure rates in acute otitis media for amoxicillin, trimethoprim plus sulfamethoxazole, erythromycin plus sulfamethoxazole, amoxicillin plus clavulanate, cefaclor, cefprozil, and cefixime. While many cases of acute otitis media will clinically resolve without any therapy, recent work suggests that antibiotic treatment, especially in cases with high fever and/or earache is more effective than placebo therapy. The use of amoxicillin or trimethoprim sulfamethoxazole as first line therapy is based primarily on cost and safety considerations. A 10 day course of antibiotic is current standard practice. However,

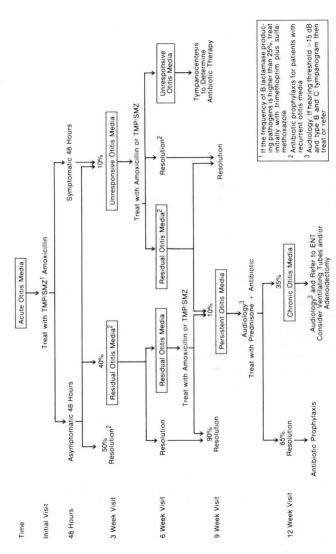

Figure 13-1. Algorithm for the management of otitis media.

439

Table 13–1. Antibiotic therapy for acute otitis media with effusion in children.

Antibiotic	Dosage[1]	Product Availability[1]
Amoxicillin	10–15 mg/kg/dose tid (bid for prophylaxis)	Liquid: 125 and 500 mg/5 mL Caps: 250, 500 mg Chewables: 125, 250 mg
Amoxicillin/ clavulanate (Augmentin)	10–15 mg/kg/dose tid	Liquid: 125, 250 mg/5 mL Chewables: 125, 250 mg Tabs: 250, 500 mg
Cefaclor (Ceclor)	10 mg/kg/dose tid	Liquid: 125, 250 mg/5 mL Caps: 250, 500 mg
Cefixime (Suprax)	8 mg/kg/day as single dose or divided bid	Liquid: 100 mg/5 mL Tabs: 200, 400 mg
Erythromycin	10 mg/kg/dose bid for prophylaxis	Liquid: 200 ml 400 mg/5 mL Chewables: 200 mg Tabs/caps: 250, 500 mg
Erythromycin/ sulfisoxazole (Pediazole)	10 mg (E)/kg/dose qid	Liquid: 100 mg (E), 600 mg (S)/5 mL
Prednisone or prednisolone	0.5–1 mg/kg/dose bid	Tabs: 5, 10, 20 mg Syrup: 1mg/1 mL
Sulfisoxazole (Gantrisin)	30–40 mg/kg/dose bid for prophylaxis	Liquid: 500 mg/5 mL Tabs: 500 mg
Trimethoprim/ sulfamethoxazole (Bactrim, Septra)	5 mg (T)/kg/dose bid or 0.5 ml/kg/dose bid	Liquid: 40 (T) mg/5 mL Tabs: 80, 160 mg T:S = 1:5 ratio

[1] T = trimethoprin component; E = erythromycin component; S = sulfisoxazole component.

it is possible that 5 days may be as effective as 10 days in the absence of a tympanic membrane perforation with drainage. Tetracyclines are contraindicated for ear infections because about 50% of pneumococci and streptococci are resistent to these drugs and because they cause staining of the tooth enamel. Trimethoprim plus sulfamethoxazole is not effective against *Streptococcus pyogenes* and should not be used if there is a suspected streptococcal pharyngitis.

Acute otitis media in infants less than 6 weeks of age who experienced a complicated neonatal course is often associated with sepsis and/or meningitis. These infants require tympanocentesis, blood culture, and a lumbar puncture and should receive intravenous ampicillin plus either gentamicin or cefotaximine in the hospital pending culture results. Acute otitis media in infants under 3 months without additional risk factors or signs of serious illness can be treated on an outpatient basis. Because of a higher frequency of *S aureus* and perhaps chlamydia, consider treatment with erythromycin plus sulfamethoxazole. Alternatives include cefaclor, cefprozil, cefixime or amoxicillin plus clavulanate. These children should be re-examined at 24 and 48 hours. If their condition worsens during this time period, they should be hospitalized.

2. Antibiotic Ear Drops–If the eardrum has been perforated, there is usually a cloudy to watery material in the ear canal, and antibiotic ear drops are usually not required. However, the child with considerable purulent drainage from the ear may profit from this adjunctive therapy. The purulent material can be removed by gentle suction, using a syringe and a short plastic tubing such as can be made by cutting a scalp vein needle set. Normal saline solution can be instilled without force and then removed. After this type of cleansing has eliminated the pus, antibiotic-corticosteroid ear drops can be instilled 3 times a day. The child should be held with head sideways and stationary for a few minutes after drops are instilled. Cotton plugs are contraindicated.

B. General Measures:

1. Analgesics and Antipyretics–An irritable child with an earache requires acetaminophen or rarely codeine in order to sleep through the first night while on treatment. However, if pain is severe consider tympanocentesis or myringotomy for pain relief. Young children can be given codeine, 0.5 mg/kg/dose, up to 4 times a day. Codeine is available in several cough medicines in a concentration of 10 mg/tsp. Antipyretics for fever control may be required during the first 1 or 2 days. Analgesic ear drops have not proved effective for the relief of pain and have the disadvantage of obscuring the field of vision if the tympanic membrane needs to be reexamined.

2. Oral Decongestants–Antihistamine-decongestant combinations are ineffective in the treatment of acute otitis media.

3. Reassurance–Some patients are overly concerned about ear infections and their complications. Reassurance should be given as required. There is little danger of permanent hearing loss as long as the prescribed medicines are taken as directed. The child can be allowed to go outside, and the ears need not be covered. Mountain travel is permitted. Swimming is permitted if perforation is not present.

4. Unwarranted Measures–Vasoconstrictor nose drops are of no value, because it is nearly impossible to deliver them to the entrance of the eustachian tube.

C. Myringotomy and Tympanocentesis: A common pitfall in therapy is not performing myringotomy or tympanocentesis when it is indicated. In a child with an acutely bulging eardrum, myringotomy is indicated if the patient has severe pain (as evidenced by inconsolable screaming) or if recurrent vomiting or ataxia is associated with the ear infection. In these circumstances, myringotomy is more effective than analgesics or antiemetics. Unfortunately, myringotomy does not appear to prevent the development of residual or persistent otitis media.

2. UNRESPONSIVE OTITIS MEDIA

General Considerations

Cases in which symptoms and otoscopic findings of tympanic membrane inflammation continue beyond 48 hours of initial antibiotic therapy have unresponsive otitis media. Approximately 10% of children treated initially with a 10 day antibiotic course will have unresponsive otitis media identified at or prior to the 3 week post therapy visit. The majority (57%) of children with unresponsive otitis media following treatment with either amoxicillin, trimethoprim plus sulfamethoxazole or erythromycin plus sulfisoxazole have sterile repeat post therapy middle ear aspirates. Therefore, failure of antibiotic therapy to eradicate the pathogen is not always the cause of unresponsive otitis media. Persistent symptoms and otoscopic findings may be related to the effects of a concomitant viral infection in the middle ear space as cases of unresponsive otitis media are associated with higher viral isolation rates from middle ear aspirates.

However, unresponsive otitis media is more common in cases when antibiotic therapy fails to eradicate pathogens than when pathogens are eradicated. Children with unresponsive otitis media treated with amoxicillin are more likely to have Beta-lactamase producing pathogens isolated in a post therapy middle ear aspirate than children who respond to an initial amoxicillin treatment. Organisms sensitive to initial therapy are identified in 24% of posttherapy aspirates. Organisms resistent to initial therapy are identified in 19% of post therapy aspirates. Eradication of a middle ear pathogen with antibiotic therapy is less likely after 2–4 days when a virus and bacteria are both isolated from a middle ear aspirate than when a bacteria is isolated alone.

Treatment of Children With Systemic Antibiotics

Unresponsive otitis media initially treated with trimethoprim plus sulfamethoxazole should receive amoxicillin or vice versa. The sequential administration of amoxicillin and trimethoprim plus sulfamethoxazole provides excellent coverage for resistent pathogens. Trimethoprim plus sulfamethoxazole covers Beta-lactamase producing organisms resistent to amoxicillin such as *H influenzae, M catarrhalis,* and most *S aureus* while amoxicillin covers organisms resistent to trimethoprim plus sulfamethoxazole such as *S pyogenes, Group B streptococcus, Enterococcus,* and resistent *S pneumoniae.* Third-generation cephalosporins, amoxicillin plus clavulanate, and erythromycin plus sulfamethoxazole offer no advantage in terms of coverage of resistent organisms. They are most useful as second line antibiotics for children who are allergic to either amoxicillin or trimethoprim plus sulfisoxazole.

If unresponsive otitis media still persists after a second course of antibiotics, myringotomy or tympanocentesis should be performed and the middle ear aspirate cultured to determine the most appropriate antibiotic therapy.

3. RESIDUAL OTITIS MEDIA

General Considerations

Residual otitis media following appropriate antibiotic therapy for acute otitis media occurs in 40% of children at a 3 week follow-up visit. These middle ear effusions clear spontaneously within 6 weeks in 75–85% of cases. Residual otitis media results when the eustachian tube dysfunction persists and the effusion present in the middle ear space fails to clear. The effusion is usually serous, resembling serum transudate, and histopathologic examination of the middle ear shows subepithelial edema. The effusion is usually associated with a low-grade (15–20 dB) conductive hearing loss.

Clinical Findings

Children with residual otitis media are usually asymptomatic and have hearing loss. The patient may complain of a feeling of fullness in the ear. An older patient may compare the feeling with ''talking inside a barrel.'' In the preverbal child, hearing loss should be suspected if irritability, inattentiveness, or increased behavior problems are noted. Unlike acute otitis media, there is minimal pain.

The tympanic membrane may appear mildly injected and dull or have a normal appearance. Mobility is diminished or absent. When fluid levels or air bubbles are visualized, the effusion is in a stage of resolution, with eustachian tube function improving. When eustachian tube dysfunction results in persistent negative pressure in the middle ear space, the tympanic membrane appears retracted, and the position of the short process of the right malleus changes from the 7 o'clock to the 9 o'clock position. Tympanic membrane mobility is altered and the membrane moves only when negative pressure is applied.

The presence of eustachian tube dysfunction and middle ear effusion predisposes the child to another episode of acute otitis media. In some children with recurrent otitis media, an effusion persists in the middle ear space between episodes and a cycle of acute otitis media alternates with residual otitis media.

Treatment

Management of residual OME is outlined in the algorithm. The efficacy of oral decongestants and antihistamines in preventing or clearing residual otitis media is controversial. In most studies, these drugs have not been shown to be effective. When residual otitis is present 3 weeks after initial antibiotic therapy, follow the patient without administering additional antibiotics. If the effusion is still present after another 3 weeks the otitis can be considered persistent and requires further antibiotic treatment.

4. PERSISTENT OTITIS MEDIA

General Considerations

Children with middle ear effusions that fail to resolve with antibiotics within 6 weeks have persistent otitis media. The rate of spontaneous resolution of middle ear effusions present at the 6 week follow-up visit varies from 6 to 51% during subsequent

4–6 week follow-up period. The majority of effusions in persistent otitis media are mucoid; about 10% are serous and less than 10% are purulent. Middle ear aspirates of persistent otitis media often grow pathogenic organisms regardless of the type of effusion. The most common pathogenic organisms isolated from these effusions are *Haemophilus influenzae* (15% of cases), *Morexella catarrhalis* (9%), *Streptococcus pyogenes* (1%). Most *H influenzae* strains and *M catarrhalis* strains are Beta-lactamase positive. *Staphylococcus epidermidis* and diphtheroids are isolated in 33% of effusions. Evidence supporting the pathogenic role of these organisms includes the findings of type-specific antibody in middle ear fluid; studies in animals also suggest that the middle ear space should be sterile.

In persistent otitis media, ongoing low grade bacterial infection of the middle ear space may persist and evoke local accumulation of leukocytes, lymphocytes, and macrophages. Antibody production, complement activation, and release of chemical mediators may all occur. The mediators, together with bacterial products such as endotoxin and neuraminidase, cause tissue edema, increased capillary leakage, and hemorrhage. In addition, the mediators stimulate the formation of goblet cells in the respiratory epithelium and these cells produce excessive secretions. The inflammatory response and/or bacterial toxins may destroy a surfactant-like substance present on the inner surface of the eustachian tube, thereby reducing surface tension and predisposing the eustachian tube to collapse.

Clinical Findings

Patients with persistent otitis media usually are asymptomatic or complain of a feeling of fullness in the ear. The tympanic membrane commonly appears dull and opaque; in severe cases, it may have a bluish tint. Tympanic membrane mobility is usually markedly diminished.

Complications

Children with persistent otitis media are at increased risk of developing retraction pockets, cholesteatoma and erosion of the ossicles. Persistent otitis media is associated with a hearing loss of 20 dB or higher, which may persist for a prolonged period of time. A persistent, moderate hearing loss early in life can result in delays in language development and adversely affect intellectual functioning.

Treatment

A. Medical Measures: Effective management should eradicate organisms involved in ongoing infection and counteract the deleterious effects of the inflammatory response. Treat children with persistent otitis media who have only received an initial course of antibiotics with a second antibiotic for 10 days. If the initial treatment was amoxicillin, give trimethoprim plus sulfamethoxazole or vice versa. At the 9-week post initial therapy visit, document persistent otitis media with tympanometry and audiology. When a type B or C tympanogram is associated with a hearing threshold of 20 dB or higher, consider a trial of prednisone 1 mg/kg/day in two divided doses for 7 days combined with a 21 to 28 day course of trimethoprim plus sulfamethoxazole or an alternative antibiotic effective against organisms that produce beta lactamase. This treatment clears the effusion in 60 to 70% of these cases. Following resolution, patients should be placed on antibiotic prophylaxis to prevent an acute otitis media episode during the next 3 to 6 months. Corticosteroids prevent the release of arachidonic acid metabolites that include prostoglandins and leukotrienes. Several studies have shown beneficial effects of combination antibiotic and corticosteroid therapy in cases of persistent otitis media. Oral decongestants and antihistamines have not been effective in treating persistent otitis media. Persistent otitis media that fails to resolve by 12 weeks despite therapy can be considered chronic otitis media and requires a referral to an otolaryngologist.

5. CHRONIC OTITIS MEDIA

General Considerations

Chronic otitis media occurs when a middle ear effusion has persisted 12 weeks or longer despite therapy or irreversible damage to middle ear structures has occurred. Damage to middle ear structures include retraction pockets, adhesive otitis, atrophy of the tympanic membrane, cholesteatoma, cholesterol granuloma and erosion of ossicles. Effusions present longer than 12 weeks frequently persist for 6 months or longer. Prolonged conductive hearing loss early in life is likely to result in a delay in language development that may adversely affect subsequent school performance and intellectual functioning.

Clinical Findings

Otoscopic examination can identify damage to the middle ear structures. Tympanosclerosis is caused by chronic inflammation and/or trauma that produces granulation tissue, hyalinization, and calcification. The appearance of a small perforation in the posteriorsuperior area of the pars tensa or in the pars flaccida suggests a retraction pocket. Retraction pockets occur when chronic inflammation and negative pressure in the middle ear space produces atrophy and atelectasis of the tympanic membrane. Continued inflammation can cause adhesions between the retraction pocket and the ossicles. This condition, referred to as adhesive otitis, predisposes to a formation of a cholesteatoma and/or fixation and erosion of the ossicles. Erosion of the ossicles results from osteitis and compromise of the blood supply. Ossicular discontinuity produces a severe hearing loss with a 50–60 dB threshold. A tympanogram with very high compliance indicates ossicular discontinuity. The presence of a greasy looking mass or debris seen in a retraction pocket or perforation suggests cholesteatoma regardless of the presence of discharge. The size of the perforation does not correlate with the extent of the cholesteatoma.

Surgical Treatment

Surgical interventions for chronic otitis media include the insertion of ventilating tubes and/or adenoidectomy or corrective surgery for adhesive otitis media, cholesteatoma, or ossicular disarticulation. The aim of surgery is restoration of normal hearing thresholds and prevention of further damage to middle ear structures.

Myringotomy followed by insertion of ventilating tubes (polyethylene flanged ventilation tubes) restore normal hearing and middle ear pressure as long as the tubes are in place. The tubes permit pressure equalization and drying of the middle ear cavity without a functional eustachian tube. Retraction pockets will resolve following insertion of ventilating tubes provided adhesive otitis media is not present. Unfortunately, insertion of ventilating tubes frequently results in damage to middle ear structures. The tubes produce a foreign body reaction that causes tympanosclerosis and/or atrophy of the tympanic membrane in approximately 50% of patients 5 to 15 years after surgery. Ventilating tubes will spontaneously extrude in 20% of children within 6 months of placement. Recurrent ventilating tube insertions accelerate the tympanosclerosis and atrophy. There is no evidence that insertion of ventilating tubes prevents retraction pockets or cholesteatoma. When a ventilating tube is placed unilaterally the subsequent incidence of retraction pockets and cholesteatoma formation is similar 5 and 15 years post surgery in the unoperated ear as compared with an ear having ventilating tube. Long term hearing may actually be better in the ear without a ventilating tube.

Studies comparing the efficacy of ventilating tubes alone, adenoidectomy alone, ventilating tubes plus adenoidectomy, and myringotomy alone have failed to resolve the controversy concerning appropriate surgical management of chronic otitis media. While ventilating tubes restore hearing loss faster than adenoidectomy alone, hearing thresholds are similar by 6 months post surgery. Adenoidectomy is associated with a 50–70% resolution rate for middle ear effusion and decrease the need for ventilating tube reinsertion. Insertion of ventilating tubes is a simpler (although not necessarily lower cost) procedure than adenoidectomy with fewer surgical risks. Younger patients may benefit from having hearing loss restored faster. Adenoidectomy is more beneficial in older children. Unfortunately the extent of benefit is not well correlated with the size of the adenoids. Adenoidectomy may also be beneficial in patients who require multiple ventilating tube reinsertions. Medical standards for ventilating tubes, adenoidectomy, or combination of both remain unclear and decisions should be made on a case by case basis.

6. RECURRENT OTITIS MEDIA

Management

A. Identification and Monitoring of Otitis-Prone Infants and Children: The criteria for identifying children with recurrent otitis media are three episodes of otitis media within a 6-month period. Because episodes of acute otitis media in infancy are frequently asymptomatic, high-risk infants with an initial episode during the first 3 months of life require close monitoring and monthly follow-up. Language development should be evaluated at 18, 24, and 36 months by use of the Early Language Milestone (ELM) scale. An appropriate home language stimulation program and guidelines for the management of behavior problems related to conductive hearing loss should be instituted for all infants and children with impaired hearing. (See Detection and Management of Hearing Deficits, below.)

B. Antibiotic Prophylaxis: Prophylaxis should be started following the resolution of the third acute otitis media episode within a 6 month period. Antibiotics shown to be effective include sulfisoxazole 70 mg/kg/d or amoxicillin 20 mg/kg/d, both given in 2 divided doses. One daily dose may also be effective.

Antibiotics should be administered daily for 3 months. During the next 3 months, it is often helpful to advise parents to restart the antibiotic at the first sign of a cold and give it for a minimum of 2 weeks or until cold symptoms resolve. However, during the winter respiratory season continuous daily antibiotic is more effective than antibiotics given only during periods with respiratory symptoms. Antibiotics can reduce the frequency of recurrent acute otitis by 50%. Failure to prevent a second new infection on continuous prophylaxis during 3 months is an indication for referral to an otolaryngologist for the insertion of ventilating tubes. Occasionally, patients with ventilating tubes continue to have recurrent acute otitis media and benefit from antibiotic prophylaxis. Children older than 2 years with recurrent otitis may benefit from receiving pneumococcal polysaccharide vaccine.

OTITIS EXTERNA
(Inflammation of the External Ear Canal)

The most common cause of otitis externa is maceration of the ear canal lining due to frequent swimming or shower bathing. Trauma, reactions to foreign bodies, and accumulation of cerumen are other contributing factors. Pyogenic (especially *Pseudomonas* or staphylococcal) and mycotic superinfections are common.

Recurrent otitis externa is usually caused by the frequent use of cotton-tipped applicators or frequent swimming in chlorinated pools (or both).

Treatment

A. Pyogenic Infections: Treatment is aimed at keeping the external ear canal clean and dry and protecting it from trauma. Debris should be removed from the ear canal by gentle irrigation. Topical antibiotics combined with a corticosteroid applied as ear drops are essential. Give systemic antibiotics (usually penicillin) in full doses for 10 days if there is evidence of extension of the infection beyond the skin of the ear canal (fever, adenopathy, or cellulitis of the pinna). During the acute phase, swimming should be avoided if possible.

B. Removal of Foreign Bodies: Removal should always be done under direct vision and never done blindly. A stream of lukewarm saline directed past the foreign body into the external canal may float it out. Vegetable matter, such as peas and beans, swells in the presence of water and should instead by removed with a wire loop; care should be taken not to push the object farther into the canal. If the object is large or is wedged in place, the patient should be referred to an otolaryngologist.

C. Removal of Impacted Cerumen: Cerumen in the external ear must be removed before the examination can continue. It may be removed with a wire loop or with cotton on the end of a thin wire applicator. Cerumen may be softened, if necessary, by instilling mineral oil or Cerumenex. (*Caution:* Cerumenex can cause contact dermatitis if left in the ear canal for over 30 minutes.) It may also be washed out with warm water or saline, using a syringe. Irrigation is contraindicated if any possibility of a perforated eardrum exists.

Prognosis

After removal of a foreign body, rapid improvement occurs.

CHRONIC PERFORATION OF THE TYMPANIC MEMBRANE

General Considerations

A perforation of the tympanic membrane can be considered chronic if it lasts for longer than 1 month. When the perforation is associated with a discharge, it is called chronic suppurative otitis media.

Clinical Findings

A. Symptoms and Signs: When a perforation is present, the condition is usually painless. If no infection is present, the middle ear cavity is seen to contain thickened, inflamed mucosa. If superimposed infection is present, serous or purulent drainage will be seen, and the middle ear cavity may contain granulation tissue or even polyps. A conductive hearing loss will usually be present depending on the size of the perforation.

The site of perforation is important. Central perforations are usually relatively safe from cholesteatoma formation. Peripheral perforations, especially in the pars flaccida, impose a risk for development of cholesteatoma because the ear canal epithelium adjacent to the perforation may invade it.

B. Laboratory Findings: Any discharge present should be cultured before treatment is initiated. Sensitivity tests are often necessary because the most common organisms are *Pseudomonas* and *S aureus*. The role of anaerobic organisms is unclear. A PPD test should be done to rule out tuberculosis.

C. Imaging: CT is helpful if a superimposed mastoiditis is suspected.

Complications

This disorder can have serious complications, but they are rare with proper therapy. They occur mainly in unattended cases of superinfected, chronically perforated eardrums. Cholesteatoma is the most common complication and can be suspected if the discharge is foul-smelling and if a white, oily mass is seen within the perforation. The associated perforation may be pinpoint in size. If the discharge does not respond to 2 weeks of aggressive therapy, mastoiditis or cholesteatoma should be suspected. Serious central nervous system complications such as extradural abscess, subdural abscess, brain abscess, meningitis, labyrinthitis, or lateral sinus thrombophlebitis can occur with extension of this process. Therefore, patients with facial palsy, vertigo, or other central nervous system signs should be referred immediately to an otolaryngologist. Otogenous tetanus is another possible sequela.

Treatment

A. Specific Measures: If a serous or purulent discharge is present, antibiotic-corticosteroid ear drops (suspensions are less irritating than solutions) should be instilled 3 times daily for 1 week. Most products contain polymyxin and neomycin. *Pseudomonas* is sensitive to the former. Gentamicin ear drops are also useful. The ear drops will not be effective unless the ear canals are aspirated free of discharge and debris before the drops are instilled. If the discharge is purulent or foul-smelling or if systemic signs are present, systemic antibiotics should also be prescribed. An antibiotic effective against Beta-lactamase-producing organisms can be given at the outset and another drug substituted depending on the culture results. This therapy can be continued for 2 weeks. If there is any recurrence of discharge, antibiotic ear drops should be instilled immediately.

Chronic suppurative otitis media with *Pseudomonas* is often resistant to outpatient therapy. If daily outpatient aspiration of discharge is unsuccessful, it may be necessary to hospitalize the patient for parenteral therapy with a antipseudomonas antibiotic.

B. Surgical Treatment: Repair of the defect in the tympanic membrane is rarely successful during the time period when children have frequent colds and recurrent auditory tube dysfunction. Therefore, tympanoplasty is usually deferred until age 9–12. The perforated eardrum can be repaired earlier if the nonperforated one remains free of infection and effusion for a year. If drainage persists despite treatment, the patient must be referred to an otologist to rule out cholesteatoma, mastoiditis, or other complication.

Prognosis

With treatment, 80–90% of perforations heal spontaneously by 1 year. The remainder require careful follow-up. With proper care, these patients will be in good condition for tympanoplasty at age 9–12.

MASTOIDITIS

Infection of the mastoid antrum and air cells may follow an episode of untreated or improperly treated acute otitis media. The most common etiologic agents are *S pyogenes, S pneumoniae,* and *S aureus. H influenzae* causes mastoiditis much less frequently than expected. Other agents that can cause this disease include *Pseudomonas, Mycobacterium* enteropathic gram-negative rods, and *B catarrhalis.* Anaerobic organisms appear to play a role in chronic mastoiditis; however, there are no data on how frequently they cause acute mastoiditis.

Clinical Findings

The principal complaints are postauricular pain and fever. On examination, the mastoid area is often swollen and reddened. In the late stage, it may be fluctuant. The earliest finding is severe tenderness upon mastoid percussion. Late findings are a pinna that is pushed forward by postauricular swelling and an ear canal that is narrowed in the posterior superior wall because of pressure from the mastoid abscess.

Mastoiditis is a clinical diagnosis. It cannot be diagnosed on the basis of x-rays alone. In the acute phase, there is diffuse inflammatory clouding of the mastoid cells as in every case of acute purulent otitis media. Only later is there evidence of bony destruction and resorption of the mastoid air cells.

Complications

Meningitis is a complication in about 9% of cases of acute mastoiditis. Brain abscess occurs in 2% of cases and may be associated with persistent headache, recurring fever, or changes in sensorium.

Treatment & Prognosis

The patient must be hospitalized because this disorder represents osteitis. Before therapy is initiated, myringotomy should be performed in order to obtain material for culture and also to relieve the pressure in the middle ear–mastoid space.

The initial management of uncomplicated acute mastoiditis includes intravenous antibiotic therapy and possibly surgery. Results of gram-stained smears taken during tympanocentesis may help in the choice of antibiotics. Ampicillin and nafcillin are a reasonable initial choice. Indications for immediate surgery include the clear evidence of a major complication such as meningitis, brain abscess, cavernous sinus thrombosis, acute suppurative labyrinthitis, or facial palsy. Some otolaryngologists consider the destruction of septal bone (osteitis) and resorption of the mastoid air cells an indication for surgery.

Oral antibiotics should be continued for 4–6 weeks after the patient is discharged.

The prognosis is good if treatment is started early and continued until the process is inactive.

DETECTION & MANAGEMENT OF HEARING DEFICITS

Hearing deficits are classified as conductive, sensorineural, or mixed (Table 13–2). Conductive hearing loss results from a blockage of the transmission of sound waves from the external auditory canal to the inner ear and is characterized by normal bone conduction and reduced air conduction hearing. In children, conductive losses are most often caused by middle ear effusion. Sensorineural hearing loss occurs when the auditory nerve or cochlear hair cells are damaged. Mixed hearing loss is characterized by components of both conductive and sensorineural loss. The criteria for normal hearing levels in children are lower than those in adults, since children are in the process of learning language. In children, a hearing loss of 15–30 dB is considered mild, 31–50 dB moderate, 51–80 dB severe, and 81–100 dB profound.

Table 13-2. Causes and types of hearing loss.

Source	Cause	Type	Degree of Loss
Congenital			
Endogenous	Hereditary (recessive, X-linked, or dominant)	Sensorineural (usually organ of Corti)	Moderate to profound
Exogenous	Asphyxia	Sensorineural (organ of Corti)	Moderate (high-frequency deficits)
	Erythroblastosis	Sensorineural (brainstem)	Mild to severe (high-frequency deficits)
	Maternal rubella and other viruses	Sensorineural (organ of Corti)	Moderate to severe
	Ototoxic drugs (aminoglycosides)	Sensorineural (usually organ of Corti)	Moderate to profound
Either endogenous or exogenous	Congenital atresia, stenosis, or ossicular deformity	Conductive (may be unilateral)	Moderate
Acquired			
	Labyrinthitis	Sensorineural (cochlear)	Mid to profound

Measles	Sensorineural (usually cochlear)	Moderate to profound
Meningitis	Sensorineural (cochlear and 8th nerve)	Moderate to profound
Mumps	Sensorineural (usually cochlear and unilateral)	Profound
Trauma	Conductive, sensorineural, or mixed	Moderate to profound
Tumors	Sensorineural (8th nerve)	Moderate to profound
Cerumen	Conductive	Mild to moderate
Cholesteatoma		
Foreign bodies		
Otosclerosis		
Perforated tympanum		
Purulent otitis media		
Repeated loud noise		
Serous otitis media		

Conductive Hearing Loss

The greatest number of conductive hearing losses during childhood are caused by otitis media and its sequelae. Other causes include atresia, stenosis, or collapse of the ear canal; furuncle, cerumen, or foreign body in the ear; aural discharge; bony growths; otitis externa; perichondritis; middle ear anomalies (eg, stapes fixation, ossicular malformation); and cleft palate.

The average hearing loss due to middle ear effusion (whether serous, purulent, or mucoid) is 27–31 dB, which is a mild hearing loss. This loss may be intermittent in nature and may occur in one or both ears, which accounts for the wide variability of the effects of ear disease on language development in children.

The American Academy of Pediatrics recommends that hearing be assessed and language development skills be monitored in children who have frequently recurring acute otitis media or middle ear effusion persisting longer than 3 months. The effects of hearing loss may be insidious and may not be discernible until the explosive phase of expressive language development occurs between 16 and 24 months of age; therefore, the optimal times for screening very young children are 18 and 24 months. An acceptable tool for language screening at these ages is the Early Language Milestone (ELM) scale. Children 3, 4, and 5 years of age should also be screened for language delays.

To mitigate the likelihood of a communication disorder developing, the physician should inform the parents of a child with middle ear disease that the child's hearing may not be normal and should instruct the parents to (1) turn off sources of background noise (eg, televisions, radios, dishwashers) when speaking to the child; (2) focus on the child's face and gain his or her direct attention before speaking; (3) speak slightly louder than usual; and (4) place the child in the front of the classroom.

Sensorineural Hearing Loss

Sensorineural hearing loss arises from a lesion in the cochlear structures of the inner ear or in the neural fibers of the auditory nerve (cranial nerve VIII). Most sensorineural losses in children are congenital, with an incidence of one in 750 live births. Causes of congenital deafness include perinatal infections, problems related to premature birth, and autosomal recessive and dominant inheritance of various deafness syndromes.

CONGENITAL MALFORMATIONS OF THE EXTERNAL EAR

Congenital malformation of the auricle is a cosmetic problem; associated abnormalities of the urogenital system or inner ear may be present. In children with congenital malformation, hearing should be tested by 6 months of age.

A small skin tag, fistula, or cystic mass in front of the tragus is a characteristic remnant of the first branchial cleft. These are best treated surgically.

Protruding auricles are a dominant hereditary characteristic. If the defect is severe, otoplasty should be performed for cosmetic purposes when the child is 5–6 years of age.

Agenesis of the external auditory canal or ear can be corrected surgically. If agenesis is bilateral, a hearing aid is fitted when the child is 2–4 weeks of age so that the child is not deprived of auditory stimulation during early development. Surgery is performed before school age in patients with bilateral agenesis and after childhood in patients with unilateral agenesis.

CERUMEN REMOVAL

Cerumen removal is an essential skill for anyone who treats ear problems. Cerumen often prevents adequate visualization of the tympanic membrane. Impacted cerumen can also cause itching, pain, hearing loss, or otitis externa. If cerumen impinges on the eardrum, a chronic cough may be triggered and will persist until the cerumen is removed. The most common cause of impacted cerumen is the use of cottontipped swabs by parents in misguided attempts to clean the ear canal. Parents should be advised that earwax protects the ear (cerumen contains lysozymes and immunoglobulins that curtail infection) and will come out by itself; therefore, they should never put anything into the ear canal to hurry the process.

The technique of removal depends on the consistency of the earwax. All the procedures described below require careful immobilization to prevent injury of the ear canal. The physician should remove cerumen under direct visualization through an operating head of an otoscope. Frequently, cerumen that obstructs a view of the tympanic membrane can be pushed aside, the pneumatic seal reestablished, and mobility assessed without removing the speculum.

(1) Very soft/average cerumen: Sticky cerumen will adhere to an ear curet. A piece of this consistency can sometimes be removed by embedding the ear curet in it. If this technique fails, irrigation as described below should be instituted.

(3) Hard cerumen: Very hard cerumen may adhere to the ear canal wall and cause considerable pain or bleeding if one attempts to remove it with a curet. This type of wax should be softened with Cerumenex or a few drops of detergent before irrigation is attempted. After 20 minutes, irrigation can be started with water warmed to 35–38°C (95–100.4°F) to prevent vertigo.

An easy-to-assemble ear syringe consists of a 12-mL plastic syringe plus a piece of small plastic tubing. The tubing can be made from any scalp vein needle set by cutting off the needle about 3 inches from the female connector. The front end of the tubing is placed in the canal, behind the cerumen if possible, and the water is ejected with maximal pressure on the syringe plunger. The advantage of this technique is that the very small tubing may be inserted into the ear canal itself and the water stream is thus directed in the proper direction without interfering with reflux.

A commercial Water Pik is also an excellent device for removing cerumen, but it is important to set it at a low power (2 or less) to prevent any damage to the intact tympanic membrane.

A perforated tympanic membrane is a contraindication to any form of irrigation.

OTOSCOPY

Removal of cerumen (see above) may be necessary for adequate visualization of the ear and for assessment of the mobility of the tympanic membrane by pneumatic otoscopy.

The tympanic membrane is divided into 4 sections, based on the position of the long process of the malleus and the umbo as shown in Fig 13–2. The anterosuperior quadrant contains the short process of the malleus; the posterosuperior quadrant, the incus and pars flaccida; the posteroinferior quadrant, the round window; and the anteroinferior quadrant, the pars tensa and light reflex. To assess mobility of the tympanic membrane, a pneumatic otoscope with a rubber suction bulb and tube is used. The speculum inserted into the patient's ear canal must be large enough to provide an airtight seal. When the rubber bulb is squeezed, the tympanic membrane will flap briskly if no fluid is present (normal finding); however, if fluid is present in the mid-

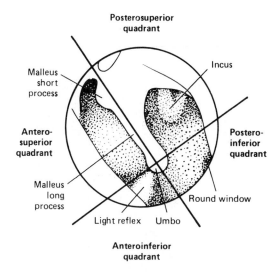

Figure 13–2. Schematic diagram of the left tympanic membrane. (Courtesy of the Department of Otolaryngology, University of Pittsburgh School of Medicine, and Eli Lilly and Co.)

dle ear space, the mobility of the tympanic membrane will be diminished.

TYMPANOMETRY

Tympanometry utilizes an electroacoustic impedance bridge to measure tympanic membrane compliance and display it in graphic form. Compliance is determined at specific air pressures (from $+200$ to -400 mm H_2O air pressure) that are created in the hermetically sealed external ear canal. The existing middle ear pressure can be measured by determining the ear canal pressure at which the tympanic membrane is most compliant. Because total visualization of the tympanic membrane is not necessary, tympanometry does not require removal of cerumen unless the canal is completely blocked.

Tympanograms can be classified into 3 major patterns, as shown in Fig 13–3. The type A pattern, characterized by maxi-

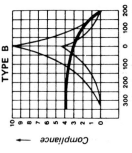

Figure 13–3. Type A tympanograms are characterized by maximum compliance at normal atmospheric pressure (0 mm H_2O air pressure). Type B tympanograms show little or no change in compliance of the tympanic membrane as air pressure in the external ear canal is varied. Type C tympanograms show near-normal compliance with significant negative middle ear pressures (typically more severe than −150 mm H_2O). (Reproduced, with permission, from Northern JL: Advanced techniques for measuring middle ear function. *Pediatrics* 1987; 61:761.

mum compliance at normal atmospheric pressure (0 mm H_2O air pressure), indicates a normal tympanic membrane, good auditory tube function, and absence of effusion. The type B pattern identifies a nonmobile tympanic membrane, which may be associated with middle ear effusion, perforation, patent ventilation tubes, or excessive and hardpacked cerumen. The type C pattern indicates an intact mobile tympanic membrane with poor auditory tube function and excessive negative pressure (> -150 mm H_2O air pressure) in the middle ear. Middle ear effusion is present in about 20% of patients with a type C pattern.

MYRINGOTOMY & TYMPANOCENTESIS

Tympanocentesis (placement of a needle through the tympanic membrane) is mainly a diagnostic procedure, because the hole closes over quickly and provides little sustained drainage. Tympanocentesis is helpful in (1) acute otitis media in a hospitalized newborn, because the pathogens may be gram-negative; (2) acute otitis media in a patient with compromised host resistance, because the organisms may be unusual; (3) painful bullae of the tympanic membrane; (4) a complete workup for presumed sepsis or meningitis; and (5) unresponsive otitis media despite courses with 2 different antibiotics.

Myringotomy involves incision of the drum with a myringotomy knife, leaving a flap through which drainage fluid may escape. This procedure is helpful for both diagnostic and therapeutic purposes. Myringotomy is indicated (1) when a patient on an initial visit with bulging acute purulent otitis media has severe pain or vomiting, because both symptoms are relieved by myringotomy; (2) when pain and fever fail to resolve after 48 hours of appropriate antibiotic treatment, because a middle ear abscess or resistant organism may exist; and (3) for acute mastoiditis, because it is important to permit drainage as well as to identify the particular organism.

Technique of Myringotomy

A. Premedication: In the conditions mentioned, the pain from a myringotomy is only slightly greater than the pain that already exists from acute inflammation of the tympanic membrane. Therefore, no premedication is generally indicated. The patient who is extremely difficult to hold may be premedicated with meperidine, 1 mg/kg intramuscularly. Some recommend applying Bonain's solution (equal parts cocaine, phenol, and menthol) to the tympanic membrane with a calcium alginate swab.

B. Restraint: The patient must be completely immobile while the incision is being made. A papoose board or a sheet can be used to immobilize the body. An extra attendant is required to hold the patient's head steady.

C. Site: With an open-headed operating otoscope, the operator carefully selects a target. This is generally in the posteroinferior quadrant. This site prevents disruption of the ossicles during the procedure.

D. Incision: The knife is lowered slowly until it touches the surface of the tympanic membrane at the chosen site. A quick 2- to 3-mm incision in the anterior direction is then made, leaving a curved flap in the area indicated (eg, from 8 o'clock to 4 o'clock on the right eardrum).

E. Culture: The myringotomy knife tip should be wiped on a cotton swab moistened with a few drops of normal saline solution. The material is then placed on a sheep blood agar plate, a chocolate agar plate, and a slide for Gram staining.

DISEASES OF THE NOSE & SINUSES

COMMON COLD

Nonbacterial upper respiratory tract infections are exceedingly common in the pediatric age group; about 2–4 such infections per year (6–8 in younger children) are considered usual in the USA.

A number of viruses are specific agents. Secondary bacterial invaders (beta-hemolytic streptococci, pneumococci, *H influenzae*) frequently contribute to prolongation of illness (beyond 4 days).

Clinical Findings

A. Symptoms: Malaise, sneezing, "stuffiness" of head, sore throat, and cough may be present.

B. Signs: Signs include serous nasal discharge and moist and boggy nasal mucous membranes. Fever is variable and may be high in an infant.

C. Laboratory Findings: The white blood cell count is normal or low.

Treatment

A. General Measures: Usually, no medications are needed. Give acetaminophen for pain or fever. Humidifying the air (vaporizer or bathroom shower water) is helpful in relieving nasal and pharyngeal discomfort and cough.

B. Local Measures: Topical vasoconstrictors, nose drops, or nasal sprays may provide symptomatic relief of nasal congestion but should not be used for more than 1 week. Overuse of any topical medication may result in irritation and "rebound" congestion. Oral decongestants cause jitters, and oral antihistamines cause lethargy; their use for treatment of the common cold is questionable.

Course & Prognosis

The usual course is of 4 days' duration. Continuation of rhinitis, regardless of whether it is serous or purulent, considerably beyond this period suggests bacterial complications or sinusitis that might respond to antibiotic therapy. Prognosis is excellent, but reinfections occur throughout life.

RECURRENT RHINITIS

A child with a chief complaint of "constant colds" is not uncommonly seen in office practice.

Differential Diagnosis & Treatment

A. Common Cold: The most common cause of recurrent runny nose is repeated viral upper respiratory tract infection. The onset is usually after 6 months of age. The bouts of rhinorrhea are usually accompanied by fever. Cultures are negative for bacteria. There is usually some evidence of contagion within the family.

Serum immunoelectrophoresis is an excessively ordered test. Children with immune defects do not have an increased number of colds.

Treatment consists of specific reassurance. The parents can be told that their child's general health is good; that the child will not have a great number of colds for more than a few years; that exposure to colds is building up the body's supply of antibodies; and that the child's problem is not the parents' fault.

B. Allergic Rhinitis: The onset of "hay fever" usually occurs after 2 years of age, ie, after the child has had adequate exposure to allergens. There is no fever or contagion among close contacts. The attacks include frequent sneezing, rubbing of the nose, and a profuse clear discharge. The nasal mucosa is pale and boggy. Smear of nasal secretions demonstrates over 20% of the cells to be eosinophils. Oral decongestants and antihistamines should be prescribed.

C. Chemical Rhinitis: Prolonged use of vasoconstrictor nose drops (beyond 7 days) results in a rebound reaction and secondary nasal congestion. The nose drops should be discontinued.

D. Vasomotor Rhinitis: Some children react to air pollution, tobacco smoke, or sudden changes in environmental temperature by manifesting prolonged congestion and rhinorrhea. Oral decongestants can be used periodically to give symptomatic relief.

PURULENT RHINITIS

Purulent yellow discharge that persists for more than 10 days usually represents purulent sinusitis, adenoiditis, or other bacterial superinfection of a common cold. The most likely organisms are *Streptococcus pneumoniae, Haemophilus influenzae,* group A β-hemolytic streptococci, and *Staphylococcus aureus.* Rare causes are diphtheria, pertussis, and syphilis. Any purulent discharge that is profuse and continuous for over 3 days probably should be evaluated, cultured for group A β-hemolytic streptococci, and considered for treatment. The common cold may also be associated with some mucopurulent discharge, but discharge is usually intermittent and worse upon awakening in the morning. The β-hemolytic streptococci are the most likely organisms if there is crusting around the nares that resembles impetigo, redness of the skin below the nares, or a blistering distal dactylitis.

Oral amoxicillin or trimethoprim-sulfamethoxazole, administered for 10 days will cure most of these patients. Occasionally, dicloxacillin will be needed because of culture results. The purulent material should be removed as completely as possible with a suction bulb or cotton-tipped applicators and a washcloth and soap.

If the problem recurs after adequate treatment, the patient should be referred to an otolaryngologist to rule out the possibility of a foreign body. If the discharge is foul-smelling and unilateral, this possibility becomes especially likely. The response to treatment is usually excellent.

SINUSITIS

1. ACUTE SINUSITIS

General Considerations

Acute inflammation of the paranasal sinuses or sinusitis may complicate up to 5% of upper respiratory tract infections. The maxillary and ethmoid sinuses are most commonly involved because of poor drainage related to anatomic features. When mucociliary clearance and drainage is further compromised by an upper respiratory infection, the risk of secondary bacterial infection increases. Sinusitis is also commonly seen during pollen season in children with allergic rhinitis. In cases in which superinfection occurs, the organisms are *S pneumoniae, H influenzae* (nontypable), *B catarrhalis*, and beta-hemolytic streptococci. Rarely, anaerobic bacterial infections can cause fulminant frontal sinusitis. Viruses can be isolated in 10% of sinus aspirates but their pathogenic role is unclear. Anerobic and staphylococcal organisms are often responsible for chronic sinusitis.

The ethmoid sinus is the only one that is significantly developed at birth. The maxillary sinus is rudimentary at birth and visible on x-ray by 6 months. The frontal sinus is not visible until 3–9 years of age. Clinical ethmoiditis does not usually occur until 6 months of age. Maxillary sinusitis is seen clinically after 1 year of age. Frontal sinusitis is unusual before 10 years of age.

Clinical Findings

A. Symptoms and Signs: The most common clinical presentation of children is persistance of nasal discharge or postnasal drip and daytime cough lasting longer than 7–10 days. Persistent low-grade fever is often present. Malodorous breath or intermittent painless morning periorbital swelling is often noted. Older patients may complain of acute onset of headache, a sense of fullness, or facial pain overlying the involved sinus. Ethmoiditis causes retroorbital pain; maxillary sinusitis causes upper molar or zygomatic pain; and frontal sinusitis causes pain above the eyebrow. These signs are often associated with a high fever.

Physical examination reveals injected nasal mucosa, usually associated with nasal or postnasal mucopurulent discharge. Occasionally there is percussion tenderness overlying the sinusitis.

B. Laboratory Findings: Sinus aspiration should be performed for diagnostic purposes in patients with complications and in those with an immunosuppressive disease. Gram stain and culture of nasal discharge is unnecessary as the type of discharge (thin, mucoid, or purulent) is not a useful predictor of sinusitis and does not correlate with cultures of sinus aspirates. If the patient is hospitalized because of complications, a blood culture should be obtained.

C. Imaging: In most cases, the clinical findings are so classic that x-rays are not needed. Positive x-rays in children over 1 year will show opacification of the involved sinus, air-fluid levels if the obstruction is intermittent, or mucosal thickening of greater than 5 mm. It is notable that x-ray findings positive for sinusitis may be found in asymptomatic patients with colds or nasal allergies. Sinus views include the anteroposterior (Caldwell) for the frontal and ethmoid sinuses, occipitomental (Waters) for the maxillary sinuses, and submento vertex and lateral for the sphenoid sinus. Sinus x-rays are mainly indicated in children with facial swelling of unknown cause; acute sinusitis that is unresponsive to 48 hours of therapy; undocumented chronic or recurrent sinusitis; and chronic asthma. A CT scan should be performed if bony erosions are present. Ultrasonography can also be used to document sinusitis.

Complications

The most frequent complication of paranasal sinusitis is preseptal periorbital cellulitis secondary to ethmoiditis. Less frequently, orbital cellulitis or abscess develops associated with decreased extraocular movement, proptosis, edema, and altered visual acuity. The most common complication of frontal sinusitis is osteitis of the frontal bone, called "Potts puffy tumor." Additional serious intracranial complications include cavernous sinus thrombosis, subdural empyema, brain abscess, and meningitis. The most common maxillary complication is cellulitis of the cheek. Rarely osteomyelitis of the maxilla can develop.

Treatment

A. Oral Antibiotics: Treat acute sinusitis with oral antibiotics for 2–3 weeks to achieve more prompt relief of symptoms and more rapid resolution of inflammation. The usual antibiotic should be amoxicillin 15 mg/kg/dose 3 times a day. In areas where beta-lactamase-positive pathogens are common or when the patient is allergic to penicillin, use trimethoprim plus sulfamethoxazole, 0.5 mL/kg/dose in 2 divided doses, erythromycin plus sulfamethoxazole 10 mg(eryth)/kg/dose in 4 divided doses, or amoxicilin clavidanate 10 mg/kg/dose in 3 divided doses. Continue antibiotic treatment for another week if the patient has improved but is not totally asymptomatic. Failure to improve after 48 hours suggests a resistant organism or potential complication. Assess the patient for a central nervous system complication. If none is found, consider hospitalization for parenteral therapy or switch antibiotics to an agent effective against beta-lactamase-producing pathogens.

B. Decongestants and Antihistamines: Topical decongestants and oral combinations are frequently used in acute sinusitis to promote drainage. Their effectiveness has not been evaluated and concern has been raised about potential adverse effects related to impaired ciliary function, decreased blood flow to the mucosa, and reduced diffusion of antibiotic into the sinuses. Patients with underlying allergic rhinitis may benefit from intranasal Cromolyn or corticosteroid nasal spray. Vasoconstrictor nose drops and sprays are all associated with rebound edema if used for more than 5 days.

Follow-up Care

The patient should be seen in 48 hours if there is no improvement with antibiotic therapy and at the end of the 2-week course. Obtain a confirmatory x-ray if symptoms persist at 2 weeks. Chronic or recurrent sinus infections suggest an underlying anatomic malformation, an allergy, cystic fibrosis, immotile cilia syndrome (Kartagener's syndrome), or an immunodeficiency disorder.

EPISTAXIS

Etiology

The most common cause of epistaxis during childhood is trauma to the nose due to nose picking or nose rubbing, which results in abrasion of the anterior inferior part of the nasal septum (Kiesselbach's area). Trauma to the nose may also be due to falls or blows. Bleeding diseases such as hemophilia, leukemia, von Willebrand's disease, and hereditary hemorrhagic telangiectasia (Rendu-Osler-Weber disease) may present as epistaxis. Other causes include presence of infection (a bloody, purulent nasal discharge is found in syphilis and diphtheria), foreign bodies, and allergic rhinitis. Severe epistaxis may occur with many tumors (eg, angiofibroma, lymphoma, sarcoma).

DISEASES OF THE THROAT

ACUTE STOMATITIS

Recurrent Aphthous Stomatitis ("Canker Sore")

The main finding is single (2 or 3 at most) small (3–10 mm) ulcers on the inside of the lips and throughout the remainder of the mouth. There is usually no associated fever or cervical adenopathy. The ulcers are very painful and last 1–2 weeks. The cause is not known, although an allergic or autoimmune basis is suspected.

Treatment consists of Topical antacids or sucralfate as a mouth coating qid. Topical corticosteroids, either in a dental paste—eg, triamcinolone acetonide, 0.1% (Kenalog in Orabase)—or in a mouthwash administered 4 times a day also have efficacy. Pain can be symptomatically improved by a bland diet, avoiding salty or acid foods, switching from a bottle to a cup in infants, 2% viscous lidocaine (Xylocaine) prior to meals, and acetaminophen or even codeine at bedtime. In children not old enough to expectorate the lidocaine, it must not be used.

Herpes Simplex Gingivostomatitis

Approximately 1% of children who have their first encounter with the herpes simplex organism develop multiple (10 or more) small (1–3 mm) ulcers of the buccal mucosa, anterior pillars, inner lips, tongue, and especially the gingiva, with associated fever, tender cervical nodes, and generalized inflammation of the mouth. The children are commonly under 3 years of age. This disorder lasts 7–10 days. Severe dysphagia interferes with eating and drinking. The primary disorder does not recur; herpes simplex recurs only in the form of cold sores that are found mainly at the labial mucocutaneous juncture. A throat culture is recommended to rule out streptococcal infection and a white blood cell count to rule out agranulocytic mucosa lesions.

Treatment is symptomatic as described for recurrent aphthous stomatitis (see above), with the exception that corticosteroids are contraindicated because they may result in spread of the infection. The patient must be followed closely. Dehydration occasionally ensues despite liberal offerings of cold fluids, in which case the patient must be hospitalized so that intravenous fluids can be administered. Herpetic laryngotracheitis is a rare complication.

THRUSH OF THE MOUTH

Oral candidiasis mainly affects bottle-fed infants and occasionally older children in a debilitated state. *Candida albicans* is a saprophyte that normally is not invasive unless the mouth is abraded. The use of broad-spectrum antibiotics may be a contributing factor. The symptoms include soreness of the mouth and refusal of feedings. Lesions consist of white curdlike plaques predominantly on the buccal mucosa. These plaques cannot be washed away after a water feeding.

Specific treatment consists of use of nystatin (Mycostatin) oral suspension, 1 mL 4 times a day for 1 week. This should be preceded by attempts to remove any large plaques with a moistened cotton-tipped applicator. The child should be fed temporarily with a spoon and cup to eliminate pain, continued abrasion, and possible contamination from nipple feedings.

ACUTE VIRAL PHARYNGITIS & TONSILLITIS

Over 90% of cases of sore throat and fever in children are due to viral infections. Most children develop associated rhinorrhea and mild cough and in fact are having a cold and nothing more. The findings seldom give any clue to the particular viral agent, but 6 types of viral pharyngitis are sufficiently distinctive to permit the clinician to make an educated guess about the specific cause.

Clinical Findings

A. Infectious Mononucleosis: The findings are an exudative tonsillitis, generalized cervical adenitis, and fever, usually in a teenage patient. A palpable spleen or axillary adenopathy adds weight to the diagnosis. The presence of more than 20% atypical lymphocytes on a peripheral blood smear or a positive mononucleosis spot test (Monospot) confirms the diagnosis. This diagnosis is often not considered until a patient with a presumptive diagnosis of streptococcal pharyngitis has failed to respond to 48 hours of treatment with penicillin.

B. Herpangina: Herpangina ulcers, 2–3 mm in size, are found on the anterior pillars and sometimes on the soft palate and uvula. There are no ulcers in the anterior mouth as seen in herpes simplex. Fever is present. The disease lasts up to a week. Herpangina is caused by several members of the coxsackie A group of viruses, and a patient can have up to 5 bouts of herpangina in a lifetime.

C. Lymphonodular Pharyngitis: The classic finding is small, yellow-white nodules in the same distribution as the small ulcers in herpangina. In this condition, which is caused by coxsackievirus A10, the nodules do not ulcerate.

D. Hand, Foot, and Mouth Disease: This entity is caused by coxsackieviruses A5, A10, and A16. Ulcers occur on the tongue and oral mucosa. Vesicles, which usually do not ulcerate, are found on the palms, soles, and interdigital areas.

E. Pharyngoconjuctival Fever: This disorder is caused by an adenovirus. Exudative tonsillitis, conjunctivitis, and fever are the main findings.

F. Rubeola: The prodrome of measles looks like any nonspecific viral respiratory infection until one closely examines the buccal mucosa and the inner aspects of the lower lip. Small white specks the size of salt granules on an erythematous base (Koplik's spots) found at these sites are pathognomonic of measles.

Treatment

The treatment of acute viral pharyngitis is strictly symptomatic. Older children can gargle with warm hypertonic salt solution. Younger children can suck on hard candy (especially butterscotch). Analgesics and antipyretics are sometimes helpful. Antibiotics are contraindicated.

ACUTE STREPTOCOCCAL PHARYNGITIS & TONSILLITIS

Approximately 10% of children with sore throat and fever have a streptococcal infection. Untreated streptococcal pharyngitis can result in acute rheumatic fever, glomerulonephritis, and suppurative complications (eg, cervical adenitis, peritonsillar abscess, otitis media, cellulitis, and septicemia). Vesicles and ulcers are suggestive of viral infection, whereas cervical adenitis, petechiae, a beefy-red uvula, and a tonsillar exudate are suggestive of streptococcal infection; the only way to make a definitive diagnosis is by obtaining a throat culture or a rapid identification test. A throat culture can be read 18 hours after being placed in an incubator. The bacteriology involved is simple, and an inexpensive office incubator is commercially available. Office throat cultures or rapid identification tests are essential for rational management of pharyngitis.

Treat cases of suspected or proved *S pyogenes* infection with a 10-day course of oral penicillin V potassium or an intramuscular injection of penicillin G benzathine. Use erythromycin for patients with penicillin allergy. Treatment failure after 10 days of penicillin V administered three times daily varies from 6% to 23%. Approximately 5% of *S pyogenes* are resistant to erythromycin. Remember that trimethoprim-sulfamethoxazole is not an effective antibiotic for *S pyogenes*.

If the child has a history of recurrent streptococcal infection, one must document the presence of *S pyogenes* in an asymptomatic patient following a course of therapy. If compliance or the antibiotic dosage was questionable, treat with intramuscular penicillin; otherwise, treat with an antibiotic effective against beta-lactamase-producing organisms (amoxicillin plus clavulanate, a cephalosporin, or erythromycin). If this therapy fails to eradicate the organism, consider a course of clindamycin for 10 days. In general, the carrier state is harmless, not contagious, and self-limited (2–6 months). An attempt to eradicate the carrier state is warranted only if the patient or another family member has frequent streptococcal infections or when a family member or patient has a history of rheumatic fever or glomerulonephritis. If the patient had three or more documented infections within 6 months, consider instituting daily penicillin prophylaxis during the winter season. Refer patients for tonsillectomy only if they continue to have frequent episodes despite antibiotic prophylaxis or when persistently enlarged tonsils cause chronic upper airway obstruction.

Other rare causes of acute nonviral pharyngitis are *Corynebacterium diphtheriae*, *Neisseria gonorrhoeae*, group C streptococci, meningococci, *Chlamydia*, *Francisella tularensis*, and *Mycoplasma pneumoniae*.

PERITONSILLAR ABSCESS
(Quinsy)

Tonsillar infection occasionally penetrates the tonsillar capsule, spreads to the surrounding tissues, and causes peritonsillar cellulitis. If untreated, necrosis occurs and a tonsillar abscess forms. This can occur at any age. The most common cause is beta-hemolytic streptococci. Other pathogens are group D streptococcus, alpha streptococcus, *S pneumoniae*, and anaerobes.

The patient complains of a severe sore throat even before the physical findings become marked. A high fever is usually present. The process is almost always unilateral. The tonsil bulges medially, and the anterior pillar is prominent. The soft palate and uvula on the involved side are edematous and displaced medially toward the uninvolved side. In severe cases, there is trismus, dysphagia, and, finally, drooling. The quality of the voice is severely impaired by the fixation of the soft palate. On palpation, the tonsil is firm and exquisitely tender.

Aggressive treatment in early cases of peritonsillar cellulitis may abort the process and prevent suppuration. The treatment of choice is penicillin or a cephalosporin. Daily follow-up is critical to detect possible abscess. If the initial swelling is marked, fluctuation develops, a neck mass develops, the patient appears toxic, or symptoms fail to respond to 48 hours of antibiotics, the patient should be hospitalized for intravenous penicillin or clindamycin. An otolaryngologist should be consulted to perform incision and drainage.

RETROPHARYNGEAL ABSCESS

Retropharyngeal nodes drain the adenoids, paranasal sinuses, and nasopharynx and can become infected. The most common cause is beta-hemolytic streptococci; less common pathogens are *S aureus* and oral anaerobes. If this pyogenic adenitis goes untreated, a retropharyngeal abscess forms. The process occurs almost exclusively during the first 2 years of life. Beyond this age, retropharyngeal abscess usually results from superinfection of a penetrating injury of the posterior wall of the oropharynx.

The diagnosis should be strongly suspected in an infant with fever, respiratory symptoms, and neck hyperextension. Dysphagia, dyspnea, and gurgling respirations are also found and are due to the impingement by the abscess. Prominent swelling on one side of the posterior pharyngeal wall confirms the diagnosis. Swelling usually stops at the midline because a medial raphe divides the prevertebral space. Lateral neck soft tissue films show the retropharyngeal space to be wider than the width of the C-4 vertebral body.

Retropharyngeal abscess is a surgical emergency. Immediate hospitalization is required. A surgeon should incise and drain the abscess under general anesthesia to prevent its extension. The head should be kept down during incision to prevent aspiration of purulent material. Intravenous hydration and antibiotics should be instituted before surgery. A penicillinase-resistant penicillin should be given. Clindamycin is an alternative.

ACUTE CERVICAL ADENITIS

General Considerations

Local infections of the ear, nose, and throat can spread to the regional node and cause a secondary inflammation there. The most commonly involved node is the jugulodigastric node, which drains the tonsillar area. The problem is most prevalent among preschool children.

A classic case involves a large, unilateral, solitary, tender node. About 70% of these cases are due to beta-hemolytic streptococci, 20% are due to staphylococci, and the remainder may be due to other bacteria and viruses.

The most common site of invasion is from pharyngitis or tonsillitis. Other entry sites for pyogenic adenitis are periapical dental abscess (usually producing a submandibular adenitis), facial impetigo (infected cuts or bug bites), infected acne, and otitis externa (usually producing a preauricular adenitis).

Clinical Findings

A. Symptoms and Signs: The patient is brought in with the chief complaint of a swollen neck or face. There is usually sustained high fever, especially in staphylococcal infections. The mass is often the size of a walnut or even an egg. It is taut, firm, and exquisitely tender. If left untreated, it may develop an overlying erythema. The exact size of the node should be measured for future follow-up. Each tooth should be examined for a periapical abscess and precussed for tenderness. A protective torticollis is sometimes present.

B. Laboratory Findings: The white blood cell count is usually about 20,000/μL with a shift to the left. The combination of leukocytosis and a positive throat culture or an elevated ASO titer identifies streptococci in about two-thirds of streptococcal cases. A tuberculin skin test should be given. Aspirated material from fluctuant nodes should be gram-stained and cultured for aerobes and anaerobes.

Differential Diagnosis

The causes of cervical adenopathy are numerous. Five general categories can be distinguished on the basis of the clinical findings.

A. Acute Unilateral Cervical Adenitis: See above.

B. Acute Bilateral Cervical Adenitis: Painful and tender nodes are present on both sides, and the patient usually has fever.

1. Infectious Mononucleosis–This diagnosis can be aided by the findings of splenomegaly, over 20% atypical cells on the white blood cell smear, and a positive mononucleosis spot test (Monospot). Toxoplasmosis and cytomegalovirus infections can imitate this disorder.

2. Tularemia–There will be a history of wild rabbit or deer-fly exposure.

3. Diphtheria–This only occurs in nonimmunized children.

C. Subacute or Chronic Adenitis: In this condition, an isolated node usually exists, but it is smaller and less tender than the acute pyogenic adenitis described previously.

1. Nonspecific Viral Pharyngitis–This accounts for about 80% of cases in this category.

2. Beta-hemolytic Streptococcal Infection–Streptococci can occasionally cause a low-grade cervical adenitis; staphylococci never do.

3. Cat-scratch Fever–The diagnosis is aided by the finding of a primary papule in approximately 60% of cases. Cat contact or scratches are present in over 90% of cases. The node is usually mildly tender. The cat-scratch skin test is helpful and relatively safe.

4. Atypical Mycobacterial Infection–The node is generally nontender and submandibular (occasionally preauricular). The nodes become fluctuant after several months. Affected patients are usually 1–5 years of age. A history of drinking unpasteurized milk is helpful. A mildly positive PPD is suggestive. A PPD-standard gives 5–10 mm of induration.

D. Cervical Node Tumors: Malignant tumors usually are not suspected until the adenopathy persists despite treatment. Classically, the nodes are painless, nontender, and firm to hard in consistency. They may occur as a single node, unilateral multiple nodes in a chain, bilateral cervical nodes, or generalized adenopathy. Cancers that may present in the neck are Hodgkin's disease, lymphosarcoma, fibrosarcoma, thyroid cancer, leukemia, and cancers with an occult primary in the nasopharynx (eg, rhabdomyosarcoma). One benign tumor that presents as enlarged cervical nodes is sinus histiocytosis.

E. Imitators of Adenitis: Several structures in the neck can become infected and resemble a node. The first 3 masses are of congenital origin and are listed in order of frequency.

1. Thyroglossal Duct Cyst–When superinfected, this congenital malformation can become acutely swollen. Helpful findings are the fact that it is in the midline, located between the hyoid bone and suprasternal notch, and moves upward on sticking out the tongue or swallowing. Occasionally, the cyst develops a sinus tract and opening just lateral to the midline.

2. Branchial Cleft Cyst–When superinfected, this can become a tender mass, 3–5 cm in diameter. Aids to diagnosis are the fact that the mass is located along the anterior border of the sternocleidomastoid muscle and is smooth and fluctuant as a cyst should be. Occasionally, it is attached to the overlying skin by a small dimple or a draining sinus tract.

3. Cystic Hygroma–Most of these lymphatic cysts are located in the posterior triangle just above the clavicle. The mass is soft and compressible and can be transilluminated. Over 60% are noted at birth, and the remainder usually present by 2 years of age. If cysts become large enough, they can compromise swallowing and breathing.

4. Mumps–Mumps crosses the angle of the jaw, is associated with preauricular percussion tenderness, and is bilateral in 70% of cases; there is frequently a history of exposure to mumps. Submandibular mumps can present a diagnostic dilemma.

5. Sternocleidomastoid Muscle Hematoma–This cervical mass is noted at 2–4 weeks of age. On close examination it is found to be part of the muscle body and not movable. An associated torticollis is usually confirmatory.

Treatment

A. Specific Measures: Unless the patient has recently been exposed to beta-hemolytic streptococci, dicloxacillin or erythromycin is usually started initially. The antibiotic can be changed to penicillin if the original antibiotic is not well tolerated and the throat culture is positive for streptococci. The patient should be referred to a dentist if a periapical abscess is suspected.

B. General Measures: Analgesics (even codeine) are necessary during the first few days.

C. Surgical Treatment: Early treatment with antibiotics prevents many cases of pyogenic adenitis from progressing to suppuration. However, once fluctuation occurs, antibiotic therapy alone is not sufficient treatment. When fluctuation or pointing is present, the primary physician should incise and drain the abscess. Hospitalization is required only if the patient is toxic, dehydrated, dysphagic, dyspneic, or less than 6 months of age.

D. Follow-up Care: The patient must be seen daily. A good response includes resolution of the fever and improvement in the tenderness after 48 hours of treatment. Reduction in size of the nodes may take several more days. The antibiotic should be continued for 10 days. If there is no improvement in 48 hours and the PPD test is negative, the node should be aspirated with an 18-gauge needle and 0.5 mL of normal saline in the syringe to obtain material for gram-stained smear, culture, and sensitivity tests. Aspirated material should be cultured aerobically and anaerobically.

The patient with a cervical node that has been enlarging for more than 2 weeks despite treatment or is still large and unchanged in size for more than 2 months should be referred to a surgeon for biopsy.

TONSILLECTOMY & ADENOIDECTOMY

Very few children require tonsillectomy and adenoidectomy. If possible, surgery should be deferred for 2–3 weeks after an acute attack has subsided.

Indications for surgery include persistent nasal obstruction, persistent oral obstruction, cor pulmonale, recurrent peritonsillar abscess, recurrent pyogenic cervical adenitis, suspected tonsillar tumor, persistent snoring, and sleep apnea syndrome. Snoring and hyponasal speech may be indications for adenoidectomy.

Contraindications to surgery include tonsillitis in the acute phase, bleeding disease, and polio epidemics. Great care must be taken in evaluating the child with cleft palate, submucous cleft palate, or bifid uvula for adenoid and tonsil surgery, because there is a risk of aggravating the defect of the short palate. Tonsillectomy and adenoidectomy do not significantly affect the later occurrence of otitis media.

Invalid reasons for surgery include "large" tonsils, recurrent colds and sore throats, recurrent streptococcal pharyngitis, parental pressure, school absence, and "chronic" tonsillitis. Over 95% of tonsillectomies and adenoidectomies are performed for these unjustified reasons.

ORAL CONGENITAL MALFORMATIONS

Cleft Lip & Cleft Palate

Cleft lip, cleft palate, or both conditions are found in one in 800 live births. They are readily diagnosed in the newborn nursery. Treatment requires a multidisciplinary team approach—plastic surgeons, otolaryngologists, audiologists, speech therapists, orthodontists, and prosthodontists. Cleft lip repair is usually performed before 3 months of age. Cleft palate repair is usually performed at about 12 months of age; this is essential to permit normal speech development, which should begin at this time. Occasionally, the palate is short and results in nasal speech.

Cleft palate causes eating problems and poor weight gain due to nasal regurgitation or lung aspiration of milk. Best results are obtained by feeding the baby with a cup or special compressible feeder. Approximately 90% of children with cleft palate have persistent and/or recurrent otitis media and must be carefully followed for this problem.

Pierre Robin Syndrome

This congenital malformation is characterized by the triad of micrognathia, cleft palate, and glossoptosis. Affected children present as emergencies in the newborn period because of infringement on the airway by the tongue. The main objective of treatment is to prevent asphyxia until the mandible becomes large enough to accommodate the tongue. In some cases, this can be achieved by leaving the child in a prone position while unattended. In severe cases, a custom-fitted oropharyngeal airway or large suture through the base of the tongue that is anchored to the soft tissue in front of the mandible is required. The child requires close observation until the problem is outgrown.

14 | Eye

Robert Sargent, MD

The most important role a pediatrician plays in the ophthalmologic care of children is to assure normal visual development. Central visual acuity sharpens until 8–9 years of age, when 20/20 vision should be attained. It is not uncommon for children to have a condition that interferes with this process, the most frequent being crooked eyes (strabismus), which occurs in 2–3% of the population.

VISION SCREENING

Vision screening should be performed as soon as a child becomes responsive to testing. Verbal responsiveness sufficient for visual screening occurs around 3–4 years of age, although some children can give feedback as early as 2–3 years of age. In children too young to respond to visual screening charts, a skilled pediatrician can sense poor fixation by one eye, by alternately covering each eye. Amblyopia, the absence of normal vision in one eye in the presence of a normal eyeball and optic nerve, needs to be detected as early as possible to assure optimal treatment.

In the preschool population, ages 3–5 years, vision screening can be performed using vision screening charts and cards. Below 4 years of age, a child is most easily tested by asking the names of objects that he or she looks at, such as an airplane, duck, hand, horse, telephone, umbrella, as found in the Allen Picture Test. By the age of 4 or 5, the Snellen letter "E" Test can be used. The "E-Game," in which a child points with his finger in the direction in which the lines of the letter E point, is appropriate. To eliminate confusion as to which item a child is to view, a particular letter can be blocked off. Most of the eye charts are designed for a distance of 20 feet from the child, for which we use the nomenclature 20/20 as the normal visual acuity.

However, a 10-foot distance with a smaller chart creates less distraction and is more convenient in many settings. A more consistent testing modality for 4-5 year old preschoolers is that of recognizing the letters H, O, T and V (Fig 14–1). The child sits with four cards with these four letters. The examiner points to one of the four letters on the wall chart and the child indicates which letter is identical to the letter on the chart. For young children, avoid the visual boxes that are mechanical where the head is placed into the viewing screen, as the instructions are too complex. In the young child, ages 3–5, it is the difference in visual acuity between eyes of one to two lines that means far more than a child who responds inattentively, but equally, in each eye.

AMBLYOPIA

Amblyopia is an abnormality of the central nervous system, in which the visual perceptual cortical cells of the occiput are not stimulated in the early years of life. As a result, the sensory portion of the brain that subserves the unused eye never learns to perceive a visual image crisply. Cellular maturation of the occipital cortex progresses until approximately 8–9 years of age. If one eye is not participating in the vision process during these formative years, the eye will never "see" normally for the remainder of the person's lifetime.

Etiology

A. Strabismus: A crooked eye is the commonest cause of amblyopia. Epicanthal skin folds which cover the white sclera nasally are common in the young child, and an infant may appear to have crossed eyes when indeed the eyes are aligned correctly.

B. Anisometropia: Anisometropia means "not the same refraction." For example, one eye has no need for glasses, while the other eye is way out of focus (either nearsighted, farsighted, or astigmatic). The brain receives clear retinal images from the normal eye, while the unfocused eye sends a blurry image to the brain. The second eye eventually becomes amblyopic, and the condition is difficult to detect unless early preschool vision screening is undertaken. A skilled pediatrician can sense poor

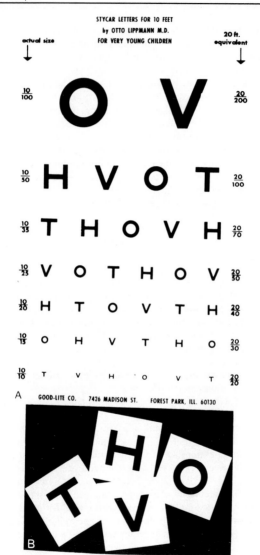

Figure 14–1.

fixation by one eye based on occlusion of the better eye, and resistance of the child to fixate with the poor eye. The diagnosis of anisometropia is made by an ophthalmologist by cycloplegic retinoscopy.

c. Ocular Pathology that Interferes with Normal Vision:
1. congenital cataract
2. corneal opacities
3. optic nerve hypoplasia
4. vitreous hemorrhage
5. chronic ocular inflammation
6. unilateral trauma or surgery during the early years of life.

Organic pathology is particularly devastating to normal visual development. One should never wait and observe these patients, but rather refer them to an ophthalmologist who is comfortable evaluating young children.

Diagnosis

Cover testing is the technique for detecting crooked eyes in pre-verbal children. This is an evaluation of shifting movements of each eye when the eyes are alternately covered (Fig 14–2). If no movement occurs, there is no misalignment of the visual axes, and therefore no strabismus is present. This is difficult to perform in young infants. The corneal light reflex from a penlight can aid in the diagnosis. The reflections should be central, or even somewhat nasal, on each side. The presence of a nasal corneal reflex is physiologic.

A. Vision Screening in the Verbal Child:
1. **Three-year-old–**Allen picture cards.
2. **Four- & Five-year-olds–**HOTV or tumbling E game (Fig 14–1).
3. **Six-year-old–**Linear alphabet.

Vision responses in children vary significantly due to differences in ability and attentiveness. If no success is obtained from a given child, utilize a simpler testing method.

The most important distinction is that of a 1–2 line difference in the vision responses rather than two eyes which are equal but poor in visual response. Amblyopia is a unilateral disease process in which one eye sees worse than the other.

At anytime in the early years of life that poor vision is suspected in one eye, the patient should be referred to an ophthalmologist.

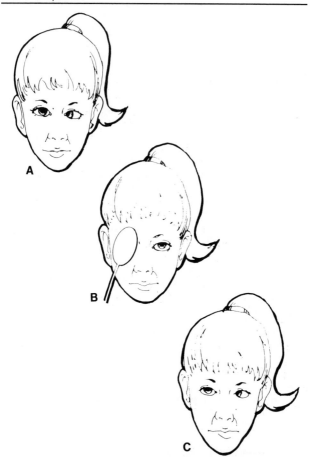

Figure 14–2. A. This girl has left esotropia. The occluder is placed over the better right eye (B), thereby forcing the child to see with the left eye. When the paddle is removed from the right eye the fixation shifts back to the dominant right eye (C). Cover-uncover testing here indicates some level of amblyopia in the left eye. An estimate of the amblyopia could be made by examining how poorly the left eye fixates when the paddle is on the right eye, and how quickly the right eye regains fixation while the left eye shifts back toward the nose. In older children a Snellen acuity test can be obtained.

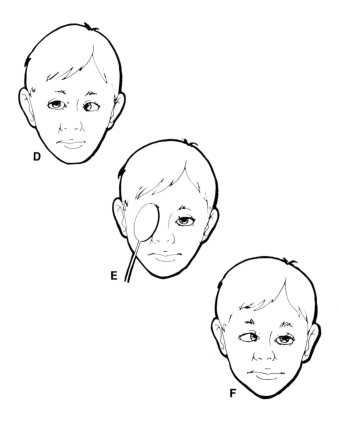

Figure 14–2. D. This boy also has left esotropia. **E.** The right eye is covered, forcing the child to use the left eye for fixation. **F.** When the paddle is removed the child maintains fixation with the left eye indicating good vision with the left eye. There is no amblyopia in this situation.

Treatment

A. Patching: This is by far the most important therapy for amblyopia. It must be undertaken vigorously in the early years of life, and, in selected cases, continued on a part-time basis, until 8–9 years of age.

B. Glasses, When Necessary: Sometimes an amblyopic eye is sufficiently out of focus that spectacle correction is of assistance in improving the visual acuity. This is particularly true when anisometropia is the cause of amblyopia.

C. Atropine Eye Drops: When a child resists occlusion, and simply pulls off the patches, one can blur the good eye by using the anticholinergic drop that paralyzes focusing. Thus, in order for the child to focus up close, there might be usage of the amblyopic eye.

STRABISMUS

Strabismus is a Greek word meaning "bent." In ophthalmology we refer to bending of the visual axis of each eye. Strabismus is significant for three reasons:

(1) Amblyopia is the most common and serious sequellae of strabismus. The first 8–9 years of life provide the only opportunity for the eyes to develop 20/20 visual acuity. All patients with strabismus should be referred to an ophthalmologist for evaluation of possible amblyopia and patching therapy.

(2) Having a crooked eye may lead to significant psychological trauma, affecting a child's self-confidence and self-esteem.

(3) Strabismus may be a sign of neurologic, ocular, or systemic pathology. Any neurologic condition that affects the third, fourth or sixth cranial nerve can lead to strabismus. Medical diseases include diabetic neuropathy, myasthenia gravis, metastatic lesions, amyloid depositions within the muscles, and other neurologic and metabolic conditions. An eye with poor vision in early infancy usually becomes esotropic. One should suspect any number of conditions within the eye when there is a persistent unilateral esotropia. These diagnoses would include retinoblastoma, chorioretinal scars from congenital viral infections, optic nerve hypoplasia, and congenital cataracts.

DEVELOPMENT OF OCULAR ALIGNMENT

0–2 Months of Age

Dysconjungate random eye movements. Strabismus is common, particularly exotropia.

2–3 Months of Age

Inattentive but intact fixation and following, best noted by mother.

3–4 Months of Age

Eyes at this stage should be straight and fixating well. Generally one waits until 6 months of age before undertaking strabismus correction.

TYPES OF STRABISMUS

Esotropia

Esotropia refers to crossed eyes (Fig 14–3A). Congenital esotropia is characterized by a large angle deviation, early infan-

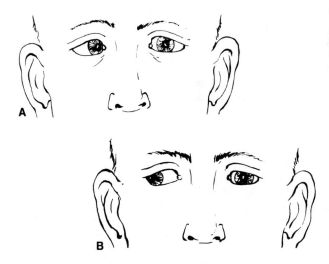

Figure 14–3. A. Right estropia. **B.** Right extropia. (Used, with permission, from Tse DT, Wright KW [editors]: *Color Atlas of Ophthalmic Surgery.* Lippincott, 1992.)

tile onset, occasional vertical imbalance such as dissociated vertical deviation in which an eye floats up with inattentiveness, or overacting inferior oblique muscles. Latent nystagmus is seen with congenital esotropia. Most congenital esotropes require surgery for correction of the deviation. Acquired esotropia is seen in individuals who have decompensation of fusional control such as an insult to the central nervous system, from a serious head injury. Diplopia is the immediate result. Children learn to suppress the diplopic image very soon, and therefore it is desirable to correct an acquired esotropia without delay in order to avoid sensory suppression or diplopia.

Accommodative esotropia may result from significant farsightedness (hyperopia) in which the act of focusing to see clearly induces accommodative convergence. It usually develops between 2 and 4 years of age. Treatment involves wearing glasses.

In cases of intermittent, non-accommodative esotropia one need not intervene early surgically; however, if the eyes are usually crossed, surgery should not be deferred.

Treatment

The purpose of "straightening eyes," whether it be by surgery or glasses, is to allow for the development of binocular fusion and depth perception. If the eyes are straight some binocular fusion may develop. If the eyes are always deviated the child has no choice but either seeing double or suppressing the image from the deviated eye.

If the eyes are fairly straight at distance fixation, but are crossed when focusing up close, bifocal glasses are sometimes indicated for excessive convergence. This type of esotropia usually improves by adolescence.

Exotropia

Exotropia is a condition of diverging visual axes (Fig 14–3B). It usually begins as an intermittent condition in which one eye or the other floats outward with fatigue, anxiety or illness. Over a period of time the frequency of diverging increases because the suppression becomes better and denser. Children with intermittent exotropia tend to squint their eyelids in bright sunlight, a peculiarity of this particular type of strabismus. Correction of the exotropia eliminates the squinting.

When exotropia presents later in childhood or at an adult age, diplopia can be experienced. The lack of diplopia usually indicates an early onset. The definitive treatment for exotropia is eye muscle surgery. Temporary measures include eye muscle exercises, or the use of glasses that induce accommodation (which in turn induces accommodative convergence that might control the exotropia). However, these therapy modalities are difficult to enforce in the young child.

Vertical Strabismus

Vertical strabismus is much less common than the horizontal deviations, and is associated with diplopia, or a compensatory face turn or head tilt. Face turning and head tilting can also be seen with torticollis, congenital jerk nystagmus, and eye muscle restrictions and palsies. An eye which is depressed is called hypotropia and an elevated eye is called hypertropia. The etiology of vertical strabismus includes congenital superior oblique palsy, Brown's syndrome involving a congenitally tight superior oblique tendon, adhesion syndromes from eye muscle surgery, and fibrosis anomalies. Treatment almost always involves eye muscle surgery or prism glasses.

EYE TRAUMA

Injuries of the eye can be divided into three broad categories:

(1) Blunt contusion and dislocation of ocular tissues.

(2) Laceration of the cornea and sclera with or without prolapse of intraocular contents.

(3) Corneal abrasion and foreign body of the cornea.

EPIDEMIOLOGY

A. Adolescent Years: Sports injuries from balls, bats, hockey pucks, and physical injuries that strike the eyes.

B. Elementary School Years: Thrown objects at the eyes including rocks, sticks, mud, snowballs, pop guns, arrows, darts, and fists.

C. Preschool Children: Accidental bumping into objects such as the corner of a table or chair posts. Of particular danger in this age group are the metallic prongs that hold items for sale in department stores, supermarkets and drug stores. These are usually placed at the eyeball level of a two to six year old child.

Males suffer eye injuries far more frequently than females. When a child loses an eye or has severely compromised vision protective lenses should be considered for the only remaining eye.

BLUNT INJURIES

A. Subconjunctival Hemorrhage: This is harmless but frightens a parent because of the blood red appearance of the bulbar conjunctiva.

B. Hyphema: This is a hemorrhage in the anterior chamber due to injury to the capillaries of the iris tissue. The amount of blood can vary from a microscopic level to complete filling of the anterior chamber. The major concern is failure of blood resorption and the development of secondary glaucoma. Re-bleeds occur most frequently on the third to fifth post-injury day. Eyeball rest is preferable to episodic visualization. Historically these children were hospitalized, but the majority of children can remain at home at eye rest. Treatment includes limitation of ocular movement. Watching television is an excellent method to reduce eye movement.

C. Fracture of the Bony Orbital Floor Between the Socket and Maxillary Sinus: This can incarcerate the fat tissue and inferior rectus muscle inferiorly leading to scarring and hypotropia. Usually diplopia is due to muscle contusion and will resolve in 1 to 2 weeks. True incarceration requires surgical intervention.

D. Disruption of the Attachment of the Peripheral Iris to the Ciliary Body: This damages the outflow trabecular meshwork, which interferes with drainage of aqueous humor into the canal of Schlemm. Secondary glaucoma can occur.

E. Cataracts: These can result from blunt injuries, but are more common from lacerating injuries.

F. Dislocated Lens: This interrupts clear vision and is of particular concern in children where amblyopia can occur.

G. Retinal or Vitreous Hemorrhage

H. Detached Retina

I. Macular Edema and Hemorrhage

J. Choroidal Rupture: This results in severe visual loss. Injuries to the posterior segment of the eye are more serious than are surface contusions and abrasions.

Treatment of Blunt Injuries

The pediatrician should obtain a visual acuity and refer when vision is not normal. Most cases resolve without a problem and are manifest by nothing more than bruised eyelids ("shiner").

LACERATING INJURIES

Lacerating injuries are ocular emergencies and require ophthalmic surgery.

Clinical Manifestations
(1) Possible history of foreign body that penetrated the globe.
(2) Pain.
(3) Red eye.
(4) Poor vision.
(5) Flat appearance to anterior chamber due to loss of aqueous humor.
(6) Irregular pupil because of incarceration of the pupil edge or peripheral iris into the lacerated area.
(7) Possible cataract.
(8) Black or pigmented opacity on the white part of the eye indicating protrusion of uvea through scleral laceration.
(9) Intravitreal or retinal foreign body.

Treatment
(1) Obtain a visual acuity, if possible.
(2) Patch or shield the eye for protection of an opened eyeball.
(3) Systemic antibiotics to get a blood level for protection of the posterior segment of the eye. Infection can occur rapidly throughout the eye (endophthalmitis), which can lead to loss of the eye itself.
(4) Refer to an ophthalmologist.
(5) Instruct patient to remain NPO for eventual anesthesia and surgical repair.
(6) Transport the patient to hospital emergency room or ophthalmologist's office.

CORNEAL ABRASION OR FOREIGN BODY

Signs & Symptoms
(1) Severe localized pain.
(2) Tearing.

(3) Blepharospasm.

(4) Reactive conjunctival hyperemia.

(5) Decreased visual acuity from the injury or copious tearing.

Sometimes a careful history will distinguish a foreign body from a surface scratch. Inspect the upper and lower cul-de-sacs between the eye and eyelids for a foreign body. The lower lid is easy to examine, but flipping the upper lid is an art, particularly in children. The easiest way to rotate the upper lid is to use a cotton applicator as a fulcrum, and then to grab the lashes and make one decisive flip-of-the-lid. This allows examination of the tarsal plate superiorly. If a foreign body is observed it can usually be removed with a cotton applicator.

If a foreign body is not observed, one applies fluorescein solution to the lower fornix (the crevice between the everted lower lid and the eye) in order to stain the corneal surface. Use the bluelight and a +10 diopter lens of the ophthalmoscope. If a scratch is observed, antibiotic ointment and tight patch is the primary treatment. If the pain is severe one can add a cycloplegic dilating drop such as Cyclogel or Homatropine, because it paralyzes the ciliary spasm that contributes to the child's pain. Sometimes a patch is necessary when a foreign body is removed from the upper or lower lids, because the object may have scratched the cornea prior to its removal. Topical anesthetic drops should not be used, because they mask the pain.

Corneal Foreign Body

If a foreign body is imbedded upon the cornea, one can instill a topical anesthetic drop. The bevelled edge of a 25-gauge needle, applied tangentially towards the eye can remove such a foreign body. Never use a sharp object directed toward the eye, because a child who thrusts forward could inadvertently suffer a perforating injury from the sharp object.

A tight patch over the scratched eye is important because it prevents blinking, minimizing pain. The prevention of blinking also allows for more rapid reepithelialization of the corneal surface. Two eye patches are placed upon the child's eye, one folded in half and the other flat upon the closed eyelid. Tape is applied from the forehead to the cheek in such a manner that the lower cheek is drawn upward before the tape is adhered to the face. When the lower cheek drops downward it flattens out the tape over the patch, applying greater pressure upon the eyeball. Additional tapes are placed nasally and temporally. Tincture of benzoin may be useful in making the skin surface sticky.

The patch can be kept on 24–48 hours, and then removed. Most all abrasions heal in this period. If there is any question about the status of the eye or vision, the child should return for a follow-up visual acuity measurement.

CHEMICAL INJURIES

Chemical injuries can be dangerous depending on the material that enters the eyes. Alkali burns soak into the corneal and ocular tissues leading to cellular necrosis and eventual corneal opacification. The loss of goblet cells of the conjunctiva lead to a dry eye and a poor prognosis, even with corneal transplantation. An alkali burn may appear white and non-painful initially, but is followed with corneal ulceration and opacity.

Acid burns such as citric acid from grapefruit juice into the eye, leads to immediate pain, irritation, tearing and conjunctival hyperemia. Other than the mechanical or chemical abrasion to the corneal surface, no serious injury usually ensues. In such cases irrigation of the eye suffices.

Organic solvents to the eye cause no serious injury to the globe but mydriasis (dilated pupil) can remain for weeks to months afterwards.

Thermal burns to the eye usually singe the lashes but do not cause serious eye pathology. If the eyes per chance are exposed to the flash of heat, a corneal abrasion results; topical antibiotics are necessary while the patient is managed for the facial skin burn. Do not apply a tight patch in these situations to loose, edematous, or sloughing skin tissue.

OCULAR INFLAMMATORY DISEASES

CONJUNCTIVITIS

Conjunctivitis is inflammation of the mucosal lining of the eye. The hallmark is a red or pink eye due to vasodilatation. Secretions can be watery, mucoid or purulent. Symptoms include burning, stinging, itching, pain, sandy, gritty and foreign body sensation.

Differential Diagnosis
  A. Allergy.
     1. Bacterial.
     2. Viral.
     3. Fungal.
  B. Unfection.
  C. Trauma.
  D. Foreign body.
  E. Dry eyes.
  F. Chemical irritation.
  G. Secondary to Other Disease:
     1. Keratitis.
     2. Uveitis.
     3. Glaucoma.
     4. Corneal abrasion.

ALLERGIC CONJUNCTIVITIS

Allergic conjunctivitis is typically itchy and often seasonal. The discharge tends to be watery and the condition bilateral. Diagnosis can be aided by conjunctival scrapings that show eosinophils.

Treatment
   (1) A decongestant-antihistamine drop is safest to use both to reduce the redness and give some relief as an astringent.
   (2) Steroids can be used for treating particularly itchy eyes. One must always use fluorescein staining of the cornea to rule out dendritic keratitis as seen with herpes simplex keratitis. Steroids are contraindicated with herpes.
   (3) Cromolyn sodium is used to inhibit mast cell degranulation and is particularly helpful in treating vernal conjunctivitis that occurs around May and June. It should be used when the patient is not responsive to steroids.
   (4) Avoid offending allergens. An allergy work-up is usually not helpful.

BACTERIAL CONJUNCTIVITIS

Bacterial conjunctivitis is more often unilateral than bilateral, and is associated with pain, mucopurulent discharge and a beefy red conjunctival injection. The most common bacteria are *Haemophilus influenzae, Streptococcus pneumoniae, S. aureus,* and other gram-positive organisms.

Treatment
Treatment includes antibiotic drops or ointment. If antibiotic drops are used, they should be administered every 2 hours while the patient is awake, and continued for at least 48 hours after signs and symptoms have disappeared. The frequent application of drops is required because tearing rapidly dilutes and eliminates antibiotic solutions from the eye. Antibiotic ointments can be used less frequently, every 4–6 waking hours; however, blurring of vision may be annoying to older children. Because spread of infection is common, topical therapy may include both eyes. A number of different antibiotic preparations can be used, including topical 10% sulfacetamide or polymyxin-bacitracin. Other options include gentamicin, tobramycin, and erythromycin. Neomycin and gentamicin opthalmic preparations can cause an allergic reaction.

VIRAL CONJUNCTIVITIS

Viral conjunctivitis is common. It is usually bilateral and is associated with a profuse watery discharge, generalized hyperemia, and nonspecific ocular irritation, burning, or itching. The diagnostic clues for viral conjunctivitis are preauricular lymphadenopathy and associated sore throat or fever.

CHLAMYDIA CONJUNCTIVITIS

Chylamydial conjunctivitis is the commonest form of infectious ophthalmia neonatorum. It is a bilateral condition with hyperacute bulbar injection with extensive mucoid discharge. The diagnosis can be made by Giemsa stain of the conjunctival scrapings or more easily with immunoflourescent monoclonal antibody stains.

Treatment of chlamydia is with topical erythromycin or tet-

racycline antibiotic. Because of the association with *Chlamydic*
pneumonia, oral erythromycin for 2 weeks should supplement
topical tetracycline medication.

HERPES SIMPLEX KERATOCONJUNCTIVITIS

Herpes simplex is the most serious viral pathogen. The
DNA virus resides in conjunctival and lacrimal tissues, and can
cause recurrent infections in susceptible individuals. The virus
invades the corneal epithelium giving a typical dendritic pattern.
One can use an ophthalmoscope with + 10 magnification, the
blue light and fluorescein staining to see the dendritic pattern.
Sometimes a slit lamp is necessary for magnification. As with
other viral conjunctivitis, preauricular lymphadenopathy is common. Vesicles on the lid margin, and a history of stomatitis are
often present.

The patient should be referred to an ophthalmologist, because blindness can be a sequellae of this desease. The mechanism of blindness is an allergic antibody response to the viral
antigen resulting in corneal opacification.

Treatment

The initial treatment of primary herpes simplex keratitis
consists of the application of topical antiviral agents. Either idoxuridine (IDU) ointment 0.5 percent or vidarabine (Vira-A) in a
3 percent ointment should be instilled five times a day, or trifluridine (Viroptic) in a 1 percent solution may be used every 2 hours
(not more than nine drops a day). The treatment should be continued until the lesions have cleared, although no longer than 10
to 12 days.

MEASLES

Rubeola typically causes a keratitis which is why photophobia is so bothersome. The disease is self-limited and no treatment
is necessary.

CHICKEN POX

Varicella infrequently involves the eyes, but can inflame
any part of the anterior segment of the eye. Most commonly

lesions involve the conjunctival surface, appearing as white blister-like domes of 1–2 mm with surrounding dilated capillaries. The lesions are asymptomatic, and clear as the varicella resolves. Occasionally there is crusting on the lid margin which can be a mechanical irritation to the cornea leading to abrasion. If so, the firm crust should be removed and sterile eye ointment applied to the eye to minimize corneal irritation.

MOLLUSCUM CONTAGIOSUM

Molluscum contagiosum is a viral disease characterized by 1–2 mm solid umbilicated lesions located near the lid margin. Virus particles are released into the eye, which cause a chronic conjunctivitis. Treatment involves debridement of the umbilicated tissue by pricking the central part of the pearl-like elevation with a sterile pin or needle. The central content is curetted, or treated with cyrotherapy.

OPHTHALMIA NEONATORUM

Ophthalmia neonatorum is a conjunctivitis occurring in the first month of life. The most common cause is chlamydia, but the most serious pathogen is *Neisseria gonorrhoeae*. The differential diagnosis also includes a spectrum of organisms that can infect the eye thorough the vaginal canal, or from nosocomial infections from the hospital setting. Silver nitrate conjunctivitis used to be the commonest cause of ophthalmia neonatorum, but because of the conversion to topical erythromycin or tetracycline to prevent chlamydia, chemical conjunctivitis is infrequently encountered. The reason for avoiding silver nitrate is that it has no effect upon chlamydia.

Treatment
Gonorrhea requires aggressive topical and systemic antibiotics. Besides diphtheria, gonorrhea is the only other organism that can penetrate the intact corneal epithelium. Once the pathogen enters the eye the disease progresses rapidly to endophthalmitis and blindness. A century ago gonorrhea was the leading cause of blindness in children. Treatment for gonococcal conjunctivitis should be started as soon as possible based on the presence of gram-negative diplococci seen on gram stain. Diag-

nosis should be confirmed by culture. Topical antibiotic therapy alone is inadequate. Neonates, older infants and children with gonococcal ophthalmia should be hospitalized and evaluated for disseminated gonococcal infection. Gonococcal ophthalmia should be treated for seven days with Ceftriaxone, 25–50 mg/kg/day IV or IM in a single dose, or Cefotaxime 25 mg/kg/day IV or IM every 12 hours. Infants should receive eye irrigations with buffered saline solutions until discharge has cleared. Because of simultaneous infection with *Chlamydia trachomatis*, the mother and infant should be tested for chlamydia infection.

ORBITAL CELLULITIS

Orbital cellulitis is characterized by a pink, violaceous swelling of the lid margins. The diagnosis is somewhat of a misnomer because the majority of cases are truly preseptal inflammation not inflammatory disease behind the eye.

Preseptal Cellulitis

There is a firm, fibrous membrane that extends from the bony orbital rim to the lid margins. This prevents extension of lid margin disease to the posterior orbital region. There are three main causes for preseptal cellulitis:

(1) Sinusitis with local extension.

(2) Local lid disease such as sties or infected chalazia.

(3) Lid trauma with secondary infection, occasionally with suppuration and abscess formation. In preseptal cellulitis, there is no proptosis, limitation of eye movement, myositic pain on eye movement, chemosis, or retrobulbar pressure upon the optic nerve or globe causing papilledema and/or vision compromise. Extension of preseptal cellulitis to the brain is rare.

In the child younger than 3 years of age, preseptal cellulitis is far more common than orbital involvement and the commonest pathogen is hemophilus influenza. In the older child, Gram-positive disease is more frequent.

A. Treatment: Periorbital, or preseptal, cellulitis is treated by aggressive intramuscular and oral antibiotics.

Orbital Cellulitis

True orbital cellulitis is an ocular emergency because the disease is located between the eye and the brain. The disease can spread posteriorly to the cavernous sinus posteriorly or anteriorly, into the eye resulting in vision loss.

Mechanism of Orbital Cellulitis

Bacterial ethmoid sinusitis extends through the thin medial bony wall into the orbital region and into the retrobulbar veins. Because these veins do not have valves, the disease can spread retrograde creating lid margin swelling that one sees with preseptal cellulitis.

Clinical Manifestations

A. Proptosis: Swelling behind the eye creates a bulgy appearance to the eye itself. One must be careful to distinguish between swollen lids per se versus a truly exophthalmic eye. The easiest way to determine this clinically is by looking over the forehead to see if the globe has a more anterior corneal protrusion on the involved side.

B. Myositic pain and limitation of eye movement.

C. Diplopia on side gaze due to inability to move the eye.

D. Chemosis: This refers to swelling of the conjunctiva with or without redness to the eye.

E. Venous dilatation and tortuosity of the retinal vascular tree on ophthalmoscopic examination.

F. Papilledema.

G. Compromise of vision.

H. CT Scan or MRI evidence of sinusitis.

Differential Diagnosis

A. Orbital Pseudotumor: This is a disease of unknown etiology involving swelling of the soft tissue and extra ocular muscles in the orbit. It is uncommon in children and diagnosed by exclusion when acute inflammatory disease does not respond to antibiotics. Unlike infectious orbital cellulitis the white count and differential are normal; the sedimentation rate is frequently elevated. Orbital pseudotumor responds to high dose oral steroids.

B. Rhabdomyosarcoma: Orbital involvement leads to rapid progression of lid swelling, pinkness, proptosis and immobility of the eye. The disease is usually asymptomatic. Diagnosis requires a biopsy, and treatment involves chemotherapy.

C. Neuroblastoma: Although metastasis can spread to the orbit, the more common finding is that of bilateral periorbital ecchymosis with minimal swelling. This is a classical sign of neuroblastoma.

D. Leukemia and Lymphoma: Either disease can have a rapid inflammatory course in the orbital region, thereby mimicking infectious orbital cellulitis.

E. Other Tumors:
  1. Neurofibroma
  2. Glioma of the optic nerve
  3. Dermoid cysts
  4. Lymphangioma
  5. Hemangioma
  6. Wilm's tumor

All of these tumors tend not to have the rapid course of infectious orbital cellulitis but must be considered in the differential diagnosis of exophthalmos.

STY (HORDEOLUM)

A sty is an acute inflammation of the oil secreting glands of the lid margin. It occurs commonly in children because they tend to rub their eyes frequently, introducing gram positive organisms from their fingers. *Staphylococcus aureus* is the most common offending organism. Some patients have a predilection for recurrent oil gland infections, just as acne tends to afflict some teenagers more than others.

The usual presentation is one of a painful, pink mass near the lid margin which occasionally spreads into an adjacent cellulitis, or encapsulates into abscess. The oil gland orifice is frequently obstructed, but pressure or moist heat therapy, can rupture the lesion causing drainage of pus. There is no serious sequelae from this infectious disease.

Treatment

Treatment involves hot soaks and topical antibiotic medication, 3–4 times a day. A useful approach with children is to have them watch TV with a warm moist wash cloth applied to the affected lid. The wash cloth requires periodic reheating. Most topical antibiotics are effective in treating the infection. Ointments last longer, and can be easier to apply. Eye drops do not blur the vision, and do not lead to a greasy appearing lid margin.

CHALAZION

A chalazion is a lipogranulomatous tumor arising from the oil secreting glands within the tarsal plate. The tarsal plate is the collagenous connective tissue condensation that forms the structural support of the eyelids. Chalazia are the sequelae of chronic lid gland inflammation. The healing process leads to granulomas that incorporate lipid material from the infected ductules. They can become secondarily infected and present with a tender pink nodule on the lid. The diagnosis can be confusing between an acute sty versus a secondarily infected chalazion. However, the treatment is the same: hot soaks and topical antibiotic medications.

Chalazia when not infected, are benign lumps that may present externally on the skin side, or internally on the tarsal conjunctiva. These usually require surgical excision.

An infected chalazion can last weeks to months, especially without treatment of hot soaks and topical antibiotics. Excision in a child requires general anesthesia. To avoid general anesthesia, one must continue hot soaks and antibiotics for 2–3 months for resolution of the lesion. Most chalazion in children eventually clear with conservative medical treatment.

UVEITIS

Iritis is inflammation of the anterior segment of the eye, whereas, uveitis is a generic term for inflammation of any portion of the uveal tract. Acute iritis in children is rare. It is usually associated with juvenile rheumatoid arthritis (JRA). Diagnosis of iritis requires a slit lamp examination. A work-up for JRA should be undertaken in children when iritis occurs. The disease is usually unilateral and treated with steroids.

PARS PLANITIS

The anatomy between the anterior iris and the posterior choroid is called the pars plana. Inflammation of the pars plana or peripheral retinal area is infrequent, but can cause blindness. Early detection of patients with poor vision, eye pain and secondary conjunctivitis requires the evaluation by an ophthalmologist. Vision below 20/40 requires retrobulbar injection of Depo-Medrol under general anesthesia. The protocol for this disease usually involves injections every two weeks for six occasions when the acuity does not improve beyond 20/40. As long as there is not damage to the macular cones, the disease usually is self limited, but can be interrupted by chronic, recurrent inflammatory episodes over a number of years.

OBSTRUCTED NASAL LACRIMAL DUCTS
(Blocked Tear Ducts)

Blocked tear ducts are the commonest cause of tearing or mucoid discharge in the neonatal period and during the first year of life. It is commonly confused with conjunctivitis because of the mucoid discharge from the eye. The serious item in the differential diagnosis is that of congenital glaucoma, both of which have watery eyes.

Seven percent of newborns are born with blocked tear ducts, but most all of the ducts clear spontaneously. The mechanism of obstruction is that of residual epithelial membranes in the tear duct passageway.

Clinical Manifestations
> (1) Watery or mucoid discharge.
> (2) White eyeballs.
> (3) Crusting on lashes.
> (4) Adherent lid margins, particularly in the morning when the watery component of tears evaporates at night.
> (5) Skin redness and maceration from chronic wetness.
> (6) Secondary infection.
> (7) Clumping of lashes instead of feathery dry lashes.
> (8) Tears dripping down the cheek.
> (9) A tendency for the infant to rub the eyes from tear crust or skin irritation.

Most blocked tear ducts are partial, which means that there is some patent passageway that allows for tear drainage when there is little stimulus for lacrimation.

Treatment
> **A. Do Nothing:** If the eyes are merely watery but there is no redness to the eyes with secondary infection, one simply can wait weeks, months or up to a year before the condition resolves spontaneously.
> **B. Massage of the Lacrimal Sac:** A downward pressure upon the lacrimal sac can push a bolus of mucous through the nasal lacrimal duct and break any membranes along the way. However, studies are not conclusive that massage is a beneficial therapy.

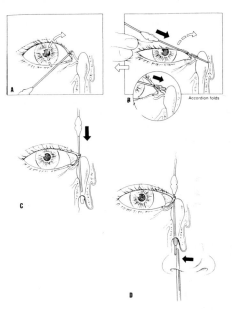

Figure 14–4. (Used, with permission, from Tse DT, Wright KW [editors]: *Color Atlas of Ophthalmic Surgery.* Lippincott, 1992.)

C. Antibiotic Medications: These should be reserved for conditions where the bulbar conjunctiva is inflamed. The tearing or mucous usually recurs after the secondary infection resolves.

D. Probing and Irrigation: This is a procedure in which the membranes are broken, followed by irrigation of saline into the nasal cavity (Fig 14–4).

Most obstructions resolve spontaneously by 1 year of age. Therefore, if a child simply has a watery eye but does not require repetitive attention or lid margin cleansing, one can wait a full year before attempting the probing and irrigation procedure.

If a child has recurrent infection or has significant discharge requiring the application of soggy tissues throughout the daytime, the obstruction can be treated by probing at anytime during the first year of life.

Most pediatric ophthalmologists are comfortable with probing in the office.

Prognosis

Most cases are successfully treated with one or two probing and irrigation procedures. If not, further surgery may be required. Down's syndrome children are particularly susceptible to failure with probing because of anomalous anatomy.

CONGENITAL CATARACT

A cataract is an opacity of the lens. Congenital cataracts are far more serious than lens opacities in adults, because dense amblyopia can result when the condition is not treated. Unilateral cataract leads to strabismus, while bilateral cataracts cause irreversible nystagmus. A neonate with dense opacites does not have visual stimulation of the central nervous system. This in turn interferes with the normal sensorimotor reflexes that maintain straight and steady eyes. It takes just a few weeks or months for permanent deterioration of vision.

Differential Diagnosis
   A. **Idiopathic.**
   B. **Familial autosomal dominant heredity.**
   C. **Ophthalmologic Conditions:**
      1. Posterior lenticonus.
      2. Microphthalmia.
      3. Aniridia.
      4. Retinopathy from congenital interuterine infections.
      5. Persistent hyperplastic primary vitreous (PHPV).
   D. **Metabolic Abnormalities:**
      1. Hyperglycemia.
      2. Hypoglycemia.
      3. Hypocalcemia.
      4. Galactosemia.
   E. **Systemic Syndromes:**
      1. Lowe's syndrome.
      2. Down's syndrome.
      3. Hallerman–Streiff syndrome.

Diagnosis
   (1) White pupil (leukocoria) due to opacity of the lens.
   (2) Unilateral strabismus, particularly esotropia, secondary to poor vision.

(3) Lack of red reflex. This may be difficult to evaluate in a black infant because of the dense melanin pigmentation of the retina. These infants may need pupil dilatation for evaluation.

(4) Clinical evidence of blindness such as poor fixation.

Treatment

If a congenital cataract is suspected either in the neonate or an older infant, the patient should be sent immediately to a pediatric ophthalmologist. The nature of the cataract dictates whether surgical intervention is necessary. For example, small dot-like anterior polar cataracts almost never interfere with vision, nor do trace remnants of the hyaloid system behind the lens. On the other hand diffuse or dense cataracts require extraction of the lens. Follow-up requires frequent changes of contact lenses or glasses prescriptions, and careful observation of vision and amblyopia.

Children with small cataracts do not require surgical removal but the cataracts may do progress with time. These children have to be followed by the ophthalmologist. Usually one considers lensectomy when the acuity is below 20/70. If the child is beyond 2–3 years of age, the eye has grown sufficiently that an intraocular lens (IOL) can be inserted. This is a new procedure in children, and is presently being investigated. An IOL obviates the need for contact lenses and puts the child's eye into optical focus immediately.

CONGENITAL GLAUCOMA

Glaucoma is a disease of high intraocular pressure associated with visual loss. The elevated pressure compresses the capillaries at the optic nerve thereby causing ischemic damage to the axons that connect the eye from the optic nerve to the brain. Glaucoma in the infant and child is very different from the silent disease seen in the older adult population.

Mechanisms of Congenital Glaucoma
  A. Primary Glaucoma:
    1. A congenital membrane between the iris and cornea obstructs the outflow of aqueous humor into the trabeculum and canal of Schlemm.
    2. Secondary Glaucomas–The mechanisms include (1) angle closure as seen with retinopathy of prematurity, micro-

phthalmos, persistent hyperplastic primary vitreous (PHPV):
(2) blood from eye trauma; (3) cellular and fibrin debris of
uveitis; and (4) abnormal trabecular cellular function as seen in
various syndromes such as neurofibromatosis, aniridia, and
Sturge–Weber syndrome.

Clinical Manifestations
(1) Tearing and watering in the first year of life. This can
mimic blocked tear ducts. Blocked tear ducts are usually associated with a mucoid discharge, while congenital glaucoma is associated with watery lacrimation.

(2) Irritability.

(3) Squeezing eyelids (blepharospasm).

(4) Severe photophobia.

The above findings precede clinical signs such as haziness
and enlargement of the cornea.

Differential Diagnosis of Cloudy Corneas
(1) Congenital glaucoma.

(2) Anterior segment dysgenesis.

(3) Congenital rubella syndrome.

(4) Interstitial keratitis, particularly syphilis and tuberculosis.

(5) Congenital hereditary endothelial dystrophy.

(6) Birth trauma from forceps injury to the cornea.

Treatment
Primary congenital glaucoma usually requires surgery in
which the membrane that obstructs aqueous humor outflow is
incised. Frequently the eye has already become enlarged prior
to surgery and therefore the larger eye becomes nearsighted.
This in turn leads to the need for tedious care for amblyopia.

PTOSIS OF THE EYELID (BLEPHAROPTOSIS)

Congenital ptosis is a muscular dystrophy of the levator
palpebrae muscle. Histopathologically, there is a lack of striated
muscle fibers. It occurs sporadically and usually has no familial
pattern. The condition can be unilateral or bilateral. The droopiness is worse later in the day with fatigue and loss of neuromuscu-

lar control. The child sometimes has to raise the chin upward to allow for visualization.

Differential Diagnosis

(1) Congenital muscular dystrophy (the commonest form).

(2) Horner's syndrome with sympathetic denervation.

(3) Congenital fibrosis syndrome involving fibrotic extraocular muscles of the eye, as well as droopiness of the eyelids.

(4) Congenital or acquired third nerve palsies.

(5) Myasthenia gravis.

(6) Chronic progressive external ophthalmoplegia.

(7) Trauma due to forceps injury to the levator muscle.

(8) Mechanical factors: large dermoid cysts, hemangiomas, and neurofibromas.

Clinical Features

(1) **Occasional anomaly** of jaw winking and twitching on attempted chewing or eating due to misdirection of innervation of the third nerve (Marcus–Gunn anomaly).

(2) **Anisometropic amblyopia.** The droopy lid sits on the cornea which distorts the shape of the eyeball. This leads to astigmatism then amblyopia. Ophthalmologists should rule out anisometropic amblyopia by performing a cycloplegic refraction in young children and repeating this procedure in the early years of life.

Treatment

Eye lid surgery. The choice of technique depends on the amount of ptosis and the degree of levator muscle function. Usually this is performed at 3–4 years of age. An exception to this rule would be the infant or toddler who raises his head excessively in order to see. In these cases a temporary fascia lata brow suspension can maintain adequate or palpebral fissure aperture to eliminate the compensatory head posture.

Prognosis

There are complications from the surgery which are intrinsic and cannot be avoided. Most lids cannot close completely and there is a lid lag on down gaze. Eye ointments are sometimes necessary to keep the eye moist, especially in the post-operative period.

RETINOBLASTOMA

Retinoblastoma is a rare malignancy of primitive retinal cells, usually seen in the first few years of life. There are two major types: (1) sporadic unilateral condition due to retinal cell mutations, and (2) hereditary autosomal dominant form that is usually bilateral and involves germinal cell mutations. In general the hereditary forms are seen earlier in the first year of life, while the sporadic form might first present after several years. The tumor can grow posteriorly through the optic nerve to the CNS and beyond. Most cases are detectable and treatable.

Clinical Manifestations
All neonates should have a red reflex check, even if the exam requires a dilating drop.

(1) White pupil (leukocoria).

(2) Strabismus.

(3) Glaucoma.

(4) Spontaneous hemorrhage (hyphema).

(5) A solid white or yellow retinal mass that extends anteriorly into the vitreous cavity.

Treatment
(1) Genetic counseling, particularly in bilateral cases with multifocal tumors, or cases with known family history of retinoblastoma.

(2) Radiation directed at the lesion. One must attempt to avoid the development of cataracts, and retinal neovascular proliferation from the radiation.

(3) Enucleation, in cases of huge tumors that are unlikely to respond to radiation, and would metastasize by direct extension.

(4) Photocoagulation.

(5) Cryoapplication.

(6) Radon plaque application to posterior lesions.

(7) Chemotherapy for extraocular extension.

(8) Involvement of "team" personnel involving oncologists, therapeutic radiologists, pediatric and retinal ophthalmologists, and geneticists.

RETINOPATHY OF PREMATURITY

Retinopathy of prematurity (ROP) is a vascular disease of the retina seen in premature infants of less than 31 weeks' gestation, particularly in those who receive high amounts of oxygen. Vascularization of the peripheral retina is a normal process between the fourth month of pregnancy to two weeks after birth.

All premature neonates undergo some degree of vessel proliferation, most of whom do not develop pathologic changes.

The abnormality is one of vessel proliferation into the vitreous cavity associated with bleeding, scarring, and ultimately complete retinal detachment and blindness. The exact mechanism is not unknown, but it is thought that a vasoproliferative substance is released in the peripheral avascular retina that leads to abnormal vessel growth. The end result is a cicatricial replacement of both the retinal and vitreous tissue.

Clinical Manifestations

The ophthalmologist usually examines the neonate 6–8 weeks after birth, when pathologic changes might be observed. There is a classification ranging from physiologic variations in the early stages to blindness at the latest stage. The following table summarizes the five stages.

Stages of Retinopathy of Prematurity

STAGE I	Demarcation line or border of dividing the vascular from the avascular retina.
STAGE II	Ridge. Line of previous stage acquires volume and rises above the surface retina to become a ridge.
STAGE III	Ridge with extraretinal fibrovascular proliferation.
STAGE IV	Subtotal retinal detachment.
STAGE V	Total retinal detachment.

Clinically, older children present with the following findings:

(1) Full recovery of central and peripheral vision.

(2) Partial visual incapacity, usually loss of central acuity due to distortion of the cones in the macula area.

(3) Cicatricial traction of the vessels and preretinal tissue drawn laterally, as can noted on ophthalmoscopy.

(4) High myopia.

(5) Anisometropia (one eye out of focus compared to the other eye).

(6) Bilateral mild microphthalmos.

(7) Deep upper lid sulcus, which means that one sees an indentation between the eyelid sitting upon the globe and the upper bony orbital rim.

(8) Secondary glaucoma.

(9) Retinal detachment.

(10) Complete scarring behind the lens, called retrolental fibroplasia (RLF).

Treatment

(1) Recognition of the disease entity by ophthalmologic examination of neonates, the first exam usually being 6 weeks after birth.

(2) Minimizing oxygen supplements, particularly long term usage rather than short high bursts of oxygen therapy.

(3) Cryoapplications to peripheral avascular retina in selected cases.

(4) Vitamin E, an antioxidant that might retard vessel proliferation. This is debatable and still being evaluated.

(5) Retinal detachment surgery, when indicated.

(6) Follow-up ophthalmologic examinations in selected cases.

EYELID DERMOIDS

Dermoids are benign tumors of the eyelid usually presenting as soft, nontender, movable masses on the outer aspect of the eyelid. It is formed at the fusion of the orbital bones, which in the early embryologic stages, incorporates ectodermal surface cells that would otherwise differentiate into skin like material; thus the term *derm*oid. Sebaceous secretions and hairs can be seen inside the capsule. These are encapsulated tumors that are benign. If the capsule is thin, the cheesy yellow contents can emerge upon traumatic impact, and cause a local cellulitis.

Treatment of dermoids involves surgical excision at some time in the early years of life. Psychologically it is easier to remove these when the child is below 2 or 3 years of age.

HEMANGIOMA

Hemangioma is a benign capillary tumor that presents as a flat pink discoloration of the skin, or as an elevated encapsulated, bluish mass. A bulky hemangioma of the upper lid can close the pupil and visual axis resulting in amblyopia.

When the hemangioma has a moderate connective tissue component there is a mottling of the red vascular tissue with gray areas giving a strawberry appearance to its surface. If the venous channels are prominent, and the tumor is subcutaneous, hemangiomas can present as a blue mass within the lid region. Characteristic of all these presentations is that of enlargement upon crying and breath holding. Hemangiomas may not be present at birth but may appear in the first 3–12 months of life. After that stage the tumor usually regresses spontaneously, thereby requiring no treatment at all.

Because of the cosmetic blemish in early life, it is a temptation to treat these lesions early on. Most therapies result in greater disfigurement and scarring. Attempts at therapy have included surgical excision, radiation, and steroids given either orally or through local injection.

When the tumor is large, intralesional steroid injections are necessary. These should be given by the ophthalmologists familiar with the specific steroids and dosages.

ANISOCORIA

Unequal pupil size (anisocoria) is a common finding in the general population, presenting in early infancy. It can worry physicians because of concern of central nervous system disease. Almost all cases of anisocoria pediatric ophthalmologists are benign congenital lesions that have no CNS implications. Anisocoria is usually a result of the sympathetic innervation to the iris dilating muscle fibers not being fully intact. The counter-balancing parasympathetic innervation to the pupil results in miosis.

Parents will indicate that the difference in pupil size is more noticeable in a dark or poorly lit room, while the pupils constrict fully in bright sunlight. From a practical point of view this has no effect upon vision at all. Only in severe cases is there a cosmetic problem. The condition is seen less with age, presumably because sympathetic innervation finally does develop in these anisocoria patients.

BLINKING

In the childhood years, blinking is almost always a functional, unconscious tic. There is often a forced component to the closure of the eyelids, atypical of the normal orbicularis closure which takes place every 5 seconds. Associated with blinking is that of "eyes rolling up." Blinking can be an unconscious tic.

Hemifacial spasm is a medical condition that is rare and associated with blepharospasm. Tourette's syndrome is a known neurologic entity.

Ocular causes for blinking include the need for glasses when a child cannot see well, diplopia in the toddler who cannot verbalize his visual discomfort, or from any form of external ocular irritation.

Respiratory Tract | 15

Steven H. Abman, MD

ACUTE RESPIRATORY EMERGENCIES

ACUTE RESPIRATORY FAILURE (ARF)

ARF is the inability of the respiratory system to provide sufficient Pao_2 or remove enough CO_2 to meet the metabolic needs of the body, because of the presence of either severe lung or airway disease or inadequate respiratory effort. In pediatrics, cardiopulmonary arrests are more commonly due to respiratory causes than to primary cardiac abnormalities. Several anatomic and physiologic factors [smaller airway diameters, easy fatigability of the diaphragm and other respiratory muscles, high chest wall compliance, and decreased intra-alveolar connections (pores of Kohn)] make young children more vulnerable than adults to ARF. ARF occurs in a wide variety of clinical settings (including all the disorders discussed in this chapter), and presents with variable physical findings depending on the exact etiology and physiologic response.

In general, early recognition of the high risk of ARF in various clinical settings is important, in order to anticipate and therefore initiate appropriate therapy prior to cardiopulmonary arrest (Tables 15–1, 15–2, and 15–3). Often the clinical severity of respiratory insufficiency may not be appreciated without arterial blood gas measurements of arterial oxygen tension (Pao_2), carbon dioxide tension ($Paco_2$), and pH. Although the use of pulse oximeter and transcutaneous Po_2 monitoring is helpful to demonstrate noninvasively serial changes in oxygenation, measurements of arterial blood gas tensions are necessary for a full assessment of acid-base balance and ventilation. $Paco_2$ is a direct reflection of alveolar ventilation; as $Paco_2$ rises, effective ventilation decreases proportionately. Determination of pH will help sort out the relative contributions of respiratory and metabolic causes of acidemia or alkalemia. A change in $Paco_2$ of 10 torr

Table 15–1. Systematic approach to acute respiratory failure.

1. Anticipate high-risk clinical setting for early monitoring and intervention prior to cardiopulmonary arrest.
2. Assessment of respiratory distress prior to arrest:
   A. *Physical examination:* mentation, cyanosis, apnea, respiratory rate, severity of distress (use of accessory muscles, grunting, retractions, paradoxical respiratory effort, breath sounds, response to oxygen administration).
   B. *Laboratory examination:* chest x-ray, monitoring with pulse oximeter and serial arterial blood gas studies.
3. Therapy dependent on clinical setting, severity of clinical findings: Intubation, ventilation, pharmacologic therapy, chest postural drainage, etc.
4. Initiate basic CPR with arrest:
   A. Airway patent? Head-tilt/chin tilt or jaw thrust; oropharyngeal/nasopharyngeal airway, endotracheal tube; cricothyrotomy.
   B. Adequacy of oxygenation? Supplemental oxygen (100%) by nasal cannula, head hood, or face mask.
   C. Adequacy of ventilation? Self-inflating bag-ventilation by face mask or through endotracheal tube.
   D. Circulation? Chest compressions if cardiac activity ineffective or absent; vascular access for fluid, drug administration; arterial and/or central venous access for monitoring.

will cause a change in arterial pH of 0.08 unit in the opposite direction. Similarly, a change in HCO_3 of 10 meq/L will cause a change in pH of 0.15 unit. The clinical approach to the patient with ARF begins with the same assessments used in CPR training: airway, breathing (effort), and circulation, with further monitoring and therapeutic interventions dependent upon the severity of distress.

Table 15–2. General indications for intubation with acute respiratory failure.

Cardiopulmonary arrest, severe shock

Apnea—frequent or prolonged episodes

Rising Pa_{CO_2} (especially if >50 mm Hg, with changes in mentation, fatigue, or in face of marked respiratory effort)

Falling Pa_{O_2} despite supplemental oxygen therapy (especially if <60 mm Hg while breathing high fraction of inspired oxygen (FiO_2)

Marked lethargy, fatigue, encephalopathy, coma

Loss of gag reflex, inability to protect airway

Severe upper airway obstruction

Table 15–3. Age-dependent changes in pediatric sizes of endotracheal tubes, laryngoscope blades, tracheostomy tubes, and chest tubes.

Age	Internal Diameter of Endotracheal Tube (mm)	Size of Laryngoscope Blade for Intubation	Tracheostomy Size (Shiley)	Chest Tube Size (French)
Premature				
1000 g	2.5	Miller 0	Neonatal 00	10
1000–2500 g	3.0	Miller 0	Neonatal 0	10–14
Newborn–6 mo	3.0–3.5	Miller 1	Pediatric 1	12–18
6 mo–1 yr	3.5–4.0	Miller 1	Pediatric 1–2	14–20
1–2 yr	4.0–5.0	Miller 1	Pediatric 3	14–24
2–6 yr	$\frac{\text{Age (yr)} + 16}{4}$	Miller 1–2	Pediatric 3,4	20–32
6–12 yr	Same as above	Miller/Macintosh 2	Pediatric 4	28–38
>12 yr	Same as above	Miller/Macintosh 3	Pediatric 6	

ADULT RESPIRATORY DISTRESS SYNDROME (ARDS)/ PULMONARY EDEMA

ARDS is a clinical syndrome characterized by the progressive development of respiratory failure associated with acute lung injury due to indirect (septic or hemorrhagic shock, head trauma, burn injury, pancreatitis, others) or direct (smoke or chemical inhalation, pneumonia, aspiration, emboli) causes. Its pathophysiologic hallmark is the presence of nonhydrostatic, or permeability, edema owing to injury to the alveolar–capillary network. This is in contrast to the pulmonary edema secondary to elevated pulmonary venous pressures more typical of congestive heart failure.

Clinical Findings

ARDS typically progresses from tachypnea, cyanosis, and retractions to ARF within 6–48 hours of an acute catastrophic event. Although the rate of progression and the severity of illness vary, early chest x-rays often appear normal. However, serial studies will reveal patchy alveolar infiltrates, air bronchograms, and loss of lung volume. Diminished breath sounds and rales are typical auscultatory findings. Although initially responsive to supplemental oxygen, hypoxemia often becomes refractory to treatment because of severe ventilation–perfusion mismatch, requiring mechanical ventilation with high mean airway pressures. Physiologically, lung compliance is low, and pulmonary artery wedge pressure (as measured with a pulmonary artery catheter) is normal.

Treatment

Therapy is currently supportive only. Along with treating the underlying disorder, the early recognition of at-risk patients allows initiation of appropriate monitoring for progressive respiratory distress, thus decreasing the risk for sudden cardiopulmonary arrest. Monitoring generally includes a systemic arterial line for frequent arterial blood gas and continuous blood pressure measurements. Pulse oximetry provides continuous assessments of oxygenation. Assessment of fluid status often requires the placement of a Foley catheter. Dependable peripheral and central venous lines provide access for administration of blood products, fluids, and medications, and for assessing volume status. In some cases, placement of a pulmonary artery catheter will allow essential measurements of cardiac output, pulmonary artery and wedge pressures, and mixed venous oxygen tension and saturation. The overall goal of therapy is to maximize tissue oxygen delivery, which is determined by the arterial oxygen content and the cardiac index. Treatment typically includes maintaining the hematocrit above 40%, cardiac index over 4.5 L/min, and oxygen saturation above 90–92%. Volume ventilators are required to ensure delivery of sufficient tidal volume in the face of changing respiratory compliance. High levels of mean airway pressure and peak end-expiratory pressures are often needed to correct the hypoxemia. Steroids have not been shown to improve the clinical course or outcome of ARDS.

Prognosis

Mortality rates of 50–60% are commonly reported, with death often due to multiple organ-system failure associated with secondary infection and progressive respiratory failure. Some patients require prolonged ventilator support and develop chronic lung disease. Most survivors, however, appear to have little sequelae at follow-up.

ACUTE AIRWAY OBSTRUCTION

The most common causes of acute airway obstruction in children include foreign body aspiration, viral croup, epiglottitis, bacterial tracheitis, peritonsillar abscess, marked adenoidal or tonsillar hypertrophy due to infection, allergy, and trauma (most commonly postextubation).

1. FOREIGN BODY OBSTRUCTION OF THE UPPER AND LOWER AIRWAY

Foreign body aspiration contributes significantly to the morbidity and mortality of early childhood, with over 3000 deaths from this cause occurring each year. Children between 6 months and 4 years are at greatest risk.

Clinical Findings

A. Symptoms and Signs: Upper airway obstruction presents as the acute onset of cyanosis and choking, with drooling, cough, and stridor (if partial) or inability to vocalize or cough (if complete). If untreated, progressive cyanosis, loss of consciousness, seizures, and cardiopulmonary arrest follow. Onset is abrupt, with a history of a small child running with food, a small toy, or other object in the mouth. Poor household "child-proofing" or an older sibling feeding the younger child age-inappropriate food are common findings.

Lower respiratory tract obstruction generally presents with the abrupt onset of cough, wheezing, or respiratory distress. These signs may decrease or disappear over time, however, and if left untreated may lead to bronchiectasis. Lower respiratory tract obstruction should be suspected in any child with chronic cough or recurrent "pneumonias." Physical examination may reveal asymmetric breath sounds or localized wheezing or rales.

B. Laboratory Findings: Foreign body obstruction is generally a medical emergency without the need for laboratory studies. If obstruction is incomplete, lateral neck x-rays may be helpful, although it generally does not replace visualization. When lower respiratory tract foreign body aspiration is suspected, inspiratory and forced expiratory (manual abdominal compression) chest x-rays should be obtained. The initial chest x-ray may show asymmetric hyperinflation or atelectasis. A positive force expiratory film will show mediastinal shift away from the side of the obstruction.

Treatment

The emergency treatment of partial upper airway obstruction due to a foreign body includes allowing the child to use his or her own cough reflex to extrude the foreign body. Acute intervention in infants less than 1 year old includes placing the child in a face-down position over the rescuer's arm, with the head positioned below the trunk. Four measured back blows are delivered rapidly between the scapulae. If still obstructed, the infant should be rolled over, and 4 chest compressions (as performed in CPR) delivered. This sequence should be repeated until the obstruction is relieved. Blind probing of the airway to attempt to dislodge the foreign body is discouraged. If the foreign body can be visualized, careful removal with the fingers or available instruments (Magill forceps) can be attempted. The abdominal thrust technique ("Heimlich maneuver") is recommended in older children.

Lower respiratory tract foreign body aspiration requires rigid bronchoscopy for removal, followed by beta-adrenergic nebulization with chest physiotherapy treatments in children with persistent symptoms.

2. INFECTIOUS CAUSES OF UPPER AIRWAY OBSTRUCTION

Several infectious agents can cause the acute onset of upper airway obstruction, and although many causes have a distinctive clinical presentation, the overlap of clinical findings must be appreciated (Table 15–4). For example, viral croup may present with high fever and marked distress, as more typically seen with epiglottitis. Upper airway obstruction from a foreign body must be considered in the different diagnosis (see above).

STATUS ASTHMATICUS

See Chapter 26, Allergic Diseases.

PLEURAL EFFUSIONS AND EMPYEMA

Pleural effusions in pediatrics are most often parapneumonic, ie, associated with a concomitant bacterial, mycoplasmal, viral, fungal, or mycobacterial lung infection. However, effusions are also associated with nephritis or nephrosis, cirrhosis, ascites, liver abscess, congestive heart failure, collagen vascular disease, pancreatitis, drug-induced lung injury, malignancy, and other causes. Clinical findings are dependent upon the underlying condition and the size of the effusion. Cough and dyspnea are common, with a secondary rise in fever often hearalding the development of pleural effusion. Breath sounds are decreased, with dullness to percussion over the involved area. Chest x-ray may show mediastinal shift; lateral decubitus or chest ultrasound studies help demonstrate the presence or absence of fluid loculation and the amount of fluid present. Thoracentesis provides helpful fluid samples for diagnostic and often therapeutic benefit. Studies should include pH determination (obtained in a small heparinized syringe, placed immediately on ice); stains and cultures for aerobic, anaerobic, and acid-fast organisms; cell count and differential; determination of glucose, lactate dehydrogenase (LDH), protein, specific gravity, hematocrit, and amylase; the cytologic examination. Serum samples from simultaneously drawn blood should be sent for protein, glucose, amylase, and LDH. These tests help differentiate transudate from exudate and may aid in providing a specific diagnosis

Table 15–4. Infectious causes of upper airway obstruction.

Disease	Clinical Signs	Ages	Season	Causes	Diagnosis and Therapy
Croup	Stridor, barky cough, mild fever, hoarseness, URI, worse at night	6 mo–3 yr	Late fall–winter	Parainfluenza (other viruses)	Cool mist, racemic epinephrine (IPPB),[1] ± brief steroid use
Epiglottitis	Abrupt onset, toxic, anxious, high fever, drooling, dysphagia, rare cough	3–7 yr	None	H influenzae B	Direct visualization,[2] nasotracheal intubation, IV antibiotics, ICU admit
Retropharyngeal abscess	Acute pharyngitis, high fever, toxic, dysphagia, hyperextension of head, drooling	Variable	None	Group A strep, S aureus, anaerobic bacteria	Visualization,[2] lateral neck x-rays, IV antibiotics, surgery
Bacterial tracheitis	Crouplike illness, high fever, toxic	<6 yr	Late fall–winter	S aureus	Visualization,[2] lateral neck x-ray, racemic epinephrine, IV antibiotics

[1] IPPB, intermittent positive pressure breathing.
[2] Visualization should be performed by experienced personnel under controlled settings (usually in the PICU or under general anesthesia). The use of lateral neck x-rays are often helpful, but do not replace direct visualization, and should not be obtained without the patient being observed by a physician capable of managing the airway in case of an abrupt obstruction.

518

for the source of the effusion and the potential need for early chest tube drainage (in the presence of a complicated parapneumonic empyema with pH < 7.15, LDH > 1000, protein > 4.5 gm/dL, and/or glucose < 40 mg/dL; Table 15–5).

APPARENT LIFE-THREATENING EPISODES (ALTE)

Marked controversy exists regarding the clinical management of infants with apnea or ALTE. As suggested by the long list of potential causes of ALTE or apnea (Table 15–6), these children are a heterogeneous group. Typically, infants with an ALTE present with an acute episode consisting of a combination of apnea (central or obstructive) with or without cyanosis or pallor, changes in muscle tone, or choking or gagging. The episode is felt to be life-threatening by the observer, with resuscitative efforts usually initiated. Whether some children truly represent "aborted" or "near-miss" sudden infant death syndrome is not known; however, there are reports of subsequent sudden death in such infants. Clinical evaluation includes obtaining a clear description of the event to determine whether the episodes are associated with being awake or asleep, with feedings, with crying, or with signs of acute infection. The duration of the episode, the resuscitative efforts, and the infant's subsequent responses are critical. Further history of developmental delays, neurologic abnormalities, signs of chronic disease, or nonaccidental trauma or neglect ("Munchausen's by proxy") are helpful. Physical examination may help direct the laboratory evaluation, which includes sleep studies to assess respiratory pattern and oxygenation (oximetry), chest x-ray, ECG, barium swallow, esophageal pH study, air laryngotracheogram, EEG, determination of serum electrolytes and hematocrit. A thorough psychosocial assessment is also an important part of the evaluation. Therapy is directed toward the identified cause. Indications for the use and duration of home apnea monitoring and respiratory stimulants, including caffeine, doxapram, and theophylline, remain controversial.

SUDDEN INFANT DEATH SYNDROME (SIDS)

SIDS, or "crib death," is a tragic but common cause of infant mortality, with an estimated frequency of 1–2 per 1000.

Table 15–5. Pleural effusions: transudate or exudate?

Type	White Blood Cell Count	Protein (g/dL)	Ratio, Pleural Fluid:Serum Protein	Ratio, Pleural Fluid:Serum LDH[1]	Glucose	pH
1. **Transudate** (CHF, nephrosis, cirrhosis)	<1000 (mononuclear)	<1	<0.5	<0.6	=serum	>7.40
2. **Exudate** (parapneumonic, inflammatory, collagen vascular diseases, etc)						
A. Uncomplicated	10,000	1.4–6.1	>0.5	>0.6	=serum	>7.30
B. Complicated[2]	20,000 (PMNs)	>4.5	>0.5	>0.6	<40 g/dL	<7.10

[1] LDH, lactic dehydrogenase.
[2] "Complicated" parapneumonic effusions are believed to require early chest tube drainage for an improved clinical response and minimize potential sequelae.

520

Table 15–6. Causes of apparent life-threatening episodes.

Infectious
    Viral (RSV, other respiratory pathogens)
    Bacterial sepsis (Group B *Streptococcus,* pertussis, others)
Gastrointestinal
    Reflux
    Aspiration
Respiratory
    Airway anomalies
    Infection
Neurologic/Metabolic
    Seizure
    Central hypoventilation
    Infection
    Leigh's syndrome
    Tumor
    Carnitine deficiency
    Medium-chain acyl dehydrogenase deficiency
    CNS hemorrhage, stroke
Cardiac/Vascular
    Cardiomyopathy
    Endocardial fibroelastosis
    Arrhythmia
    Malformations
    Pulmonary hypertension, A-V malformation
Nonaccidental Trauma
Unknown
    (Apnea of infancy)

Although its cause is unknown, SIDS generally occurs in children between 1 and 6 months of age (peak incidence, 2 months), with most deaths occurring between midnight and 8 A.M. Mild upper respiratory tract infection symptoms may be present, but whether infection plays an important role is not known. Risk factors include low birth weight; teenage, drug addicted, or smoking mothers; and a family history of previous SIDS deaths. There are still no known predictors to identify at-risk newborns. The diagnosis is based on the clinical setting and a postmortem examination that rules out other causes of death, and may include such findings as intrathoracic petechiae, mild respiratory tract congestion, brainstem gliosis, and extramedullary hematopoiesis. Therapy is directed toward providing family support during the immediate crisis as well as follow-up counseling by local resources. The National SIDS Foundation is an excellent resource for providing this support.

ACUTE BRONCHIOLITIS

Bronchiolitis is one of the most common causes of acute hospitalizations in young infants, especially during the winter months. Although respiratory syncytial virus (RSV) is the most common cause, other agents include parainfluenza, influenza, adenovirus, *Mycoplasma,* and *Chlamydia.*

Clinical Findings

A. Symptoms and Signs: The usual course of RSV-bronchiolitis is 1–2 days of fever, rhinorrhea, and cough, followed by tachypnea, wheezing, and retractions. Some young infants, especially preterm newborns, may present with apnea and few ausculatory findings, but may later develop rales, rhonchi, and wheezing. Otitis media and superimposed bacterial pneumonia (especially pneumococcus may develop).

B. Laboratory Findings: Chest x-ray findings include hyperinflation with mild interstitial infiltrates or segmental atelectasis. The peripheral white blood cell count may be normal or show a mild lymphocytosis.

Treatment

Although most children infected with RSV are readily managed as outpatients, hospitalization is frequently required for children less than 2 years of age. Indications for admission include hypoxemia in room air, apnea, moderate tachypnea with feeding difficulties, or marked respiratory distress. Admission is more frequent in children with underlying chronic cardiopulmonary disorders, such as congenital heart disease, bronchopulmonary dysplasia, or cystic fibrosis. Arterial blood gas assessments or noninvasive measurements of oxygenation with a pulse oximeter or transcutaneous PO_2 monitor should be used to assess oxygen requirements and the response to therapy. Supportive therapy includes supplemental oxygen, intravenous hydration, beta-adrenergic nebulization, theophylline, or steroids. Mechanical ventilation may be required in infants with apnea or marked distress. Ribavirin therapy is currently recommended for children with coexistent cardiopulmonary disease or immunodeficiency (eg, recent transplant recipients and children undergoing chemotherapy for malignancy). Its efficacy, however, remains unproven.

Prognosis

Whereas the acute outcome is generally excellent, children with pulmonary hypertension, bronchopulmonary dysplasia, or cystic fibrosis my have prolonged courses with high morbidity and mortality. In addition, recurrent episodes of wheezing may follow acute infection in almost half of hospitalized patients, suggesting either a predisposition to acute bronchiolitis or an important role in the pathogenesis of chronic reactive airways disease.

CHRONIC RESPIRATORY DISORDERS

General Considerations

The diagnostic evaluation of children with chronic respiratory disease can be approached in a staged work-up, which includes consideration of the age at onset of symptoms, the predominant clinical respiratory signs, and related findings (Table 15–7). Because of the wide diversity of etiologies, the pace of the work-up should be based on the severity or rate of progression of clinical findings. In addition, since normal, healthy children often have 6–8 respiratory infections during infancy, it is important to distinguish several different infections in a thriving child from a chronic lung disorder in which there are intermittent exacerbations superimposed on persistent respiratory signs. Also, evaluations should seek to determine whether exposure to environmental factors, such as passive smoking, gas heat and stoves, wood-burning stoves, or pollution, plays any role.

ASTHMA

See Chapter 26, Allergic Diseases.

BRONCHOPULMONARY DYSPLASIA (BPD)

BPD is a significant chronic lung disease that may be defined clinically by the following criteria. (1) Acute respiratory distress in the first week of life (mostly in preterm infants with hyaline membrane disease). (2) Past or ongoing treatment with mechanical ventilation and oxygen therapy. (3) Persistent signs of chronic respiratory distress, including physical signs, chest x-ray findings, and oxygen requirement after the first month of life. Imma-

Table 15–7. Work-up of chronic lung disease.[1]

Initial Laboratory Studies
1. Review previous course, lab data, and radiologic studies.
2. Obtain: Chest x-ray (PA and lateral)
   CBS with differential
   Sweat test (pilocarpine iontophoresis)
   Skin testing (TB, coccidioidomycosis, histoplasmosis, etc, depending on history)
   Pulmonary function testing (if age-appropriate)
   Sputum or nasal washings for culture

Follow-up ("Second Stage") Studies
1. More extensive pulmonary function testing (response to bronchodilator, exercise, or methacholine challenge).
2. Additional imaging studies:
   Air laryngotracheogram
   Barium swallow
   Chest CT or ultrasound
3. Serologic studies.
4. Screening immunologic testing (serum immunoglobulin levels, including IgE and IgG subclasses, antistreptolysin, isohemagglutinin, and titers assessing response to past immunizations, T cell subsets, HIV status, etc).

"Third Stage" Studies
1. Flexible or rigid laryngoscopy/bronchoscopy (with or without bronchoalveolar lavage, brush sampling, biopsy, or bronchography).
2. More specialized immunologic or serologic testing.
3. Esophageal pH monitoring.
4. Cardiac catheterization, angiography.
5. Lung biopsy.

[1] Reproduced, with permission, from Taussig LM, Lemen RJ: Chronic obstructive lung disease. In: *Advances in Pediatrics*. Year Book, 1979.

turity, oxygen toxicity, barotrauma, and inflammation are considered to be the major risk factors for developing BPD. The exact definition and cause of BPD remain controversial. Factors such as excessive fluid administration, patent ductus arteriosus, pulmonary interstitial emphysema, pneumothorax, infection, and inflammatory stimuli appear to play important roles in its pathogenesis and pathophysiology. The differential diagnosis based on radiographic findings includes Wilson-Mikity disease, meconium aspiration syndrome, congenital infection (especially cytomegalovirus and perhaps *Ureaplasma*), cystic fibrosis, cystic adenomatoid malformation, recurrent aspiration, pulmonary lymphangiectasia, total anomalous pulmonary venous return, overhydration and idiopathic pulmonary fibrosis.

Clinical Course & Treatment

The clinical course of BPD is widely variable, ranging from patients with mild oxygen requirements who improve steadily over a few months to more severely affected children who require chronic tracheostomy and mechanical ventilation. Airways hyperreactivity is common in infants with BPD, leading to frequent treatment with beta-adrenergic agonists (such as terbutaline, salbutomol, and metaproterenol), theophylline, steroids and cromolyn. Part of the rationale for steroids use is to decrease lung inflammation and enhance responsiveness to the beta-nebulization treatments. Recurrent atelectasis, tracheomalacia, subglottic stenosis, and other structural airway problems frequently contribute to the severity of the underlying BPD. Recurrent pulmonary edema, perhaps owing to increased vascular permeability, pulmonary hypertension, left ventricular dysfunction, or fluid overload, leads to the frequent use of long-term diuretic therapy, including furosemide, hydrochlorothiazide, and aldactone. Severe volume contraction, hypokalemia, hyponatremia, and alkalosis are common side effects of the diuretics. To minimize the development or progression of pulmonary hypertension, infants with BPD are carefully monitored with serial pulse oximeter and blood gas tension measurements to maintain Pao_2 or O_2 saturations above 55–60 torr or 92%, respectively. Serial ECG and echocardiogram studies monitor for the development of right ventricular hypertrophy (cor pulmonale) and left ventricular hypertrophy. Along with the cardiopulmonary abnormalities of BPD, clinical management requires close monitoring of growth, nutrition, metabolic status, development, neurologic status, and related problems.

Prognosis

Although mortality is high for advanced ("stage 4") BPD, the long-term outlook is generally favorable for most infants with BPD. However, more time and further study are needed to better determine the long-term impact of such sequelae as persistent airways hyperreactivity (asthma), exercise intolerance, and perhaps abnormal lung growth.

CYSTIC FIBROSIS (CF)

CF is the most common lethal genetic disease (autosomal recessive) occurring in Caucasians, with an estimated incidence of 1 in 2000 births. Although CF is found in black (1:17,000) and oriental children (1:100,000), the incidence is far less than in Caucasians. Genetic studies have demonstrated the CF gene to be on the long arm of chromosome 7 (7q31). Deletion of phenylalanine at the 508 position (delta F508) accounts for most CF mutations (70–80%). This results in an abnormal protein called the CF transmembrane conductance regulator (CFTR). The CFTR may have several cellular functions, but appears to be a chloride channel. This defect is believed to cause the characteristic abnormalities in sweat electrolytes and secretions in the lung, pancreas, intestine, liver, and other sites, which subsequently cause multiple organ dysfunction. The clinical manifestations of CF are diverse, and children with CF may present with a wide variety of clinical abnormalities (Table 15–8). As 90% of children with CF have pancreatic insufficiency, many present with severe failure to thrive, steatorrhea, and malabsorption. These signs may present with or without respiratory disease in young infants. Diagnosis is primarily based on elevated sweat chloride levels by pilocarpine iontophoresis. The leading cause of morbidity and mortality, however, is progressive respiratory failure due to chronic endobronchial infection and inflammation. *Pseudomonas aeruginosa*, especially in its mucoid form, is the major bacterial pathogen of CF; *Staphylococcus aureus* and nontypable *Haemophilus influenzae* are other common isolates. Although clinical courses are variable, recurrent hospitalizations for respiratory exacerbations and gastrointestinal and nutritional problems are common. Prognosis has improved over the past decade but is variable; the current median age of survival is 26 years. Management approach to CF is presented in Table 15–9.

RECURRENT ASPIRATION

Although a history of breathing difficulties that occur during or shortly after a feeding, awake apnea, or vomiting can be elicited in patients with chronic aspiration, some patients present with recurrent wheezing, "recurrent pneumonia," or chronic cough, in the absence of such a history. Disorders associated with recurrent aspiration include abnormal sucking or swallowing owing to neuromuscular immaturity, brain injury, or other primary neurologic and muscle abnormalities; structural lesions of the mouth, tongue, pharynx, or jaw; esophageal dysfunction

Table 15–8. Presenting signs of patients with cystic fibrosis.

1. **Respiratory**
   Chronic cough, wheezing
   Persistent atelectasis
   "Recurrent pneumonia"
   Staphylococcal pneumonia
   Pseudomonas aeruginosa pneumonia, sinusitis, or bronchitis
   Clubbing
   Bronchiectasis
   Nasal polyps
   Hemoptysis
2. **Gastrointestinal/nutritional**
   Meconium ileus or plug syndrome
   Small bowel atresia
   Meconium peritonitis
   Direct hyperbilirubinemia
   Unexplained hepatomegaly, cirrhosis
   Failure to thrive
   Steatorrhea
   Chronic diarrhea
   Rectal prolapse
   Bowel obstruction
   Hypoalbuminemia
   Vitamin A, E, or K deficiency
3. **Other**
   Family history of CF
   Aspermia
   "Tastes salty"
   Metabolic alkalosis
   Hypoelectrolytemia
   Heat stroke, exhaustion
   Elevated intracranial pressure (vitamin A deficit)
   Intracranial hemorrhage (vitamin K deficit)

owing to vascular ring, severe reflux, achalasia, hiatal hernia, or other causes; or aspiration owing to tracheoesophageal fistula or cleft. Chest x-ray findings of migratory asymmetric infiltrates are suggestive of recurrent aspiration. Barium swallow, esophageal pH studies, and the presence of significant numbers of lipid-laden alveolar macrophages in tracheal aspirates or bronchial washings may help with the diagnostic evaluation. The decision to undergo surgical (fundoplication) intervention depends upon the severity and frequency of aspiration, as well as on its underlying cause.

Table 15–9. General clinical management of CF.

1. **General:** Frequent clinical assessments, every 2–4 months (depending on age, disease severity); extensive history and physical, especially growth parameters, respiratory and GI systems; psychosocial issues related to chronic disease.
2. **Nutrition:** Pancreatic enzyme supplements; caloric supplements; vitamin supplements (especially vitamin E, often A, D, and K); monitoring liver function and nutritional indices (including trace element, protein and vitamin levels, glycosylated hemoglobin).
3. **Respiratory:** Physiotherapy (conventional, autogenic drainage, PEP treatments); monitoring of oxygenation (pulse oximeter); chest x-ray; pulmonary function testing, including exercise studies; EKG; influenza vaccine (fall); Medications: aerosolized bronchodilators (if responsiveness proven), cromolyn, steroids, antibiotics (oral, IV, or aerosolized; generally directed against *S aureus*, *P aeruginosa*).
4. **Promising interventions currently under investigation:** DNase therapy; amiloride; IV gammaglobulin therapy; protease inhibitors; anti-*Pseudomonas* vaccines.

INTERSTITIAL LUNG DISEASES

Pediatric interstitial lung diseases include a diverse group of clinical disorders (Table 15–10), which can be characterized by persistent inflammation and edema of the lung interstitium, alveoli, and bronchiolar walls, which may lead to mild dysfunction or cause progressive pulmonary fibrosis.

The clinical presentation is highly variable, but generally tachypnea is the earliest manifestation, with cough, dyspnea, retractions, and cyanosis often found. Weight loss, clubbing, hemoptysis, chest pain, and other signs may be present. Often respiratory symptoms develop insidiously. Fine rales and diminished breath sounds are heard on chest auscultation. Chest x-ray findings are highly variable, with diffuse reticular, reticulonodular, or nodular infiltrates present. Peribronchial cuffing, hilar adenopathy, and other abnormalities are present depending on the underlying cause. Pulmonary function tests often indicate a restrictive pattern, with low lung volumes and compliance and a widened gradient of alveolar–arterial oxygen tensions, especially with exercise. Diagnostic assessments include bronchoalveolar lavage and lung biopsy. Treatment and prognosis depend on the specific abnormality.

Table 15–10. Causes of pediatric interstitial lung disease.

Infectious
    Viral (CMV, HIV, RSV, adenovirus, influenza, parainfluenza, measles, EBV, varicella)
    Mycoplasma
    Protozoal (*Pneumocystis carinii*)
    Mycobacterial
    Fungal
    Bacterial (*Haemophilus influenzae, Legionella, Bordetella pertussis*)
Postinfectious
    Bronchiolitis obliterans
Inhalational
    Inorganic dusts (silica, asbestos, talcum powder)
    Organic dusts (hypersensitivity pneumonitis)
    Fumes (sulfuric acid, hydrochloric acid)
    Gases (chlorine, nitrogen dioxide, ammonia)
    Aerosols
Drug-induced
    Cytotoxic (cyclophosphamide, BCNU, CCNU, methotrexate, azothioprine, vinblastine, bleomycin, cytosine arabinoside)
    Others (nitrofurantoin, penicillamine, gold salts)
Radiation
Neoplastic
    Leukemia
    Lymphoma
    Histiocytosis
Lymphoproliferative disorders
    Pseudotumor
    Others
Metabolic
    Cystic fibrosis
    Lipidoses
    Storage disorders
Idiopathic interstitial fibrosis
Associated with collagen vascular disease, systemic vasculitis
Associated with neurocutaneous syndromes
Sarcoidosis
Pulmonary hemosiderosis
Pulmonary alveolar proteinosis
Pulmonary infiltrates with eosinophilia
Cardiac failure
Renal disease

BRONCHIECTASIS

Bronchiectasis generally refers to chronic, irreversible airways injury that leads to fixed dilatation. It is most commonly due to recurrent lower respiratory tract infections, often in association with a primary chronic disease, including CF, immune deficiency, immotile cilia syndrome, anatomic airway obstruction, congenital deficiency of bronchial cartilage, foreign body, chronic aspiration pneumonitis, or sequelae of severe acute infections (including such agents as tuberculosis, pertussis, adenovirus, measles, influenza, or *Staphylococcus aureus*). Bronchiectasis can be classified as cylindric, varicose, or saccular, depending on its radiologic, bronchographic, or histologic appearance. With cylindric lesions, there is slight but uniform dilatation of the larger bronchi. Varicous bronchiectasis has irregular dilatation and constriction of bronchi, and the saccular form is described as having a progressively larger bronchial diameter, with gross destruction of more peripheral airways.

Clinical Findings

A. Symptoms and Signs: In 80–95% of patients with bronchiectasis, a chronic suppurative cough is present, which is generally worse in the early morning or with exercise. Purulent sputum production, hemoptysis, wheezing, and severe sinusitis can be present. Auscultation frequently reveals localized wheezing or moist rales over the bronchiectatic lung. Digital clubbing may be present.

B. Laboratory Findings: Although chest x-ray findings are often insensitive and not specific for the presence of bronchiectasis, the typical appearance of "tram lines," increased localized bronchovascular markings, or cystic changes may be found. The left lower lobe, right middle lobe, and lingula are the most common sites. Chest CT-scan may be helpful to confirm the presence of bronchiectasis, as well as to evaluate the rest of the lung for diffuse lesions. Bronchography can be performed in centers with experience in this technique if surgical removal is under consideration. Diagnostic evaluation depends on the clinical setting, but often includes sweat test; immunologic work-up; PPD skin test, sputum cultures and stains for bacteria, fungi, and mycobacteria; barium swallow and esophageal pH study; CBC; and bronchoscopy.

Treatment

In addition to specific therapy to treat an underlying primary disease, aggressive chest physiotherapy after beta-adrenergic nebulization therapy is undertaken for at least 2–4 weeks. Antibiotics (based on culture results) are often used. Indications for surgical resection include the presence of localized disease producing severe symptoms or pulmonary hemorrhage. In the presence of diffuse lung involvement, surgery is generally not indicated.

HEMOPTYSIS, PULMONARY HEMORRHAGE, & HEMOSIDEROSIS

Acute pulmonary hemorrhage can occur with or without overt hemoptysis, and is usually accompanied by alveolar infiltrates on chest x-ray. Hemosiderin-laden macrophages are found within the sputum and tracheal and gastric aspirates. Many cases are secondary to infection (bacterial, mycobacterial, parasitic, viral, or fungal), lung abscess, bronchiectasis (CF, immune deficiency), foreign body, coagulopathy, elevated pulmonary venous pressure (congestive heart failure), structural lesions (arteriovenous fistula, telangiectasia, sequestration, bronchogenic cyst), lung contusion, tumor, pulmonary embolus, or collagen-vascular diseases (lupus, Wegener's granulomatosis, rheumatoid arthritis, polyarteritis nodosa, Shönlein-Henoch purpura, Goodpasture's syndrome, others). Idiopathic pulmonary hemosiderosis refers to the accumulation of hemosiderin in the lung (alveolar macrophage). It may be related to cow's milk allergy ("Heiner's syndrome").

Clinical findings are often nonspecific, and include cough, tachypnea, retractions, hemoptysis, poor growth, and fatigue. Some patients may present with massive hemoptysis. Auscultation reveals decreased breath sounds, wheezing, or rales. The presence of iron-deficiency anemia and hematuria should be sought. Chest x-ray findings are variable; fluffy alveolar or interstitial infiltrates may be transient, with or without atelectasis and mediastinal adenopathy. Pulmonary function testing generally reveals restrictive impairment with low lung volumes and poor compliance. Diagnostic evaluation depends upon the age of the patient and the associated signs (for example, serum precipitins to cow's milk proteins in infants and young children). Treatment and prognosis are dependent on the underlying etiology. Steroids or cytotoxic agents are frequently used.

CONGENITAL STRUCTURAL LESIONS

Congenital extrathoracic respiratory abnormalities cause inspiratory stridor or poor air movement despite increased respiratory effort from birth or within the first months of life. Congenital causes of airway obstruction that present in early infancy include choanal atresia; macroglossia; micrognathia (Pierre–Robin); laryngeal atresia, cleft, web, stenosis, or cyst; subglottic hemangioma; and others. Laryngomalacia is one of the most common causes, accounting for perhaps more than half the cases. The epiglottis and arytenoid cartilages collapse into the airway during inspiration, causing laryngeal stridor. Diagnosis is readily made by flexible laryngoscopy. Although tracheostomy may be required, most children resolve their stridor within the first 2 years of life.

Congenital intrathoracic lesions are diverse and have variable clinical presentations, ranging from severe neonatal respiratory distress to mild chronic cough in older adolescents.

Tracheomalacia

Tracheomalacia consists of dynamic collapse of the trachea, often associated with other conditions, such as vascular rings, tracheoesophageal fistula, BPD, and others. It may be primary. Diagnosis can be made by air laryngotracheogram or flexible bronchoscopy.

Vascular Rings

The clinical signs of vascular rings or slings vary considerably, depending on the type of lesion and the severity of compression of central airways or the esophagus. Most commonly, stridor, wheezing, or obstructive apnea are the initial presenting signs within the first months of life. Some children may have a more delayed presentation after long-term therapy for presumed asthma. The most common type of vascular abnormality is double aortic arch, in which persistence of left- and right-sided embryologic fourth aortic arches leads to esophageal and tracheal compression. Aberrant innominate artery, right aortic arch with aberrant left subclavian and left ligamentum arteriosum, and pulmonary sling (distal take-off of the left pulmonary artery) are other common vascular anomalies. Laboratory evaluation includes a chest x-ray, especially noting which side the aortic arch is on and the tracheal caliber. Barium swallow may reveal persistent indentation of the esophagus, suggesting an aortic arch anomaly (posterior esophageal compression) or pulmonary vascular sling or aberrant subclavian artery (anterior esophageal compression). A normal barium esophagogram is found with aberrant innominate artery compression; however, anterior tracheal compression about 2 centimeters above the carina may be noted on lateral chest film in these patients. Further evaluation generally includes bronchoscopy to assess tracheal or bronchial compression, and, often, angiography to more precisely define the anatomy. Surgical intervention is required for children with significant airway obstruction. Tracheomalacia may persist at the site of compression following surgery.

Mediastinal Masses

Mediastinal masses present with stridor, wheezing, chronic cough, or as incidental findings on chest x-rays obtained for other purposes. The differential diagnosis is dependent upon the mediastinal compartment in which the mass is located (Table 15–11). Although some of the lesions are congenital, others develop later in childhood. Work-up includes barium swallow, chest CT scan, bronchoscopy, or exploratory thoracotomy. Skin testing for mycobacterial disease with related controls should be performed as well.

Tracheoesophageal Fistulas (TEF)

Tracheoesophageal fistulas are caused by the failure of septation of the esophagus and trachea. Distal TEF with esophageal atresia is the most common type (90%), and includes a proximal esophagus that ends in a blind pouch, with the distal esophagus connected to the trachea. Clinically, TEF may be associated with polyhydraminios, and with congenital abnormalities (35%), such as vertebral anomalies, imperforate anus, congenital heart disease, and genitourinary lesions. Cough, choking, and respiratory distress present shortly after birth. Lung injury can occur from gastric secretions entering the airway. Diagnosis is suggested by attempts to pass an esophageal catheter. Chest x-ray will confirm the position of the nasogastric tube curled in the proximal esophagus. Treatment includes suctioning secretions from the esophageal pouch to prevent aspiration; ultimate treatment is surgical repair in the newborn period. Tracheomalacia

Table 15–11. Mediastinal masses.

Compartment	Cause
Superior	Cystic hygroma
	Hemangioma
	Thymic tumors
	Teratoma
Anterior	Thymoma
	Thymic hyperplasia
	Thymic cyst
	Teratoma
	Intrathoracic thyroid
	Lymphoma
	Pericardial cyst
Posterior	Neurogenic tumors
	Neurenteric anomaly
	Anterior meningocele
	Bronchogenic cyst
Middle	Lymphoma
	Lymphadenopathy
	Bronchogenic cyst
	Pericardial cyst
	Cardiac tumors
	Anomalies of the great vessels

often persists as a clinical problem after surgical repair. Late complications include leakage at the anastomosis site, mediastinitis, esophageal stricture, diaphragm paralysis, hiatal hernia, poor esophageal motility, and recurrent fistulas.

Pulmonary Hypoplasia

Pulmonary agenesis or hypoplasia represent imcomplete lung development, generally reflecting an intrauterine interruption or alteration of the normal sequence of embryologic events. It may be associated with other congenital anomalies. Lungs are considered hypoplastic when their size is decreased as assessed by weight (ratio of lung to body weight is below 0.15 in premature infants less than 28 weeks' gestation, or 0.012 in older newborns). Etiologies include the presence of an intrathoracic mass resulting in the lack of space for lung growth (eg, diaphragmatic hernia, fetal hydrops, extralobar sequestration, thoracic neuroblastoma), decreased size of the thoracic cage (eg, asphyxiating thoracic dystrophy, achondrogenesis), decreased fetal breathing movements or diaphragmatic elevation (eventration, phrenic

nerve agenesis, fetal ascites, abdominal masses), oligohydramnios (urinary outflow tract obstruction, polycystic kidneys, prolonged amniotic fluid leak); trisomies 13, 18 and 21; severe musculoskeletal disorders (arthrogryposis, osteogenesis imperfecta),
and cardiac lesions (Ebstein's anomaly, pulmonic stenosis, hypoplastic right heart, scimitar syndrome). Clinical presentation
is highly variable, and is related to the severity of hypoplasia as
well as to associated abnormalities. Some newborns present with
spontaneous pneumothorax, perinatal stress, and persistent pulmonary hypertension. Children with milder degrees of hypoplasia may present with tachypnea and related chronic respiratory
signs. Chest x-ray findings include variable degrees of volume
loss with a small hemithorax and mediastinal shift. Ventilation-
perfusion scans, angiography, and bronchoscopy are often helpful with the clinical evaluation. Outcome is dependent on the
severity of hypoplasia or related clinical problems.

Pulmonary Sequestrations

Pulmonary sequestrations are localized masses of pulmonary parenchyma that may be anatomically separate from the
lung. Extralobar sequestrations have a distinct pleural invest-
ment and intralobar are located within the lung pleura. Extralobar sequestration receives its blood supply from the systemic
circulation, pulmonary vessels, or both, and rarely communicates with the stomach or esophagus. The arterial supply to intralobar lesions is from the aorta or systemic branches. Intralobar lesions are often found in lower lobes (98%), are rarely
associated with congenital lesions (less than 2% versus 50% with
extralobar), are rarely seen in the newborn period (unlike extralobar), and may represent acquired lesions (ie, postinfectious). Clinically, sequestrations can present as chronic cough,
wheezing, recurrent pneumonias, or hemoptysis. Treatment is
by surgical resection.

Congenital Lobar Emphysema

This usually presents in the newborn period as severe respiratory distress, or during the first year of life as progressive
respiratory impairment. Rarely, there is a delayed diagnosis because of mild or intermittent symptoms in older children. Chest
x-ray shows overdistention of the affected lobe, with wide separation of bronchovascular markings, collapse of adjacent lung,
shift of the mediastinum away from the affected side, and a depressed diaphragm on the affected side. Diagnostic studies often

include fluoroscopy, ventilation–perfusion scans, chest CT, angiography, and exploratory thoracotomy. Bronchoscopy may be helpful to examine whether extrinsic or intrinsic compression of the bronchus is present. The differential diagnosis includes pneumothorax, pneumatocele, ateletasis with compensatory hyperinflation secondary to ball-valve mechanism, and cystic adenomatoid malformations. Management is usually surgical resection.

Cystic Adenomatoid Malformations (CAM)

These are unilateral hamartomatous lesions that generally present with marked respiratory distress within the first days of life. This lesion accounts for 95% of cases of congenital cystic lung disease. These space-occupying lesions are gland-like ("adenomatoid"), and have intercommunicating cysts of various sizes. Classification of the 3 types of CAM is based on the size of the cysts. Type 1 consists of large cysts; it is the most common (75%), and has the best survival (98%). Type 2 lesions consist of smaller cysts, and are often associated with other congenital anomalities (renal, cardiac, intestinal), leading to a lower (40%) survival. Type 3 CAM presents as a bulky, firm mass, and has a 50% survival rate. Treatment is by surgical resection.

Bronchogenic Cysts

These are middle mediastinal masses of variable sizes, which are usually located near the carina and major bronchi. These cysts usually do not communicate with the airway, and can present with acute respiratory distress and chronic cough and wheezing, or may be incidental findings on chest x-ray. Chest CT scan or ultrasound can differentiate solid from cystic mediastinal mass. Surgical excision is required.

Pulmonary Lymphangiectasia

This is a rare and usually fatal disorder that presents as acute or persistent respiratory distress in the newborn period. It may be accompanied by generalized lymphangiectasis, Noonan syndrome, asplenia, cardiovascular lesions (especially total anomallous pulmonary venous return), chylothorax, or renal malformations. Chest x-ray findings include a "ground glass" appearance, prominent interstitial markings, and hyperinflation. Therapy is largely supportive, and prognosis is poor, with most deaths occurring within the first months of life. There are isolated reports of its diagnosis and survival later in childhood.

Heart | 16

Elizabeth M. Shaffer, Lee Ann Pearse, MD, &
Michael S. Schaffer, MD

Cardiovascular disease in children is a significant cause of morbidity and mortality throughout the world. Congenital heart defects are a major cause of these illnesses, while acquired heart diseases also play an important role. We also recognize that the precursors of adult heart disease begin in in childhood and its prevention needs to be addressed at these early ages.

DIAGNOSTIC EVALUATION

History

The history of patients suspected of cardiac disease is extremely important. Information surrounding the perinatal period including prenatal exposure to potential teratogens and the birth history provide clues to particular types of heart disease. The timing of events such as neonatal distress, cyanosis, and the appearance of murmurs is particularly helpful in the differential diagnosis of heart disease. Symptoms suggestive of congestive heart failure such as feeding difficulties and diaphoresis are important and must be sought. Family history is crucial in this group of patients because some forms of congenital heart disease are hereditary and may not be apparent at the initial evaluation of a child (Table 16–1).

Physical Examination

The cardiac examination is done in stages including inspection, palpation, and auscultation. The examination begins with a general inspection of the patient noting peripheral perfusion, color, attitude, and dysmorphic features. Vital signs, including four limb blood pressures are imperative. Growth parameters must be assessed. The chest should be inspected for signs of dyssymmetry. Cardiac palpation and auscultation should be done with the patient in various positions (ie, standing, sitting,

Table 16–1. Genetic and environmental associations.

A. CHROMOSOMAL ABNORMALITIES

Autosomal

Trisomy 13	VSD, PDA, dextrocardia
Trisomy 18	VSD, PDA, PS
Trisomy 21	Endocardial cushion defect, VSD, ASD
Pericentric inversion of chromosome 8	TOF, DORV, PDA

Sex Chromosome

XO (Turner's)	Coarctation of the aorta, AS, ASD
XXXXY	PDA, ASD
Fragile X	Aortic root dilatation, MVP

B. GENE ABNORMALITIES

Autosomal Recessive

Ellis–van Crevald	ASD, single atrium
Friedreich ataxia	Cardiomyopathy
Glycogen storage disease, type II	Cardiomyopathy
Jervell–Lange–Nielson	Prolonged QT interval
Hurler	Coronary artery disease, AI, MR, conduction defects
Seckel	VSD, PDA
Smith–Lemli–Opitz	VSD, PDA

Autosomal Dominant

Ehlers–Danlos	Rupture of the large blood vessels
Holt–Oram	ASD, VSD
Marfans	Great artery aneurysm, AI, MR
Neurofibromatosis	PS, coarctation of the aorta
Osler–Weber–Rendu	Pulmonary AV fistulas
Romano–Ward	Prolonged QT interval
Tuberous sclerosis	Myocardial rhabdomyoma, aortic aneurysm
Ullrich–Noonan	PS, ASD, IHSS

X-Linked Recessive (X-R) and X-Linked Dominant (X-D)

Hunter (X-R)	Coronary artery disease, valve disease
Duchenne muscular dystrophy (X-D)	Cardiomyopathy

(continued)

Table 16–1. Genetic and environmental associations. *(continued)*

C.	**TERATOGENS**	
	Alcohol	VSD, PDA, ASD
	Phenytoin	PS, AS, coractation of the aorta, PDA
	Trimethadione	TGA, TOF, HLHS
	Lithium	Ebstein's anomaly, TGA, ASD
	Thalidomide	TOF, VSD, ASD, truncus arteriosus
	Rubella	PPS, PDA, VSD, ASD
	Maternal DM	ASH, TGA, VSD, coarctation of the aorta
	Maternal phenylketonuria	TOF, VSD, ASD
	Maternal SLE	Complete heart block

[1] AI, aortic insufficiency; AS, aortic stenosis; ASD, atrial septal defect; ASH, assymetric septal hypertrophy; AV, arteriovenous; DORV, double outlet right ventricle; HLHS, hypoplastic left heart syndrome; IHSS, idiopathic hypertrophic subaortic stenosis; MR, mitral regurgitation; MVP, mitral valve prolapse; PDA, patent ductus arteriosus; PPS, peripheral pulmonic stenosis; PS, pulmonary stenosis; SLE, systemic lupus erythematosus; TGA, transposition of the great arteries; TOF, tetralogy of Fallot; VSD, ventricular septal defect.

and supine) because physical findings may be position dependent such as the click in mitral valve prolapse. The peripheral arterial pulses must be palpated noting any discrepancy in caliber or timing. Palpation of the chest includes locating the point of maximal impulse and noting its intensity. Frequently in patients with right sided cardiac pathology, right ventricular preponderance is present. Thrills may be present and should be noted. Auscultation must be done in an orderly fashion. Each component of the cardiac cycle (ie first heart sound, second heart sound, systole and diastole) must be evaluated from the left upper sternal border, right upper sternal border, left sternal border and apex. It is also important to auscultate the axilla and back for murmurs. When characterizing murmurs, the timing of the murmur along with its location, intensity, and quality must be described.

LABORATORY INVESTIGATION

Electrocardiography

The electrocardiogram (ECG) is a graphic representation of myocardial electric activity: the P wave represents atrial depolarization, the QRS wave represents ventricular depolarization, and the T wave represents ventricular repolarization. The QRS wave is a summation of both left and right ventricular activity. Throughout childhood, the heart continues to mature with a shift from right to left ventricular predominance. Thus, normal electrocardiographic criteria are dependent on the age of the subject (Figure 16–1). Increased myocardial muscle mass creates

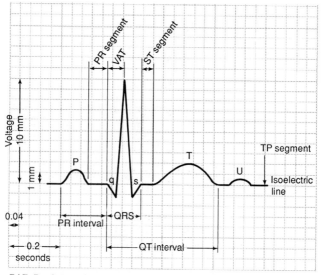

RAE: P > 2.5 mm in any lead; peaked

LAE: P > 0.08 sec; terminal deep inversion V_3R, V_1 notched

RVH: RV_1	0–24 h	> 20 mm
	1–7 d	> 29 mm
	1 wk–16 yr	> 20 mm
SV_6	0–7 d	> 14 mm
	8–30 d	> 10 mm
	1–6 mo	> 7 mm
	0.5–16 yr	> 5 mm

LVH: SV_1	0–1 d	> 28 mm
	1 d–1 yr	> 19 mm
	1–16 yr	> 25 mm
RV_6	0–6 m	> 16 mm
	6–12 m	> 19 mm
	1–16 yr	> 21 mm

Figure 16–1. The pediatric electrocardiogram. LAE, left atrial enlargement; LVH, left ventricular hypertrophy; RAE, right atrial enlargement; RVH, right ventricular hypertrophy; VAT, ventricular activation time.

an imbalance of forces and is depicted as ventricular hypertrophy. In the presence of hypoplastic chambers, the balance of forces will be shifted and represented as hypertrophy of the opposite ventricle (eg, right ventricular hypertrophy in hypoplastic left heart syndrome).

Chest Radiography

The chest x-ray is critical for evaluating heart size and pulmonary blood flow. The cardiothoracic ratio is increased in neonates, with 0.55 being the upper limit of normal in neonates and 0.5 the maximum in normal older children. The presence of increased and enlarged pulmonary arteries or the paucity of pulmonary vascular markings suggests increased or decreased pulmonary blood flow, respectively (Figure 19–2).

Echocardiography

Echocardiography is used extensively in the evaluation and follow-up of pediatric patients with cardiac pathology. Two-dimensional imaging can supply anatomic details while Doppler provides pressure and flow data (Fig 16–2).

Cardiac Catheterization

The role of cardiac catheterization is rapidly evolving from a diagnostic tool to one of therapeutic intervention. Anatomic definition and intracardiac pressures are evaluated via catheterization when noninvasive means fail to produce the desired information.

Balloon dilation valvuloplasty has become the treatment of choice for stenotic valves and coarctation of the aorta. Catheter occlusion of PDA, ASD, systemic collaterals and surgically placed shunts is available at some centers.

Many pediatric patients with dysrhythmias are routinely evaluated by intracardiac electrophysiologic studies to determine the mechanism of their dysrhythmias and potential therapies. Transcatheter ablation of accessory pathways can now be performed in the electrophysiologic laboratory and obviate the need for surgery.

CONGESTIVE HEART FAILURE

Congestive heart failure (CHF) is a clinical syndrome in which the heart cannot generate sufficient cardiac output to sup-

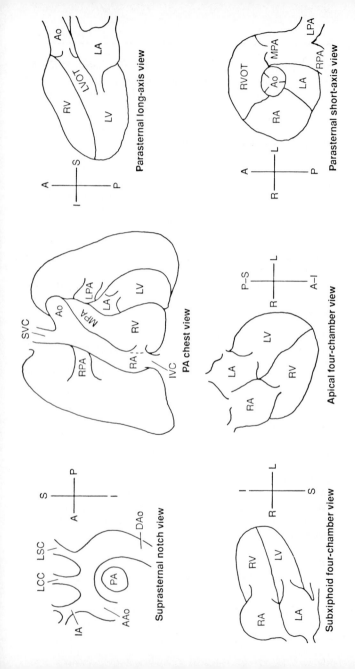

Parasternal long-axis view

Ao · LVOT · LA · RV · LV

PA chest view

SVC · RPA · Ao · MPA · LPA · LA · RA · IVC · RV · LV

Suprasternal notch view

LCC · LSC · IA · AAo · PA · DAo

Parasternal short-axis view

RVOT · Ao · MPA · LPA · RPA · LA · RA

Apical four-chamber view

LA · LV · RA · RV

Subxiphoid four-chamber view

RA · RV · LV · LA

ply the needs of the body. The syndrome is the result of one of 4 circumstances: 1) dysfunctional myocardium, eg, myocarditis or cardiomyopathy; 2) congenital cardiac malformations that decrease systemic perfusion, eg, critical aortic stenosis or large left to right shunts with pulmonary overcirculation; 3) normal cardiovascular systems in the face of an abnormal demand, eg, thyrotoxicosis or severe anemia and; 4) dysrhythmias that fail to produce an adequate cardiac output.

Clinical Findings

Tachycardia, tachypnea, and hepatomegaly characterize the clinical findings in CHF. Despite the numerous underlying mechanisms, the clinical findings are surprisingly similar in all cases. Additional clinical findings include diaphoresis, jugular venous distention, peripheral edema (periorbital edema in infants), cardiomegaly and, in severe, advanced cases, cyanosis.

Treatment

The treatment of CHF should be directed at the underlying cause; however, nonspecific treatment will generally improve the patient's condition. 1) Oxygen should be administered even in the absence of cyanosis as it will increase systemic oxygen delivery and also reduce reactive pulmonary vasoconstriction. 2) Digitalization will improve myocardial contractility and increase cardiac output and produce a diuresis. 3) Diuretics decrease preload and reduce pulmonary edema. 4) Afterload reduction will decrease systemic vascular resistance and increase cardiac output (for medication doses, see Table 16–2).

Figure 16–2. Standard chest x-ray and echocardiographic views. A, anterior; AAo, ascending aorta; Ao, aorta; DAo, descending aorta; I, inferior; IA, innominate artery; IVC, inferior vena cava; L, left; LA, left atrium; LCC, left common carotid artery; LPA, left pulmonary artery; LSC, left subclavian artery; LV left ventricle; LVOT, left ventricular outflow tract; MPA, main pulmonary artery; P, posterior; PA, pulmonary artery; R, right; RA, right atrium; RPA, right pulmonary artery; RV, right ventricle; RVOT, right ventricular outflow tract; S, superior; SVC, superior vena cava.

Table 16–2. Commonly used medications.[1]

Drug	Route	Dose	Onset	Mechanisms of Action[2]	Precautions/ Complications
Diuretics					
Bumetanide	PO	0.015–0.1 mg/kg/d	30–60 min	Inhibits sodium reabsorption in the ascending loop of Henle	Hypotension, hypokalemia, hypocalcemia, hyperuricemia
	IV	Dose not established	15–30 min		
Ethacrynic acid	PO	25 mg/dose max 2–3 mg/kg/d	30 min	Inhibits sodium reabsorption in the ascending loop of Henle and proximal and distal tubules	Hypotension, hypokalemie
	IV	1 mg/kg/dose, repeat dose not recommended	5 min		
Furosemide	PO	2 mg/kg/dose	30–60 min	Inhibits sodium reabsorption in the ascending loop of Henle	Ototoxicity in renal disease, hypokalemia, hypocalcemia, dehydration, nephrocalcinosis in premature infants
	IV	1 mg/kg/dose	Minutes		
Hydrochlorothiazide	PO	2–3 mg/kg/d	1–2 h	Inhibits renal tubular absorption of sodium	Hyperbilirubinemia, hypokalemia, hypoglycemia, hyperuricemia
Spironolactone	PO	1–3 mg/kg/d	4–5 d	Aldosterone inhibitor	Hyperkalemia, GI distress
Inotropic Agents					
Digoxin Therapeutic Level: 0.6–2.0 ng/ml	PO	Total digitalizing dose (TDD ½, ¼, ¼ q 6–8 hr) Premature—20–40 μg/ kg Newborn–2 yr—50 μg/ kg >2 yr—40 μg/kg Maintenance: ¼ TDD divided bid	1–2 h	CHF–contractility Dysrhythmia–atrial conduction, AV node refractoriness	Anorexia, nausea vomiting, headache, diarrhea, excitement, disorientation, abdominal pain, bradycardia, atrial fibrillation, ventricular tachycardia
	IV	75–80% po dose	15–60 min		
	IM	75–80% po dose	5–15 min		

Drug	Route	Dose	Onset	Action	Adverse Effects
Dobutamine	IV	2.5–20 µg/kg/min	Minutes	Low dose: alpha+, beta1++, beta2++; Medium dose: alpha++, beta1++, beta2+++; High dose: alpha++, beta1+, beta2+	Tachydysrhythmias, ectopy, hypertension; contraindicated in hypertrophic cardiomyopathy
Dopamine	IV	1–4 µg/kg/min; 4–8 µg/kg/min; 8–20 µg/kg/min	Minutes	Dopaminergic +++, alpha+; Dopaminergic ++++, alpha+, beta1+, beta2+; Dopaminergic alpha+++, beta1+++, beta2++	Tachydysrhythmias, hypertension
Amrinone lactate	IV	.75 mg/kg bolus over 2–3 minutes maintenance infusion neonate—3–5 mcg/kg/min child—5–10 mcg/kg/min note: Dose should not exceed 10 mg/kg/24 hrs	Minutes	Vasodilator increased contractility	Hypotension, thrombocytopenia, hepatotoxicity
Epinephrine	IV	0.1–0.5 µg/kg/min	Minutes	Alpha, beta1, beta2	Tachycardia, hypertension, headaches, nausea, vomiting
Isoproterenol	IV	0.05–0.5 µg/kg/min	Minutes	Beta agonist	Tachycardia, ventricular ectopy

Table 16-2. Commonly used medications (*continued*).

Drug	Route	Dose	Onset	Mechanisms of Action[2]	Precautions/ Complications
Antihypertensives					
Captopril	PO	1–4 mg/kg/d divided q 8–12h $\frac{1}{10}$ dose for premature infants, increasing with caution	1 hr	Angiotensin converting enzyme inhibitor	Hypotension, decreased renal perfusion
Diazoxide	IV	3–5 mg/kg/dose	1–2 min	Arterial vasodilator	Hypotension, hyperglycemia
Hydralazine	PO	0.75–7.0 mg/kg/d divided q 6–8 hr	Hours to days	Arterial vasodilator	Hypotension, tachycardia lupuslike syndrome
	IV	0.8–3.0 mg/kg/d divided q 4–6 hr	10–30 min		
Nitroprusside	IV	0.5–6.5 µg/kg/min IV drip	Minutes	Peripheral vasodilator (arterial and venous)	Hypotension, cyanide toxicity (discontinue if thiocyanate level >12 mg/dL)
Propranolol	PO	0.5–1.0 mg/kg/dose q 6 hr	30 min	Beta blockade	Decreased cardiac output, bradycardia, hypoglycemia, asthma
	IV	0.01–0.1 mg/kg/dose q 6–8 hr	2–5 min		
Antidysrhythmics					
Atropine	IV	0.01–0.03 mg/kg/dose q 4–6 hr, maximum dose 0.4 mg/dose	Seconds	Parasympathetic blockade	Tachycardia
Bretylium tosylate	IV	5 mg/kg then 1–2 mg/ min	Minutes	Inhibits norepinephrine release	Hypotension
Digoxin (see above)					
Lidocaine Therapeutic Level: 2–5 µg/mL	IV	1.0 mg/kg then 30–50 µg/kg/min	15–90 sec	Local anesthetic Decreases myocardial irritability	Dysrhythmia

Drug / Therapeutic Level	Route	Dose	Onset	Mechanism	Side Effects / Contraindications
Phenytoin Therapeutic Level: 10–20 µg/mL	PO	2–5 mg/kg/d, divided q 8–12 hr	2–4 hr	Elevates fibrillation threshold	Bradycardia, hypotension with rapid IV infusion, blood dyscrasias, gingival hyperplasia
Procainamide Therapeutic Level:	IV PO	3–5 mg/kg loading dose 40–60 mg/kg/d divided q 6–8 hours 10–20 mg/kg/dose	5–10 min 30–60 min 1–5 min	Slows myocardial conduction and prolongs repolarization	Hypotension, blood dyscrasias, lupuslike syndrome, acquired long QI syndrome, GI upset
Adenosine	IV IV	Rapid IV bolus 37.5–100 mcg/kg If no response, 72–225 mcg/kg Dose may be repeated once if no effect	Seconds	Purinergic agonist	Contraindicated in patients with second or third degree AV block, atrial fibrillation flutter and sick-sinus syndrome
Flecainide	PO	2–6 mg/kg/d in 2–3 divided doses	2–3 hrs	Fast sodium channel blockade (IC)	Contraindicated in patients with second or third degree AV block, bifascicular or fascicular block, sick sinus syndrome and myocardial depression. May be proarrhythmic
Propranolol (see above)					
Quinidine gluconate Therapeutic Level: 1–6 µg/mL	PO	10–30 mg/kg/d divided q 12 hr	Minutes	Slows myocardial conduction and prolongs repolarization	Hypotension, blood dyscrasia, tinnitus, GI upset
Verapamil	PO IV	3–6 mg/kg/d divided tid 0.1–0.15 mg/kg over 1 min	Minutes	Calcium antagonist	Exacerbates heart failure; have colloid and calcium available during rapid infusion
Ductal-Related					
Indomethacin	IV	0.2 mg/kg q 12 hr (0.1 mg/kg for 2nd and 3rd dose if infant <48 hr old)	Minutes	Prostaglandin inhibitor	GI bleeding, infection, transient renal impairment; discontinue if urine output <0.6 mL/kg/hr
Prostaglandin E1	IV	0.01–0.1 µg/kg/min	Minutes	Smooth muscle relaxation especially ductal tissue Maintain systemic or pulmonary perfusion in ductal-dependent CHD	Apnea, fever, hypotension

1 AV, atrioventricular; CHD, congenital heart disease; CHF, congestive heart failure; TDD, total digitalizing dose.
2 Plus signs indicate degree of activity.

HYPERCYANOTIC SPELLS

Hypercyanotic or "tetralogy spells" are sudden episodes of increasing irritability, tachypnea, and intense cyanosis that may progress to syncope and seizures. They may last from minutes to hours and are frequently seen in patients with tetralogy of Fallot, tricuspid atresia, or any cardiac anomaly with reduced pulmonary blood flow and unobstructed intracardiac communication. The spells are caused by 1) infundibular hypercontractility, 2) decreased systemic vascular resistance, or 3) decreased systemic venous return.

Hypercyanotic spells are a medical emergency. Treatment of the spells is directed at correcting the underlying problem. Frequently, soothing the child and placing the child in a knee–chest position will break the cycle. Oxygen should be administered. Morphine sulfate 0.1–0.2 mg/kg subcutaneously will quiet the child and reduce the tachypnea. Intravenous propranolol 0.05–0.10 mg/kg may be given in acute cases and oral propranolol 1.0–4.0 mg/kg/d may be used chronically until palliative or definitive surgery can be arranged.

CONGENITAL HEART DISEASE

Congenital heart disease (CHD) occurs in approximately 6–8/1000 live births; in the USA alone 25,000–35,000 children with CHD are born each year. Palliative or corrective surgery is now available for well over 90% of these children, with successful intervention dependent upon an early, accurate diagnosis. When a child presents with cyanosis or CHF, a rapid, orderly sequence of evaluation and intervention must begin immediately.

ACYANOTIC HEART DISEASE

Ventricular Septal Defect (VSD)
   A. General Considerations: VSD is the most common form of CHD, excluding bicuspid aortic valves. It occurs in 25% of all cases of CHD, and is more common in males than in females.

It is the most common lesion found in chromosomal abnormalities.

B. Anatomy: The most common location is in the perimembranous ventricular septum. VSDs can also be found in the muscular, outlet, and inlet portions of the septum. The size ranges from pinpoint to involving most of the septum. VSDs may be singular or multiple. They are frequently associated with other cardiac defects.

C. Symptoms and Signs: The physical presentation depends largely on the size of the defect, pulmonary vascular resistance and associated lesions. In a small to moderate sized defect there will be a normal P2 and a grade II–VI/VI harsh, pansystolic murmur (PSM) at the lower left sternal border. In a large shunt without pulmonary hypertension the P2 is normal, a grade II–III/VI PSM is heard at the lower left sternal border, a mid diastolic flow rumble is appreciated at the apex, and CHF is present. In the presence of marked pulmonary hypertension, a right ventricular lift is present, P2 is loud, a short systolic ejection murmur is present along the left sternal border, and the patient may be cyanotic if Eisenmenger's syndrome has developed.

D. Laboratory Findings: In a small shunt, the heart size will be normal on the chest x-ray and the ECG will be normal. In moderate-sized defects, the chest x-ray may show mild cardiac enlargement and increased pulmonary blood flow, and the ECG will be variable. Large defects result in marked cardiomegaly with increased pulmonary vascularity; the ECG demonstrates right ventricular hypertrophy (RVH), left ventricular hypertrophy (LVH), or both. The echocardiogram is useful in defining the position and size of the defect. Doppler echocardiography can be used to estimate the pulmonary artery systolic pressure.

E. Treatment: Small defects rarely need any surgical or medical management other than subacute bacterial endocarditis (SBE) prophylaxis. There is a significant spontaneous closure rate indirectly related to the size of the defect. Anticongestive heart failure medications are used in the presence of CHF. Surgery is recommended for patients with refractory CHF, failure to thrive in spite of adequate medical and nutritional management, repeated episodes of pneumonia or reversible pulmonary hypertension. Surgery involves closure of the VSD, usually through the right atrium, by suture or synthetic patch.

Patent Ductus Arteriosus (PDA)

A. General Considerations: PDA is a common form of CHD, accounting for 12% of all cases of CHD; it occurs in

20–60% of all premature infants. Females are affected twice as often as males and there appears to be an increased incidence at higher altitudes.

B. Anatomy: The ductus arteriosus is a vessel located between the pulmonary artery and the descending aorta, found in all fetuses and generally closing shortly after birth in full-term infants. It is commonly located on the left side but may be right-sided or occasionally bilateral.

C. Symptoms and Signs: In premature infants, depending on the size of the PDA, the precordium may be hyperactive and a variable systolic murmur may be present. The absence of a murmur does not correlate with the absence of a PDA. The pulses are often bounding. In the older child a continuous murmur can be heard at the left upper sternal border below the clavicle, with radiation to the back. The pulses are bounding.

D. Laboratory Findings: In a small PDA the chest x-ray and ECG are normal. Moderate to large PDAs will show LVH on the ECG with cardiomegaly and increased pulmonary markings on the chest x-ray. If pulmonary hypertension is present the ECG will show RVH or biventricular hypertrophy. The two-dimensional and doppler echocardiogram can demonstrate the PDA. In large shunts, the left atrium will be enlarged secondary to increased pulmonary venous return.

E. Treatment: Premature infants are urgently treated either medically (indomethacin) or surgically. In the absence of pulmonary vascular obstructive disease, effective surgical ligation or transvenous occlusion in the catheterization lab is indicated for older children.

Atrial Septal Defect (ASD)

A. General Considerations: There are 3 types of ASDs—ostium secundum, ostium primum, and sinus venosus. Ostium secundum make up 10% of cases of CHD and have a 2:1 female:-male ratio. Ostium primum defects comprise 2% of cases of CHD and occur approximately equally among males and females. Five percent of ASDs are made up of sinus venosus ASDs.

B. Anatomy: Ostium secundum defects involve the area around the fossa ovalis. Ostium primum anomalies result from deficiencies in the atrial septum primum during the embryonic period. The sinus venosus defect is located posteriorly to the fossa ovalis and is often associated with partial anomalous pulmonary venous return of the right upper pulmonary veins.

C. Symptoms and Signs: In general, there is a right ventricular heave and the S2 is widely split and fixed. A grade II/VI systolic ejection murmur is heard at the left upper sternal border, followed by a mid diastolic flow rumble in the tricuspid valve region.

D. Laboratory Findings: The chest x-ray demonstrates cardiomegaly with increased pulmonary markings. The ECG shows RVH with an rsR' in V1. Left axis deviation (LAD) and RVH with an rsR' in V1 is seen in ostium primum defects. The echocardiogram reveals a dilated right atrium and right ventricle plus paradoxical septal motion. The defect itself can be visualized in the atrial septum with intracardiac shunt flow detected by Doppler.

E. Treatment: Spontaneous closure has been reported, although it is not as common as in VSDs. Anticongestive medications are used for CHF. Where there is a large left to right shunt, CHF, or pulmonary congestion, surgical closure is recommended. Transvenous closure in the catheterization lab with an occluding device is now an alterative to surgical closure.

Atrioventricular Septal Defect

A. General Considerations: This disorder, common in Down syndrome, is found in approximately 4% of patients with CHD. Males and females are affected equally. Pulmonary hypertension and irreversible pulmonary vascular obstructive disease are major risks.

B. Anatomy: In complete atrioventricular septal defect, there is a large AV septal defect and a common AV valve that arises from both the right and left atria. The partial form has an ostium primum ASD and an abnormal mitral valve, with mitral regurgitation.

C. Symptoms and Signs: In the newborn period the murmur may be inaudible and P2 will be loud. A nonspecific systolic murmur along with a mid diastolic flow rumble at the apex is usually heard in later infancy.

D. Laboratory Findings: The chest x-ray demonstrates cardiomegaly and increased pulmonary vascular markings. The ECG will show LAD with RVH, LVH, or both. Fifty percent of cases will have first-degree heart block. The echocardiogram is useful in assessing the AV valve structures and the atrial and ventricular septal defects.

E. Treatment: Anticongestive medication is used to control CHF. Surgery is performed prior to the development of irreversible pulmonary vascular disease, usually before 6–12 months.

Aortic Stenosis (AS)

A. General Considerations: AS accounts for 5% of cases of CHD, with a 2:1 male predominance. AS can be classified as valvar, subvalvar, or supravalvar. Supravalvar AS is associated with William's syndrome (elfin facies and hypercalcemia of infancy).

B. Anatomy: In valvar AS, the valve is usually bicuspid and the leaflets are dysplastic and thickened with decreased mobility. In severe cases the anulus itself is frequently hypoplastic.

C. Symptoms and Signs: Infants may present with CHF and weak pulses. Older children are usually asymptomatic. A systolic ejection click will be heard at the apex and a grade II–VI/VI systolic ejection murmur will be heard at the upper right sternal border with radiation to the carotids. In moderate to severe disease a thrill is often palpable at the suprasternal notch and the base. The click is absent in subvalvar and supravalvar disease. Subaortic stenosis is frequently associated with aortic regurgitation.

D. Laboratory Findings: The chest x-ray shows a normal heart size and a dilated aortic root. The ECG is similar to CoA with RVH in infancy and LVH in older children. Echocardiography demonstrates the abnormal aortic valve and the left ventricular outflow tract abnormalities. Doppler flow studies can precisely estimate the pressure gradient.

E. Treatment: The gradient can be relived by balloon valvuloplasty or surgery. Indications for surgery are symptoms, a gradient greater than 60 mm Hg, an abnormal blood pressure response to exercise, or electrocardiographic evidence of myocardial strain.

Coarctation of the Aorta (CoA)

A. General Considerations: CoA accounts for 6% of cases of CHD, with a 1.7:1 male predominance. CoA is commonly seen in association with Turner's syndrome.

B. Anatomy: CoA is defined as a constriction of the aorta typically in the region adjacent to the ductus arteriosus (juxtaductal). It may involve a discrete narrowing or a long segment. Bicuspid aortic valves are associated in 50% of cases. The CoA syndrome consists of coarctation. PDA, tubular hypoplasia of the aortic isthmus, and VSD and is frequently complicated by CHF.

C. Symptoms and Signs: Hypertension and decreased femoral pulses with a brachial-femoral pulse lag herald the diagnosis.

In neonates the decreased femoral pulses can be masked in the presence of a large PDA. Severe CoA can present in the first weeks of life with CHF and absent femoral pulses.

D. Laboratory Findings: The chest x-ray shows cardiomegaly with pulmonary venous congestion in infants with CHF. The ECG will show RVH (LV hypoplasia). In older children the chest x-ray may be normal or show rib notching or poststenotic dilatation of the aorta. LVH is seen on the ECG. The echocardiogram shows a dilated right ventricle and possibly a hypoplastic left ventricle during infancy. The aortic arch and coarctation site can be visualized; in addition, aortic doppler studies will demonstrate the disturbed arterial flow.

E. Treatment: Infants with CHF need stabilization and urgent surgery. In neonates, administration of PGE_1 to reopen the ductus arteriosus will improve systemic perfusion and resolve acidosis. Several surgical options are currently available. The most commonly used approaches are subclavian flap repair and end to end anastomosis with resection. Both of these techniques have excellent results. Recoarctation may occur. Balloon angioplasty in the catheterization laboratory is highly successful at relieving the obstruction.

Hypoplastic Left Heart Syndrome (HLHS)

A. General Considerations: HLHS occurs in 1.5% of patients with CHD, with a male predominance. Without surgery it virtually 100% fatal.

B. Anatomy: Aortic and mitral atresia with small left ventricular cavity.

C. Symptoms and Signs: The patients usually present in the first week of life with CHF and weak pulses. There is a single S2, and a pulmonary ejection click is associated with a nonspecific systolic ejection murmur at the left sternal border.

D. Laboratory Findings: The chest x-ray shows cardiomegaly and interstitial pulmonary edema. The ECG shows RVH with absence of left-sided forces. The echocardiogram demonstrates the hypoplastic left ventricle and aorta.

E. Treatment: In the recent past, the outlook for this group of patients has changed drastically. With the advent of neonatal cardiac transplant and complex surgical repairs (Norwood procedure), several options are available for this lethal lesion. Currently, neonatal cardiac transplant has a one year survival rate of 85%. Preliminary long-term results of morbidity and mortality studies are encouraging.

Mitral Valve Prolapse (MVP)

A. General Considerations: The incidence of MVP is from 2–20% and most often occurs in slender females over the age of 6 years. Significant symptoms are rare.

B. Anatomy: Focal or diffusely redundant (myxomatous) valve tissue exists involving one or both leaflets with or without associated lengthening of the chordae tendinea.

C. Symptoms and Signs: A mid systolic click is heard at the apex and possibly the left sternal border. A mid to late systolic murmur may follow the click if mitral regurgitation is present.

D. Laboratory Findings: The chest x-ray is normal. Electrocardiographic findings vary from normal to nonspecific ST-T wave changes and/or dysrhythmias. The echocardiogram demonstrates abnormal posterior displacement of the mitral valve leaflets in systole.

E. Treatment: SBE prophylaxis is recommended if mitral regurgitation is present. Patients with significant chest pain are treated with beta blockade.

Pulmonary Stenosis (PS)

A. General Considerations: PS occurs in 10% of cases of CHD, with a male predominance.

B. Anatomy: The valve is conical or dome-shaped and is formed by fusion of the valve leaflets. Twenty percent of autopsy cases show bicuspid-valves and 10–15% cases have dysplastic valves.

C. Symptoms and Signs: In mild to moderate PS the P2 is soft and there is a systolic ejection click. The click is followed by a grade I–III/VI systolic ejection murmur at the left upper sternal border that radiates to the back. In severe PS, P2 becomes silent and the murmur becomes longer and louder and peaks later in systole. In severe PS, cyanosis will be evident.

D. Laboratory Findings: The chest x-ray in mild PS shows a normal-sized heart and dilatation of the main pulmonary artery. The degree of pulmonary artery dilatation does not correlate with the severity of the stenosis. The ECG is normal. In moderate to severe pulmonary stenosis, the ECG shows RVH and RVH with strain in critical PS. The echocardiogram demonstrates the abnormal pulmonary valve and the associated degree of right ventricular hypertrophy. Doppler echocardiography defines the transvalvular gradient precisely.

E. Treatment: Transcatheter balloon valvuloplasty is the recommended procedure for moderate and severe cases. It is now being performed in small infants, thus avoiding the high risks of neonatal surgery.

CYANOTIC HEART DISEASE

Cyanotic heart disease describes those children who have right to left shunts and are *usually,* but not always, cyanotic. Cyanosis is determined by the presence of at least 4–5 grams of unsaturated hemoglobin in the capillary bed. With this in mind, therefore, a child with a cyanotic heart lesion with anemia may not appear cyanotic. It is important to also remember that cyanotic infants may appear ashen in color rather than blue. Evaluation of the cyanotic infant is presented in Figure 16–3.

Tetralogy of Fallot (TOF)

A. General Considerations: TOF is the most common form of cyanotic cardiac malformation, accounting for 10–15% of all cases of CHD. There is a slight predominance of males over females.

B. Anatomy: TOF consists of infundibular PS, a large unrestrictive VSD, an aorta overriding the VSD, and RVH. Associated anomalies may include a right aortic arch in 25%, an ASD in 15%, absent pulmonary valve, pulmonary atresia, atrioventricular septal defect, and a left superior vena cava to the coronary sinus.

C. Symptoms and Signs: Depending on the degree of left-to-right shunting, the patient may either by acyanotic (ie, pink tetralogy) or cyanotic. The degree of right ventricular outflow tract obstruction largely determines the degree of cyanosis. Auscultation reveals a single S2 and a grade I–III/VI systolic ejection murmur at the mid to high left sternal border. During a hypercyanotic spell the murmur diminishes in intensity and the patient becomes more cyanotic and irritable.

D. Laboratory Findings: The ECG commonly shows right axis deviation and RVH. The chest x-ray reveals a normal or small heart, often with the apex upturned, and a narrow mediastinum. The pulmonary markings are normal to decreased. The aortic arch is right sided in approximately 25% of cases. The echocardiogram demonstrates the overriding aorta, VSD, pulmonary infundibular stenosis, and the hypertrophied right ventricle. An arterial blood gas demonstrates a normal pH and P_{CO_2} at rest, with a variable degree of hypoxemia.

E. Treatment: Beta blockade may prevent hypercyanotic spells. Surgical palliation is provided with creation of a systemic

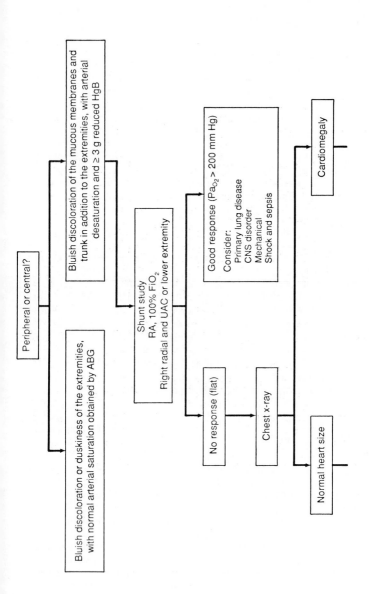

Peripheral or central?

Bluish discoloration of the mucous membranes and trunk in addition to the extremities, with arterial desaturation and ≥ 3 g reduced HgB

Bluish discoloration or duskiness of the extremities, with normal arterial saturation obtained by ABG

Shunt study
RA, 100% FiO₂
Right radial and UAC or lower extremity

Good response (Pa$_{O_2}$ > 200 mm Hg)

Consider:
Primary lung disease
CNS disorder
Mechanical
Shock and sepsis

No response (flat)

Chest x-ray

Cardiomegaly

Normal heart size

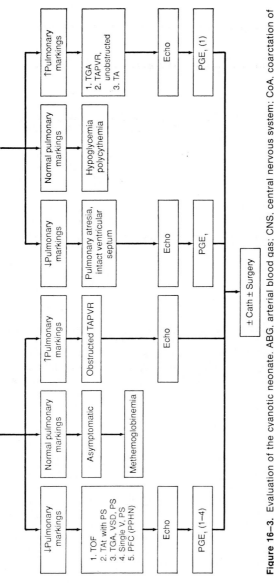

Figure 16–3. Evaluation of the cyanotic neonate. ABG, arterial blood gas; CNS, central nervous system; CoA, coarctation of the aorta; FiO₂, % inspired oxygen; PFC, persistent fetal circulation; PGE, prostaglandin; PPHN, persistent pulmonary hypertension of the newborn; PS, pulmonary stenosis; RA, room air; TAt, tricuspid atresia; TA, truncus arteriosus; TAPVR, total anomalous pulmonary venous return; TGA, transposition of the great arteries; TOF, tetralogy of Fallot; UAC, umbilical artery catheter; V, ventricle; VSD, ventricular septal defect.

artery to pulmonary artery anastomosis to increase pulmonary blood flow (Blalock–Taussig shunt). Later, total correction is completed with VSD closure and patch augmentation of the right ventricular outflow tract or the placement of a conduit from the right ventricle to the pulmonary artery.

Transposition of the Great Arteries (TGA)

A. General Considerations: TGA is the second most common cyanotic heart lesion and accounts for 5–7% of all cases of CHD. There is a 3:1 male predominance.

B. Anatomy: The aorta arises from the right ventricle and the pulmonary artery arises from the left ventricle. Associated anomalies may include a VSD (30–35%), PS and VSD (10%), PS alone (5%), or CoA (5%).

C. Symptoms and Signs: The infants are cyanotic at birth and generally comfortable appearing and well developed. The first heart sound is normal and S2 is single. The systolic murmur of PS or VSD is heard when those associated lesions are present.

D. Laboratory Findings: The ECG may be entirely normal or show right-axis deviation and RVH. In the first few days of life, the chest x-ray can be normal or show the diagnostic triad of an oval or egg-shaped cardiac silhouette, a narrow mediastinum, and increased pulmonary markings. The echocardiogram will demonstrate the aorta arising from the right ventricle and the pulmonary artery from the left ventricle. Associated anomalies such as VSD and PS can be ascertained. The arterial blood gas shows Pao_2 rarely higher than 35 mm Hg with little or no response to supplemental oxygen and a normal Pco_2.

E. Treatment: Medically, the infant is started on PGE_1. At cardiac catheterization, a balloon atrial septostomy is performed to enlarge an ASD and improve systemic and venous mixing. Surgically, the systemic and pulmonary venous return may be rerouted at the atrial level (Mustard or Senning procedure) or a supravalvar arterial switch with coronary artery relocation may be performed.

Total Anomalous Pulmonary Venous Return (TAPVR)

A. General Considerations: TAPVR describes a group of disorders in which no pulmonary venous return enters directly into the left atrium. This heart lesion accounts for 2% of cases of CHD and is seen equally in males and females except when the veins enter the portal system, in which case there is an approximate 3:1 male predominance.

B. Anatomy: The pulmonary veins generally form a confluence and then enter the heart (1) via vertical vein into the left innominate vein; (2) directly into the coronary sinus, the right atrium, or the right superior vena cava; or (3) across the diaphragm and into the inferior vena cava or the portal system. They may or may not be obstructed.

C. Symptoms and Signs: Patients without pulmonary venous obstruction are usually mildly cyanotic and asymptomatic at birth; CHF develops later. A right ventricular heave may be present. S1 is loud, followed by a widely split S2 and usually an S3 at the apex. A grade II/VI systolic ejection murmur is usually, but not always, heard in the pulmonic region, with a mid diastolic flow rumble in the tricuspid valve region. Patients with obstruction to pulmonary venous return usually develop signs and symptoms within 24 hours of birth, including respiratory distress, feeding problems, and cardiac failure. They are cyanotic. S1 is normal and S2 splits with an increased P2. A murmur may be barely audible.

D. Laboratory Findings: In *unobstructed* TAPVR, the ECG shows right-axis deviation, right atrial enlargement (RAE), and RVH. The chest x-ray will demonstrate increased pulmonary flow, an enlarged right heart, and occasionally a "snowman" figure when the return is supracardiac. The echocardiogram shows an enlarged right atrium and ventricle. The anomalous pulmonary veins can usually be demonstrated. With *obstructed* pulmonary venous return the ECG will show RVH. The chest x-ray reveals a normal heart size and diffuse interstitial edema. The echocardiogram shows a large right ventricle, and Doppler flow studies will demonstrate the pulmonary venous obstruction.

E. Treatment: Surgical correction with reanastomosis of the pulmonary veins to the left atrium is mandatory in early infancy and is emergent when the veins are obstructed.

Tricuspid Atresia

A. General Considerations: This lesion occurs in 2% of cases of CHD and is slightly more common in males.

B. Anatomy: There is complete atresia of the tricuspid valve and, therefore, no direct communication between the right atrium and the right ventricle. The right ventricle has varying degrees of hypoplasia. There is a mandatory ASD. The great vessels may be normally related or transposed and a VSD may or may not be present. The pulmonary valve is normal, stenotic, or atretic.

C. Symptoms and Signs: The infants are cyanotic at birth. S1 is normal and S2 is single. A grade I–III/VI harsh systolic ejection murmur is heard along the lower left sternal border and there may be CHF when the pulmonary blood flow is increased.

D. Laboratory Findings: The ECG shows LAD, RAE, and LVH. The chest x-ray reveals a slightly to markedly enlarged heart with variable pulmonary artery markings, depending on the associated lesions. The echocardiogram demonstrates the absence of the tricuspid valve and the right ventricular hypoplasia. The relationship of the great vessels can be determined and the status of the pulmonary valve and ventricular septum identified.

E. Treatment: A balloon atrial septostomy is performed in the catheterization lab to allow unobstructed flow to the left heart. For those patients with high pulmonary blood flow, anticongestives are utilized followed by an atriopulmonary anastomosis (Fontan procedure) at a later date. Pulmonary artery banding may be required to protect the pulmonary vascular bed prior to the Fontan repair. Low pulmonary blood flow indicates the need for a systemic-to-pulmonary shunt followed later by the Fontan procedure.

Pulmonary Atresia, Intact Ventricular Septum

A. General Considerations: Pulmonary atresia with an intact ventricular septum accounts for approximately 1% of cases of CHD.

B. Anatomy: The pulmonary valve does not form and the right ventricle is either small with a hypertrophied wall or of relatively normal size. The ventricular septum is intact. The tricuspid valve shows varying degrees of hypoplasia. Fistulous communication between the right ventricle and coronary arteries may occur.

C. Symptoms and Signs: The infants are cyanotic from birth. S1 is normal and S2 is single. A grade I–II/VI continuous murmur (PDA) may be heard at the left upper sternal border as may a grade I–III/VI harsh pansystolic murmur at the left lower sternal border (tricuspid regurgitation).

D. Laboratory Findings: The ECG shows a normal axis, RAE, and LVH. The chest x-ray reveals a large heart with decreased pulmonary blood flow. The echocardiogram shows the atretic pulmonary valve plus an intact ventricular septum. The size of the right ventricular cavity can be ascertained as well as the presence and degree of tricuspid regurgitation.

E. Treatment: Prostaglandins are utilized to keep the ductus arteriosus open while awaiting intervention. A balloon atrial septostomy is performed in the catheterization lab. If the right ventricle is small a systemic-to-pulmonary shunt procedure is created. If the right ventricle is of adequate size a pulmonary valvulotomy is performed. Right ventricular outflow tract reconstruction is performed at a later date if necessary.

Truncus Arteriosus

A. General Considerations: Approximately 0.7% of children with CHD have truncus arteriosus, which is equally distributed between males and females. DiGeorge's syndrome with thymic aplasia is frequently present.

B. Anatomy: One large vessel giving rise to the aorta, pulmonary artery, and coronary arteries arises from the heart. It overrides a VSD. The truncal valve may be stenotic and/or incompetent. A right aortic arch is common.

C. Symptoms and Signs: When there is unobstructed pulmonary blood flow the child presents with CHF. If there is decreased flow to the lungs the infant will be cyanotic. S1 and S2 are loud, and a systolic ejection click is present. A grade II–IV/VI systolic ejection murmur is heard at the left lower sternal border. A diastolic decrescendo murmur of truncal valve insufficiency may be audible.

D. Laboratory Findings: ECG usually demonstrates right ventricular or biventricular hypertrophy and ST-T wave depression. The chest x-ray reveals a large boot-shaped heart with absence of the pulmonary artery segment, often a right aortic arch, and variable pulmonary markings. The echocardiogram identifies the single truncal root and the large VSD.

E. Treatment: Anticongestive medications are needed for patients with high pulmonary blood flow. Early total correction is performed by closing the VSD to include the truncal root. The pulmonary arteries are detached from the root and then reanastomosed to the right ventricle, with or without an interposed conduit.

ACQUIRED HEART DISEASE

Acquired heart disease includes infectious, immunologic, and metabolic involvement of the endocardium, myocardium, or pericardium. It frequently presents in all age groups as a life-threatening illness.

ACUTE RHEUMATIC FEVER (ARF)

See Chapter 27, Collagen Diseases.

KAWASAKI DISEASE

A. General Considerations: Kawasaki disease, or mucocutaneous lymph node syndrome, is an inflammatory disorder of unknown etiology; it has multisystem involvement, most notably the heart. Eighty percent of the cases involve children less than 4 years of age, with a 1.5:1 male to female ratio. Asians are affected more frequently than blacks, who are more frequently affected than whites.

B. Symptoms and Signs: As with acute rheumatic fever, the physical findings depend on the particular criteria present, 5 of which are needed to make the diagnosis.

1. Fever—longer than 5 days, not responsive to antibiotics.

2. Mucous Membrane Involvement—cracked, fissured lips and tongue—''strawberry tongue.''

3. Conjunctivitis—nonpurulent.

4. Polymorphous Rash—generally involving the trunk and extremities.

5. Lymphadenopathy

6. Digital Swelling and Desquamation

Examination of the cardiovascular system may reveal findings consistent with myocarditis, pericarditis, and peripheral arteritis.

C. Laboratory Findings: The WBC, ESR, and CRP will be elevated, as will the platelet count. A normochromic anemia can be present, as can a sterile pyuria. The ECG often shows a prolonged PR interval, ST-T wave changes, and low voltage. The chest x-ray may show cardiomegaly. The echocardiogram is vital in Kawasaki disease since 20% of patients will develop coronary artery aneurysms or dilatation. A pericardial effusion may be present.

D. Treatment: Current therapy includes aspirin and intravenous gamma globulin. Serial ECGs and echocardiograms should be obtained since Kawasaki disease has acute and chronic phases and some findings, most notably coronary involvement, may not be present on the initial examination.

ENDOCARDITIS

A. General Considerations: Infective endocarditis is an infection of the endocardium in patients with structural heart disease or in immunocompromised hosts. It is rarely seen in a normal population. The most common organisms include *Streptococcus viridans* and *Staphylococcus aureus*, along with fungal infections.

B. Symptoms and Signs: The patient may have a history of persistent fever and weight loss. The physical examination will be positive for changing murmurs and splenomegaly (70%), petechiae, and peripheral embolic phenomenon.

C. Laboratory Findings: The ESR and WBC are often elevated and the urine can be heme positive. Cultures of the blood may or may not be positive. Cardiomegaly will be present on the chest x-ray and heart block will be seen on the ECG when the aortic anulus is involved. The echocardiogram will identify large endocardial vegetations, but may be normal.

D. Treatment: Appropriate antibiotics should be administered for both culture-positive and culture-negative endocarditis. Treatment for CHF and valve replacement may be necessary.

E. Prophylaxis: Many children with congenital or acquired heart disease are at increased risk for infective endocarditis; therefore, prophylaxis is recommended. Prophylaxis is recommended at times when there is a known increased risk for bacteremia, such as with certain dental or surgical procedures. Antibiotics are given around the time of the procedure in sufficient doses to assure adequate antibiotic concentrations in the serum during and after the procedure. The recommended antibiotic is that which is more likely to be effective against bacteria that commonly cause endocarditis. Children with valve dysfunction who take chronic penicillin for secondary prevention of rheumatic fever require infective endocarditis prophylaxis with an alternative regimen because of potentially resistant oral pathogens. Children with repaired ventricular septal defects, atrial septal defects, and patent ductus arteriosus who do not have cardiac residua require endocarditis prophylaxis for 6 months following surgery. Infective endocarditis prophylaxis is not recommended for children with functional murmurs or isolated secundum atrial septal defect. For specific indications and dosing regimens refer to the American Heart Association recommendations (*JAMA* **264**:2919–2922, 1990).

MYOCARDITIS

A. General Considerations: In a majority of cases the cause is unknown. Viral etiologies are common and include Coxsackie A & B, rubella, cytomegalovirus, mumps, adenovirus, and herpes.

B. Symptoms and Signs: In the newborn period the onset is rapid with CHF and vascular collapse. Mitral and tricuspid regurgitation may also be present. The onset is more insidious in the older child.

C. Laboratory Findings: The WBC is variable and both bacterial and viral cultures are usually negative. A chest x-ray will show cardiomegaly with moderate to marked venous congestion and possibly pneumonia. Decreased voltage, ST-T wave changes, and dysrhythmias may be seen on the ECG. Decreased contractility and dilation of the heart are seen by echocardiography.

D. Treatment: CHF is treated with digitalis, diuretics, and afterload reduction. Care is taken with digitalization, using two-thirds the total digitalizing dose owing to an increased risk of toxicity.

PERICARDITIS

A. General Considerations: Pericarditis may be nonpurulent, secondary to rheumatic fever, viral infection, collagen vascular disease, and uremia; or purulent, caused by *Haemophilus influenzae*, *S aureus*, and streptococcus pneumoniae. It is rarely an isolated event. Tamponade may occur and may lead to rapid deterioration and death.

B. Symptoms and Signs: Fever is present along with retrosternal chest pain. Dyspnea and grunting respirations may be present in infants. There may be jugular venous distention and pulsus paradoxus. Cardiac examination may reveal muffled heart sounds and a pericardial friction rub.

C. Laboratory Findings: In nonpurulent pericarditis, the WBC and ESR may be elevated with negative blood cultures.

In purulent pericarditis the blood culture is positive and the WBC and ESR may be elevated. In the presence of an effusion, the cardiac silhouette has a "water-bottle" shape. ST-T wave changes can be seen on the ECG. The echocardiogram can document the presence of a pericardial effusion and evidence of purulent loculation.

D. Treatment: Aspirin and other anti-inflammatories are used for nonpurulent pericarditis. Antibiotics and pericardiectomy are indicated in purulent pericarditis. Cardiac tamponade requires an emergent pericardiocentesis.

DYSRHYTHMIAS

Recognition and management of cardiac dysrhythmias in childhood is growing rapidly. This growth is due partly to increased awareness secondary to the availability and improving technology in cardiac monitoring equipment, eg, continuous heart rate monitoring in intensive care units and the 24-hour Holter monitor. Also, there is a true increase in the incidence and prevalence of dysrhythmias as more patients are surviving open heart surgery, and dysrhythmias are frequently seen in these survivors. Understanding the basic underlying mechanism of dysrhythmias helps in establishing a diagnostic and treatment approach.

SINUS DYSRHYTHMIAS

Sinus Arrhythmia
Sinus rhythm with a variable heart rate. This is a normal variant with an increase in rate with inspiration and a decrease with expiration. No treatment is required.

Sinus Bradycardia
Sinus heart rate less than the lower limits of normal for age (60 BPM in newborns, 40 BPM in older children). This may be a normal finding in athletes and at rest. Other causes include sick sinus syndrome, hypertension, and central nervous system abnormalities. Asymptomatic patients need only to be watched,

while treatment should be directed at correcting the underlying cause.

Sinus Tachycardia

Sinus heart rate greater than the upper limits of normal for age (220 BPM in newborns, 190 BPM in older children). This is found in fever, anemia, hypovolemia, and CHF. Treatment should be directed at the underlying cause.

CONDUCTION ABNORMALITIES

First-Degree Heart Block

Prolonged PR interval that is greater than the upper limits of normal for age. No treatment is required.

Second-Degree Heart Block

Mobitz Type I (Wenckebach) is progressive lengthening of the PR interval until a nonconducted P wave occurs. Mobitz Type II has a consistent PR interval with an occasional nonconducted P wave. Type I may be seen in normal persons while Type II implies advanced conduction system disease. Type I seldom requires treatment, while Type II may need temporary or permanent pacing.

Third-Degree Heart Block (Complete AV Block)

This may be congenital or acquired after cardiac surgery, myocarditis, or drug ingestion. Seventy-five percent of patients with congenital third-degree block *without structural heart disease* have mothers with systemic lupus erythematosus.

Treatment of acute complete block includes isoproterenol or temporary pacing. Long-term treatment requires a permanent pacemaker if the patient is symptomatic, has exercise intolerance, or has a sleeping heart rate less than 40.

PREMATURE DEPOLARIZATIONS

Premature Atrial Contraction (PAC)

Premature atrial depolarizations—P waves—that may or may not be conducted through the AV node. It is usually idiopathic (normal variant) but may be secondary to hypokalemia, hypoxia, hypoglycemia, atrial enlargement, or digitalis toxicity. No treatment is required unless supraventricular tachycardia (SVT) is present.

Premature Junctional Contraction (PJC)

Premature QRS waves of normal morphology not preceded by a P wave. The beats originate in the AV nodal region and have the same significance as PACs.

Premature Ventricular Contraction (PVC)

Premature QRS complex with a prolonged duration and a morphology different from the preceding normal QRS complex. It is not preceded by a P wave. PVCs may be found in a normal heart or may be secondary to hypokalemia, hypocalcemia, cardiomyopathy, or myocarditis. In asymptomatic patients with no underlying heart disease, no treatment is necessary. Treatment should be directed at correcting the underlying cause. Suppression with antidysrhythmic agents should be initiated in a hospital setting.

TACHYDYSRHYTHMIAS

Supraventricular Tachycardia (SVT) (Fig 16–4)
Atrial Flutter

Saw-tooth configuration of atrial flutter waves with atrial rates varying from 300 to 600. There may be variable AV node conduction. This rhythm is seen in right or left atrial enlargements, sick-sinus syndrome, hypokalemia, hypoxia, hypoglycemia, atrial septal aneurysm, and following cardiac surgery. Acute treatment includes DC cardioversion, overdrive atrial pacing, and intravenous digitalis or procainamide.

Atrial Fibrillation

Rapid irregularly-irregular atrial rate with irregular QRS rhythm. This is a rare entity in children but can occur in right and left atrial enlargement, hypokalemia, hypoxia, hypoglycemia, hyperthyroidism, and following atrial surgery. Acute treatment includes DC cardioversion and intravenous digitalis.

Ventricular Tachycardia

Three or more consecutive PVCs at rates of greater than 120. The PVCs may be unifocal and multifocal. The ventricular

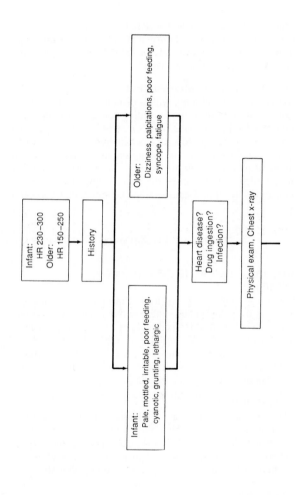

Infant:
HR 230–300
Older:
HR 150–250

History

Older:
Dizziness, palpitations, poor feeding, syncope, fatigue

Infant:
Pale, mottled, irritable, poor feeding, cyanotic, grunting, lethargic

Heart disease?
Drug ingestion?
Infection?

Physical exam, Chest x-ray

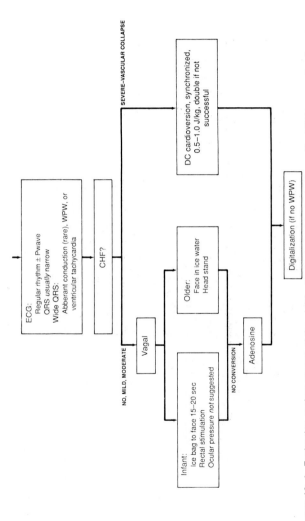

Figure 16–4. Evaluation and treatment of the child with supraventricular tachycardia. CHF, congestive heart failure; CXR, chest x-ray; DC, direct current; ECG, electrocardiogram; HR, heart rate; WPW, Wolff-Parkinson-White syndrome.

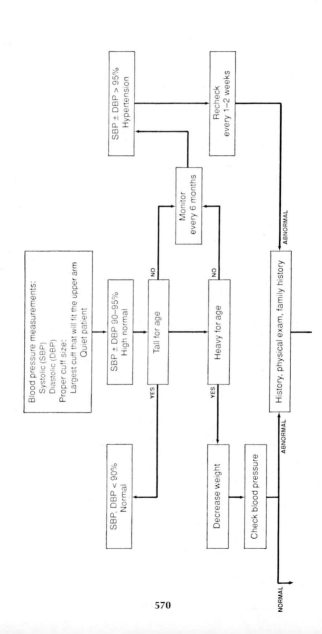

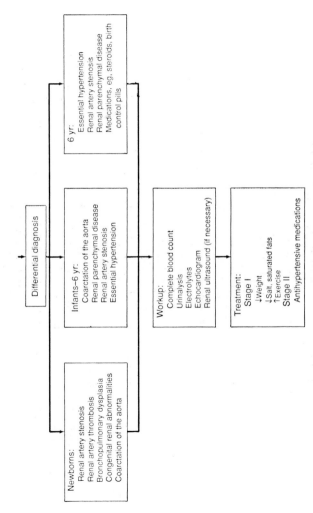

Differential diagnosis

Newborns:
Renal artery stenosis
Renal artery thrombosis
Bronchopulmonary dysplasia
Congenital renal abnormalities
Coarctation of the aorta

Infants–6 yr:
Coarctation of the aorta
Renal parenchymal disease
Renal artery stenosis
Essential hypertension

6 yr:
Essential hypertension
Renal artery stenosis
Renal parenchymal disease
Medications, eg, steroids, birth
control pills

Workup:
Complete blood count
Urinalysis
Electrolytes
Echocardiogram
Renal ultrasound (if necessary)

Treatment:
Stage I
↓Weight
↓Salt, saturated fats
↑Exercise
Stage II
Antihypertensive medications

Figure 16–5. Evaluation of the child with hypertension.

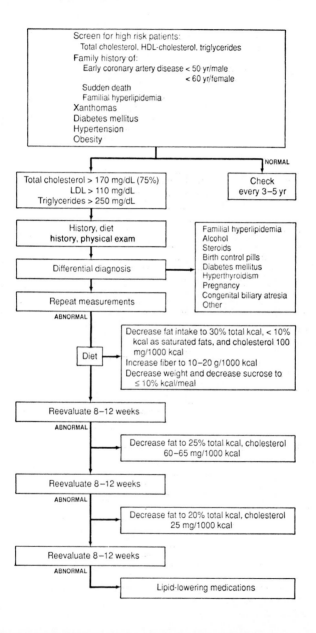

origin of the tachycardia is substantiated by the presence of fusion beats. Ventricular tachycardia can be seen in myocarditis, cardiomyopathy, digitalis toxicity, long QT syndrome, hypertrophic cardiomyopathy, myocardial tumors, and following cardiac surgery. Treatment includes DC cardioversion when the patient is hemodynamically unstable. Antidysrhythmic agents are used to suppress recurrences and must be initiated in a hospital setting.

PREVENTIVE CARDIOLOGY

Hypertension (Fig 16–5) and hyperlipidemia (Fig 16–6) are well recognized as risk factors for atherosclerotic heart disease. Long-range population-based studies have shown elevations of these risk factors to persist from childhood throughout adolescence and adulthood. Screening and intervention programs are now being offered in most pediatric centers.

Figure 16–6. Screening and evaluation of the child with hyperlipidemia. HDL, high density lipoproteins; Hx, history; LDL, low density lipoproteins; PE, Physical Examination.

17 | Gastrointestinal Tract

Judith M. Sondheimer, MD

RECURRENT ABDOMINAL PAIN

Recurrent abdominal pain of childhood is characterized by at least 3 discrete episodes of abdominal pain in a 3-month period in a child whose physical examination is normal. It occurs in 10–15% of children between 4 and 12 years of age. The pain may be severe, is sometimes associated with pallor and emesis (30%), and frequently interferes with school attendance. Less than 10% of such children will prove to have organic disease. The incidence of organic disease increases in children under 3 years and in the presence of other symptoms such as diarrhea, weight loss, dysuria, fever, or neurologic symptoms. The pain is variable in intensity, duration, and sometimes location. The presence of nighttime pain does not rule out the diagnosis. Headache, constipation, and limb pains are common findings. Overt emotional stress related to family or school may be found in 30–50%. Laboratory evaluations are usually negative and should be used sparingly. Abdominal examination is usually negative except for voluntary guarding, which may be out of proportion to the apparent pain.

Treatment is directed toward relieving anxiety surrounding the symptom by providing both parent and child with a clear explanation of the frequency and benign nature of the complaint. Return to school is important. Antispasmodics and fiber supplements are sometimes used. A lactose-free diet is occasionally helpful in the child with associated lactase deficiency.

VOMITING

Vomiting is a common symptom throughout childhood and may be associated with a wide variety of diseases of all degrees of severity. Organic disease must always be considered if vomiting is protracted or severe. Bilious emesis must always be investigated. A list of the causes and characteristics of vomiting is given in Table 17–1.

DIARRHEA

(See Tables 17–2, 17–3.)

Diarrhea (>20 mL of stool/kg/d) is a common symptom in children. When it occurs acutely, it is usually infectious. In the infant under 2 years of age, it may be the first or only symptom of infection outside the gastrointestinal tract, eg, pneumonia, sepsis, or meningitis. The physician should always consider diarrhea seriously because of the risk of dehydration, and must begin general treatment measures as soon as diagnostic studies are obtained. Because diarrhea may gradually become severe, the patient should be under careful observation. If the child is being kept at home, parents should be instructed to observe and report signs of dehydration.

The following information should be routinely obtained: (1) Duration, frequency, and description (consistency and color) of diarrheal stools. The parents may interpret watery stool as urine. (2) Incidence and character of vomiting. (3) Incidence, volume, and frequency of urination. Dehydration will decrease the volume and frequency of urination. (4) Estimate of weight loss. In the infant or young child, weighing at the onset of diarrhea will provide an index with which subsequent weights can be compared. (5) Incidence of other cases of diarrhea or vomiting in the family, nursery, or school.

Examine the abdomen for tenderness and abnormal masses. Examine rectally for further localization and to obtain stool for microscopic examination and culture.

GENERAL TREATMENT MEASURES FOR DIARRHEA

General Considerations

Loss of more than 5% of body weight through emesis or diarrhea must be replaced immediately. Dehydration from acute viral gastroenteritis is often accompanied by metabolic acidosis (decreased serum HCO_3) and sometimes by hyper- or hyponatremia, depending upon the concentration of electrolyte in the stool. Potassium content of stool may be as high as 30–40 meq/L, and the dehydrated infant may be depleted of intracellular

Table 17–1. Causes and characteristics of vomiting.

	Emesis	Other Characteristics
Gastric Outlet Obstruction:		
Pyloric stenosis	Forceful emesis, gastric contents.	4–12 wk infant; alkalosis, weight loss, palpable mass in right upper quadrant (see Pyloric Stenosis section).
Gastric web, duplication, annular pancreas	Emesis of variable force, usually gastric contents.	Presents at any age; x-ray diagnosis.
Duodenal stenosis/ atresia	Emesis of variable force depending upon severity of obstruction; usually gastric contents.	Duodenal atresia presents at birth; common in Down's syndrome.
Malrotation with mesenteric bands	Often bilious.	May be associated with intestinal volvulus.
Intestinal Obstruction:		
Volvulus	See Malrotation section.	See Malrotation section.
Intussusception	See Intussusception section.	See Intussusception section.
Superior mesenteric artery syndrome	Emesis of variable force; may be bilious.	Associated with sudden weight loss; often follows body casting after scoliosis repair; x-ray shows obstruction of transverse duodenum.
Peptic Disease:		
Gastric, duodenal ulcer, gastritis, esophagitis	Emesis is especially common in young infants; may contain bright red or dark blood.	Pain, irritability; weight loss in small infants; endoscopy most accurate diagnostic test.
Motility:		
Hypokalemia	Distention, ileus and emesis.	Generalized weakness.
Hypercalcemia, hypermagnesemia	Forceful emesis, constipation.	
Pseudo obstruction	Distention, ileus, emesis of gastric contents and bile.	Cause unknown; may be present at birth or present later; sometimes familial; may spare segments.

(continued)

Table 17–1. Causes and characteristics of vomiting *(continued)*.

	Emesis	Other Characteristics
Irritants:		
Aspirin, alcohol	Gastric contents; may contain gross blood.	History of ingestion but not necessarily overdose.
Erythromycin, theophylline	Gastric contents.	Many drugs are direct gastric irritants.
Opiates	Gastric contents.	Stimulation of medullary vomiting center.
Infections:		
Gastroenteritis	Usually precedes diarrhea.	Mediated by toxin or secondary to ileus.
UTI and obstructive uropathy	Usually gastric contents, sometimes bilious.	Common in infants; probably centrally mediated.
Otitis media	Usually gastric.	Common in infancy; probably centrally mediated.
Pneumonia, pertussis bronchiolitis	Usually gastric; often post tussive.	
Central Nervous System:		
Meningitis, tumor, pseudotumor; vascular anomalies	Usually gastric; often upon change of position.	Stimulation of medullary vomiting center.
Metabolic:		
Galactosemia, fructosemia, hyperammonemia, congenital adrenal hyperplasia, organic acidemia, phenylketonuria	Usually gastric, occasionally bilious.	Ill infant; seek specific diagnostic indicators for these diseases.
Gastroesophageal Reflux:	Gastric contents; variable force; often postprandial.	Most common under 6 months.

Table 17-2. Causes, characteristics, and treatment of acute enteritis.

Cause	Stool Examination	Symptoms	Treatment
Bacterial:			
Salmonella	Liquid, foul, + WBC + gross or occult blood.	Fever, abdominal pain.	None unless signs of extraintestinal infection or sepsis; ampicillin, amoxicillin, amoxicillin + trimethoprim-sulfamethoxazole.
Shigella	Small, grossly bloody, frequent.	Fever, tenesmus, abdominal pain.	None or trimethoprim-sulfamethoxazole.
Campylobacter jejuni *Yersinia enterocolitica* *Aeromonas hydrophila*	Similar to *Salmonella*. Gross blood and mucus. Watery; mild to moderate.	Few systemic symptoms. Similar to *Salmonella*.	None or erythromycin.
Pleisiomonas shigelloides	Watery.	Nausea, vomiting; probably enterotoxin-mediated.	Usually self-limited; trimethoprim-sulfamethoxazole.
Escherichia coli		Nausea, vomiting; possible enterotoxin.	Usually self-limited; trimethoprim-sulfamethoxazole.
Invasive	Small, grossly bloody, + WBC.	Abdominal pain, tenesmus.	Trimethoprim-sulfamethoxazole; ampicillin; gentamicin.
Enterotoxic	Liquid, green, voluminous.	Nausea, vomiting; heat labile toxin-mediated.	Usually self-limited.
Enteropathogenic	Liquid, green, voluminous.	Nausea, vomiting; adherence factors important.	Usually self-limited.
Hemorrhagic 0157:H7	Small, grossly bloody, + WBC.	Fever, tenesmus, organism produces shigella-type toxin; may precede hemolytic-uremic syndrome.	Trimethoprim-sulfamethoxazole.

Viral:			
Rotavirus	Liquid, few WBC.	Emesis, nausea.	None; fluid management.
Others—Norwalk, enteric, adenovirus, enteroviruses	Same as above.	Same as above.	None; fluid management.
Parasitic:			
Giardia lamblia	Very foul, liquid; cysts present in 30–60%.	Vomiting, nausea, abdominal distention, gas.	Furazolidone (5 mg/kg/d × 7 d); Metronidazole (15mg/kg/d × 5 d); Quinacrine (6 mg/kg/d × 5 d).
Entamoeba histolytica	Blood and mucus, trophozooites on fresh stool exam.	Abdominal pain, tenesmus.	Metronidazole (35–50 mg/kg/d × 10 d).
Cryptosporidium	Watery or bloody depending upon site of infestation.	Often in immunodeficient patients but occasionally in healthy children; history of animal exposure.	Spiramycin or metronidazole may be tried.
Other Toxic Diarrhea:			
E coli (see above)			
Clostridium difficile	Bloody, + WBC, cytotoxin present in stool.	Abdominal pain, fever, history of prior antibiotic use is typical.	Vancomycin (30–40 mg/kg/d × 7 d); metronidazole (25 mg/kg/d × 7 d); oral bacitracin (1500 U/kg/d × 7 d).
Staphylococcus aureus	Explosive, watery, + WBC.	Nausea, emesis, history of group outbreaks.	Fluid management.
Clostridium perfringens	Explosive, watery, + WBC.	Emesis, abrupt onset, history of meat ingestion.	Fluid management.

Table 17–3. Chronic diarrhea—guide to differential diagnosis.

	Age	Type of Diarrhea	Associated Features
Disease:			
Bacterial infections	Any age	Mucoid bloody stool.	Rarely chronic except in immunocompromised hosts; *Salmonella* and *Yersinia* most likely.
Viral infection	Any age	Watery.	Rarely chronic except in immunocompromised hosts; CMV, adenovirus, rotovirus.
Parasitic infestation	Any age	Depends on organism.	Amoeba, giardia, cryptosporidium.
Dietary Factors:			
Overfeeding—especially starches	<6 m	Watery.	Colicky behavior without weight loss.
Protein allergy	<2 m	Watery ± malabsorption of fat; at times blood and mucus.	Colic, emesis, anemia, hypoproteinemia.
Acrodermatitis enteropathica	<12 m	Voluminous with steatorrhea.	Malnutrition, skin rash; low serum Zn; usually genetic; sometimes secondary to severe dietary Zn deficiency.
Primary bile acid malabsorption	<1 m	Voluminous with steatorrhea.	Malnutrition; defective ileal transport of bile acids.
Irritable colon/chronic nonpecific diarrhea	6–36 m	Watery, frequent, with mucus, undigested food; no steatorrhea.	Healthy child; often starts with bout of gastroenteritis.

	Age	Stool	Clinical Features
Toxic diarrhea (antibiotics, cancer chemotherapy, radiation)	Any age	Loose; sometimes steatorrhea, occult blood or pus.	Vomiting; anorexia.
Functional tumors (neuroblastoma, carcinoid, pancreatic cholera, Zollinger-Ellison syndrome)	Any age	Secretory diarrhea, watery, persists when patient fasting.	Hypokalemia; other symptoms depend upon tumor.
Carbohydrate malabsorption:			
Sucrase—isomaltase	<6 m	Watery; low pH; reducing substance positive after acid hydrolysis; volume varies with sucrose intake.	Abdominal distension; poor growth; deficiency present in 0.8% North Americans, 10% Alaskan natives.
Glucose galactose malabsorption	<1 m	Intractable diarrhea with feeding; stool pH low; watery; reducing substances present.	Poor growth; defect in glucose transport.
Genetic Deficiencies:			
Lactase	<4 yr	Watery diarrhea with lactose; low pH; reducing substances present.	Deficiency develops at about 4 years of age in 100% Orientals; 80% American blacks, 15% American whites.
Acquired Deficiencies:			
Lactase and sucrase	Any age	Watery; low pH; reducing substances present.	Follows intestinal injury or infection.
Monosaccharide transport	<6 m	Watery; low pH; reducing substances present.	Rare; follows infection; made worse by malnutrition.

581

Table 17–3. Chronic diarrhea—guide to differential diagnosis (*continued*).

	Age	Type of Diarrhea	Associated Features
Pancreatic Disorders:			
Cystic fibrosis	<6 m	Steatorrhea; bulky, foul, pale.	Respiratory infection; poor weight gain.
Shwachman syndrome	<2 yr	Steatorrhea; bulky, foul, pale.	Neutropenia; short stature; bacterial infections; metaphyseal dysostosis.
Chronic pancreatitis	Any age	Steatorrhea; bulky, foul, pale.	Rare in children; usually associated with alcoholism.
Celiac disease	<12 m	Steatorrhea; bulky, foul, pale.	Emesis, distention, irritability, anorexia.
Intestinal lymphangiectasia	3 m	Voluminous, steatorrhea.	Lymphedema, lymphopenia, hypoalbuminemia.
Immune defects:			
Hypogammaglobulinemia; IgA deficiency	Any age	Watery; sometimes steatorrhea.	Recurrent cutaneous and respiratory infection.
Combined immunodeficiency, AIDS, cellular defect	<1 m Any age <2 yr	Severe; watery; steatorrhea.	Stomatitis, skin rash, recurrent infection, opportunistic infection.
Genetic-Metabolic:			
Chloride losing diarrhea	<1 m	Watery.	Alkalosis; growth failure.
Hypobetalipoproteinemia and a-betalipoproteinemia	<3 m	Profuse; steatorrhea.	Progressive neurologic symptoms; low serum cholesterol; acanthocytosis.
Wolman's disease	<1 m	Profuse; steatorrhea.	Emesis; severe growth failure; adrenal calcification; hypercholesterolemia.
Folate malabsorption	<1 m	Watery.	Anemia; stomatitis, seizures, retardation.

	Age	Stool	Comments
Anatomic:			
Blind (stagnant) loop/ bacterial overgrowth	Any age	Watery; fat and carbohydrate malabsorption.	Caused by surgical adhesions, intestinal duplication, abnormal GI motility, partial obstruction.
Short bowel	Any age	Watery; malabsorption of all nutrients.	Rarely congenital, usually secondary to surgical resection.
Intestinal pseudoobstruction	Any age	Watery; malabsorption of all nutrients.	Distention; may be acquired or congenital; diarrhea secondary to bacterial overgrowth.
Inflammatory Bowel Disease:			
Crohn's disease		See Table 17–6.	
Ulcerative colitis		See Table 17–7.	
Eosinophilic gastroenteritis	Any age	Watery or bloody depending upon site of disease.	Intestinal or gastric obstruction, eczema, asthma, increased blood eosinophiles.
Hirschsprung's disease with enterocolitis	<1 yr	Foul, liquid with WBC and RBC.	Abdominal distention, fever, history of constipation.
Malnutrition	<1 yr	Loose, steatorrhea, sometimes with carbohydrate malabsorption.	Becomes temporarily worse with refeeding.
Endocrine:			
Hyperthyroidism	Any age	Frequent, loose stool without malabsorption.	Other signs of hyperthyroidism.

potassium with normal serum potassium. Serum electrolytes should be checked in any child with more than 5% dehydration.

Treatment

A. Parenteral Fluid Therapy: Parenteral fluid therapy is indicated in the following circumstances: (1) if vomiting or weakness prevents oral therapy; (2) in the presence of shock because of severe dehydration and acidosis; or (3) if surgical procedures are contemplated (see Chapter 4).

B. Oral Rehydration:

1. Replacement of Fluid Deficit–Commercially available oral solutions for replacement of fluid deficits resulting from viral gastroenteritis usually contain 75 meq Na/L, 20 meq K/L, 65 meq Cl/L, 30 meq citrate or bicarbonate/L, and 25 g dextrose/L. Fluid deficit should be calculated by comparing weights or by physical signs. The desired volume should be administered by mouth over 12–24 hours.

2. Ongoing Fluid Needs–Commercially available oral solutions for maintenance during acute viral enteritis contain slightly less sodium (45 meq/L) and chloride (35 meq/L) than replacement solution. As the calorie content of these solutions is only 100 kcal/L, they should not be used as the sole fluid intake for more than 48 hours.

3. Return to Normal Caloric Intake–This should be fairly rapid in uncomplicated viral gastroenteritis. Intestinal lactase levels may be depressed for 7–14 days after acute gastroenteritis, and a lactose-free formula is advisable. Gastric retention and diminished bile salt secretion may temporarily decrease fatty food tolerance. High-fat solids should be reintroduced into the diet only after the child has demonstrated tolerance for carbohydrates.

4. Symptomatic Therapy–Symptomatic treatment of acute gastroenteritis is rarely indicated and may seriously complicate fluid management. Diphenoxylate with atropine (Lomotil) should not be used in any infant under 3 years. Kaolin and pectin preparations are usually ineffective in acute gastroenteritis.

5. Specific Therapy for Infectious Gastroenteritis–See Table 17–2.

CONSTIPATION

Normal frequency of defecation in children ranges from 3 per day to 1 per week. In healthy infants, stooling frequency is generally higher, but some normally defecate only 2–3 times per week. If stools are unusually hard or large, if pain or excessive straining is associated with defecation, if stooling frequency is less than once per week, if impaction of the rectum with fecal leakage occurs (this is a common manifestation of retentive constipation in school children) or if abdominal distention, emesis, or failure to thrive accompany infrequent stooling, symptomatic treatment and a careful assessment of possible organic causes should be undertaken.

Etiology

See Table 17–4.

Treatment

A. Disimpaction:

1. If the Impacted Stool is Soft or Puttylike–disimpaction can be accomplished with oral laxatives such as Senokot or Milk of Magnesia given 2–3 days in a row.

2. If the Impacted Stool is Very Large or Firm–enemas may be required. Rectal instillation of mineral oil (30–90 mL) will lubricate the impaction and a subsequent hypertonic phosphate enema (Fleet) or normal saline enema (20–40 mL per kg) will stimulate evacuation. It is rarely necessary to use more than 1000 mL of normal saline. Tap water enemas or soapy water enemas are not recommended because of the risk of water intoxication and colitis, respectively.

3. Rectal Suppositories–glycerine or bisacodyl (Dulcolax) are useful occasionally.

B. Long-term Therapy:

1. Increased Fluid and Fiber Intake.

2. Addition of Nonabsorbable Carbohydrate to Formula–Karo syrup.

3. Stool Softeners–Mineral oil (2–3 mL/kg/d) may be used in ambulatory patients. The risk of aspiration and lipid pneumonia must be considered in infants and in recumbent patients, particularly those with psychomotor retardation. Detergent agents (Colace) may also function to soften stools.

4. Fiber Supplements

5. Stimulant or Osmotic Laxatives–Laxatives such as Senokot, Dulcolax, or Milk of Magnesia may be used for short periods of time to prevent reimpaction while retraining of habit constipation is taking place.

Table 17—4. Constipation.

	Agents
Infancy:	
Mechanical obstruction	Imperforate anus, anal stenosis. Intestinal obstruction.
Abnormal intestinal motility	Hirschsprung's disease: Lack of ganglion cells in the colon wall causes failure of peristalsis through affected areas. Intestinal pseudoobstruction. Hypothyroidism, congenital or acquired. Hypokalemia, hypercalcemia, hypermagnesemia.
Somatic weakness or incoordination	Hypotonia, acquired or congenital; cerebral palsy; sacral agenesis; spina bifida.
Pain on defecation	Anal fissure, perianal skin disease, or abscess.
Drugs	Narcotics, antihistamines, calcium salts, aluminum hydroxide antacids, vincristine.
Dehydrating conditions	Diabetes mellitus, diabetes insipidus, following acute gastroenteritis.
Childhood:[1]	
Retentive constipation	This is the most likely cause of constipation in healthy toddlers or school-age children. Boys are more commonly affected. Fecal leakage around an impaction is present in 60%. Urinary tract infection or obstruction may be associated, especially in females.

[1] All of the above conditions may present in childhood.

COLIC

Colic in small infants is characterized by lengthy bouts of crying totaling more than 3 hours per day and apparent discomfort. It usually occurs in the firstborn infant, starting at around 10 days of age and lasting through the third month. It is a source of great anxiety for the parents whose ineffective attempts to calm the infant may exacerbate the condition. The causes of colic are poorly understood. Some of the following factors may be of importance.

A. Gastrointestinal Distention with Air: Prolonged crying may fill the stomach and intestines with air. This may lead to crampy pain and the expulsion of gas per rectum. Continuous sucking on a pacifier or frequent breast or bottle feeding may do the same. A vicious cycle of crying, air swallowing, and more crying may be established.

B. Food: Overfeeding with large volumes of formula in an effort to quiet the infant may cause gastric distention and discomfort. Paradoxically, genuine hunger may initiate this cycle.

C. Emotional Factors: Colic occurs most often in a first-born infant during the first weeks at home. The hyperactive, tense infant is likely to have colic. Family tension and parental anxiety may be aggravating factors.

D. Allergy: Intestinal allergy to cow's milk protein, especially in families with a history of allergy in other members, may be associated with colic, emesis, and diarrhea.

Treatment

The most important first step is a careful physical examination and history to look for organic causes of fussiness such as otitis media, urinary infection, central nervous system disorders (tumors, seizures, infections), intestinal disease (ulcer, esophagitis, gastritis, infection or obstruction), and other problems such as osteomyelitis or traumatic injury secondary to child abuse.

If careful evaluation indicates no cause for fussiness, the following conservative measures are sometimes helpful:

(1) Supportive, sympathetic instruction of parents regarding colic and its benign nature.

(2) Regular schedule for feedings and naps to avoid chaotic routines, overfeeding, or underfeeding.

(3) Low-level sound in the infant's sleeping area such as a radio or vacuum cleaner may be soothing.

(4) Gentle movement in a swing or rides in the automobile. There are even crib vibrators that simulate the sound and movement of an automobile.

(5) Trial of milk-free diet may help an infant with true protein allergy. Avoid frequent formula changes.

(6) Rest and assistance for the infant's caretakers is essential to prevent exhaustion.

(7) Medications are only occasionally useful and include antihistamines, antispasmodics, and antacids. Bentyl has been shown effective, but there is a risk of respiratory depression.

Table 17–5. Peptic ulcer—primary vs. secondary.

	Primary	Secondary
Location	Duodenal > gastric.	Gastric = duodenal.
Age	More common > 5 yr.	Any age.
Cause	Hypersecretion; *Helicobacter pylori* infections; genetic factors (+ family history in 30%).	Burn, CNS trauma, local irritants, shock, decreased mucosal defenses.
Symptoms	Pain, emesis, irritability, bleeding.	Emesis, bleeding.
Diagnosis	Endoscopy.	Endoscopy.
Treatment	Histamine receptor antagonist; antibiotics for *H pylori;* antacids; local mucosal protective agents (sucralfate).	Remove primary stress; all other modalities noted for primary ulcer.

The use of beer, wine or other alcoholic beverages for sedation is not recommended.

PEPTIC ULCER DISEASE

See Table 17–5.

INFLAMMATORY BOWEL DISEASE

See Table 17–6.

The two major inflammatory bowel diseases in children are Crohn's disease (regional enteritis) and ulcerative colitis. A comparison of the two conditions is found in Table 17–6. The etiology of both is unknown, but autoimmune factors are suspected. A family history of inflammatory bowel disease is obtained in 25% of cases. Ulcerative colitis and Crohn's disease may occur in the same family, suggesting some common etiology for the two conditions.

DISEASES OF THE LIVER

See Tables 17–7 and 17–8.

Cholestasis

Many newborns have elevated total serum bilirubin levels. This is secondary to physiologic jaundice or hemolytic disease for the most part. If the direct reacting fraction of bilirubin (conjugated fraction) is greater than 15% of the total, cholestatic liver disease should be suspected and thoroughly evaluated. Conjugated hyperbilirubinemia is *never* physiologic.

PANCREATIC DISEASE

See Table 17–3.

Cystic Fibrosis

In pediatrics, the most common cause of exocrine pancreatic insufficiency is cystic fibrosis (CF). Malabsorption, present from birth in 85% of persons with CF, is a result of obstruction of the ductular system and progressive destruction of the exocrine pancreas. Exogenous pancreatic enzymes must be provided with meals to improve digestion of complex carbohydrate, protein, and fat. Other gastrointestinal problems associated with CF include peptic ulcer, pancreatitis, cholecystitis, cholelithiasis, biliary cirrhosis, meconium ileus (in the newborn), meconium ileus equivalent (in older cystics, a result of large-volume fatty stool obstructing the distal small bowel or proximal colon), and rectal prolapse.

Shwachman Syndrome

This is a rare condition of unknown etiology (probably genetic) characterized by exocrine pancreatic insufficiency (because of fatty replacement of acinar tissue), neutropenia (either cyclic or continuous), growth failure, and metaphyseal dysostosis. Recurrent severe bacterial infections occur in some patients. Diarrhea and malnutrition are common. Sweat test is normal.

Pancreatitis

Pancreatitis is usually an acute viral infection in childhood. It is sometimes associated with overwhelming bacterial infection, connective tissue diseases, Reye's syndrome, drug toxicity, hyperlipidemia, and rarely (in pediatrics) alcohol. Forty percent of cases are idiopathic. Trauma may cause pancreatitis and/or pancreatic pseudocyst. Abdominal tenderness, high serum amylase, and enlarged pancreas on abdominal ultrasound with ascites are diagnostic findings. Hypocalcemia may occur. Hemorrhagic pancreatitis carries a very high morality.

Table 17–6. Features of Crohn's disease and ulcerative colitis.

	Crohn's Disease	Ulcerative Colitis
Age at onset	10–20 yr	10–20 yr
Incidence (general population)	4–5/100,000	3–15/100,000
Relative incidence in children	2	1
Area of bowel affected	Oropharynx, esophagus, and stomach—rare Small bowel only, 25–30% Colon and anus only, 15% Ileocolitis, 40% Diffuse disease, 5%	Total colon, 90% Proctitis, 10%
Distribution	Segmental; disease-free skip areas common.	Continuous.
Pathology	Full thickness; acute and chronic inflammation; noncaseating granulomas (50%); fistulas, abscesses, strictures, and fibrosis may be present.	Superficial acute inflammation of mucosa with microscopic crypt abscess.
X-ray	Segmental lesions; thickened circular folds; cobblestone appearance of bowel wall secondary to longitudinal ulcers and transverse fissures; fixation and separation of loops; narrowed lumen "string sign"; fistulae.	Superficial colitis; loss of haustra; shortened colon and pseudopolyps (islands of normal tissue surrounded by denuded mucosa) are late findings.

Intestinal symptoms	Abdominal pain, diarrhea, perianal disease; enteroenteric/enterocutaneous fistula, abscess, anorexia	Abdominal pain, bloody diarrhea, urgency, and tenesmus.
Extraintestinal Symptoms:		
Arthritis/arthralgia	15%	9%
Fever	40–50%	40–50%
Stomatitis	9%	2%
Weight loss	90% (mean 5.7 kg)	68% (mean 4.1 kg)
Delayed growth and sexual development	30%	5–10%
Uveitis/conjunctivitis	15% (in Crohn's colitis)	4%
Sclerosing cholangitis	rare	4%
Renal stones	6% (oxalate)	6% (urate)
Pyoderma gangrenosum	1.3%	5%
Erythema nodosum	8–15%	4%
Laboratory findings	High ESR; microcytic anemia; low serum iron and total iron binding capacity; increased fecal protein loss; low serum albumin.	High ESR; microcytic anemia, high WBC with "left shift."
Treatment	Corticosteroids, azulfidine, metronidizole (especially for perianal disease); surgical resection as last resort.	Corticosteroids, azulfidine, azathioprine, or 6-mercaptopurine, colectomy for toxic megacolon, resistant symptoms, intractable pain or bleeding.

Table 17–7. Causes of neonatal cholestasis.

	Associated Findings
Infection:	
Bacterial (UTI, sepsis, meningitis)	+ Bacterial cultures.
Viral-intrauterine (rubella, CMV, herpes, toxoplasmosis)	+ Cultures; infant often SGA with DIC and other abnormalities secondary to infection.
Viral-acquired (HAV, HBV, HCV, EBV, herpes, Enterovirus)	+ serologic tests; enterovirus associated with encephalitis; cutaneous lesions in herpes.
Idiopathic (giant cell) hepatitis	Negative cultures; giant cells on liver biopsy.
Metabolic:	
Cystic fibrosis	+ Sweat test; pale, fatty stools, large gallbladder with viscid bile.
Galactosemia	Emesis, acidosis; reducing substances in urine while taking lactose; decreased RBC gal-1-PO_4-uridyl transferase.
Alpha-1-antitrypsin deficiency	Baby may be SGA; variable degrees of hepatitis and cirrhosis at presentation; serum α-1-antitrypsin <70 mg%.
Tyrosinemia	Hypoalbuminemia, coagulopathy, and hepatitis, increased urinary succinyl acetone.
Parenteral nutrition	Gradual onset; jaundice a late finding occurring after several weeks of IV nutrition.
Extrahepatic biliary atresia, choledochal cyst	Acholic stools, firm large liver, generally healthy appearance.
Paucity of intrahepatic bile ducts:	
Alagille syndrome	Odd facies, growth failure. Hypogonadism. Peripheral pulmonic stenosis. Vertebral anomalies.
Other nonsyndromatic paucity	More rapidly progressive liver disease.

GLUTEN ENTEROPATHY-CELIAC DISEASE

In celiac disease, malabsorption of all nutrients occurs owing to the diminished absorbing surface in the small intestine. Villous atrophy occurs in response to gluten present in wheat,

Table 17–8. Liver disease of older children.

	Agents
Acute infection (usually viral)	Cytomegalic inclusion virus
	Epstein-Barr virus
	Hepatitis A, hepatitis B, hepatitis C, hepatitis E
	Other systemic viral infections
	Bacterial agents include *N gonorrhea* (causes perihepatitis)
Fatty liver	Malnutrition
	Storage (Wolman's disease)
	Reye's syndrome
	Mitochondrial dysfunction (eg, carnitine deficiency)
Tumors	Hepatoblastoma
	Hemangiomatosis
	Metastatic Wilms' tumor
	Neuroblastoma
	Gonadal tumor
	Leukemic infiltration
	Histiocytosis
Parasitic disease	*E histolytica*
	Visceral larva migrans
	Shistosoma mansoni
	S japonicum
Metabolic/genetic/ storage diseases	Cystic fibrosis—fatty liver/biliary cirrhosis
	Glycogen storage disease
	Galactosemia
	Tyrosinemia
	Alpha-1-antitrypsin deficiency
	Neiman–Pick disease
	Gaucher's disease
	Amyloidosis
	Congenital hepatic fibrosis
	Wilson's disease
Chronic inflammatory disease	Autoimmune chronic active hepatitis
	Chronic active hepatitis B or C
	Sclerosing cholangitis, or chronic active hepatitis associated with inflammatory bowel disease

rye, barley, and oats. It is thought that gliadin is bound by entero-cytes in the intestine and that a local immune reaction ensues, which destroys the absorbing cells. Diarrhea and malabsorption usually appear in the second year of life, often after an acute viral illness. Weight loss, fatty stools, anorexia, and irritability are common. Occasionally, severe diarrhea, dehydration, electrolyte deficiency, and prostration occur (celiac crisis).

Diagnosis rests on typical villous atrophy and plasma cell infiltrate in small intestinal biopsies. Antigliadin antibodies are present. Diagnosis by trial of gluten-free diet is not recommended. Treatment is by gluten-free diet. Lactose tolerance is poor until intestinal recovery occurs. Vitamin and iron supplements may be necessary if diarrhea has been long-standing.

Full recovery is expected. The sensitivity to gluten is lifelong. Ten percent of first-degree relatives will be affected in this genetically determined disease.

DISACCHARIDASE DEFICIENCIES

Diminished levels of disaccharidase enzymes on the microvillous surface of the small intestine cause malabsorption of disaccharides and watery, acid, osmotic diarrhea upon ingestion of the offending sugar. Stools contain undigested disaccharide and their fermentation by-products. Symptoms also include nausea, vomiting, and flatulence. Disaccharidase deficiency may be primary (genetic) or secondary to bowel injury. Disaccharide tolerance tests or breath hydrogen assay after an oral disaccharide test meal may be diagnostic. Direct measurement of enzyme levels in intestinal biopsies can be performed (see Table 17–3). Treatment of deficiency is by avoidance of the offending sugars. Tolerance in genetic forms sometimes improves with age.

COW'S MILK ALLERGY

Cow's milk protein allergy is more often suspected than proved. The onset is usually in patients under 3 months of age, and the symptoms are diarrhea, vomiting, and, in older children, a malabsorption syndrome compatible with small bowel injury. Early introduction of milk into the diet, especially following gastrointestinal infection, may predispose to this condition. Laboratory findings include eosinophilia demonstrated in a smear of rectal mucus, eosinophilic mucosal infiltrate, proctitis at sigmoidoscopy, and occasionally an atrophic small bowel lesion.

Diagnosis must be confirmed by a response to elimination of cow's milk followed by recurrence of symptoms after reintroduction of milk.

Treatment depends upon the elimination of cow's milk and cow's milk products from the diet for 6 months to 1 year. Soy-based or protein hydrolysate formulas may be substituted. Concomitant soy protein allergy is seen in up to 30% of these infants.

Cow's milk protein allergy usually resolves after 6–12 months.

ESOPHAGEAL ATRESIA WITH OR WITHOUT TRACHEOESOPHAGEAL FISTULA

Most infants with tracheoesophageal fistula (TEF) present at birth with cough, vomiting and apparent excessive salivation. Aspiration pneumonia is common. In about 90% of cases, the upper esophagus ends in a blind pouch while the lower esophageal segment communicates with the lower trachea. In about 10% of cases, there is upper esophageal atresia without an associated distal tracheoesophageal fistula. Maternal polyhydramnios is common in these patients. In about 5% of cases there is an H-type fistula between an intact esophagus and the trachea. These infants usually present later, after repeated bouts of aspiration pneumonia or choking with feedings. Thirty percent of infants with TEF have associated anomalies, usually cardiac or gastrointestinal. Imperforate anus is common. Careful barium esophagram is necessary to make the diagnosis. The H-type fistula, usually located in the lower cervical esophagus, is often tiny and may not be demonstrated by standard barium esophagram. Endoscopy or bronchoscopy may be necessary. Early diagnosis, normal birth weight, absence of lung disease, and a short distance between the proximal and distal esophageal segments improve the prognosis. The treatment is surgical. Stricture and fistula formation at the site of esophageal repair may occur, especially in high atresias. Gastroesophageal reflux occurs in 75% of patients postoperatively. Esophageal peristaltic function is always abnormal.

ESOPHAGEAL OBSTRUCTION

Partial obstructions of the esophagus cause a variety of feeding problems during infancy or childhood including vomiting, aspiration, and malnutrition. Vascular ring may cause external compression, especially double aortic arch. Esophageal strictures develop after correction of tracheoesophageal fistula, ingestion of corrosive chemicals (eg, lye), or as a result of chronic peptic esophagitis from gastroesophageal reflux. Congenital strictures are rare, as is congenital achalasia. Globus hystericus, or a sensation of esophageal obstruction in the absence of obstructing lesions, may be seen even in preschool children. These children often refuse food but usually have no difficulty swallowing their own secretions.

Diagnosis

The upper GI series is the most informative study when symptoms suggest esophageal obstruction. Vascular ring causes characteristic external compression of the esophageal outline. Location and length of stricture, esophageal dysmotility, and hiatus hernia are easily seen. Endoscopy adds more information regarding esophagitis.

INGUINAL HERNIA & HYDROCELE

The testis forms cephalad to the kidney and descends into the scrotum during the last trimester of pregnancy. As it descends, the peritoneum descends with it to form the tunica vaginalis. The peritoneal connection between the abdominal cavity and the scrotum (the processus vaginalis) is normally obliterated. All hernias, hydroceles, and ectopic testes relate to abnormalities in this process.

Inguinal Hernia

A hernia is seen as an intermittent bulge lateral to the pubic tubercle; the bulge appears when the patient is crying, straining, or standing and usually reduces spontaneously when the patient is relaxed or supine. The hernia usually contains bowel or mesentery. In females the ovary may herniate.

The incidence of hernia in the general population is 1%, and in premature infants, 5%. Males are affected most commonly (85% of cases). One half of cases of inguinal hernia during childhood occur in infants under 6 months of age. Right-sided hernias are more frequent than left (2:1). Twenty-five percent of patients have bilateral hernias. The percentage is higher in females. Elective repair of inguinal hernia is recommended and repair of the asymptomatic side is often performed in children less than 2 years of age, especially in females.

Incarceration (failure to reduce) occurs in about 10% of cases, most often in children under 1 year of age. The hernia becomes tender and erythematous. The abdomen becomes distended, with vomiting and signs of bowel obstruction. Pressure on testicular vessels in the inguinal canal by an incarcerated hernia can cause testicular infarction. Incarcerated hernia can often be reduced by gently squeezing the bowel back into the abdomen along the axis of the inguinal canal. Sedation (pentobarbital, 4 mg/kg, and meperidine, 1 mg/kg) is necessary in most cases. Reduction should not be attempted after 12 hours of incarceration because of the risk of bowel perforation. Immediate surgical repair is indicated.

Hydrocele

Hydrocele is very common in newborns. Spontaneous regression by age 6 months is the rule. Frequent and rapid change in size of the hydrocele indicates a patent processus vaginalis with communication to the peritoneal cavity. Since hernia may develop, communicating hydroceles should be repaired.

Acute hydrocele may develop about the testis or in the spermatic cord and may be difficult to differentiate from incarcerated hernia. Examination at the internal ring level, with one finger in the upper rectum and another feeling the abdomen from the outside, may aid in differentiation. Acute hydrocele in the canal of Nuck presents as an oblong, firm swelling in the groin of a female infant and may be confused with a groin node. Exploration is required in doubtful cases.

GASTROESOPHAGEAL REFLUX
(Chalasia)

Gastroesophageal reflux occurs in 40% of healthy infants less than 6 months. Postprandial spitting and vomiting are the most common symptoms. Infants usually remain healthy, but aspiration pneumonia, esophagitis, esophageal stricture, and malnutrition may occur if vomiting is severe. Reflux is common in physically and neurologically handicapped children, in those with severe scoliosis, and after tracheoesophageal fistula repair.

Diagnosis is based upon characteristic history, upper GI series, sometimes esophageal scintiscan, and esophageal pH monitoring in atypical cases.

Conservative measures often suffice in healthy infants as the condition is usually self-limited. Infants are given small-volume, frequent feedings thickened with cereal and are kept in the prone position as much as possible to reduce reflux. Medication includes antacids, H_2 receptor antagonists, and smooth muscle stimulants such as bethanechol. In more resistant cases, gastric fundoplication may be necessary.

CONGENITAL HERNIA OF THE DIAPHRAGM

The most common area of herniation is in the left posterolateral portion, the foramen of Bochdalek. Foramen of Morgagni hernias rarely present during the newborn period and rarely cause significant respiratory symptoms.

Clinical Findings
A. Symptoms and Signs: Cyanosis and dyspnea in a newborn infant suggest the diagnosis. Chest movements are asymmetric with dullness on the affected side. Breath sounds may be absent. The abdomen is scaphoid and feels less full on palpation than usual. The mediastinum shifts away from the affected side. There is usually hypoplasia of the lung on the affected side with persistent pulmonary hypertension, which makes ventilatory management difficult.

B. Imaging: Chest x-ray usually shows a portion of the gastrointestinal tract in the thorax and displacement of the mediastinum.

Treatment
Diaphragmatic hernia is a surgical emergency. The viscera are reduced from the thorax through a subcostal incision. The diaphragm is closed or patched if the defect is large and a chest tube left in place to water-seal drainage. If abdominal closure requires tension, close only the skin to prevent undue pressure on the diaphragm or inferior vena cava.

Persistent pulmonary hypertension and pulmonary hypoplasia are the commonest causes of mortality. Pulmonary vasodilators are sometimes helpful. Recently, extracorporeal membrane oxygenation has been used with success in some of these infants.

Course & Prognosis
Survival depends on the degree of pulmonary hypoplasia; survival rate is about 50%. Lung weights of infants who do not survive are about half those of normal infants of the same gestational age and birth weight. The morphology of the lung on the

side of the hernia is immature. Long-term survivors have normal
lung weights, although they may have some degree of emphysema and decreased blood flow.

PYLORIC STENOSIS
(Congenital Hypertrophic Pyloric Stenosis)

Pyloric stenosis is more apt to occur in firstborn infants
and is more common in males than in females (4:1 ratio). In
most cases, the diagnosis is made between 3 and 12 weeks of
age.

There is a marked increase in the circular musculature of
the pylorus, causing obstruction of the lumen.

Clinical Findings

A. Symptoms and Signs: Vomiting begins in most cases
after the 14th day of life. It is usually mild at first but becomes
progressively more projectile over 3–7 days. Vomiting occurs
within one-half hour of feeding and does not contain bile. The
infant appears hungry. Stools are small. Weight loss, dehydration, and hypochloremic alkalosis may be severe. Jaundice develops in 2–5% of cases. Gastric stasis results in gastritis and
hematemesis in some cases. On examination, the infant is alert,
irritable, dehydrated, and hungry. The epigastrium may be distended and the gastric outline obvious. Gastric peristalsis passing from left to right during feeding can be seen on the abdomen.
An olive shaped mass is palpable in the right upper quadrant,
especially directly after vomiting. Inguinal hernias develop in
10% of cases secondary to forceful emesis. Tetany as a result
of alkalosis and reduction of free serum calcium may occur.

B. Laboratory Findings: Findings include metabolic alkalosis, hypokalemia, and variable hyponatremia. Urine is alkaline
and concentrated. Hemoglobin and blood urea nitrogen may be
high secondary to dehydration. The indirect bilirubin (unconjugated) may be elevated.

C. Imaging: If the typical mass in the right upper quadrant
is not palpable, the pyloric muscle may be demonstrated by ultrasonography. The upper gastrointestinal series shows an enlarged
stomach with a narrow, elongated pyloric channel and prolonged
gastric retention of barium. The impression of the pyloric muscle
on the antrum can be seen.

Treatment

A. Preoperative Care:

1. Rehydration– Rehydration by the intravenous route is preferred. The rate of infusion will depend on the severity of dehydration.

2. Nasogastric Intubation– Before operation, a nasogastric tube may be inserted to preclude regurgitation and aspiration of stomach contents during anesthesia.

B. Surgical Measures: Ramstedt pyloromyotomy divides the hypertrophied muscle bundles that obstruct the pylorus. Surgery should not be performed until rehydration and correction of alkalosis are complete.

Prognosis

Complete relief is to be expected following surgical repair. Mortality is low.

MECONIUM ILEUS

Meconium ileus with small bowel obstruction is the presenting sign in 15% of newborn infants with CF. Lack of pancreatic trypsin causes unusually thick meconium, which obstructs the lower 10–20 cm of ileum. The ileocecal valve and the entire colon are normal albeit small.

Clinical Findings

A. Symptoms and Signs: Intestinal obstruction in the newborn is characterized by progressively more severe vomiting, beginning within the first day or two of life. The vomitus contains bile. The abdomen is distended, and loops of bowel may be seen through the abdominal wall. Firm masses within the loops strongly suggest meconium ileus. In most cases, no meconium will have been passed per rectum.

B. Laboratory Findings:

If meconium appears in stools, it can be shown to contain no trypsin. The sweat test shows an increase in the chloride concentration of sweat (> 60 meq/L). Serum immunoreactive trypsinogen (a screening test for CF in the newborn) may be falsely normal in CF patients with meconium ileus, probably because of the severe reduction in exocrine pancreatic secretion.

C. Imaging: Marked intestinal dilatation may be seen. A granular, mottled appearance to the intestinal content especially in the right lower abdomen is characteristic. Microcolon may be seen on barium enema. Free air seen in the peritoneal cavity or the presence of fluid between the loops of bowel indicates perforation. Calcification of the peritoneum, when present, represents antenatal perforation and meconium peritonitis.

Treatment

A. Preoperative Care: Provide continuous gastric suction through a nasogastric tube. Administer diatrizoate (Gastrografin) enemas but only when the infant is adequately hydrated. The hypertonic contrast medium draws water into the bowel and may "float out" the inspissated meconium. This procedure must be done under fluoroscopy by a radiologist familiar with newborn infants.

B. Surgical Measures: Surgery is required if obstruction is not relieved by enemas. The ileum is opened and meconium removed. The portion of distal ileum containing the greatest amount of meconium may have to be resected. The ends are brought out and sutured to the skin. Postoperatively, the terminal ileum and colon are cleansed with pancreatic enzyme suspension. Closure of the enterostomy is performed 2–3 weeks later.

Prognosis

There is no relationship between meconium ileus and the severity of the respiratory symptoms of CF.

CONGENITAL ATRESIA OR STENOSIS OF INTESTINES & COLON

Congenital intestinal atresia and stenosis probably result from vascular obstruction in the mesenteric vessels during fetal development. Atresia designates a complete block, while stenosis indicates narrowing of the intestinal lumen. Atresia or stenosis of the duodenum is frequently associated with Down's syndrome.

Meconium ileus must be considered in any child with intestinal atresia (see above).

Clinical Findings

A. Symptoms and Signs: Atresia of the intestinal tract or colon causes vomiting on the first day of life. Intestinal stenosis may not come to the physician's attention for weeks or months.

The vomitus contains bile. Depending on the level of involvement, abdominal distention is often present and becomes progressively worse. Peristaltic waves are often seen. Intestinal loops may be outlined on the abdominal wall. Dehydration is common because of persistent vomiting.

B. Imaging: Upright abdominal x-ray shows air and fluid levels with dilatation of the duodenum and the proximal loops of small bowel. The distal loops will be free of gas if the obstruction is complete. In partial obstruction, there may be gas without distention distal to the point of obstruction. Presence of free air in the abdominal cavity means that perforation has occurred. A granular, mottled appearance in the small bowel as a result of gas and meconium suggests meconium ileus.

Barium enema is an important part of the preoperative x-ray study. In low-intestinal atresia, it will often demonstrate the markedly decreased caliber of the unused portion of the gastrointestinal tract—the so-called microcolon. The chief indication for barium enema is to rule out Hirschsprung's disease and malrotation with volvulus, which can present with symptoms identical to those of intestinal atresia.

Treatment

Resection of the dilated, hypertrophic intestine proximal to the atresia and end-to-end anastomosis, where possible, are usually preferred for the surgical correction of atresia or stenosis. In all cases of atresia and marked stenosis, early intervention is essential to prevent perforation. If the infant is debilitated or if perforation has occurred, intestinal contents proximal to the stenosis may be diverted via an intestinal enterostomy and delayed resection with anastomosis.

Course & Prognosis

The mortality rate in infants with atresia or marked stenosis is increased by delay in diagnosis. Postoperative hypomotility of the dilated proximal bowel may compromise enteral feedings, necessitating parenteral nutrition.

MALROTATION OF INTESTINES & COLON

Malrotation is the result of incomplete rotation of the gut and lack of attachment of the mesentery of the small intestine during intrauterine development. It may result in a volvulus of the midgut or obstruction of the second part of the duodenum by peritoneal bands. It may be associated with no symptoms.

Clinical Findings

A. Symptoms and Signs: If malrotation is accompanied by an intrinsic obstruction of the second portion of the duodenum (eg, atresia, stenosis), vomiting occurs within 48 hours of birth. Midgut volvulus may occur at any time but is most common in the first 3 months. In the early stages of midgut volvulus, the general condition is good. Bilious emesis is the significant symptom, followed by shock and acidosis secondary to bowel infarction. Abdominal distension may not be prominent.

B. Laboratory Findings: Hematocrit and red blood cell counts are elevated owing to dehydration. Slight leukocytosis is usually present. Marked leukocytosis suggests impending or actual gangrene of the bowel.

C. Imaging: Plain films of the abdomen may or may not show dilatation of the stomach and duodenum. Barium examination may show that the cecum and ascending colon are displaced to the left. Upper gastrointestinal barium studies are preferred by some pediatric radiologists for diagnosing malrotation.

Treatment

The goal of surgery is to relieve extrinsic compression in the duodenum by dividing the bands that bind the second and third portions to the retroperitoneum and by straightening the duodenojejunal junction. The midgut always twists in a clockwise fashion in North America; thus, the mass of bowel loops must be unwound in a counterclockwise direction. The small bowel is then placed in the right side of the abdomen and the colon to the left.

Course & Prognosis

Recurrences after surgical correction are uncommon.

MECKEL'S DIVERTICULUM

Meckel's diverticulum may be asymptomatic throughout life or may be associated with any of the following: hemorrhage; Meckel's diverticulitis, with symptoms identical to those of acute appendicitis; perforation; intussusception, with the diverticulum as the leading point; patent omphalomesenteric duct, with a diverticulum opening at the umbilicus; and intestinal obstruction from a vestigial band connecting the diverticulum to the umbilicus. It is found in 2% of the population and is usually located in the distal ileum.

Clinical Findings

Bleeding from a Meckel's diverticulum is a result of peptic ulceration of the diverticulum itself or of adjacent intestinal mucosa. Bleeding is massive but usually painless. Diverticula containing no gastric mucosa do not usually bleed. Foreign bodies occasionally impact in a diverticulum.

Treatment

Treatment of a diverticulum which has bled is excision. Meckel's diverticula discovered incidentally at laparotomy may be removed, especially if they contain gastric mucosa.

Course & Prognosis

The prognosis is excellent following surgery. If perforation through a gangrenous diverticulum has occurred, massive peritonitis may follow and is a serious threat to life.

DUPLICATIONS OF THE GASTROINTESTINAL TRACT

Cysts of enteric origin may occur anywhere from the upper esophagus to the anus and are often intimately associated with the adjacent areas of the gastrointestinal tract, usually sharing a common muscular wall. There may be communication between cyst and bowel lumens. The nature of the mucosal lining varies considerably and may not necessarily correspond with the level of the gastrointestinal tract to which the cyst is adjacent. There is considerable variation in the size and shape of these cysts.

A duplication may present as an asymptomatic mass, with gastrointestinal bleeding, as an intestinal obstruction resulting from volvulus or intussusception, with localized peritonitis or with malabsorption secondary to bacterial overgrowth. Special types of duplications include neurenteric cysts and hindgut duplications. Neurenteric cysts usually arise from the proximal small bowel and extend toward the vertebral column; they are associated with a bony defect in the vertebral column and extension through the diaphragm and into the chest. Hindgut duplications actually represent a double colon and are often associated with doubling of the anus and the perineal structures.

Diagnosis can sometimes be made by use of radioactive technetium perchlorate to demonstrate ectopic gastric mucosa in the duplication.

Treatment consists of resection of the duplication and, in most cases, of the adjacent bowel also. The prognosis is good.

BILIARY ATRESIA

Biliary atresia is a progressive extrahepatic biliary obstruction in the newborn. The extrahepatic biliary tree is fibrotic, involved in an intense inflammatory reaction suggesting infection. If untreated, it eventually compromises the intrahepatic biliary system and results in cirrhosis, portal hypertension, ascites, and liver insufficiency.

Clinical Findings

Progressive jaundice, hepatomegaly and acholic stools develop, usually after week two of life. Failure to thrive and nutritional deficiencies secondary to steatorrhea develop in the first few months of life.

Neonatal hepatitis is the condition most often confused with biliary atresia. This and other causes of jaundice (see table 17–7 & 17–8) must be ruled out.

Treatment

Laparotomy and operative cholangiogram should be performed to confirm the diagnosis. The liver biopsy gives an indication of long-term prognosis, based upon the degree of hepatic cirrhosis.

Bilioenteric drainage (portojejunostomy) procedures must be performed between the first and second months of life. The condition cannot be surgically palliated after 12–16 weeks, and death from liver failure or complications of portal hypertension usually occurs between 2 and 3 years.

Course & Prognosis

The average survival of patients with untreated biliary atresia is 18 months. Progression of hepatic fibrosis is common even after surgical palliation, although 30–50% of patients may remain anicteric. The short-term transplant survival rate is about 75%.

CHOLEDOCHAL CYST

Choledochal cyst is less common than biliary atresia. The manifestations consist of intermittent jaundice, fever and chills (when infection is present), and a mass in the right upper quadrant. X-ray examination may show a mass on a plain film and indentation of the duodenum on an upper gastrointestinal series. Ultrasonography is the preferred method to confirm the diagnosis. The cyst should be excised rather than simply drained into the gastrointestinal tract. The overall prognosis is excellent if operative excision is done early. Newborns with symptomatic choledochal cysts have a poorer prognosis, with a course similar to that of extrahepatic biliary atresia.

INTUSSUSCEPTION

Intussusception is one of the most dangerous surgical emergencies in early childhood. It is characterized by the telescoping of a proximal portion of the intestine into a more distal portion, resulting in impairment of the blood supply and necrosis of the involved segment of bowel. In 95% of cases, no cause of intussusception can be found, but viral infections have been implicated. The condition is most common in infants between the ages of 5 months and 1 year. Telescoping occasionally occurs from a Meckel's diverticulum.

Intussusception most commonly involves the telescoping of the ileum into the colon (ileocolic type). Gangrene of the intussusception occurs if the incarcerated bowel loses its blood supply.

Clinical Findings

A. Symptoms and Signs: A sudden onset of recurrent, paroxysmal, sharp abdominal pain in a healthy child suggests intussusception. The child perspires and draws up the legs to ease the pain. The child may appear well or merely lethargic in the pain-free intervals. Vomiting frequently occurs after the onset of the abdominal pain but is not universally present. Fifteen percent of patients do not have pain.

After 1 or 2 hours of recurrent pain, there is pallor, sweating, and lassitude with each attack of pain. After 5 or more hours, dehydration and listlessness are noted, and the eyes are sunken and soft. A low-grade fever is usually present as a result of dehydration and obstruction.

Careful palpation usually reveals a nontender, firm, sausage-shaped mass in the abdomen. Its location varies, but it frequently is in the upper midabdomen. The right lower quadrant is characteristically less full than usual. If the leading point of the intussusception has reached the rectum, it may be possible to palpate a mass by rectal examination. Blood frequently is found on rectal examination. A ''currant jelly'' stool (blood and mucus clot) may be evacuated in a bowel movement.

B. Laboratory Findings: Depending on the duration of symptoms, dehydration may be found, requiring replacement fluid and electrolyte therapy.

C. Imaging: A plain film of the abdomen will frequently show absence of bowel gas in the right lower quadrant. Dilated loops of small bowel, when present, suggest partial or complete obstruction of the small intestine. When barium enema examination is performed, the intussusception is outlined as an inverted cap, and an obstruction to the further progression of the barium is noted. Barium enema may also be used to reduce the intussusception (see Treatment, below).

Treatment

A. General Measures: After intravenous fluids are given, nonoperative reduction by barium enema administered by a skilled radiologist under fluoroscopic control will safely reduce intussusception in two thirds of cases. The enema must reflux through the ileocecal valve, and unless the ileum is filled, it may be impossible to tell whether complete reduction has occurred. Subsequent laparotomy is necessary if reduction is not accomplished. If too much hydrostatic pressure is employed or if the bowel wall has been weakened owing to impairment of its vascular supply, perforation can occur. Hydrostatic reduction (barium enema) should *not* be attempted if there are physical findings of peritonitis.

B. Surgical Measures: Surgical reduction is possible in most cases of early diagnosis. The bowel is usually found to be viable. If not, resection and anastomosis should be done.

Course & Prognosis

With adequate early treatment, the prognosis is excellent and recurrences are uncommon. For this reason, no attempt is made to do anything more than reduce the intussusception unless some condition that caused the obstruction such as a polyp or Meckel's diverticulum is discovered at surgery.

Table 17–9. Differential diagnosis of rectal bleeding in infants and children.

Cause	Usual Age Group	Additional Chief Complaints	Amount of Blood	Type of Blood	Treatment
Allergy	Colon	Colicky abdominal pain.	Moderate to large.	Dark or bright	Eliminate allergen.
Anal fissure	<2 yr	Pain.	Small	Bright	Soften stool; anal dilatation.
Bacterial enteritis	All ages	Diarrhea, cramps.	Small	Usually bright with diarrhea	See Table 17–2.
Duplication of bowel	All ages	Variable.	Usually small	Usually dark	Surgery.
Esophageal varices	>4 yr	Bloody emesis; signs of portal hypertension; signs of chronic liver disease.	Variable	Usually dark	Reduce portal hypertension; sclerose varices.
Hemangioma or telangiectasia	All ages	Usually none.	Variable	Dark or bright	None.
Hemorrhagic disease of the newborn	Newborns	Other evidence of bleeding.	Variable	Dark or bright	Vitamin K, transfusion.

Condition	Age	Symptoms	Amount	Appearance	Treatment
Inserted foreign body	Children	Pain.	Small	Bright	Removal.
Intussusception	<18 m	Abdominal pain; mass; bilious emesis.	Small to large	Red jelly-like	Barium enema or surgery.
Meckel's diverticulum	Young children	None or anemia.	Small to large	Dark or bright	Surgery.
Peptic ulcer	All ages	Abdominal pain, emesis, hematemesis.	Usually small	Dark	Antacid.
Swallowed maternal blood	Newborns	None.	Variable	Dark, resists alkaline hemolysis	None.
Volvulus	Infants or young children	Abdominal pain, intestinal obstruction.	Small to large	Dark	Surgery.
Ulcerative colitis; Crohn's colitis	>3 yr	Pain, fever.	Small to large	Bright, with diarrhea	See Table 17–6.
Juvenile polyps	>3 yr	None.	Small	Bright	May be removed endoscopically.

Children more than 4 years of age who have intussusception frequently have a small bowel lymphosarcoma, polyp, or other leading point for the intussusception.

POLYPS OF THE INTESTINAL TRACT

See Table 17–10.

Juvenile Polyps

Most juvenile polyps are located in the colon (60% in the recto-sigmoid), but they may be found anywhere in the intestine. They may be single or multiple. They are usually soft, and they may show ulceration of the surface.

In most cases, colonoscopic removal of juvenile polyps from the colon is possible. Single juvenile polyps have no malignant potential. Occasionally, adenomatous changes develop in patients with multiple juvenile polyps. Laparotomy is never indicated unless massive bleeding or intussusception develops. Most juvenile polyps will slough in time without complication.

Multiple polyps in the older child suggest the possibility of Peutz-Jegher's syndrome, Gardner's syndrome, or familial adenomatous polyposis. Family history, excisional biopsy of the lowest polyp, and examination for cutaneous manifestations will rule out these rare causes of polyps. A colectomy with ileorectal pull-through operation is usually the procedure of choice for children with Gardner's syndrome or adenomatous polyposis because of the high cancer risk.

HIRSCHSPRUNG'S DISEASE

Infants with Hirschsprung's disease lack normal development of Meissner's and Auerbach's plexuses in the distal bowel. The defect always begins at the anorectal junction and may involve all or most of the large bowel. In most cases, only the rectosigmoid is involved. The disease is 5 times more common in males and usually causes symptoms soon after birth.

Clinical Findings

A. Symptoms and Signs: Obstipation, abdominal distension, and vomiting may begin in the first days of life. Ninety percent of patients with aganglionosis fail to pass meconium dur-

Table 17-10. GI polyposis syndromes.

	Location[1]	Number	Histology	Associated Findings	Malignant Potential
Juvenile polyps	Colon.	Usually single; rarely multiple.	Hyperplastic, hamartomatous.	None.	None in single polyps; rare in multiple polyps.
Familial polyposis	Colon (stomach and small bowel).	Multiple.	Adenomatous.	None.	95–100%.
Peutz–Jegher syndrome	Small bowel, stomach, colon.	Multiple.	Hamartomatous.	Pigmented cutaneous and oral macules; ovarian cysts and tumors; bony exostoses.	2–3%.
Gardner syndrome	Colon (stomach, small bowel).	Multiple.	Adenomatous.	Cysts, tumors, and desmoids of skin and bone; other tumors.	95–100%.
Cronkhite–Canada syndrome	Stomach, colon (esophagus, small bowel).	Multiple.	Hamartomatous.	Alopecia, onychodystrophy, hyperpigmentation.	Rare.
Turcot syndrome	Colon.	Multiple.	Adenomatous.	Thyroid and brain tumors.	Possible.

[1] Parentheses indicate less common locations.

ing the first 24 hours of life. Obstipation may alternate with watery diarrhea. Complete obstruction, perforation, or acute enterocolitis may develop. Poor weight gain is common.

The abdomen is distended, often with palpable loops of bowel. Rectal examination shows no stool in the ampulla. There may be an explosive release of feces and flatus when the examining finger is withdrawn.

B. Imaging: An upright abdominal x-ray may show massive distention of the colon with gas and feces. In advanced cases, there may be air-fluid levels. Look carefully for air in the wall of the bowel, a sign of enterocolitis.

Barium enema should be performed *without* the usual bowel preparation. Use only sufficient barium to study the colon up to the junction of the anganglionic and the stool-filled ganglionic segment. The transitional segment is spastic, with an irregular, saw-toothed outline. This may be best seen on a lateral view. In the newborn, this may not be striking, and the only positive finding may be retention of barium in the proximal bowel for more than 24 hours after the examination.

C. Rectal biopsy: This should be performed if there is doubt in the diagnosis. A biopsy specimen shows absence of ganglion cells in both Meissner's and Auerbach's plexuses. Marked hypertrophy of nerve trunks may be seen.

D. Rectal Manometry: Rectal manometry demonstrates loss of the normal reflex relaxation of the internal anal sphincter upon rectal distention.

Treatment

Colostomy is usually performed early and must be done as an emergency procedure if perforation or enterocolitis is suspected. Resection of the aganglionic segment, with reestablishment of continuity (Swenson, Duhamel, or Soave procedure), may be performed when the patient is 6 months or older.

ANORECTAL MALFORMATIONS
(Imperforate Anus)

Most males with an anorectal malformation have a fistula to the membranous urethra and no connection between the hindgut and the perineal skin. Most females have a fistula to the perineum at the posterior junction of the labia (posterior fourchette). In the female, communication between the rectum and the urinary tract is rare.

Clinical Findings

A. Males: There is no opening where the anus should be. The intergluteal fold may be well developed, with good sphincter response to perineal stimulation. Look for a fistula along the median raphe. Watch for meconium in urine. There is a significant incidence of associated tracheoesophageal fistula. Absence of a perineal fistula means that the patient probably has a communication to the urethra and requires a diverting colostomy. In doubtful cases, this communication (fistula) can sometimes be seen on urethrogram.

B. Females: Look for a fistula in the posterior fourchette and perineum. Gentle dilation of the fistula with a sound will often relieve obstipation temporarily. A high vaginal fistula cannot be handled by dilation; the patient should have a colostomy.

C. General Findings: Since there is a high incidence of absence of kidneys and strictures of the ureteropelvic and ureterovesical structures, all infants with imperforate anus require thorough study of the urinary tract.

Treatment

A. Surgical Measures: Perineal fistulas in males and females require only dilation during the newborn period; anoplasty can be done later. Diverting colostomy is necessary if no perineal fistula is present. Pull-through operations for patients with a high imperforate anus should be done after the age of 6 months. The best results are reported when a transcoccygeal approach is used. The results are poor if the child has myelomeningocele or a significant malformation of the lumbosacral spine.

Prognosis

All infants with perineal fistulas should be continent since bowel passes normally through the levators. Infants with a high proximal pouch and no perineal fistula have only a fair chance for complete rectal continence as anal musculature and levators may be absent.

APPENDICITIS

Appendicitis is the most common pathologic lesion of the intestinal tract requiring surgery in childhood. Most cases are seen in children between the ages of 4 and 12 years and may be associated with other illnesses, especially measles. The cause is not clear, although some cases seem to result from impaction of a fecalith in the lumen of the appendix. Pinworms may occasionally cause appendicitis.

Clinical Findings

A. Symptoms: Acute periumbilical or generalized abdominal pain is usually constant. After 1–5 hours, the pain becomes localized in the right lower quadrant. Urinary pain or frequency may be present if the appendix lies near the bladder or ureters. When vomiting occurs, it is usually only after prolonged pain. Constipation occurs frequently, but diarrhea is only occasionally seen.

B. Signs: Fever is low-grade, varying from 37.8 to 38.4°C (100 to 101.6°F), or may be absent early in the course. Very high fevers are suggestive of appendiceal perforation, with peritonitis, or of the simultaneous presence of bacterial enteritis, especially if accompanied by diarrhea.

The child usually is anxious and may be "doubled up" (with hips flexed) or walk bent over, often holding the right side.

Palpation may reveal a difference in muscular tension between the 2 sides of the abdomen. The hand should be warm and palpation gentle. Localization of tenderness may be difficult, but an opinion about whether the pain is greater on the right or left side may be formed by observing the child's expression while palpating each area and noting the involuntary spasm of the abdominal musculature. Most children tend to flex the right thigh in an effort to decrease the spasm of the psoas muscle. However, the elicitation of a positive psoas sign is of doubtful value in small children.

There may be rectal tenderness, a mass consisting of peritoneal fluid, or an indurated omentum wrapped around an inflamed appendix.

C. Laboratory Findings: Two or 3 consecutive determinations of white blood cells will frequently show a rise in the total white blood cell count, with an accompanying shift to the left in the neutrophilic series. It is imperative that a careful urinalysis be made in order to rule out infection of the kidney or bladder.

D. Imaging: In uncomplicated appendicitis, plain films of the abdomen may show a fecalith, scoliosis, or an abnormal gas pattern. When exudate has formed, evidence of peritoneal inflammation may cause disappearance of the preperitoneal fat line along the right wall of the abdomen or obliteration of the psoas shadow.

A barium enema may be of value if the diagnosis is not clear. Normal filling of the appendix tends to exclude the diagnosis of appendicitis. In well-established cases of appendicitis, persistent pressure defects and other abnormalities of the cecum may be noted.

In the presence of perforation, fluid may accumulate between loops of the bowel. However, free intra-abdominal air is rare except in children under 2 years of age. With abscess formation, there may be evidence of a soft tissue mass in the region of the perforation. In atypical cases, a plain film of the chest is of value to rule out reflex pain and abdominal spasm of an undiagnosed pneumonitis.

Differential Diagnosis

Differential diagnosis includes mesenteric adenitis, pyelitis, cystitis, pneumonitis (especially pneumococcal), gastroenteritis, peritonitis, constipation, Meckel's diverticulitis, and acute onset of inflammatory bowel disease (especially Crohn's ileitis/ileocolitis).

Treatment

Appendectomy should be done as soon as the child has been prepared by adequate fluid and electrolyte administration. If there is doubt as to diagnosis, an exploratory laparotomy, with removal of the appendix and culture of peritoneal fluid, should be performed. Intravenous antibiotic therapy may be indicated if peritoneal contamination has occurred. Penrose drains are indicated for localized abscesses.

For patients with ruptured appendix, prolonged gastric suction may be required until intestinal peristalsis is normal. Fowler's position (semi-sitting) should be maintained in order to permit drainage into the pelvic region. Parenteral fluid therapy is administered as indicated (see Chapter 4). Antibiotics (see Chapter 31) are given as determined by peritoneal culture.

FOREIGN BODIES IN THE GASTROINTESTINAL TRACT

The incidence of foreign bodies in the gastrointestinal tract is highest in children 1–3 years of age. Coins, toys, and marbles may lodge in the esophagus and should be removed by esophagoscopy. If passed into the stomach, they usually pass through the entire gastrointestinal tract without incident. If x-rays are taken for presumed ingestion, be sure to include the esophagus and pharynx if the foreign body is not in the abdomen.

Pointed foreign bodies (eg, pins, nails, screws) usually pass without incident. Remove endoscopically if the patient has pain, fever, vomiting, or local tenderness. Only 2–4% of such cases require surgery. X-ray examination is required only if the foreign body has not passed in 4 or 5 days. If a pin or other sharp object remains in the same location for 4 or 5 days, the point may have penetrated the bowel, and endoscopic removal or surgery is then indicated.

Kidney & Urinary Tract | 18

Gary M. Lum, MD

CLINICAL FINDINGS

Clinical manifestations of diseases of the kidneys or urinary tract include those symptoms that suggest (1) infection (eg, urgency; frequency; dysuria; and abdominal, suprapubic, or costovertebral angle pain); (2) urolithiasis (abdominal pain, colic); (3) voiding problems (frequency, straining, incontinence); and (4) chronic renal failure (CRF) from abnormal renal development (polyuria, enuresis, failure to thrive). The inability of the kidneys to elaborate a concentrated urine is one of the first signs of inadequate renal development (if urinary concentrating ability is the *only* renal abnormality noted, the diagnosis of diabetes insipidus must be entertained as well).

Renal inflammation, such as glomerulonephritis, is often asymptomatic unless it produces an immediate, severe compromise in renal function. Subsequent disease progression can produce symptoms of CRF, including anorexia, nausea and vomiting, malaise and easy fatigability, and bone pain.

Renal compromise should be suspected in newborns with congenital absence of the abdominal musculature; presence of a single umbilical artery; abdominal masses; or abnormalities of the spinal cord, sacrum, perineum, or external genitalia. Renal anomalies may also be seen in association with ear deformities, aniridia, hemihypertrophy, chromosomal disorders, hepatic cysts or fibrosis, pulmonary hypoplasia, and congenital ascites. The presence of oligohydramnios and spontaneous pneumothorax should also raise the question of renal disease. With the application of prenatal ultrasonography, abnormalities of the urinary tract may be demonstrated early in pregnancy.

Findings such as hypertension; edema; skeletal deformity; pallor or anemia; hematuria; proteinuria; bacteriuria; crystalluria; acidosis; and elevations in BUN, creatinine, potassium, and serum phosphate may be encountered in various renal disease states.

DIAGNOSTIC STUDIES

Laboratory assessment of renal function begins with a carefully performed urinalysis. The urinary dipstick is a helpful screening tool. The detection of hematuria, leukocyturia, and/or bacteruria, however, should be followed by microscopic inspection of the urinary sediment. Abnormal amounts of urinary protein should be quantitatively measured. If infection is suspected, the urine is sent for culture and sensitivity. A reliably performed mid-stream, clean-catch urinary specimen is adequate for culture. If this cannot be obtained with confidence a bladder catheterization or suprapubic bladder tap may be performed. Bacterial colony counts of less than 10,000/mL, or multiple flora, are usually considered contaminants unless obtained by catheterization or bladder tap (provided proper technique is followed). Appropriate diagnostic work-up should follow to exclude genitourinary abnormalities or conditions predisposing to infection (eg, obstruction, reflux, foreign body, trauma, hygiene, infestations such as pinworms).

Abnormalities or disease resulting in functional renal disturbance is demonstrated and monitored by the serum BUN and creatinine (Cr). Serum creatinine is a reflection of muscle metabolism and therefore is related to total body muscle mass. In general in pediatrics the normal range is from 0.3–0.8 mg%. Since normal renal function maintains the serum level in a "steady-state," a doubling of the serum creatinine reflects approximately a 50% reduction in renal function. Thus, even a level of 0.8 mg% is of concern, if normal serum creatinine for a given-sized child is 0.4 mg%. Calculation of the renal creatinine clearance (CrCl) can be useful in estimating renal function; however, it requires the reliable collection of a timed (12–24 h) urinary specimen. The calculation is as follows:

$$\frac{\text{Urine Cr mg\%} \times \text{Volume mL/min}}{\text{Serum Cr mg\%}}$$

Verification of reliability can be demonstrated by determination of the creatinine index (24-h creatinine excretion in mg/kg body wt = 12–20). The difficulties encountered in obtaining such a specimen are avoided by estimating glomerular filtration rate with the serum creatinine. The following formula derives creatinine clearance:

in serious compromise to renal parenchymal development and function. Antenatal US can provide information on the developing kidneys and urinary tract enabling anticipation of postnatal renal functional disturbances. Some degree of hydronephrosis is a common finding in utero, but postnatal US can easily dispel concern. In cases where concern is founded, timely urologic intervention to reduce further deleterious effects on remaining renal tissue is of paramount importance.

Clinical & Laboratory Findings

Delays or abnormalities in voiding patterns may signal poor renal function and/or urinary tract obstruction. Abdominal masses, absence of abdominal musculature, and anomalies of the external genitalia or lower spine suggest urinary tract maldevelopment. Renal functional capacity will vary according to severity of the abnormality and its effect on renal parenchyma. Laboratory findings reveal the level of renal function, and diagnostic work-up proceeds as mentioned above.

URINARY TRACT INFECTION

Acute urinary tract infection may be limited to the lower urinary tract, but persistent or recurrent cases often result in reflux nephropathy, and at times one may observe acute pyelonephritis. Newborns of both sexes and females of all ages seem at highest risk of developing urinary tract infections.

Infection may be caused by a variety of organisms, particularly *Escherichia coli* and other organisms commonly found in the intestinal tract. Kidney involvement often results from ascending infection. Congenital abnormalities associated with obstruction and ureterovesical reflux may be important predisposing factors.

Clinical Findings

A. Symptoms and Signs: Symptoms may be mild or absent. Common symptoms, however, are fever and chills, urinary urgency and frequency, incontinence, dysuria, and abdominal pain. Occasionally, there may be complaints of anorexia and nausea or vomiting. With acute pyelonephritis, these symptoms may be more obvious. Asymptomatic bacteriuria occurs in 1% of schoolgirls.

Signs include dull or sharp pain and tenderness in the kidney area or abdomen. Hypertension and evidence of chronic renal failure may be present. Jaundice may occur, particularly during early infancy.

B. Laboratory Findings: Pyuria is characteristic, but it may be absent in the majority of patients during some phase of the disease. Slight or moderate hematuria occasionally occurs. There may be slight proteinuria. Pathogenic organisms and casts of all types may be present in the urine, but the urine may be normal for long periods of time. Anemia may be found in cases of long-standing infection. Leukocytosis is usually in the range of $15,000-35,000/\mu L$. The diagnosis of urinary tract infection should be suspect if it is based on examination of a single voided urine specimen. A reliably performed mid-stream, clean-catch urine specimen is suitable for culture. If that cannot be obtained with confidence, suprapubic bladder tap or catheterization may be performed.

C. Urologic Studies: Intravenous urography and voiding cystourethrography are recommended by many investigators for all children after the initial infection. Others feel that these procedures should be performed after the first urinary tract infection only for newborn infants, boys of all ages, and girls with symptoms suggestive of pyelonephritis; otherwise, they should be performed after second infections. Referral to a urologist and the need for further urologic evaluation depends on the nature and severity of any abnormalities noted.

Treatment

A. Specific Measures: Eradicate infection with appropriate chemotherapeutic or antibiotic therapy (see Chapter 8), usually for at least 10 days and particularly with drugs to which the patient has not recently been exposed. A prolonged course of urinary tract antisepsis (2–6 months or longer) may be indicated, especially for repeated infections. Repeat urinalyses at intervals of 1 or 2 months for at least a year is recommended.

B. General Measures: Force fluids during the acute stage. If possible, have the patient shower instead of bathing. Discontinue "bubble baths." Avoid constipation. Look for evidence of pinworms, which are often associated with repeated episodes of cystitis. Sexual activity may also play a role.

C. Surgical Measures: There is no clear evidence that routine surgical correction—by either bladder neck revision, dilation, urethrotomy, or meatotomy—alters the course of recurrent urinary tract infections to any significant degree, but clearly obstructive lesions , severe ureteric reflux or bladder dysfunction or abnormalities warrant urologic intervention.

D. Prophylactic Measures: After control of the infection, a prophylactic regimen using trimethoprin sulfa is of value. If methenamine is used, the urine should be kept acid. Nalidixic acid is an effective substitute for methenamine. The dipstick nitrite test is a useful adjunct to home screening. Urine cultures should be repeated as clinically indicated or suggested by urinalysis.

In some cases, it is not sufficient to institute treatment only for clinical exacerbations, since asymptomatic bacteriuria may persist and be associated with progressive severe renal damage.

Reinfection in females, regardless of the absence of obstruction or reflux, is not uncommon. In such cases, the child should be checked periodically for at least 5 years.

HEMATURIA

The finding of abnormal numbers of red blood cells (RBCs) in the urine, especially if asymptomatic, suggests the possible presence of glomerular disease. Other "nonrenal," and largely symptomatic, problems (eg, trauma, bleeding diathesis, infection, lithiasis, hypercalciuria, history of sickle cell disease, renal tumors, cystic diseases) should be excluded. Work up is depicted in Fig 18–1. If presentation is one of acute glomerulonephritis the differential diagnosis includes: postinfectious GN (most common), the GN of systemic lupus erythematosus (SLE), Henoch-Schönlein purpura (HSP), IgA nephropathy, and membranoproliferative GN (histologic types I, II, and III). Occurring rarely in children are the entities of antiglomerular basement membrane (anti-GBM) disease (eg, Goodpasture's syndrome) and idiopathic, rapidly progressive GN. Hereditary forms of glomerulonephritis (eg, Alport syndrome) do not present as acute GN.

Laboratory Findings (Fig 18–1)

Since preceding streptococcal disease is most frequently the cause of acute, postinfectious forms of GN, the search for evidence of recent exposure may reveal elevations in antistreptolysin O titer and/or streptozyme. Such data are of little relevance in "nonacute" GN or purely nephrotic syndrome presentations.

Other helpful laboratory data in evaluating GN include the

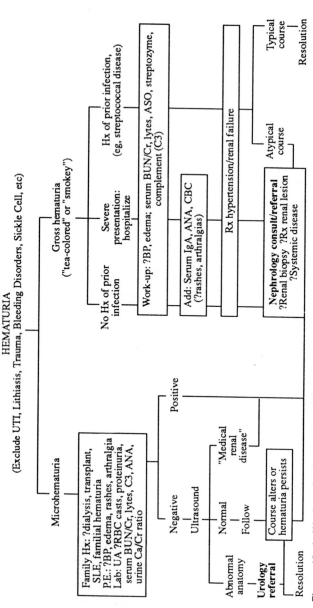

Figure 18–1. Work-up for hematuria. UTI = urinary tract infection; SLE = systemic lupus erythematosis; ANA = antinuclear antibody; ASO = antistreptolysin O titer.

serum complement. Complement may be found to be depressed in postinfectious GN, membranoproliferative GN, and SLE-GN. Normalization of serum complement is expected rapidly (1–30 days) in typical poststreptococcal GN. Intermittent or persistent depression suggests chronic GN (eg, membranoproliferative GN varieties), or SLE, where complement depression and antinative DNA elevations, hallmarks of disease activity, can be used to guide therapy.

Treatment

There is no specific therapy for poststreptococcal GN. Treatment is aimed at controlling hypertension and following the effect of disease on GFR. Depending on the degree of associated renal failure (usually at >50% reduction of GFR), measures can be taken to reduce protein, salt, and potassium intake; phosphate binders can be used to reduce dietary phosphate; and dialysis can be used as indicated in severe renal failure until (and if) renal recovery occurs. Such extreme measures would be instituted earlier in the more severe forms of GN, in which acute renal failure (ARF) progresses at a more rapid rate.

There are, of course, specific therapeutic measures that can be taken in the more severe or chronic forms of GN. Corticosteroids are useful in membranoproliferative GN and SLE. High dose, intravenous corticosteroids, cytotoxic agents, anticoagulation, and plasmapheresis have been used alone and in combination with variable results in these and other GNs (eg, anti-GBM disease, rapidly progressive GN). Some cases of HSP GN and IgA nephropathy, when severe (usually with excessive proteinuria and/or marked reduction in renal function) have also prompted attempts at treatment intervention, although there is no universally accepted therapy for these clinical entities. The likelihood of ARF or CRF progressing toward end stage renal disease (ESRD) requiring chronic dialysis treatment and/or transplant is of considerable concern in all such cases.

PROTEINURIA

Like hematuria, the presence of abnormal amounts of protein in the urine suggests renal or urinary tract abnormalities. Excretion of more than 250 mg of protein in 24 hours should raise the suspicion of significant proteinuria. Urinary dipstick can estimate the amount of protein in a given specimen, but total 24-hour quantitation should be undertaken (apply creatinine index to verify collection). The albumin:creatinine ratio in a spot urine specimen provides a practical screening tool. Although there is some variation with age, it is convenient to think of a ratio of less than 0.1 as normal, 0.1–1.0 as slight, 1.0–10 as moderate, and greater than 10 as heavy proteinuria. Some children will excrete abnormal amounts of protein only while maintaining an upright posture (orthostatic or postural proteinuria). This phenomenon can be documented by measuring the protein content of urine produced during the day (upright) and comparing it with the urine formed overnight (recumbent). In such cases more than 80% of the protein lost in the urine will be demonstrated in the upright specimen. The total quantity should not exceed 1.5 g in 24 hours. The work-up is depicted in Fig 18–2.

Laboratory Findings (Fig 18–2)

Urinalysis is expected to be otherwise unrevealing in cases of isolated proteinuria (although the presence of significant quantities of RBCs would suggest glomerular disease). However, as many as 20 RBCs per high-power field (no RBC casts) can be seen in the urine of children with idiopathic nephrotic syndrome of childhood (INSC) where no glomerular lesion is expected. If NS is present, lipid droplets (maltese crosses) can be seen in the urine with the use of Polaroid filters.

Glomerular lesions can also produce reductions in GFR; thus, serum BUN and creatinine may be elevated. However, keep in mind that in NS, whether or not glomerular injury is responsible, circulatory volume contraction can lead to renal underperfusion ("prerenal" insufficiency) also resulting in elevations of BUN (primarily) and creatinine.

Furthermore, in NS, serum albumin will be decreased (as will measured total calcium) and serum lipids will be increased. Hyponatremia may be present. Although total body sodium is high owing to renal affinity for sodium in this state, the kidney is also avidly reabsorbing water (vasopressin) in defense of circulating volume. Factitious hyponatremia is also created by measurement of serum sodium in lipemic sera.

Treatment

The complications of NS may require immediate attention while awaiting the response, if any, to therapy directed at reducing or eliminating proteinuria. Restoration of life-threatening volume depletion should be accomplished with the administration of

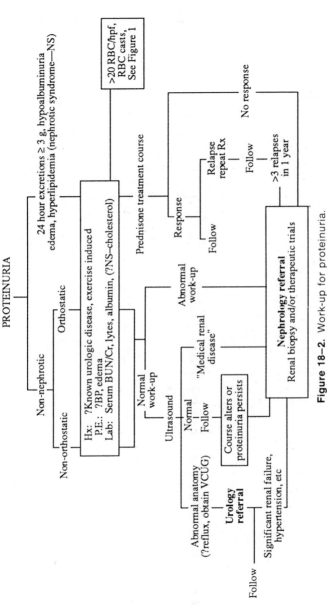

Figure 18–2. Work-up for proteinuria.

627

albumin. Care must be taken if hypertension is also paradoxically present. Administration of diuretics can lead to further circulating volume contraction, but can aid in mobilization of problematic edema and urine production, if administered while replenishing serum albumin. Infections should be promptly treated. The tendency to increased intravascular thrombosis can also be a threat.

Therapy directed against specific renal lesions will first demand documentation by renal biopsy except in the cases where clinical presentations favor "minimal change" disease (INSC). If the clinical presentation strongly supports the diagnosis of INSC, corticosteroids are the treatment of choice. Approximately 85% of children with this disease respond to prednisone. A dose of 2 mg/kg of body weight (maximum 60 mg) is given as a single daily dose until the urine is protein-free (negative to trace by dipstick) for a maximum of 4 weeks. After remission has been maintained for 3–5 days, the same dose is administered every other day for 4 weeks and then is slowly tapered over another 4–6 weeks and discontinued. Of patients who do not respond to this treatment, a few will still reveal no significant histopathology on renal biopsy, but the rest will likely have either focal glomerular sclerosis (most prevalent), mesangial nephropathy, or membranous lesions. Even some of initial responders may prove "steroid-dependent" or "steroid-resistant" with time.

When prolonged steroid exposure poses the risks associated with steroid toxicity, cytotoxic drugs such as chlorambucil and cyclophosphamide can induce longer, if not permanent, remission. They must be administered judiciously as they are not without significant side effects. Diagnostic confirmation of renal morphology with steroid resistance is again needed. Cyclosporine A is also now being used in steroid-dependent or resistant NS. Certainly the application of therapeutic trials with the immunosuppressive class of drugs requires the participation of a nephrologist.

Prognosis

INSC, despite multiple relapses and the use of cytotoxic agents, is expected to resolve without sequelae. The most concerning aspects of the entity relate to the complications of the nephrotic condition, which have been previously addressed. Complications of NS are likewise of considerable concern in the other glomerular lesions capable of producing it. Of these, mesangial nephropathy has a guarded prognosis relative to progressive renal failure, whereas as many as 15–20% of children with focal glomerular sclerosis develop CRF, although improved results with attempts at various treatment regimens have been reported. Corticosteroid therapy is reported to improve the prognosis of membranous nephropathy.

ACUTE RENAL FAILURE

Renal insufficiency, or acute renal failure (ARF)—"the clinical appearance of the inability of the kidneys to maintain their role in body homeostasis"—may be practically divided into causes resulting from compromise in renal perfusion (prerenal), obstruction to urinary flow (postrenal), or renal parenchymal disease (renal). Examples of each of these entities are listed in Table 18–1.

Clinical Findings
A. Symptoms and Signs: Depending on the degree of reduction in GFR and urine production, symptoms will range from those associated with fluid overload (eg, shortness of breath) to those of uremia (anorexia, nausea and vomiting, lethargy, etc).

Clinical signs vary from mild to severe edema, hypertension, congestive heart failure, pulmonary edema, anemia, and encephalopathy.

B. Laboratory Findings: Serum BUN and creatinine are increased and must be monitored. Serum analysis will reveal disturbances in electrolytes, most importantly potassium and bicarbonate (acidosis). Serum calcium generally decreases while phosphate increases. Anemia may be noted.

Table 18–1. Causes of acute renal failure in children.

Prerenal:	Dehydration, congestive heart failure, renal arterial thrombosis, nephrotic syndrome.
Postrenal:	Urinary tract obstruction (eg, ureteropelvic and ureterovesical junctional stenoses and posterior urethral valves), urolithiasis, clot, foreign body.
Renal:	Glomerulonephritis, hemolytic uremic syndrome, systemic vasculitis, acute tubular necrosis (asphyxia, hypotension, ischemia), drugs, interstitial disease.

Treatment

All immediately correctable causes (usually prerenal or postrenal) should be addressed. Renal glomerular or interstitial diseases, once identified, are treated accordingly. The complications of ARF should be carefully monitored and controlled. Timely intervention with dialysis is important in reducing morbidity. Recovery is largely dependent on the nature of the renal lesion and its response to therapy.

The Hemolytic Uremic Syndrome (HUS) (see Chapter 19) is responsible for many cases of ARF in children. Management is directed at the consequences of the renal failure (dialysis in severe cases), although there have been reported improvements seen with plasma infusion or plasmapheresis in isolated cases.

Acute tubular necrosis (ATN)—or vasomotor nephropathy—is the disturbance in renal function usually suspected in clinical settings where renal ischemia or nephrotoxicity (hemoglobin, myoglobin, drugs, etc) is implicated and no other immediately identifiable cause is elucidated. Precipitating factors should be quickly identified and eliminated. The urinary indices (Table 18–2) are helpful in assessing oliguria when a distinction must be made between diminished renal perfusion and ATN. Rapid restoration of renal perfusion and induction of diuresis (furosemide, up to 5 mg/kg IV) may avert ATN or at least establish nonoliguric ATN, which by virtue of reasonable urinary output is considerably easier to manage. The treatment for this entity is otherwise largely supportive, including dialysis as indicated. Renal recovery is expected unless renal ischemia is of the degree producing cortical necrosis, or unless metabolic toxins have caused irreversible injury. Recovery from oligoanuric ATN generally includes a nonoliguric or "diuretic" phase, and thus careful attention is directed toward preventing severe volume depletion during this period.

Table 18–2. Urinary findings in oliguria-prerenal vs ATN.

Test	Prerenal	ATN
Sodium (meq/L)	<20	>20
Fractional Na excretion[1]	<1	>1
Urine/serum creatinine	>40	<40
Osmolality (mosm/L)	>400	<400

[1] FENa $\dfrac{\text{U/P Na}}{\text{U/P Cr}} \times 100.$

Overall management of prolonged ARF with oliguria includes careful attention to fluid balance. Measurement of input and output as well as daily weight is advised. Central venous pressure monitoring may be indicated. Urinary bladder catheterization may be helpful in assessing the clinical situation early in ARF, but if oliguria is established the presence of a foreign body in the bladder invites infection.

Hypertension should be controlled with appropriate antihypertensive medications and normalization of intravascular volume. Intake of water, sodium, potassium, and phosphate should be restricted. Dietary phosphate binders, eg, calcium carbonate, should be administered as well. Reduced protein intake and adequate calories to decrease catabolism will minimize the rate of rise in serum BUN. On the other hand, such restrictions can be greatly modified or eliminated with the use of dialysis.

Metabolic acidosis may be treated with bicarbonate, intravascular volume permitting. Likewise, correction of pH will aid in the intracellular movement of serum potassium, thus bicarbonate administration should be one of the first steps in treating life-threatening hyperkalemia.

Other temporizing measures to combat hyperkalemia include the infusion of dextrose and insulin. Calcium administration is "cardioprotective" in this situation; moreover, hypocalcemia itself may be a problem, and may be clinically manifest in tetany with correction of acidosis—alkalinization increases protein-bound calcium. Such temporizing treatment of life-threatening hyperkalemia must be followed by the removal of excess potassium with either $Na-K^+$ exchange resins (Kayexalate) or dialysis. Again, most, if not all, of the complexities of management and consequences of uremia may be easily handled with the institution of dialysis.

RENAL TUBULAR DEFECTS

As previously mentioned in the discussion concerning juvenile nephronophthisis, there are renal disorders that are expressed primarily, if not solely, by abnormal function of the renal tubule. The most commonly encountered abnormality of this type is isolated renal tubular acidosis (RTA). Although this is a "renal" acidosis, it is to be distinguished from the acidosis seen in CRF, which is primarily the result of decreasing renal mass. The De Toni-Fanconi-Debré syndrome describes the more extensively malfunctioning nephron that produces not only renal bicarbonate losses but also phosphaturia, glycosuria, and amino-aciduria. This abnormality is most frequently encountered in metabolic diseases such as cystinosis, renal developmental conditions such as juvenile nephronophthisis, and acquired conditions of either unknown etiology or renal toxin exposure. Some of the acquired conditions may resolve but the usual course in untreated cystinosis, for example, is progressive CRF to end-stage disease.

Depending on the type of isolated RTA, however, the prognosis varies. Type 1 RTA (distal tubule—hydrogen ion gradient defect/bicarbonate loss) is generally associated with more complex metabolic disorders and nephrocalcinosis. Type 2 RTA (proximal tubule—lowered ''threshold'' for bicarbonate reabsorption bicarbonate wasting) is most frequently encountered as a transient form in infancy (suggesting delayed renal development of normal proximal bicarbonate reclamation). If this type is an isolated tubular problem it is expected to spontaneously resolve by age 2–4 years. Type 3 can be said to be a combination of types 1 and 2, and type 4 (deficiency in the renal physiologic effect of aldosterone) is primarily seen in adults with renal tubulo-interstitial disease.

1. RENAL TUBULAR ACIDOSIS

Clinical Findings

A. Symptoms and Signs: Failure to thrive is the most common presenting symptom. Polydypsia and polyuria may be noted. Anorexia, vomiting, constipation, and general listlessness may also be prominent features depending on the severity of systemic acidosis and extent of urinary losses. Skeletal pain associated with rickets (usually in more severe forms of type 1 and Fanconi syndrome) can also occur. There may be associated hypokalemia, producing symptomatic muscle weakness.

B. Laboratory Findings: Non–anion gap acidosis (hyperchloremic) is demonstrated with inappropriate urine pH (nonacidified). Hypokalemia may be present, or may come about with the administration of alkali therapy. Glycosuria, phosphaturia, and aminoaciduria are noted in Fanconi syndrome. Normal urinalysis should help exclude tubulo-interstitial disease. Demonstration of normal renal architecture with ultrasonography is advisable.

Treatment

Administration of alkali is the mainstay of treating the metabolic abnormality. Sodium citrate solution (Bicitra, 1 meq each Na and HCO_3 per mL, or Polycitra, 1 meq each Na and K and 2 meq HCO_3 per mL) is commonly used. Type 1 RTA will require 1–3 meq/kg body wt/d in 3 divided doses. Type 2, owing to the magnitude of proximal tubular bicarbonate losses, will generally require 5–15 meq/kg/d.

Course & Prognosis

Genetically transmitted or sporadic type 1 (with or without associated systemic disease) disorders resulting in nephrocalcinosis, or autoimmune diseases associated with type 1, are likely to be permanent defects. Drug-induced type 1 may resolve with discontinuation of the offending agent, as should RTA secondary to reflux nephropathy or obstruction if there is satisfactory recovery with correction of the urinary tract abnormality. Transient forms of type 2 are expected to resolve, as are those associated with drugs. Familial type 2 or that associated with the Fanconi syndrome are permanent defects, or are at least a significant management problem until CRF occurs in those entities with progressive renal interstitial and glomerular deterioration.

2. NEPHROGENIC DIABETES INSIPIDUS

Another tubular disorder less frequently encountered is this inherited (primarily X-linked) disorder, in which there is impaired or absent renal response to antidiuretic hormone.

Clinical Findings

A. Symptoms and Signs: Nephrogenic diabetes insipidus occurs early in infancy with irritability, failure to thrive, and poor feeding. Polyuria, polydypsia, dehydration, and rapid weight loss are remarkable, and fever may be noted.

B. Laboratory Findings: Urine output is increased and the osmolality is low, but urinalysis is otherwise unremarkable. Urinary concentration does not respond to vasopressin administration. Hypernatremia is marked (serum osmolality high) and metabolic acidosis develops with severe dehydration.

Treatment

Intake should be reduced in solutes (which obligate urinary water excretion) but appropriate in caloric content. However, care must be taken to assure adequate protein intake for growth, and to avoid hyponatremia. Thiazide diuretics are useful as they decrease sodium reabsorption in the cortical diluting segment of the renal tubule, resulting in increased sodium loss, while the resulting volume contraction leads to enhanced proximal tubule absorption of fluid. A dose of 30 mg/kg of chlorthiazide per day in 3 divided doses is helpful in treating this abnormality.

Hematologic Disorders | 19

Taru Hays, MD

CHILDHOOD ANEMIAS

Anemia is a common blood disorder in children and differs from that in adults in that the anemia may be more pronounced. This is due in part to the fact that growth in childhood is associated with an increased need for blood-building substances. Furthermore, infections, which are so common in childhood, have a more profound effect on blood formation in early life than in adulthood. A classification of childhood anemia based on mean corpuscular volume (MCV) is presented in Table 19–1.

PHYSIOLOGIC "ANEMIA" OF THE NEWBORN

A gradual drop in red cells and hemoglobin occurs normally during the first 10–12 weeks of life, owing to shortened red cell survival time, expanded intravascular volume, and improved oxygenation. The red blood count is reduced to 3.5–4.5 million/ μL, and the hemoglobin level may reach a low of 10 g/dL in full-term infants and 7 g/dL in premature infants. This is followed by a gradual increase in the number of red cells, with a correspondingly slower rise in hemoglobin level.

ANEMIA OF PREMATURITY

Although at birth the red cell count and hemoglobin levels of a premature infant are only slightly lower than those of a full-term one, the subsequent reduction that occurs is greater in premature infants. The magnitude of the drop of red cell count and hemoglobin level is inversely proportionate to the size of the infant. In very small infants (<1 kg at birth), a reduction of hemoglobin to 7–8 g/dL and a reduction of red cells to 2.5–3

Table 19–1. Classification of anemias based on mean corpuscular volume (MCV).

Microcytic	Normocytic	Macrocytic
Iron deficiency	Hemolytic anemias	Folate deficiency
Thalassemia	Chronic disease anemia	Vitamin B_{12} deficiency
Lead poisoning	Acute blood loss	Congenital hypoplastic anemia (Diamond-Blackfan)
Pyridoxine deficiency	Anemia of infection/inflammation	Fanconi's anemia
Copper deficiency	Infiltrative process	Preleukemia
Hemoglobin E	Aplastic process	Other bone marrow failure states

million/μL may occur. Lowest levels are reached at about the end of the second month of life. More severe anemia occurs in premature infants than in full-term infants, because premature infants undergo a greater growth in body size and a correspondingly greater increase in blood volume. Furthermore, the total iron stores are smaller in the premature infant, since most of a newborn's iron is acquired during the last 3 months of gestation and erythropoietin production in response to anemia is less than in the term infant.

Pallor is the principal manifestation. The anemia generally is normochromic and normocytic early in the course of the disease and relatively hypochromic and microcytic late in the course.

The initial drop in hemoglobin level or red blood cell count cannot be prevented by early treatment with iron. After the second month of life, supplemental iron should be given.

IRON DEFICIENCY ANEMIA

Because expansion of blood volume is part of the growth process, the need for iron in children is greater than that in adults. In the average full-term infant, the stores of iron available at birth are adequate for 3–6 months. In the premature infant, twin, or child born of a mother with severe iron deficiency, the iron reserves will be expended earlier, placing these children at increased risk of developing iron deficiency anemia.

Iron deficiency anemia may result from inadequate storage, deficient intake, chronic blood loss, poor absorption and utilization of iron, or milk protein sensitivity. Iron deficiency anemia is uncommon in breast-fed infants.

Clinical Findings

A. Symptoms and Signs: Pallor may be the only early finding. Weakness, listlessness, and irritability appear later. Interference with growth may occur in long-standing cases, and delayed development (reversible) may occur in anemia of short duration. Congestive heart failure occurs occasionally; generalized edema, rarely.

B. Laboratory Findings: In hypochromic microcytic anemia, hemoglobin values are decreased, and there is relatively less reduction in red cells. Anisocytosis and poikilocytosis may be marked. The reticulocyte count may be low, normal, or slightly elevated. The serum ferritin concentration is reduced; serum iron level is low, iron-binding capacity is increased; transferrin saturation is reduced; and the level of free erythrocyte protoporphyrin is elevated. Blood may be present in stools. Histologic abnormalities of the bowel may be present. Severe iron deficiency may be associated with copper deficiency, a decreased serum albumin level, and thrombocytosis.

Treatment

Iron is specific therapy. Other blood-building elements are not necessary.

A. Medicinal Iron: Iron should be given as the ferrous salt. Elemental iron, 5–6 mg/kg/d in 3 divided doses, should be given before meals. Therapy should be continued for several months after the concentration of hemoglobin returns to normal in order to build reserves of iron.

Intramuscular iron (iron dextran injection [Imferon]) should be used only when treatment with oral iron is not feasible.

B. Dietary Iron: Food contains insufficient iron for effective therapy of iron deficiency anemia. Absorption of iron from most foods is generally good; phytates (oatmeal, brown bread) may inhibit absorption. Good sources of iron include red meats; liver; dried fruits such as apricots, prunes, and raisins; and pinto beans. Fair food sources of iron include carrots, beans, spinach, peas, sweet potatoes, and peaches.

C. Transfusions: Transfusions of packed red cells are reserved for patients with severe symptomatic anemia in whom a rapid rise in hemoglobin concentration is desired. If evidence of heart failure is present, transfuse very slowly. Parenteral diuretics and partial exchange transfusion may be of value.

Course & Prognosis

Progressive anemia will result unless medicinal or dietary therapy is instituted and the underlying abnormality, if any, corrected. Improvement is then prompt, with a significant rise in the reticulocyte count appearing in 4–7 days and a rise in the hemoglobin concentration of approximately 0.1–0.2 g/dL/d. Simple iron deficiency anemia due to a low intake of iron should clear rapidly, but the presence of other deficiencies, congenital malformation, infection, or poor compliance with therapy may alter this favorable outcome.

Administration of iron, 2 mg/kg/d for full-term infants and 4 mg/kg/d for premature infants at high risk for developing iron deficiency during the first year, either in infant formulas or in a medicinal form, has been recommended to prevent iron deficiency.

ANEMIA OF CHRONIC INFECTION & INFLAMMATION

Chronic infection or inflammation is often accompanied by anemia. These chronic conditions may inhibit iron exchange by blocking the release of catabolized iron from the red cells to the reticuloendothelial system. This form of anemia is often confused with iron deficiency anemia because the red cells may be slightly hypochromic (although they are often normal) and the reticulocyte count is low. However, in anemia of chronic infection, serum ferritin and serum iron levels are normal but total iron binding capacity is low, and the anemia does not respond to iron therapy. Anemia may be an important clue to an underlying inflammatory condition; it resolves when the primary disease process is controlled or resolves.

HYPOPLASTIC & APLASTIC ANEMIAS

Congenital hypoplastic anemia (Diamond-Blackfan anemia, aregenerative pure red blood cell anemia) is associated with decreased hemoglobin concentration and reticulocyte counts and increased MCV. Erythroid precursors are decreased or absent from the marrow. Patients usually respond well to corticosteroids; transfusions may be necessary. They are short children with some skeletal malformations.

Children may develop transient erythroblastopenia, with a temporary halt in red cell production manifested by normochromic normocytic anemia, reticulocytopenia, and the absence of red cell precursors in otherwise normal bone marrow. Erythroblastopenia is usually preceded by viral or bacterial infection and can be differentiated from congenital hypoplastic anemia by the presence of normal MCV. Recovery is spontaneous without treatment, often within a few weeks.

Fanconi's anemia (hypoplastic anemia, often with pancytopenia) presenting after the age of 2 years may occur as an autosomal recessive disorder in association with abnormal pigmentation, skeletal anomalies (eg, absent, hypoplastic, or supernumerary thumb; hypoplastic or absent radius), retarded growth, hypogonadism, small head, renal anomalies, micro-phthalmos, strabismus, and abnormalities of the reproductive tract (Fanconi's syndrome). The anemia usually responds to tes-tosterone. Bone-marrow transplantation, using a nonrelated HLA donor, may be considered.

Acquired aplastic anemia, characterized by pancytopenia and hypoplasia of the bone marrow, is rare in childhood. The peak incidence is 3–5 years of age. Acquired aplastic anemia may occur as a toxic reaction to drugs or chemicals (chloramphenicol, phenylbutazone, sulfonamides, solvents, insecticides), as a com-plication of infection, or in association with early manifestations of leukemia. Although anemia appears to be acquired in most cases, no causative agent can be identified in as many as 50% of patients (idiopathic aplastic anemia). Children with aplastic anemia present with pallor, fatigue, fever, and an increased ten-dency to bleed. Hepatosplenomegaly and adenopathy do not re-sult. The prognosis of aplastic anemia without treatment is ex-tremely poor; fewer than 10% of patients recover fully within 5 years, and 50% of patients die from hemorrhage or infection within the first 6 months. Bone marrow transplant from a sibling with HLA-compatible marrow may increase survival to 50–70% and is presently the treatment of choice. When bone marrow transplant is not feasible, the use of immunosuppressive therapy with high-dose corticosteroids and antithymocyte globulin (ATG) may be of value in up to 50% of patients.

HEMOLYTIC ANEMIAS

GENERAL CONSIDERATIONS

Anemias associated with shortened red cell survival are known as **hemolytic anemias.** Symptoms and signs may include pallor, jaundice, and splenomegaly. Gallstones may develop after many episodes of hemolysis.

Anemia, reticulocytosis, hyperbilirubinemia, and hapto-globinemia are the hallmarks of hemolytic anemia. The urine and feces contain increased amounts of urobilinogen. With severe chronic hemolysis, erythroid hyperplasia of the bone marrow often results in widening of the marrow spaces, and hemosid-erosis may occur.

Classification of Congenital Hemolytic Anemia

 A. Membrane Defects: Congenital spherocytosis, congenital elliptocytosis, congenital stomatocytosis, pyropoikilocytosis.

 B. Hemoglobinopathies: Sickle cell anemia, sickle syndromes (S-thalassemia, SC hemoglobinopathy), thalassemias, unstable hemoglobins.

 C. Enzyme Defects: Glucose-6-phosphate dehydrogenase (G6PD) deficiency, pyruvate kinase deficiency, hexokinase deficiency.

Classification of Acquired Hemolytic Anemia

 (1) Autoimmune process.

 (2) Infections.

 (3) Toxins and drugs.

 (4) Thermal injury.

 (5) Disseminated intravascular coagulation (DIC).

 (6) Hemolytic-uremic syndrome.

 (7) Transfusion reactions.

AUTOIMMUNE HEMOLYTIC ANEMIA

In autoimmune hemolytic anemia, hemolysis occurs when IgG or IgM antibodies are directed against and cause damage to the red cell membranes. IgG-mediated disease is primarily an extravascular process, with hemolysis occurring in the spleen or other reticuloendothelial organs, while IgM-mediated disease is generally intravascular. The cause of anemia cannot be identified in about half of affected patients (idiopathic autoimmune hemolytic anemia). Anemia in other patients may be associated with immunoproliferative disorders (lupus erythematosus, Hodgkin's disease, and other malignant diseases), infection (especially Epstein-Barr virus, cytomegalovirus, other viral infections, and *Mycoplasma*), and chronic inflammatory conditions (ulcerative colitis).

The clinical presentation may be indolent (IgG-mediated) or fulminant (complement and IgM-mediated), with symptoms of anemia (pallor, malaise, and congestive heart failure); jaundice (common), with increased amounts of urobilinogen in the urine; and splenomegaly, which is more common with the IgG-mediated form of the disease. Laboratory findings include reticulocytosis and the presence of microspherocytes. Results of direct Coomb's tests are positive for IgG antibody in sera from patients with IgG-mediated anemia; negative for IgG antibody in sera from those with IgM-mediated anemia; and positive for complement fixation with IgM and, occasionally, with IgG.

If hemolysis is mild, treatment may not be necessary. Most patients respond to prednisone administered for 7–10 days; an initial larger dose is decreased over the next few days. Splenectomy is reserved for patients with severe hemolysis that is unresponsive to an adequate trial of corticosteroids. Other immunosuppressive therapy may be used in refractory cases. Transfusions are given if signs of congestive heart failure are present.

ISOIMMUNE HEMOLYTIC ANEMIA

Isoimmune hemolytic anemia is seen primarily in the newborn and is due to incompatibility with maternal Rh, ABO, or other antibodies. It may also occur with transfusion reactions in patients of all ages. Findings are similar to those of autoimmune hemolytic anemia. After the source of exogenous antibody has been discontinued, the anemia is usually self-limited. However, exchange transfusion may be required, especially in infants with Rh incompatibility.

CONGENITAL (HEREDITARY) SPHEROCYTOSIS

Congenital spherocytosis is a hereditary (dominant) disease caused by excessive destruction of abnormally shaped cells (spherocytes). The disease may be discovered during a "hypoplastic" crisis, when the reticulocyte count may be very low and the degree of anemia more profound than usual. Crises may occur at periodic intervals.

Other members of the family may have overt or subclinical disease with slight spherocytosis and increased osmotic fragility of red blood cells (demonstrated in hypotonic saline solution). In a small percentage of cases, no family involvement can be determined.

Findings include spherocytosis, increased osmotic fragility, and reticulocytosis. The osmotic fragility test will show abnormal findings if the blood is incubated (at 37°C for 24 hours) prior to testing. The autohemolysis test results are also abnormal. Maturation arrest of all elements in the marrow may be present at times of aplastic crises. Neonates may show early and exaggerated jaundice. Cholelithiasis may develop in the second or third decade.

Treatment is by splenectomy, ideally performed in patients after the age of 5 years. Until the time of splenectomy, folic acid, 1 mg/d, should be given. Pneumococcal vaccine provides additional protection.

Following removal of the spleen, the underlying defect of the red cells persists, but most patients will have a complete remission of hemolysis and anemia.

HEREDITARY ELLIPTOCYTOSIS

Hereditary elliptocytosis (ovalocytosis) is a congenital disease characterized by numerous elongated or oval cells. It is usually asymptomatic, but some patients may have mild to severe hemolysis. In the latter, splenectomy may be of value.

NONSPHEROCYTIC HEMOLYTIC ANEMIA ASSOCIATED WITH DEFICIENCIES OF VARIOUS ENZYMES

Glucose-6-phosphate dehydrogenase (G6PD) deficiency is the most common red cell enzyme deficiency. It is inherited as an X-linked recessive trait and primarily affects males. It occurs in high frequency in Africa, the Mediterranean region, the Arabian peninsula, the Middle East, and Southeast Asia. Approximately 15% of black males in the USA are affected. Chronic anemia usually is not present, but acute episodes of severe hemolysis occur with exposure to certain drugs and foods, including primaquine, sulfonamides, aspirin, acetanilide, phenacetin, nitrofurans, synthetic vitamin K, compounds containing naphthalene, and fava beans. The deficiency is less severe in blacks, and hemolysis usually occurs only with use of antimalarials and nitrofurans. Hemolysis is occasionally precipitated by infections. A screening test and assay are available, although the results may be normal if the reticulocyte count is high. With drug exposure, there is a rapid development of hemolytic anemia with hemoglobinuria and subsequent reticulocytosis. Blood transfusion may be required for treatment.

A number of other red cell enzyme deficiencies have been reported as causes of chronic nonspherocytic hemolytic anemia.

They are usually autosomal recessive disorders and hence symptomatic only in the homozygous state. These disorders are very rare except for pyruvate kinase deficiency. Specific diagnosis is made by red cell enzyme assays. Patients with pyruvate kinase deficiency show a partial response to splenectomy. Transfusions may be needed for hemolytic or aplastic crises.

HEMOLYTIC-UREMIC SYNDROME

Hemolytic-uremic syndrome (HUS), occurring mainly in children between the ages of 6 months and 6 years, is characterized by (1) a sudden onset of Coomb's negative hemolytic anemia; (2) thrombocytopenic purpura; and (3) nephropathy (with renal insufficiency, azotemia, and acute renal necrosis). Occasionally, there is central nervous system involvement, with drowsiness and convulsions. Clinical manifestations of the syndrome are frequently preceded by diarrhea (commonly due to enterovirus infection or *Escherichia coli*) or, less often, by an upper respiratory tract infection, with an intervening symptom-free period of 1–10 days. Helmet-shaped and fragmented red cells are the hallmark of HUS. Fibrinogen and platelet deposition in the arterioles may play a very significant role in the pathophysiology of HUS.

Packed red blood cell transfusions and peritoneal dialysis are often required as supportive measures. Heparin, inhibitors of platelet function, or activators of fibrinolysin have been used in treatment, with very little effect on the course of the renal disease. Complete recovery from hematologic manifestations usually occurs, but permanent impairment of renal function is not uncommon.

HEMOGLOBINOPATHIES

BETA-THALASSEMIA

Beta-thalassemia is a relatively common anemia that is due to an inherited defect in the synthesis of the beta chains of hemoglobin. It may occur in a severe homozygous form, characterized by pronounced changes in the blood and in various organ systems; or it may occur as the "trait," with little or no anemia and no systemic changes. It is most common in Italians, Greeks, and Southeast Asians and occurs occasionally in other persons of non-Mediterranean background. A mild beta-thalassemia gene (β^+) also occurs in blacks of African descent and may be seen in association with the sickle gene.

Beta-Thalassemia Major
(Cooley's Anemia)

The homozygous form is a severe hypochromic microcytic anemia with hemolysis in the bone marrow that starts in the first year of life. Both parents will be carriers of the "trait." Symptoms are secondary to the anemia and include pallor, characteristic facies due to widening of the tabular bones of the skull, jaundice of varying degrees, and hepatosplenomegaly. Laboratory findings (Table 19–2) include hypochromic microcytic anemia, anisocytosis, poikilocytosis, basophilic stippling, and decreased fragility of the red cells, with the presence of target cells, nucleated erythrocytes, and an increased number of reticulocytes in the peripheral blood. Levels of hemoglobin F and A_2 are elevated; hemoglobin A is usually absent. Findings on x-ray include changes in the bones due to extreme marrow hyperplasia. These changes include widening of the medulla, thinning of the cortex, and coarsening of trabeculation (the so-called hair-on-end appearance).

Beta-Thalassemia Minor
(Thalassemia Trait)

In the heterozygous form, evidence of mild anemia and splenomegaly may be present. Blood smears show hypochromic microcytosis, target cells, anisocytosis, and poikilocytosis. The diagnosis may be confirmed by finding elevated levels of F or A_2 hemoglobin on hemoglobin electrophoresis.

Treatment

Transfusions are the only effective means of temporarily overcoming the anemia in severe cases, but they do not alter the underlying disease. Other hematopoietic agents are entirely ineffective and should not be used. Iron chelation with deferoxamine combined with hypertransfusion (maintaining hemoglobin at levels greater than 11 g/dL) are very beneficial. Chronic hypoxia and iron loading are the significant factors in the production of myocardial and hepatic damage.

Table 19–2. Summary of findings in abnormal hemoglobin diseases and thalassemia.

	Hemoglobin Type	Anemia	Spleno-megaly	Pain Crises	Increased Blood Destruction	Target Cells	Sickling (Solubility) Test	Microcytosis	Hypochromia
Normal adult and child	AA (A2↑ F⁺)	0	0	0	No	0	0	0	0
Normal newborn	AF↑	0	0	0	No	0	0	0	0
Iron deficiency anemia	AA (A2⁺ F⁺)	+ to + + + +	±	0	No	±	0	+ to + + + +	+ to + + +
β⁰-Thalassemia major	F↑ A2↑	+ + + +	+ + + +	0	Yes	+ +	0	+ + + +	+ + + +
β⁰-Thalassemia minor	A (S2↑ F↑)	±	0 to +	0	±	+	0	+ +	+ +
β⁺-Thalassemia-hemoglobin C disease	CA (F⁺)	+	0	0	Yes	+ + +	0	+	+
β⁰-Thalassemia-hemoglobin E disease	EF↑	+ + +	+ + +	0	Yes	+ +	0	+ +	+ + +
Sickle cell trait	AS (A2⁺ F⁺)	0	0	0	No	+	+	0	0
Sickle cell anemia	SS (A2⁺ F↑)	+ + +	±	+ + +	Yes	+ +	+	0	0 to +
Sickle-β⁺-thalassemia	SA (A2↑ F↑)	+	±	+	Yes	+ +	+	+	+ +
Sickle-β⁰-thalassemia	S (A2↑ F↑)	+ + +	+ + +	+ + +	Yes	+ +	+	+	+ +
Sickle-hemoglobin C disease	SC (F↑)	+	+ +	+ +	Yes	+ + +	+	0	0

Sickle-hemoglobin D disease	SD (A_2* F†)	++	++	Yes	+	+	+
Hemoglobin C trait	AC (F*)	0	0	No	+++	0	0
Homozygous hemoglobin C disease	CC (F*)	+	0 to ++	Yes	+++++	0	0
Hemoglobin D trait	AD (A_2* F*)	0	0	No	0	0	0
Hemoglobin E trait	AE (F*)	0	0	No	±	0	0
Homozygous hemoglobin E disease	EE (F†)	+	±	Yes	+++	0	++
α-Thalassemia "carrier"	A (A_2* F*)‡	±	0	0	±	0	+
α-Thalassemia-hemoglobin H disease	AH (A_2* F*)‡	++	++	++	+++	0	+++
α-Thalassemia-fetal hydrops	Bart's	++++	++++	++	+++	0	+++

* A_2 is usually <4% and F <2% of the total hemoglobin.
† Elevated levels.
‡ Hemoglobin Bart's is also present at birth.

Splenectomy may be necessary when the spleen is so large as to produce discomfort or if an acquired hemolytic component is superimposed on the primary disease. However, the risk of infection in splenectomized children with thalassemia is great, and prophylactic penicillin and pneumococcal vaccine should be given.

Course & Prognosis

In the past, in spite of repeated transfusions, children with thalassemia major generally died within the first 2 decades of life from intercurrent infections or from hemochromatosis. However, with hypertransfusion and iron chelation, the outlook is greatly improved. Gallbladder stones frequently develop in patients surviving to the early teens. Thalassemia trait is associated with a normal life span.

ALPHA-THALASSEMIA

Alpha chains of the hemoglobin molecule are genetically determined by 4 genes, and thus gene deletions can result in 4 degrees of alpha-thalassemia.

Type 2 is always mild, and its incidence is high in Africa, Arabia, the Middle East, and Southeast Asia. The heterozygote with one gene deletion (—α/$\alpha\alpha$) is called the "silent carrier" and is clinically and hematologically normal, while the homozygote with 2 deletions (—α/—α) is called the "carrier" and has microcytosis, hypochromia, and mild or borderline anemia.

Type 1 alpha-thalassemia occurs primarily in Southeast Asians. The heterozygote, or "carrier," with 2 gene deletions (—/$\alpha\alpha$) also shows microcytosis, hypochromia, and mild anemia, while the homozygous state (—/—) results in fetal hydrops and is incompatible with life.

In the double heterozygous state for type 1 and type 2 alpha-thalassemia, genes are deleted (—/—α); this is known as hemoglobin H disease and occurs in people of Southeast Asia. It is characterized by splenomegaly and a moderate hemolytic anemia with microcytosis, hypochromia, and elevated reticulocyte count.

Diagnosis is made in the mild forms by ruling out iron deficiency (by documenting a normal serum iron or ferritin level) and beta-thalassemia minor (A_2 and F hemoglobin levels are normal in alpha-thalassemia). Hemoglobin Bart's (4 gamma globins) is present in varying degrees in all forms in the newborn infant, while hemoglobin H (4 beta globins) is present in the older child with the 3-gene deletion disease.

Treatment is not needed in the mild forms. Hemoglobin H disease may require transfusions, but most patients maintain hemoglobin levels of 9–10 g/dL.

SICKLE CELL ANEMIA

Sickle cell anemia is an inherited abnormality of hemoglobin (hemoglobin S). It has a high incidence in blacks but is also common in people of the Arabian peninsula, Sicily, and certain parts of Greece, Turkey, and India. In hemoglobin S, the amino acid valine replaces glutamic acid in the beta chain. Although the sickle trait occurs in about 8% of the black population in the USA, the disease with anemia occurs in only fewer than 1% of blacks.

Clinical Findings

A. Symptoms and Signs: Onset of clinical manifestations may be at any time in the first decade. Findings include fever, headache, "pain crises" in the long bones, osteopathy (particularly of metacarpals and phalanges), abdominal pain and tenderness, pallor, jaundice, splenomegaly (in the very young), hepatomegaly, cardiomegaly, and hemic heart murmurs. The spleen ceases to function normally early in childhood, and "autosplenectomy" occurs as a result of repeated infarctions. Patients with sickle cell anemia have an increased resistance to malarial infection; an increased susceptibility to bacterial sepsis, osteomyelitis, pneumonia, and meningitis [in particular with encapsulated organisms (eg, pneumococcus)]; and an increased risk of anesthetic complications. Enuresis and nocturia may be present. Strokes are commonly seen in young teens. In the severe form, the general picture is of poor health, development, and nutrition. Folic acid deficiency is common. During a pain crisis, the disease may mimic acute surgical abdomen or osteomyelitis. Aplastic crises may occur, with diminished red cell production superimposed on rapid destruction. In young infants, acute anemia and hypovolemia can be seen with splenic sequestration.

B. Laboratory Findings: Sickle-shaped red blood cells are seen in peripheral blood smears. Other findings include normochromic anemia, reticulocytosis, nucleated red blood cells in the peripheral blood, leukocytosis, hyperbilirubinemia, increased excretion of urobilinogen, increased lactate dehydrogenase levels, and an abnormal electrophoretic pattern, with 75–100% hemoglobin S and increased amounts of fetal hemoglobin. There is excretion of excessive quantities of urine of low specific gravity. Severe hyponatremia may occur during a crisis. Zinc deficiency has been described and may contribute to short stature and delayed onset of puberty.

Heterozygotes (carriers of sickle trait) may be identified by use of a screening test (Sickledex Test; sodium metabisulfite test) and hemoglobin electrophoresis. Characteristically, 25–45% hemoglobin S is found. Heterozygotes are not anemic and—except for conditions with extreme hypoxia—are asymptomatic. Hematuria has rarely been associated with sickle trait.

Treatment

Parenteral fluid therapy, analgesics, and transfusion for severe anemia and crises are the only consistently effective methods of treatment. Placing the patient in oxygen during the crisis and giving bicarbonate have been recommended.

Adequate hydration of the patient at the onset of a crisis sometimes obviates the need for transfusions. Because infection exacerbates sickling of the patient's red blood cells, all infections should be treated promptly and vigorously. Sepsis and meningitis should be suspected in the febrile infant.

Folic acid, 1 mg/d, should be given. The routine administration of prophylactic penicillin has been advocated, and pneumococcal vaccine should be given at 2 years of age.

Course & Prognosis

The course is determined by the severity of the sickling tendency and resulting hemolysis, the frequency and duration of crises, and the age of the patient. Interference with growth, nutrition, and general activity is common, although many patients lead active lives with persistent hemoglobin levels of 7–9 g/dL.

Repeated transfusions in conjunction with iron chelation using deferoxamine, designed to maintain hemoglobin levels above 11 g/dL and thus decrease bone marrow production of S hemoglobin, is recommended for patients with strokes and heart failure.

SICKLE-HEMOGLOBIN C DISEASE

Sickle-hemoglobin C disease is caused by the inheritance of hemoglobin S from one parent and hemoglobin C from the other. It occurs almost exclusively in the black population.

The clinical manifestations are similar to those of sickle cell anemia but tend to be less severe. Splenomegaly may be present and acute enlargement may occur with splenic sequestration crises. Proliferative retinopathy is common after the age of 15 years. Diagnosis is suspected by the presence of mild to moderate anemia, elevated reticulocyte counts, many target cells on blood smear, and positive results in the sickling (solubility) test. It is confirmed by hemoglobin electrophoresis.

Treatment is similar to that for sickle cell anemia and is primarily symptomatic. Patients should receive annual retinal examinations and be treated with laser therapy if retinopathy is detected.

BLEEDING DISEASES IN CHILDHOOD

GENERAL CONSIDERATIONS

Family History

A family history of easy bruising and excessive bleeding is valuable in the following disorders: (1) hemophilia (males only), (2) von Willebrand's disease (both sexes), (3) congenital thrombocytopenia or platelet dysfunction syndromes, (4) hereditary hemorrhagic talangiectasia, and (5) deficiencies of factor II, V, VII, X, or XI (Table 19–3), which may be hereditary and not X-linked.

Physical Examination

Bleeding disorder should be considered in patients with abrupt changes in the pattern or severity of bruising and bleeding, unexplained bleeding from a circumcision, or excessive bleeding at the site of surgery.

Bruises on the extremities are found in many normal children following trauma and usually have no clinical significance.

Table 19–3. Blood clotting factors and hemorrhagic disorders.

	Clotting Factor[1]	Deficiency Disease
I	Fibrinogen	Afibrinogenemia
II	Prothrombin	Prothrombin deficiency disease
III	Tissue thromboplastin	None
IV	Calcium (Ca^{2+})	None
V	Proaccelerin; labile factor	Factor V deficiency disease
VII	Proconvertin; stable factor	Factor VII deficiency disease
VIII	Anthihemophilic factor (AHF)	Hemophilia A, AHF deficiency disease, factor VIII deficiency disease
IX	Plasmin thromboplastin component (PTC); Christmas factor	Hemophilia B, PTC deficiency disease, Christmas disease, factor IX deficiency disease
X	Stuart factor; Stuart-Prower factor	Stuart-Prower factor deficiency disease, factor X deficiency disease
XI	Plasma thromboplastin antecedent (PTA)	Hemophilia C, PTA deficiency disease, factor XI deficiency disease
XII	Hageman factor	None
XIII	Fibrin-stabilizing factor	Fibrin-stabilizing factor deficiency disease, factor XIII deficiency disease
	α_2-Antiplasmin	α_2-Antiplasmin deficiency disease

[1] Factor VI is not considered a separate entity.

In infants and young children, petechiae can occur in the head and neck areas in association with crying, vomiting, or coughing without an underlying bleeding disorder. Mucocutaneous bleeding usually signifies an abnormality in the number or function of the platelets or a defect of the blood vessels. Hemarthrosis is uncommon except in patients with hemophilia.

Laboratory Examination

Recommended basic screening tests include bleeding time, platelet count, partial thromboplastin time (PTT), prothrombin time (PT), thrombin time, and fibrinogen level.

HEMOPHILIA

Hemophilia is an X-linked bleeding disorder transmitted by females to their male offspring. Hemophilia A (factor VIII deficiency, or classic hemophilia) accounts for 75% of cases of hemophilia. It occurs with an incidence of 1 per 10,000 population. Affected family members generally have equally severe disease. Hemophilia B (factor IX deficiency, or Christmas disease) is much less common. It may demonstrate the same levels of severity.

Clinical Findings

A. Symptoms and Signs: Symptoms vary greatly in severity; many cases are mild. Severely affected patients are usually identified at circumcision or in the first year of life and show signs of increased bruising and hemarthrosis (most commonly of the knees, ankles, or hips) as they begin to walk. In older patients, bleeding may occur in the large muscle groups, the genitourinary tract, or the skin. Mucous membrane bleeding, usually of the mouth, is also a problem after even a minor laceration or contusion. Mildly affected patients rarely have bleeding into the joints and may present with hemophilia only at the time of a surgical procedure.

B. Laboratory Findings: See Table 19–4. The PTT should be determined and other screening tests performed in any suspected case of hemophilia. If the PTT is prolonged, a specific-factor assay should be carried out to confirm the diagnosis.

Treatment

A. Specific Measures: The specific treatment of hemophilia consists of replacing missing clotting factors. In hemophilia A, only fresh frozen plasma, factor VIII concentrates, or cryoprecipitates of fresh plasma should be used. In younger children, this can be achieved with cryoprecipitates (100 units of factor VIII per plastic pack); for dosage, see Therapeutic Blood Fraction Products, below. Older children with hemophilia A may be given factor VIII concentrates (250 units per vial). The use of concentrates carries a higher risk of hepatitis and HIV than does use of cryoprecipitates. In hemophilia B, use of stored or fresh blood, fresh frozen plasma (200–250 units per plastic pack), or a concentrate or factor IX (Konyne; 550 units of factor IX per vial) is effective; for dosage, see Therapeutic Blood Fraction

Table 19-4. Differentiation by laboratory findings of coagulation defects.

Disease[1]	Bleeding Time	Platelet Count	One-Stage Prothrombin Time	Partial Thromboplastin Time	Thrombin Time
Afibrinogenemia	N or ↑	N	↑	↑	↑
Factor II deficiency disease	N	N	↑	N or ↑	N
Factor V deficiency disease	V[2]	N	↑	↑	N
Factor VII deficiency disease	N	N	↑	N	N
Factor VIII deficiency disease	N	N	N	↑	N
Factor IX deficiency disease	N	N	N	↑	N
Factor X deficiency disease	N	N	↑	↑	N
Factor XI deficiency disease	N	N	N	↑	N
Factor XIII deficiency disease	N	N	N	N[3]	N
Thrombasthenia (Glanzmann's syndrome)	↑	N	N	N	N
Thrombocytopenia	↑	↓	N	N	N
Von Willebrand's disease	↑	N	N	↑	N

[1] See Table 19-3 for synonyms of factor deficiency diseases.
[2] Variable.
[3] Diagnosis should be suspected in a congenital bleeding state when results of all screening tests are normal. Diagnosis is confirmed by showing instability of fibrin clot in urea.
[4] Associated with factor VIII deficiency in most cases.

654

Products, below. In mild cases, because of the danger of hepatitis and other infections, frozen plasma should be used instead of pooled plasma when possible. Dosage is determined by the severity of the bleeding to be treated. Hypervolemia may be avoided by the use of antihemophilic factor (AHF) or factor VIII concentrates. Adjuncts to transfusion therapy include (1) aminocaproic acid (Amicar), 100 mg/kg every 6 hours, for oral mucosal bleeding; and (2) desmopressin acetate (DDAVP, Stimate), 0.3 μg/kg given intravenously in 20 mL of saline over a 20-minute period, in mild cases of hemophilia A.

B. Special Problems:

1. Head Injuries–Head injuries can be life-threatening in severe hemophiliacs. Raise the factor VIII level to over 50% as soon as possible. Patients with head injuries often require repeated factor replacement initially and, if intracranial hemorrhage is documented, for several weeks.

2. Hemarthroses–In patients with bleeding into the joints or muscles, raise the factor VIII levels to 20–40% every day until the pain becomes less severe. Bed rest and a short period of immobilization (usually for no longer than 24 hours) are indicated. This is followed by a slow increase in the level of physical therapy, with an active range of motion to regain full use of the joint. Acetaminophen is usually sufficient for analgesia if the patient receives transfusion early. Aspirin should not be used. Subsequent therapy includes exercises (passive and then active) and prevention of ankylosis in the unphysiologic position. Repeated episodes of joint effusion may be treated by corticosteroids.

3. Sutures–If suturing is necessary, raise the factor VIII levels to 20–40% every other day until the sutures are removed, including the day of removal.

4. Hematuria–Patients with hematuria may be treated with a short course of corticosteroids.

5. Open Wounds–In patients with bleeding from open wounds (skin, tooth socket), follow the measures outlined above, as indicated. Do *not* cauterize the wounds. Use sutures as necessary. Use pressure bandage and application of cold to accessible areas.

Prognosis

The prognosis has been much improved since the institution of home care programs of prophylactic therapy. Many of the problems of chronic joint disease have been avoided. Major problems of repeated administration of blood products include the increased risk of hepatitis, HIV infection, and the development of inhibitors (IgG antibody) to factor VIII in 10–15% of patients. With home transfusion programs, most patients are successful in leading independent and nearly normal lifestyles.

VON WILLEBRAND'S DISEASE

Von Willebrand's disease is a mild to severe familial bleeding disorder characterized by abnormalities of the factor VIII molecule. In severe classic von Willebrand's disease, the factor VIII procoagulant activity (VIIIc), the portion of the molecule that corrects the bleeding time defect and supports ristocetin-induced aggregation of platelets (VWF), and the factor VIII measured by heterologous antibodies (VWF antigen) are reduced. Variants of the disorder are seen in which combinations of the above portions of the factor VIII molecule are defective.

Patients with von Willebrand's disease show skin and mucous membrane bleeding (epistaxis, menorrhagia). The disorder is usually inherited as an autosomal dominant trait. The bleeding time is usually prolonged, as is the PTT, although in mild cases measurements of VIIIc, VWF antigen, and VWF must be made to establish the diagnosis.

Treatment consists of infusions of fresh frozen plasma, 10–15 mL/kg; cryoprecipitate, one plastic pack per 5 kg; or desmopressin acetate (DDAVP, Stimate), 0.3 µg/kg in 20 mL of saline, given intravenously over a 20-minute period.

DISSEMINATED INTRAVASCULAR COAGULATION

Disseminated intravascular coagulation (DIC) is characterized by intravascular consumption of plasma clotting factors (factors I, II, V, and VIII) and platelets; fibrinolysis, with production of fibrin split products; widespread deposition of fibrin thrombi that produce tissue ischemia and necrosis in various organs (principally the lungs, kidneys, gastrointestinal tract, adrenals, brain, liver, pancreas, and skin); generalized hemorrhagic diathesis; microangiopathic hemolytic anemia, with fragmented, burred, and helmet-shaped erythrocytes; and shock and death. The disorder has been found in association with infections, surgical procedures, burns, neonatal conditions (especially sepsis and respiratory distress syndrome), neoplastic diseases, severe hypoxia and acidosis, other metabolic disorders, and a variety of miscellaneous causes (eg, hemangioma, transfusion reactions, drugs, hemolytic-uremic syndrome). The clinical manifestations depend on the systems involved. Laboratory findings include proglonged PT and PTT, elevated levels of monomers and fibrin split products, decreased levels of fibrinogen, and decreased platelet counts.

Therapy consists of treating the underlying cause (sepsis, acidosis, hypoxia) and replacing clotting factors with fresh frozen plasma, 10 mL/kg, or platelet transfusions. In the newborn with severe DIC, exchange transfusion may be of value. Indications for use of heparin include severe meningococcemia, associated large vessel thrombosis, purpura fulminans, and promyelocytic or monoctic leukemia.

THERAPEUTIC BLOOD FRACTION PRODUCTS

When therapeutic blood fractions are given, there is a risk of transmitting the virus of serum hepatitis; this risk is greater when pooled blood fraction products are given than when single donor products are used. There appears to be an increased risk of acquired immune deficiency syndrome (AIDS) with the use of factor VIII concentrates or other blood components; however, this risk is decreased by use of heat-treated concentrates and screening of donors.

AHF or Factor VIII Concentrates (Cryoprecipitates)

Cryoprecipitates are a blood bank product made from fresh frozen plasma. One pack of cryoprecipitate contains 100 units.*

A dosage of one pack per 5 kg usually gives a factor VIII level of 40%. The usual level desired is 40%; however, 20% is the minimal hemostatic level.

Factor VIII Concentrate (Monoclate)

A. Indications: For therapy of factor VIII deficiency (hemophilia A or von Willebrand's disease).

B. Dosage and Administration: Reconstitute lyophilized material (stored at 4°C) and inject by intravenous push. Dose is calculated as follows:

---

* A unit of clotting factor is the amount contained in the equivalent of 1 mL of fresh plasma with 100% clotting activity.

Units* of factor VIII = Desired level in percent × 0.5 × Weight (kg)

Factor IX Complex
Factor IX complex (Konyne, Profilnine, Proplex) is a lyoph-ilized product containing factors IX, II, VII, and X in vials of 500 units.*

A. Indications: For therapy of congenital factor IX defi-ciency (hemophilia B, or Christmas disease) or severe liver disease.

B. Dosage and Administration: Dosage is calculated as follows:

Units* of factor IX = Desired level in percent × Weight (kg)

PURPURAS

Purpura is defined as large, multiple, raised hematomas due to a reduced number of platelets, abnormal function of platelets, or to a defect in or abnormality of the vascular system.

Purpuras are classified by the clinical picture, the quantity and quality of platelets.

Classification of Common Purpuras
A. Quantitative Defect of Platelets (Thrombocytopenia):
1. Idiopathic thrombocytopenic purpura.
2. Disseminated intravascular coagulation.
3. Hemolytic uremic syndrome.
4. Familial thrombocytopenia.
B. Qualitative Defect of Platelets (Platelet Dysfunction):
1. Congenital.
2. Acquired: secondary to drugs, infection, inflammation, or uremia.

---

* A unit of a clotting factor is the amount contained in the equivalent of 1 mL of fresh plasma with 100% clotting activity.

C. Non-thrombocytopenic Purpura:
1. Henoch-Schönlein purpura.
2. Vasculitis.
3. Vitamin C deficiency (scurvy).
4. Drug and toxins.
5. Collagen disorders (Ehlers-Danlos syndrome, Marfan's syndrome).
6. Psychogenic purpura.

IDIOPATHIC THROMBOCYTOPENIC PURPURA

Idiopathic thrombocytopenic purpura (ITP) of childhood is a relatively common bleeding disorder associated with antiplatelet antibodies. It usually occurs in patients between 2 and 10 years of age and commonly follows an infection by 2–3 weeks. In the neonatal period, ITP may follow infection or exchange transfusion or may be due to maternal isoantibodies to the infant's platelets.

Clinical Findings
A. Symptoms and Signs: Bleeding into the skin or from the nose, gums, and urinary tract is the most common symptom. Bleeding into joints or from the bowel is uncommon. Central nervous system bleeding occurs rarely but may be fatal. Petechiae are usually present. Splenomegaly is rare.
B. Laboratory Findings: The platelet count is decreased, and large platelets are seen. Red and white blood cell counts are normal unless severe hemorrhage has occurred. Megakaryocytes in the bone marrow are normal or increased in number. Antiplatelet antibodies may be demonstrated. Coagulation studies are usually normal.

Treatment
A. Specific Measures: There is no specific treatment for ITP. Corticosteroids are useful in 60–70% of children. Indications include patients with severe thrombocytopenia with bleeding and patients at increased risk for central nervous system bleeding. More recently, intravenous gamma globulin has been useful in acute bleeding episodes and also in steroid-refractory thrombocytopenia.
B. General Measures: Pressure and application of cold packs help in arresting bleeding. Eradicate infection, if present.

Antibiotics and chemotherapeutic agents are not contraindicated unless the thrombocytopenia is the result of the administration of these drugs. All medications should be given either orally or intravenously. Avoid intramuscular injection.

Other measures include red cell transfusions to maintain hemoglobin level, prevention of trauma, institution or maintenance of regular diet with vitamins, and avoidance of aspirin. Watchful waiting for 6–8 months is appropriate for many cases.

C. Surgical Measures: Splenectomy is indicated (preferably after age 5 years) if conservative therapy has been carried out for 12 months without improvement, if the disease process is very severe, if the patient is becoming progressively worse in spite of other therapy, if the patient develops a sudden intracranial hemorrhage, or if the patient is having recurrent bouts of severe ITP for which no definite cause can be determined. Splenectomy is also indicated in an adolescent girl with severe menorrhagia. Splenectomy should be avoided, if possible, in children under 5 years of age.

Course & Prognosis

Symptoms may continue to be evident for 2 weeks to several months, but significant improvement usually occurs within 4–6 weeks. Eighty-five percent of children who have ITP with normal or elevated numbers of megakaryocytes in the bone marrow will have a spontaneous and complete recovery within 6 months even without therapy, but spontaneous recovery may occur after a period of as long as 3 to 5 years. A few will need splenectomy.

Adolescents tend to have a more chronic course, often associated with the presence of other antibodies. ITP during adolescence may be associated with subsequent development of subacute lupus erythematosus.

ANAPHYLACTOID OR "VASCULAR" PURPURA

Anaphylactoid purpura (Henoch-Schönlein purpura) is a disease of unknown cause. Many patients have a history of allergic manifestations. Some cases of anaphylactoid purpura follow infections; a causal relationship with group A streptococcal infections has been suspected. The disease tends to recur, and it may persist over a span of many years.

Clinical Findings

A. Symptoms and Signs: Abdominal and joint pains are present in most children, but the pain may occur only in the abdomen (Henoch type) or only at the joints (Schönlein type). The pain may precede the development of skin lesions. Either small or large joints may be involved. The joints are painful and swollen. Ecchymoses, petechiae, or bullous hematomas may be present. The initial lesions may resemble urticaria, but these soon become hemorrhagic. They often appear first around the elbows and ankles and over the buttocks. Gastrointestinal hemorrhage is common in children. Nephritis may occur early or after the acute phase in over one-third of cases. Intussusception may develop. Associated group A beta-hemolytic streptococcal infections are frequent.

B. Laboratory Findings: Platelet counts and most hemotologic test results are normal. Eosinophilia may be present in some cases. Serum IgA levels may be elevated.

Treatment

In many cases, treatment is either unnecessary or ineffective.

A. Specific Measures: Therapy includes eradication of infection, using appropriate antibiotics, and elimination of allergens (if known). Antihistamines may be given if allergy is suspected. Anti-inflammatory agents are useful.

B. General Measures: Corticosteroids may relieve joint and abdominal symptoms. They do not appear to benefit patients with renal complications.

Course & Prognosis

The disease may vary in degree from mild to quite severe. Complete recovery eventually occurs in most cases, but recurrences are not infrequent and nephritis occasionally persists and may become chronic.

HYPERCOAGULABILITY

Hypercoagulability describes an increased tendency toward thrombosis in patients with certain underlying conditions. Patients at risk include those with a deficiency of antithrombin III, protein C, protein S, or plasminogen; newborns and older children with central plastic catheters or prosthetic heart valves;

postsurgical patients who required prolonged periods of bed rest and thus are susceptible to venous stasis; and patients with vasculitic processes (eg, systemic lupus erythematosus, nephritis, hemolytic-uremic syndrome) in which damaged endothelium provides a nidus for clot formation and occasionally for progression to a more generalized thrombotic process.

The patient may present with pain and swelling of the involved extremity or with symptoms of a stroke. Homozygous protein C deficiency can present as purpura fulminans in neonates. The diagnosis of thrombosis is made by physical examination. Supporting laboratory findings may include decreased levels of fibrinogen, antithrombin III, protein S, or protein C; decreased platelet counts; or elevated levels of fibrin split products or monomers. However, laboratory findings may be normal even in the face of significant thrombosis.

Treatment involves interruption of the triggering process. Heparinization should be instituted at once, with the goal of increasing the PTT to 1½ times that of normal. Plasma heparin level is better correlated with therapeutic heparinization, so if available heparin levels should be followed. Give a loading dose of heparin, 100 units/kg, followed by a continuous intravenous infusion of 15–20 units/kg/h. Newborn infants may require an increased dosage. Prolonged anticoagulation for 4–6 months with warfarin (Coumadin) may be indicated once the initial thrombosis is controlled. Antiplatelet agents (aspirin, sulfinpyrazone, dipyridamole) may be indicated in cases in which a prosthetic heart valve or arterial malformation is the inciting agent for thrombosis. The use of fibrinolytic agents (streptokinase, urokinase) in children is reserved for extensive and life-threatening thrombus. Local urokinase therapy is very useful in catheter-induced thrombosis.

ABSENCE OF THE SPLEEN

Absence of the spleen, whether the absence is congenital, postsurgical, or functional (secondary to an underlying disease such as sickle cell anemia), places the child at significant risk for infection with encapsulated bacteria. The overall incidence of infection is 5–10%, with the fatality rate 30–50%. Those at greatest risk are children under 2 years of age and children with recent splenectomy (ie, for the first 2 years following splenectomy). The classic hematologic finding is the presence of Howell-Jolly bodies on the peripheral blood smear.

The tendency to develop life-threatening infections is markedly decreased in older children when the spleen is removed for trauma, ITP, portal vein thrombosis, local tumors, or hereditary spherocytosis. The risk is significant in those with histiocytosis, inborn errors of metabolism, hepatitis with portal hypertension, thalassemia, and Wiskott-Aldrich syndrome.

The use of prophylactic antibiotics remains controversial. Some physicians use continuous penicillin prophylaxis in the younger child, while others treat at the first sign of fever. Polyvalent pneumococcal vaccine (Pneumovax 23), which protects against infection with many of the common pneumococci, should be given to all children prior to splenectomy and repeated in early childhood if given to infants under 2 years of age. Prompt therapy with antibiotics in any child with fever has been recommended.

SPLENOMEGALY

Splenomegaly is generally an indicator of systemic disease. The tip of the spleen may normally be felt in 30% of newborn infants and 5% of young children. Splenomegaly may be associated with other signs of systemic disease, particularly adenopathy, hepatomegaly, petechiae, ecchymoses, and jaundice. Less common causes of splenomegaly include acute viral infections (particularly infectious mononucleosis and cytomegalovirus), hematologic disorders (eg, congenital or acquired hemolytic anemias, red cell membrane defects, disorders of hemoglobin synthesis), metabolic diseases (eg, Gaucher's disease, Niemann-Pick disease), vascular abnormalities (eg, portal hypertension), and, rarely, cysts (eg, splenic cysts). When leukemia or other malignant neoplastic disease presents with splenomegaly, it is usually accompanied by adenopathy, pallor, and other signs of systemic illness.

Evaluation of patients with splenomegaly should include an assessment of the complete blood count, platelet count, peripheral blood smear, and reticulocyte count. Other studies may include tests for viral infection, liver-spleen scan, work-up for hemolytic anemias, and bone marrow examination for evaluation of storage diseases.

NEUTROPENIA

Neutropenia, a total granulocyte count below 1000 μL, may result from poor release of granulocytes from the bone marrow, decreased survival of granulocytes in the circulation, or abnormalities of granulocyte production and development. The congenital forms of neutropenia include (1) cyclic neutropenia, occurring at 2- to 4-week intervals in association with mucous membrane ulcers, cervical lymphadenopathy, and stomatitis; (2) benign chronic neutropenia, which may be genetically transmitted (as a dominant or recessive trait), with manifestations of mild infection; (3) severe congenital neutropenia, transmitted as a recessive trait, with life-threatening infection in early infancy; (4) Shwachman-Diamond syndrome, with metaphyseal chondrodysplasia, dwarfism, pancreatic exocrine insufficiency, anemia, and thrombocytopenia; (5) cartilage-hair hypoplasia, with short limb dwarfism, abnormally fine hair, and T cell deficiencies; and (6) Chédiak-Higashi syndrome. Acquired neutropenias are the most common forms of childhood neutropenia and are induced by an autoimmune mechanism. Viral infections are the commonest reason for neutrophil antibodies causing both leukopenia and neutropenia. Atypical lymphocytosis and monocytosis are common associated findings. Drugs and toxins may cause neutropenia.

Benign forms of neutropenia may not require therapy. In other forms, infections should be treated with appropriate antibiotics. Patients with neutropenia associated with acute suppression of the bone marrow from cytotoxic drugs should be treated with broad-spectrum antibiotics; growth factors such as G-CSF or Gm-CSF are useful in some forms of neutropenia. Leukocyte transfusion has a limited value.

IMMUNOLOGIC DEFICIENCY SYNDROMES

Immunologic deficiency diseases are characterized by (1) increased susceptibility to bacterial, viral, and fungal infections; (2) a generalized or selective deficiency in the serum immunoglobulins; (3) a diminished capacity (in varying degrees) to form circulating antibodies or to develop cellular immunity (delayed hypersensitivity) after an appropriate antigenic stimulus; and (4) clinical and immunologic variability. Several broad categories are definable based upon whether the defect originates with a disturbance of antibody-producing lymphoid cells (B cells) or with thymus-derived cells that mediate cellular immunity (T cells).

Classification of Immunologic Disorders
A. Immunoglobulin Deficiencies:

1. Infantile X-linked agammaglobulinemia (IgG, IgA, or IgM deficiency).

2. Selective immunoglobulin deficiency (dysgammaglobulinemia).

3. Acquired hypogammaglobulinemia.

4. Transient hypogammaglobulinemia of infancy.

B. Cellular Immune Deficiency with "Normal" Immunoglobulins:

1. Thymic dysplasia (Nezelof type).

2. DiGeorge's syndrome (congenital absence of thymus and parathyroids; third and fourth pharyngeal pouch syndrome).

C. Combined Immunoglobulin and Cellular Immune Deficiencies:

1. Congenital–

a. Severe combined immunodeficiency (Swiss type agammaglobulinemia, thymic dysplasia).

b. Wiskott-Aldrich syndrome (dysgammaglobulinemia and progressive cellular immunity deficiency).

2. Acquired–

a. Lymphoid neoplasms.

b. Iatrogenic conditions (steroid or antimetabolite therapy).

c. Acquired immune deficiency syndrome (AIDS).

Clinical Findings
A. Signs and Symptoms: In patients with immunoglobulin deficiency disease, recurrent pyogenic bacterial infections predominate, and chronic otitis media, sinusitis, and bronchiectasis are especially common. In agammaglobulinemia, viral infections (such as measles, varicella, and mumps) are weathered without incident. In individuals with cellular immunity defects, progressive vaccinia has been a frequent complication, and vaccination should be avoided. Candidal infections are not uncommon in such patients, and unusually severe infections with cytomegalovirus, herpesvirus, and *Pneumocystis* occur as well. In the acquired forms, malignant disorders of the lymphoreticular system occur with increased frequency. AIDS, which has been reported in children with hemophilia and in infants born to infected moth-

ers (eg, IV drug abusers), is often difficult to distinguish from congenital deficiency disease.

Laboratory Findings

Diagnosis is based on results of the following.

(1) Quantitative immunochemical determination of the serum levels of IgG, IgM, and IgA.

(2) Isohemagglutinin determination. These antibodies to the blood group substance belong for the most part to the IgM class. They are normally present after about 1 year of age in all individuals of blood groups A, B, and O. Therefore, their absence is presumptive evidence of IgM deficiency.

(3) Absolute lymphocyte count. The count is 4000–6000/μL in normal children but reduced in patients with cellular immunity deficiency (especially in patients with severe combined immunodeficiency).

(4) Examination of bone marrow for plasma cells.

Confirmatory tests include the following:

(1) Results of immunization with well-characterized antigens (eg, diphtheria toxoid, tetanus toxoid) in terms of specific antibody production and plasma cell development.

(2) Presence of germinal center formation, plasma cells, and small lymphocytes in a biopsy of the regional lymph node taken 1 week after antigenic stimulation.

(3) Reaction to *Candida* and mumps skin tests.

(4) Induction of contact dermal hypersensitivity with dinitrochlorobenzene.

(5) Results of in vitro tests of lymphocyte function [common mitogens: phytohemagglutinin (PHA), concanavalin A (ConA), and pokeweed mitogen].

Treatment

Treatment for patients with immunoglobulin deficiency consists of replacement therapy with immune globulin, which is chiefly IgG. Give loading dose of 200 mg/kg intravenously and then 100 mg/kg every 3 or 4 weeks. Preparations consisting solely of IgM and IgA are not yet available. Preparations suitable for intravenous use (Gamimune, Sandoglobulin) are now available.

Each individual has genetically determined differences in gamma globulins, and isoimmunization can occur as a result of giving genetically foreign gamma globulin. Since isoimmunization may have some deleterious effects, injudicious administration of immune globulin should be avoided.

Therapy of cellular immune deficiencies with bone marrow transplant is still experimental, but results are improving.

Neurologic & Muscular Disorders | 20

Joanne Janas, MD, & Alan R. Seay, MD

SEIZURES

Seizure is defined as a sudden, transient disturbance of brain function usually manifested by involuntary motor, sensory, autonomic, or psychic phenomena, alone or in any combination. Often an alteration or loss of consciousness occurs. These alterations in neurologic function are accompanied by abnormally synchronized electrocerebral discharges. The term "epilepsy" denotes recurrent seizures that are not caused by identifiable, correctable metabolic disturbances. "Convulsion" refers to seizures that consist of generalized muscular rigidity or rhythmical jerking.

Seizures occur in approximately 2 to 4% of children and most childhood seizure disorders remit spontaneously. Factors that increase the probability of seizure recurrence when antiepileptic drugs are discontinued include the presence of preexisting neurologic deficits or mental retardation, age of onset less than 2 years, and an abnormal EEG at the time of discontinuing medication. Seizures that were difficult to control initially or that required multiple antiepileptic drugs for control are more likely to recur than seizures that were quickly suppressed by monotherapy.

Seizures and epilepsy are often classified as symptomatic (the cause is known) and idiopathic (the cause is unknown). When "idiopathic" is used to describe seizures, it usually implies a genetic etiology or predisposition. The younger the infant or child, the more likely the etiology for the seizure can be identified. Genetically determined epilepsy usually begins between ages 4 and 16 years. Seizures and epilepsy should not be considered idiopathic or genetic in origin until a thorough history, neurologic examination, and appropriate laboratory evaluation have excluded other possible causes.

Status epilepticus, neonatal seizures, and their therapy are discussed in other sections of this book (see Chapters 7 and 28). Table 20–1 lists the major types of childhood seizures along with their most prominent clinical manifestations and their treatment. Table 20–2 lists several of the most common antiepileptic drugs and outlines their dosages and most frequent, potential side effects.

Clinical Findings

The history provides the most important information upon which to make the diagnosis of seizures or epilepsy. Some seizures, complex partial seizures for example, may be preceded by an aura. An aura usually consists of transient subjective symptoms such as numbness, tingling, visual disturbances, or a vague feeling of fear and anxiety. Although the patient may remember the aura, they are amnestic for the remaining portion of the seizure. Some patients with generalized seizures experience a more vague prodrome to their seizure. They may feel tired or have a recognizable malaise for several minutes or hours before the seizure occurs.

Proper classification of seizures depends upon an accurate and detailed account of the sequence of events leading to and during the spell. Did the patient become pale or cyanotic before he or she fell, began to jerk, or lost consciousness? Was the patient able to respond to any type of stimulation during the episode? Did the patient lose consciousness completely? Did the patient fall, become rigid, jerk rhythmically, or go limp? How long did the stiffening or jerking last? What parts of the body were involved by the stiffness or rhythmical jerking? What was the patient's behavior like after the episode was over?

A careful analysis of all factors related to an episodic event or spell will aid in determining if the patient had an epileptic seizure, possibly a pseudo-seizure, or some other nonepileptic type of event. The proper classification of the seizures is necessary to make an accurate diagnosis, prognosis, and appropriate management decisions.

Febrile Seizures

Febrile seizures are very common, occurring in 2 to 3% of children. Simple febrile seizures are generalized and brief usually lasting less than 5 minutes. They are typically triggered by viral-like infections of the ear, pharynx, or gastrointestinal tract. Febrile seizures probably reflect a genetically determined lowered

Table 20–1. Common seizure types in children.

Seizure Type	Age at Onset	Clinical Manifestations	Treatment
Partial			
Simple partial (focal motor, sensory, autonomic)	Any age	No disturbance of consciousness. May involve any part of the body. May spread in fixed pattern (Jacksonian) and become generalized.	Carbamazepine, phenytoin, phenobarbital or primidone; valproic acid may be a useful adjunct.
Complex partial	Any age	Associated with impairment of consciousness. The aura may be sensation of fear, epigastric discomfort, odd smell or taste, visual or auditory hallucination. Proceeds to period of altered behavior which may be characterized by walking in a daze, facial movements such as eye blinking, lip smacking, chewing or other automatisms. If the seizure consists solely of an aura, it is classified as a partial seizure. Complex partial seizures may also generalize.	Carbamazepine, phenytoin, phenobarbital or primidone. Valproic acid may be a useful adjunct.
Generalized			
Tonic–Clonic	Any age	Loss of consciousness, ± bladder/bowel incontinence, postictal confusion.	Phenobarbital, carbamazepine, phenytoin, valproic acid, primidone.
Absence	3–15 years	Lapses of consciousness lasting about 10 seconds. Often in clusters. May see automatisms of face and hands.	Ethosuximide or valproic acid.
Myoclonic	Any age (usually 2–7 years)	Abrupt contractions of one or more muscle groups, singly or irregularly repetitive. Usually no or only brief loss of consciousness.	Valproic acid, clonazepam, ethosuximide. Imipramine is adjunct. Diazepam. Ketogenic or medium chain triglyceride diet. ACTH or corticosteroids in West's Syndrome.

Table 20-2. Common antiepileptic drugs.

Drug	Preparation	Therapeutic Plasma Concentration	Dose (Initial & Maintenance)	Laboratory Monitoring	Side Effects	Drug & Clinical Interactions
Carbamazepine (Tegretol)	Tabs: 200 mg Chewable Tabs: 100 mg Suspension: 100 mg/5 mL	6–12 μg/mL	*Under 6 yrs:* Initial: 10 mg/kg/24h PO—QD or BID or 100 mg/dose BID Increment: up to 20 mg/kg/24h *6–12 yrs:* Initial: 10 mg/kg/24h PO—QD or BID up to 100 mg/dose BID Increment: 100 mg/24h at intervals of 1 day (TID or QID) until best response Maintenance: 20–30 mg/kg/24h—PO, TID or QID **Max. dose:** 1000 mg/24 h *Adolescent & Adult:* Initial: 200 mg BID Increment: 200 mg/24h at intervals of 1 day using TID or QID schedule until best response. Maintenance: 600–1200 mg/24h —TID or QID **Max.** 12–15 yr: 1000 mg/24h **Max.** Adult: 1200 mg/24h	Baseline CBC, LFTS, electrolytes. Monitor for hematologic and hepatic toxicity.	*Acute:* Diplopia, drowsiness, vertigo, blurred vision, dry mouth, stomatitis, SIADH, dehydration, headache, diarrhea, constipation, paresthesia *Chronic:* Enzyme induction, aplastic anemia, leukopenia, hepatic enzyme elevation, nervousness	*Increased by:* INH Propoxyphene Erythromycin Hepatic disease *Decreased by:* Phenobarbital Phenytoin Primidone Pregnancy

Drug	Dosage Forms	Serum Level	Dose	Comments	Interactions
Clonazepam (Klonopin)	Tabs: 0.5, 1.0, 2.0 mg Suspension: 80 µg/5 mL or 0.1 mg/mL	0.013–0.072 µg/ml	*Children:* Up to 10 yr or 30 kg: Initial: 0.01–0.05 mg/kg/24h —Q8h PO Increment: 0.25–0.5 mg/24h Q3 days, up to **maximum** maintenance dose of 0.1–0.2 mg/kg/24h —Q8h *Adolescent & Adult:* Initial: 1.5 mg/24h PO—TID Increment: 0.5–1 mg/24h Q3 days **Max. dose: 20 mg/24h**	CNS depression, drowsiness and ataxia common. May cause behavioral changes, and other CNS symptoms: increased bronchial secretions. GI, CV, GU and hematopoietic toxicity may occur. Use with **caution** in renal impairment.	*Increased by:* Phenytoin *Decreased by:* Phenobarbital
Diazepam (Valium)	Tabs: 2, 5, 10 mg Oral solution: 1.5 mg/mL Injection: 5 mg/mL		*Status Epilepticus:* *Neonate:* 0.5–1.0 mg/kg/dose IV Q15–30 min × 2–3 doses *1 mo–5 yr:* 0.2–0.5 mg/kg/dose IV Q15–30 min (**max. total dose: 5 mg**) *>5 yrs:* 0.2–0.5 mg/kg/dose IV Q15–30 min (**max. total dose: 10 mg**). *Adolescent & Adults:* 5–10 mg/dose IV Q10–15 min (**Max. total dose: 30 mg**)	Hypotention and respiratory depression may occur. Use with caution in glaucoma, shock, and depression. Give undiluted no faster than 2 mg/min. **Do not** mix with IV fluids. Not recommended for use in neonates. In status epilepticus, diazepam must be followed by long-acting anticonvulsants.	

(continued)

Table 20-2. Common antiepileptic drugs *(continued)*.

Drug	Preparation	Therapeutic Plasma Concentration	Dose (Initial & Maintenance)	Laboratory Monitoring	Side Effects	Drug & Clinical Interactions
Ethosuximide (Zarontin)	250 mg tabs 250 mg/5 mL elixir	40–100 µg/mL	*3–6 yr:* Initial: 250 mg/24h —QD—BID PO Increment: Increase 250 mg/24h every 4–7 days Maintenance: 20–40 mg/kg/24h—QD *>6 yr:* Initial: 500 mg/24h —QD—BID PO Increment: Same as above Maintenance: Same as above *Adolescents & Adults:* Initial: 750 mg/24h —QD Increment: Same as above Maintenance: Same as above **Max. children's dose:** 1500 mg/24h	Baseline CBC and LFTS. Monitor for hematologic and hepatic changes.	*Acute:* Nausea, vertigo, loss of appetite, vomiting, hiccups, headache *Chronic:* Loss of sleep, nervousness, occasional psychotic behavior, hiccups, headache, reported exacerbation of major seizures. May also see lupus-like syndrome, dystonia.	
Lorazepam (Ativan)	Tabs: 0.5, 1, 2 mg Injection: 2, 4 mg/mL		*Status Epilepticus:* *Infants and Children:* 0.03 to 0.05 mg/kg/ dose IV up to **max.** of		May cause respiratory depression, especially in combination with other sedatives. May	

672

| Phenobarbital (Luminal) | Tabs: 8, 15, 16, 30, 32, 60, 65, 100 mg
Caps: 16 mg
Elixir: 15, 20 mg/5 mL
Injection: 30, 60, 65, 130 mg/mL | 15–40 µg/ml | 4 mg/dose. May repeat in 15 to 20 min. × 1.
Adolescents & Adults: 2.5–10 mg/dose IV. May repeat in 15–20 min.
Children: 10–20 mg/kg/dose IV × 1, then 5–10 mg/kg/dose Q20 min PRN
Max. total dose: 40 mg/kg
Adolescents & Adults: 300–800 mg IV × 1, then 120–240 mg/dose Q20 min PRN
Max. total dose: 1–2 g
Chronic
Anticonvulsant:
Neonates:
Initial: 2–4 mg/kg/24h—QD—BID × 2w
Maintenance: 5 mg/kg/24h—QD—BID
Infants: 5–8 mg/kg/24h—QD—BID
Children: 3–5 mg/kg/24—QD—BID
Adolescents & Adults: 120–250 mg/24h—QD—BID (1–3 mg/kg/24h) | Baseline CBC
Folate/B12 if anemic | also cause sedation, dizziness, mild ataxia, mood changes, rash and GI symptoms. Injectable product may be given rectally. IV administration may cause respiratory arrest or hypotension. **Do not exceed** push of 1 mg/kg/mn.
Acute: Sedation, behavior disturbances, ataxia
Chronic: Difficulty with concentration, cognitive deficit, loss of initiative, hemorrhage in newborn. | *Increased by:*
Valproic acid
Phenytoin
Lasix
Amphetamines
Renal disease
Hepatic disease
Decreased by:
Clonazepam
Alkaline urine |

(continued)

Table 20-2. Common antiepileptic drugs *(continued)*.

Drug	Preparation	Therapeutic Plasma Concentration	Dose (Initial & Maintenance)	Laboratory Monitoring	Side Effects	Drug & Clinical Interactions
Phenytoin (Dilantin)	Chewable Tabs: 50 mg (Infatab) Prompt Caps: 30, 100 mg Extended Release Caps: 30, 100 mg Susp.: 30, 125 mg/5 mL Injection: 50 mg/mL	10–20 µg/mL	*Status Epilepticus:* 15–20 mg/kg IV **Max. dose:** 1000 mg/24h *Maintenance for Seizure Disorders: Infants/Children:* 4–7 mg/kg/24h—QD—BID IV or PO *Adolescents & Adults:* 300–400 mg/24h— QD—BID IV or PO	Baseline CBC, LFTS	*Acute:* Drowsiness, ataxia, diplopia, nystagmus, gastrointestinal complaints, choreoathetosis, nausea, hypotension (after injection). *Chronic:* Gingival hyperplasia, hypertrichosis, coarse facies, Dupuytren's contractures, folate deficiency, megaloblastic anemia, osteomalacia with vitamin D deficiency, peripheral neuropathy, encephalopathy, cerebellar dysfunction, endocrine dysfunction (adrenal, thyroid, diabetogenesis), pseudolymphoma, immunosuppression, agranulocytosis, hemorrhage in the newborn.	*Increased by:* Phenobarbital Valproic acid Ethosuximide Chloramphenicol Disulfiram Isoniazid Dicumarol Amphetamines Tolbutamide Chlordane Phenylbutazone Alcohol (acute) Aminosalicylic acid Chlorpromazine Estrogens Methylphenidate Prochlorperazine Sulfaphenazole Hepatic disease *Decreased by:* Phenobarbital Carbamazepine Clonazepam Chronic ETOH Reserpine ? Theophylline Pregnancy Renal disease

Drug	Preparations	Levels / Labs	Dosing	Toxicity	Interactions / Notes
Primidone (Mysoline)	Tabs: 50, 250 mg Susp.: 250 mg/5 mL	Phenobarbital: 15–40 mg/L Mysoline: 8–12 mg/L Follow both (?)	*<8 yrs:* Initial: 125 mg/24h QD PO Increment: 125 mg/24h weekly PO Maintenance: 10–25 mg/kg/24h—TID—QID PO *>8 yrs–Adults:* Initial: 250 mg/24h QD PO Increment: 250 mg/24h weekly PO Maintenance: 0.75–1.5 g/24h—TID—QID PO	Metabolizes to Phenobarbital, so at risk for same toxicities. *Acute:* Sedation, vertigo, nausea, unsteadiness *Chronic:* Behavior disturbances in the young, loss of libido, difficulty with concentration, hemorrhagic disease in newborn.	Mononucleosis Acute Hepatitis May decrease effectiveness of OBC pills. Induces liver enzymes. *Increased by:* Valproic Acid Clonazepam *Decreased by:* Phenytoin
Valproic acid	Caps: 250 mg Syrup: 250 mg/5 mL Sprinkles: 125 mg caps	Baseline CBC, LFTS	*PO:* Initial: 10–15 mg/kg/24h—QD—TID Increment: 5–10 mg/kg/24h at weekly intervals to max. of 60 mg/kg/24h Maintenance: 30–60 mg/kg/24h QD—TID *PR:* Syrup diluted 1:1 may be given PR using the same doses as those given PO.	*Acute:* Drowsiness, gastrointestinal disturbances (nausea and vomiting) *Chronic:* Alopecia, weight gain, weight loss, tremor, ankle swelling, amenorrhea, hyperammonemia, unexplained stupor, granulocytopenia, hepatic enzyme elevation, thrombocytopenia, occasional psychosis	*Increased by:* Hepatic disease *Decreased by:* Carbamazepine Phenytoin Phenobarbital Primidone

Table 20–3. Febrile seizures: Risk factors for non-febrile epilepsy.

- Seizure >15 minutes
- More than 1 seizure in a day
- Focal seizure
- Abnormal neurologic status preceding the seizure (eg, cerebral palsy)
- <1 year of age
- Positive family history for epilepsy

seizure threshold to the stress of fever. Risk factors for the later development of non-febrile epilepsy are presented in Table 20–3. Even with these factors, the risk of epilepsy in later life is only about 15 to 20%. After a single febrile seizure, the probability of recurrence is estimated to be 20 to 40%. In general, recurrence of febrile seizures does not alter the longterm, uniformly good outlook.

After the child with a febrile seizure is examined and the history reviewed, laboratory studies including CBC, electrolytes, glucose, calcium, EEG, and brain imaging studies may be done selectively and tailored to the needs of each child. Bacterial meningitis must be excluded either by careful clinical observation or by spinal fluid examination. Because signs of bacterial meningitis are often absent in young infants, a lumbar puncture is recommended in most instances.

Most neurologists elect not to use antiepileptic drugs after one or a few simple febrile seizures. The benign nature of febrile seizures and their natural tendancy to spontaneously remit must be balanced against the potential side effects and risks of antiepileptic drugs. Fever control with sponging and antipyretics and appropriate use of antibiotics for suspected bacterial infections constitute the major treatment approach. In addition, the family is reassured about the benign nature of simple febrile seizures. In some cases, an electroencephalogram is obtained, but in patients with simple febrile seizures the results are normal. In about 10% of patients, an EEG done within a few days of the seizure will show nonspecific, sometimes asymmetric occipital slowing. These changes resolve within two weeks after the seizure. In young infants, EEG results seldom aid in predicting the likelihood of future seizure recurrence, either febrile or non-febrile.

Differential Diagnosis of Seizures

Several conditions closely resemble seizures and should be considered in the differential.

A. Breatholding Spells: These episodes occur in children between the ages of 6 months and 3 years and are precipitated by trauma, fright, anger, frustration, or emotional upset. After beginning to cry, the child holds his breath and then passes out. During these spells the child may become cyanotic or pale. The child may have a few rhythmical clonic jerks, but he or she rapidly regains consciousness. Family history for similar spells is positive in about 30% of cases. The EEG is typically normal. No medical therapy is effective at preventing recurrences, and treatment is reassurance to parents about the benign nature of these spells. These spells spontaneously remit by 4 to 6 years.

B. Sleep Disturbances: Night terrors most frequently affect children between 3 and 10 years old. The episodes occur 30–90 minutes after the child falls asleep. The child begins to cry and appears fretful, agitated, and frightened. The child may be noted to have small, dilated pupils and profuse sweating. The spell lasts several minutes, then the child becomes quiet again. The child has no memory for the spell upon awakening. Results of polysomnography and EEGs are normal. No therapy is indicated. The spells spontaneously cease.

Nightmares are vivid, frightening dreams that usually occur in the early morning hours. All or only a portion of the dream is remembered. Occasionally, bizarre behavior may occur during nightmares that resembles a complex partial seizure. In selected cases, an over-night EEG may help to differentiate seizures from nightmares and other sleep disturbances.

C. Migraine: Migraine attacks can result in a variety of motor and sensory deficits that resemble partial or generalized seizures. The presence and location of a throbbing headache helps to differentiate migraine attacks from seizures. Migraine episodes in general last longer than seizures and are less likely to be followed by amnesia. Family history is positive for migraine in about 65 to 75% of children with migraine. Propranolol, amitriptyline, and cyproheptadine are useful prophylactic agents for migraine.

Confusional migraine attacks most often affect children in late childhood and early adolescence. These attacks may occur in a child with a previous history of migraine or as the initial presentation of migraine. The child has sudden onset of delirium, confusion, agitation, and combative behavior. Throbbing headache is usually present when the child's sensorium begins to clear. Symptoms can last from 1 to 2 hours or occasionally as long as 20 to 24 hours. Resolution usually occurs after a short period of sleep. Fortunately, these types of spells are typically infrequent and do not require prophylactic drug therapy.

D. Syncope: Syncope is often precipitated by identifiable factors, and the patient remembers the initial symptoms of lightheadedness, dim vision, generalized weakness, and nausea. Observers notice extreme pallor and profuse sweating. The heart rate and blood pressure may be quite low. Patients regain consciousness rapidly. Occasionally, brief tonic posturing or clonic jerking occurs as a result of generalized, transient cerebral ischemia. Incontinence is rare. EEGs between attacks are normal. The family history is frequently positive for similar syncopal episodes.

E. Shuddering Spells: Shuddering or shivering attacks occur in infancy and may be the early manifestation of a familial, essential tremor. The attacks are brief, lasting several seconds, and are not associated with any impairment of consciousness. Shuddering spells may occur frequently and they tend to occur as the patient awakens from sleep. EEGs are normal and the family histories frequently positive for similar spells as well as for essential tremor.

F. Gastroesophageal Reflux: Reflux of acidic gastric contents can lead to severe abdominal pain and can be accompanied by unusual posturing and movements of the head, neck and trunk. Barium swallow radiographs and gastric pH probe studies are the most frequently used and reliable tests to confirm the diagnosis.

G. Pseudoseizures: Many patients with unquestionable epileptic seizures also have non-epileptic pseudoseizures. These episodes may consist of tonic posturing, bizarre nonrhythmical jerking and thrashing movements, and impaired responsivity. The triggers for such attacks are usually obscure. In many patients, simultaneous EEG/video tape monitoring helps to clarify which spells are epileptic and which are not. A normal or non-epileptiform EEG during a spell usually confirms that a spell is a pseudoseizure.

H. Staring Spells: School teachers often make referrals for suspected seizures in youngsters who have brief staring spells. Non-epileptic inattentiveness may not be observed at home and usually does not cluster in the early morning hours as might be seen in patients with absence seizures. The child can generally be brought out of this spell by verbal or tactile stimulation. An EEG is sometimes used to reassure parents and teachers that the child is not having seizures. Longterm EEG/video tape monitoring may be needed to provide unequivocal distinction between absence seizures and brief non-epileptic staring spells.

ABNORMAL HEAD SIZE & SHAPE

Microcephaly

Microcephaly is defined as a head circumference that is 2 standard deviations or more below the mean for age and sex. The etiology may be primary (malformation, chromosomal anomaly, genetic syndrome) or secondary (infections, birth asphyxia, trauma, malnutrition, systemic disease). Microcephaly at birth indicates that the etiological process affected brain growth in utero. Babies with neonatal asphyxial brain damage will have normal head sizes at birth, but head growth rate will be slower than normal. A family history of small heads may aid in the diagnosis of familial trait microcephaly or, more rarely, autosomal dominant microcephaly. An outline of some common causes of microcephaly is provided in Table 20–4.

Microcephaly may be discovered when the child is evaluated for developmental or neurologic problems. There may be a marked backward slope of the forehead with narrowing of the bitemporal diameter. The fontanelle may be closed earlier than expected and suture lines excessively prominent.

Based on the history and clinical findings, congenital infec-

Table 20–4. Disorders associated with microcephaly.

Genetic/Chromosomal	Trisomy 13, 18, 21
	Lissencephaly
	Rubenstein-Taybi
	Cornelia de Lange
	Familial microcephaly
Toxins	Maternal alcohol
	Antiepileptic drugs
	Maternal PKU
Infections	Congenital viral (CMV, HSV, Toxo)
	AIDS
	Bacterial meningitis
	Viral meningoencephalitis
Metabolic	Perinatal asphyxia
	Hypoglycemia
	Aminoacidopathies
Birth injury	

tions are evaluated by measuring serum antibody titers against CMV, HSV, toxoplasmosis, and rubella virus. The presence of organism-specific anti-IgM antibodies are the most specific diagnostic findings. The comparison of maternal antiviral IgG titers with the infant's antiviral IgG titers or the demonstration of rising IgG titers in the infant postnatally are important alternative ways of documenting probable congenital infections. Serum and urine organic acid screens are occasionally diagnostic. Infants born to women with untreated PKU may suffer severe microcephaly and mental retardation. Karyotyping may be considered in selected cases.

Skull films are rarely helpful in the evaluation of microcephaly. Head CT or MRI scans may aid the diagnosis by demonstrating intracranial calcifications, cerebral malformations, or cerebral atrophy.

The treatment of children with microcephaly is usually supportive and directed at associated motor and sensory deficits and any associated endocrine disturbance, such as diabetes insipidus. Catch-up growth after correction of an underlying metabolic disturbance can occur. Perhaps as many as 80% of children with microcephaly are mentally retarded to some degree.

Macrocephaly

Macrocephaly is defined as a head circumference that is 2 or more standard deviations above the mean for age and sex. A large head may be due to hydrocephalus, true megalencephaly, thickening of skull bone, or the presence of extra-axial fluid accumulations. As with microcephaly, it is important to review familial head circumferences, the onset and progression of the abnormal head size, and the child's developmental progress. A careful family history of abnormal skin pigmentation, cafe-au-lait spots, cutaneous tumors, or neurologic disorders should be obtained that might indicate neurofibromatosis.

A. Hydrocephalus: Hydrocephalus is characterized by increased volume of cerebrospinal fluid in association with progressive ventricular dilatation and may result from impaired reabsorption of CSF (communicating hydrocephalus) or from obstruction of CSF flow through the ventricles and into the subarachnoid space (non-communicating hydrocephalus). A wide variety of disorders, such as hemorrhage, infection, tumors, and congenital malformations can play an etiologic role in development of hydrocephalus.

Clinical features of hydrocephalus include macrocephaly

and excessive head growth rate. Increased intracranial pressure causes irritability, vomiting, loss of appetite, impaired upward gaze, impaired extraocular movements, lower extremity hypertonia, and generalized hyperreflexia. Papilledema may not occur in young infants but usually is present in older children. Without treatment, hydrocephalus can result in progressive loss of vision, loss of consciousness, autonomic failure, and ultimately death.

Hydrocephalus is suspected by the clinical course and physical examination findings and is confirmed by head CT or MRI scans. Treatment of hydrocephalus is directed at providing an alternative outlet for CSF from the intracranial compartment, usually by ventriculoperitoneal shunting. Treatment should also be directed, if possible, at any underlying etiology.

B. Megalencephaly: A large brain may be normal or may be secondary to abnormal neuronal migration or cerebral organization. Hamartomatous proliferation of cerebral tissue is found in patients with neurocutaneous disorders, such as neurofibromatosis, tuberous sclerosis, and hypomelanosis of Ito. Large brains are also characteristic of some storage and neurometabolic disorders, for example, Alexander's disease, Canavan's disease, Krabbe's disease, Tay-Sachs disease, and the mucopolysaccharidoses.

Craniosynostosis

Craniosynostosis, or premature closure of cranial sutures, is usually a sporadic, idiopathic disorder. However, some patients have syndromes such as Apert's and Crouzon's that are inherited and that are associated with characteristic abnormalities of the digits, extremities, and heart. Rarely, craniosynostosis may be associated with an underlying metabolic disturbance such as hyperthyroidism and hypophosphatasia. The most common form of craniosynostosis involves the sagittal suture and results in scaphocephaly, an elongation of the head in the anterior-to-posterior direction. Premature closure of the coronal sutures causes brachycephaly, an increase in cranial diameter from left to right. Unless multiple sutures close prematurely, intracranial volume is not compromised, and the brain's growth potential is not impaired. Neurologic functions are not affected. Surgical management of craniosynostosis is directed at preventing cosmetically unsatisfactory distortions in skull shape.

Arnold–Chiari Malformation

This malformation results from abnormal, incomplete closure of the neural tube during the first month after conception.

The malformation is characterized by elongation and kinking of the brainstem and protrusion of cerebellar tonsils into the foramen magnum. This malformation is usually classified into three types.

Type I consists of elongation and displacement of the caudal end of the brainstem into the spinal canal with protrusion of the cerebellar tonsils through the foramen magnum. Minor to moderate abnormalities of the base of the skull including basilar impression, platybasia, and small foramen magnum may be present. Type I may remain asymptomatic for years, but may cause progressive ataxia, lower cranial nerve paresis, and progressive vertigo in adolescents and adults.

Type II is the most commonly recognized variant and consists of any combination of Type I abnormalities plus a lumbosacral meningomyelocele. Hydrocephalus is present in 90% of cases. Aqueductal stenosis, hydromyelia, and syringomyelia are frequent, associated anomalies.

Type III consists of any combination of Type I or Type II abnormalities plus occipital cranium bifidum with encephalocele or cervical spinal bifida. Hydrocephalus is frequently present and is secondary to aqueductal stenosis, atresia of the fourth ventricle, or narrowing of the foramen magnum.

Dandy–Walker Malformation

Dandy–Walker malformation is characterized by vermal aplasia, cystic enlargement of the fourth ventricle, rostral displacement of the tentorium, and absence or atresia of the foramina of Magendie and Luschka. Although hydrocephalus is usually not present at birth, it often develops within the first few months of life. In those patients who develop hydrocephalus, 90% do so by 1 year of age. On physical examination, there is often a rounded protuberance or exaggeration of the occiput. In the absence of hydrocephalus and increased intracranial pressure, there may be few or no abnormal neurologic findings. An ataxic syndrome, if it develops, usually appears late, but occurs in fewer than 20% of patients. Many of the long-term neurologic deficits result directly from hydrocephalus. Diagnosis of Dandy–Walker malformation is confirmed by head CT or MRI scanning. Treatment is directed at the management of hydrocephalus.

Agenesis of the Corpus Callosum

Agenesis of the corpus callosum, once thought to be a rare cerebral malformation, has been seen frequently with modern neuroimaging techniques. Occasionally agenesis of the corpus callosum appears to be inherited in an autosomal dominant or autosomal recessive pattern. X-linked patterns have also been described. Agenesis of the corpus callosum may be found in conjunction with metabolic defects (pyruvate dehydrogenase deficiency, nonketotic hyperglycinemia). Most cases, however, are sporadic and idiopathic. Maldevelopment of the corpus callosum may be partial or complete. Many patients with agenesis of the corpus callosum have associated seizures, developmental delay, microcephaly, or mental retardation although this malformation may be found coincidentally in normal people. In Aicardi's syndrome, agenesis of the corpus callosum is associated with infantile spasms, mental retardation, lacunar chorioretinopathy, and vertebral body abnormalities. Aicardi's syndrome is inherited in an X-linked dominant pattern.

Lissencephaly

Lissencephaly is a severe malformation of the brain characterized by an extremely smooth cortical surface with minimal development of sulci and gyri. There is primitive cytoarchitectural construction of the cerebral mantle. Pachygyria and agyria are defects in cerebral development that are closely associated with lissencephaly but which represent more restricted forms of migrational abnormalities. Patients with lissencephaly usually suffer from severe neurodevelopmental delay, microcephaly, and infantile spasms. Patients with lissencephaly frequently have additional associated malformations, dysmorphic features, or metabolic abnormalities, as in Walker-Warburg syndrome, Miller–Dieker syndrome, and Zellweger syndrome. Deletion defects of chromosome 17 have been found in some patients. It is particularly important to identify genetic syndromes so that families can be counselled appropriately regarding prognosis and recurrence risk.

DISORDERS AFFECTING MUSCLES

Progressive Spinal Muscular Atrophy

Progressive deterioration of the anterior horn cells is usually inherited in an autosomal recessive pattern and is characterized by severe progressive weakness, hypotonia, and areflexia. Muscle wasting and fasciculations are present in distal extremity, facial, and tongue muscles.

Early infantile onset and rapid progression is characteristic of Werdnig–Hoffman disease, while later onset and slow progression is typical of Kugelberg–Welander disease. Many intermediate forms are also seen. Steady progression and eventual incapacitation are common with early onset forms. Diagnosis is aided by electromyography, which provides evidence of denervation. Serum creatine kinase levels are usually normal. Muscle biopsy confirms the neurogenic nature of the illness. Therapy is supportive only. Death in later childhood results from secondary infections, pulmonary insufficiency, and congestive heart failure.

Muscular Dystrophies

The most common muscular dystrophy in childhood is Duchenne dystrophy. This X-linked recessive disorder becomes symptomatic in young boys by the age of 2 to 3 years. Weakness is first evident in proximal muscles of the lower extremities. The child displays a waddling gait, has progressive difficulty running and walking, and soon becomes unable to stand from a sitting position without using his upper extremities to push or pull the body up. All skeletal muscles and cardiac muscle are affected by the dystrophic process. Enlargement of calf muscles occurs in 70 to 80% of patients. The serum creatine kinase level is 50 to 100-fold above normal. Abnormal EKG findings are present in 75% of patients. The diagnosis is confirmed by the presence of myopathic abnormalities on the EMG and dystrophic changes on muscle biopsy. The recent development of dystrophin staining of muscle biopsies provides the most definitive diagnostic information. No specific therapy is available. Affected boys are wheelchair confined by 12–14 years, and death occurs between 20–30 years.

Myotonic dystrophy is an autosomal dominant form of muscular dystrophy that is characterized by weakness, progressive distal muscle wasting, and inability to relax contracted muscle. When newborns and infants are symptomatic, they may display generalized hypotonia of all extremities as well as facial and tongue muscles. More than 90% of symptomatic neonates inherit the disorder from their mothers. In older patients, frontal balding, cataracts, endocrinopathies, diabetes mellitus, and immunologic disorders are common, non-muscular manifestations, and cardiac dysrrhythmias and cardiomyopathy are frequent. Serum levels of creatine kinase are normal or only mildly elevated. The EMG demonstrates diagnostic myotonic discharges, though these findings may be absent in the neonate and very young infant. Muscle biopsy findings include excess numbers of central nuclei, ring fibers, and excessive proliferation of connective tissue. No specific therapy is available. Painful myotonic contractions can be partially relieved by the use of phenytoin or procainamide. Prognosis is excellent for long survival, but many patients eventually require assistance to walk, and others become confined to a wheelchair.

Congenital Myopathies

Several inherited disorders of muscle structure (nemaline myopathy, central core disease, centronuclear myopathy, and myotubular myopathy) result in generalized hypotonia and nonprogressive or very slowly progressive weakness in children. Many, though not all, of these disorders are symptomatic at birth or during early infancy. Typical features include facial diplegia, weak suck, poor swallow, weak cry, extraocular movement disorders, and respiratory insufficiency. Some infants with these disorders improve with age if they are given early supportive care. Serum levels of creatine kinase are normal or mildly elevated. The EMG confirms nonspecific myopathic changes. Muscle biopsy with light and electronmicroscopic studies are necessary to accurately diagnose these disorders. Specific therapy is not available.

Dermatomyositis

Generalized progressive weakness is the hallmark of dermatomyositis in childhood. Skin rashes on the face and extensor surfaces of joints are typical, but may be fleeting and absent at the time of medical evaluation. Fever, muscle pain, and muscle tenderness are not reliable signs of inflammatory myopathy. Erythrocyte sedimentation rate and serum levels of creatine kinase may be normal or elevated moderately. EMG shows nonspecific signs of a myopathic process, occasionally mixed with fibrillations. Muscle biopsy is necessary and confirms the inflammatory nature of the process. Dermatomyositis is treated with corticosteroids or other anti-inflammatory drugs. Occasionally, therapy with cytoxan, plasmapheresis, and intravenous gammaglobulin is beneficial. Prognosis is variable. Some patients have spontaneous resolution without therapy while other patients are refractory to all modes of therapy. Death can occur from cardiac involvement, associated gastrointestinal hemorrhage, or secondary complications of immunosuppressive therapy.

Myoneural Junction Disorders

Myasthenia gravis is uncommon in early childhood with fewer than 25% of all patients having their onset before 10 years. The disorder is characterized by generalized weakness, dysphagia, dysphonia, easy fatigability, and external ophthalmoplegia. The typical disorder that affects older children and adults is due to defective function of the post-synaptic membrane. IgG antibodies directed against acetylcholine receptors impair the ability of acetylcholine released from the presynaptic nerve terminal to attach to receptor sites in the clefts of the post-synaptic muscle membrane. Approximately 12% of infants born to mothers with this form of IgG antibody-mediated myasthenia gravis develop passively acquired, transient myasthenia gravis that spontaneously resolves in 2–6 months. These infants may be profoundly weak as neonates, but their prognosis is excellent for full recovery if they receive aggressive supportive care, including mechanical ventilation, and anticholinesterase therapy. Other rare forms of non-immune mediated myasthenia gravis have been described in neonates. These forms of congenital, persistent myasthenia gravis also produce generalized weakness. Their diagnostic separation from IgG-mediated myasthenia may require elaborate biochemical and ultrastructural studies of nerve terminals and post-synaptic membrane.

Diagnosis of myasthenia gravis rests upon the patient's response to test doses of acetylcholinesterase inhibitors such as edrophonium and neostigmine. Repetitive nerve stimulation studies provide evidence of defective myoneural junction transmission. Serum levels of anti-acetylcholine receptor antibodies are increased in adults and some children with the immune-mediated forms of myasthenia gravis. Although chest CT scans are often done, thymomas and thymic hyperplasia are uncommon in young children with myasthenia gravis.

Treatment involves general support and administration of anticholinesterase medications. Pyridostigmine is the most commonly used anticholinesterase and it is begun at about 5 mg per kg per day in 4 to 6 divided doses. The dosage is adjusted to the patient's response and to the occurrence of adverse, cholinergic side-effects. Atropine can be used to control some of the cholinergic side-effects. Cholinergic crisis occurs when the patient is overdosed with anticholinesterase medications. The patient becomes weaker and has copious salivation, excessive lacrimation, abdominal cramping, diarrhea, miosis, and hypotension. Distinguishing between a cholinergic crisis and a myasthenic crisis can usually be accomplished by giving the patient an intravenous test dose of edrophonium (0.1 mg per dose, not exceeding a total of 10 mg per dose). The patient will improve if the weakness is from worsening myasthenia, but he or she will worsen if the weakness is the result of cholinergic crisis. Cholinergic crises are managed by discontinuing anticholinesterase medications and using atropine judiciously. In addition to anticholinesterase medications, other treatment options for myasthenia gravis include use of corticosteroids and early thymectomy. Prognosis for full recovery is excellent for infants with passively acquired, transient neonatal myasthenia gravis. The prognosis of the later onset, IgG-mediated myasthenia is generally good for improvement with therapy, and about 10 to 15% of young children with myasthenia eventually have spontaneous remission. For some infants with congenital, non-immune myasthenia, weakness may remain unimproved but stable while others become progressively weaker.

Infant botulism represents another disorder of myoneural junction function important in pediatrics. Typically, infants between 2 and 4 months of age, ingest *Clostridium botulinum* bacteria. The neurotoxin formed by the bacteria in the child's intestinal tract is absorbed systemically, and then attaches with high affinity to the membrane of the presynaptic nerve terminal. The toxin interferes with release of acetylcholine and results in weakness, hypotonia, impaired pupillary light reflexes, impaired extraocular movements, and decreased frequency of stooling. The diagnosis is confirmed by finding abnormalities on repetitive nerve stimulation tests indicative of presynaptic, myoneural junction dysfunction and by identifying botulinum toxin in stool and serum. Treatment is supportive and prognosis excellent for full recovery. Complete recovery, however, can take many months.

Other Disorders

In addition to the neuromuscular disorders described above, acute weakness and flaccidity may result from other diseases. Guillian-Barré syndrome (post-infectious polyradiculoneuritis), acute spinal cord compression, and acute transmyelitis can cause an acute clinical picture of weakness, flaccidity, and hyporeflexia. Associated clinical features such as low back pain, Babinski signs, bowel and bladder dysfunction, and sensory deficits can be used to separate these disorders diagnostically. Spinal fluid examination, nerve conduction studies, and imaging tests will provide additional diagnostic separation.

STROKE IN CHILDHOOD

Stroke is uncommon in children occurring in 2.5 to 2.75 children per 100,000 per year. The onset of symptoms may be acute or subacute and may consist of hemiplegia, aphasia, vertigo, diplopia, or sensory deficits. The differential diagnosis of acute onset focal or lateralized neurologic deficits should include trauma, infection, seizure, and migraine. A thorough evaluation should be done to determine the etiology of stroke so that appropriate therapy and preventive measures can be taken. Congenital cyanotic heart disease is the most common underlying systemic disorder predisposing children to stroke. A search for underlying cardiopulmonary, hematologic, systemic vascular, and intracranial vascular disorders should be undertaken (Table 20–5).

Laboratory investigations are guided by the history and physical findings. Blood studies include CBC, platelet count, sedimentation rate, ANA, electrolytes, BUN, creatinine, coagulation studies, lipid profile, and lactate levels. A urinalysis is performed, and the presence of homocystine in urine determined. An EKG and echocardiogram are indicated for all children suspected of having stroke. Head CT and MRI scans are helpful in defining the location and extent of cerebral infarctions and hemorrhages and may identify abnormal intracranial structures that are etiologically important. The development of MR angiography has drastically reduced the need for invasive, contrast angiography. EEGs frequently show nonspecific abnormalities, but rarely shed light on the cause of stroke.

Initial treatment is directed at correcting the underlying etiology if possible. In patients for whom no etiology is found, stroke recurrence is uncommon, but aspirin or other drugs that inhibit platelet aggregation may be given for several months in an attempt to reduce recurrence risks to a minimum. Anticoagulation therapy is seldom used in children unless a specific coagulopathy is diagnosed. The prognosis for neurologic recovery is excellent for most children. Seizures occur in about 30% of patients at some point in their clinical course and may require antiepileptic medications.

Table 20–5. Conditions associated with stroke children.

Cardiac
  Cyanotic heart disease
  Valvular heart disease
  Cardiomyopathy
  Dysrhythmias
Hematologic disorders
  Polycythemia
  Thombocytopenia
  Thrombocythemia
  Hemoglobinopathies
  Coagulopathies
  Hypercoagulable states
  Leukemia
Systemic vascular disorders
  Carotid dissection
  Vasculitis
  Fibromuscular dysplasia
  Diabetes
  Familial hyperlipidemia
  Hypertension
  Homocystinuria
  Mitochondrial cytopathy
Intracranial vascular anomalies
  Carotid-cavernous fistula
  Venous sinus and cortical vein thrombosis
  Arteriovenous malformation
  Arterial aneurysms
  Moyamoya disease

HEADACHE

Headaches are common in children occurring in nearly 40% of all children under 7 years of age. Migraine occurs in 2.7% of children by 7 years of age and gradually increases to 11% by 14 years. Onset of migraine by age 4 years is not uncommon. In later childhood, migraine affects twice as many girls as boys. A careful description of the headaches, associated circumstances, and associated neurologic and systemic symptoms will usually differentiate migraine from other types of headache (Table 20–6). Potential emotional problems that might trigger headaches should be identified and discussed in detail. A careful, detailed history together with complete general and neurologic examinations will allow correct classification of the headache and will

Table 20–6. Features of common headaches in childhood.

Muscle contraction/tension
Chronic and protracted
Diffuse squeezing or pressure sensation
Band distribution around head
No prodrome
Associated anxiety and depression
Environmental triggers prominent
Migraine
Acute, paroxysmal
Unilateral or bilateral
Temporal, retro-orbital, or frontal
Throbbing or pulsating quality
May have prodrome
Positive family history (75%)
Environmental triggers occasionally
Increase intracranial pressure/traction headache
Intermittent or chronic
Progressively increasing severity or frequency through time
Positional pain
Diffuse pressure
No prodrome
Associated focal or lateralized neurologic deficits

almost always identify those patients whose headaches are caused by an underlying systemic or progressive neurologic illness. If there is evidence of a specific intracranial condition or systemic illness, diagnostic testing and therapy should be directed at the primary disorder.

Migraine headaches usually last 2–6 hours, but many patients have both longer and shorter attacks. The frequency of headaches can vary from 1 or fewer per year to more than 1 headache a day. Between attacks the child is normal. Migraine headaches in children are commonly accompanied by loss of appetite, gastric discomfort, nausea, vomiting, light-headedness, vertigo, and photophobia. Motion sickness is prominent in about 45% of children with migraine. It is uncommon for children to experience or describe scotomata, visual field cuts, sensory and motor disturbances, dysphasia, or hemiplegia. Older children and adolescents may experience acute confusional episodes or subjective distortions of space, time, and body image perceptions (termed the "Alice-in-Wonderland" syndrome) as part of their migraine attack.

EEGs done during or shortly after an attack of migraine are

abnormally slow or mildly dysrhythmic in up to 80% of patients. Between attacks the EEG is normal. Neuroradiologic studies, such as head CT or MRI scans, are usually not indicated unless the history suggests atypical features or unless there are definite neurologic deficits.

Sleep or rest and simple analgesic therapy are the mainstays of therapy for childhood migraine. Acetaminophen alone is often effective and sufficient for children. In children over 12 years of age, severe migraine can usually be controlled with ibuprofen or capsules containing a mixture of acetaminophen, butalbital, and caffeine. If these medicines are ineffective, especially in older children, ergotamine containing medications may be useful. Parenteral doses of chlorpromazine may help patients become calm, relieve their nausea, allow them to fall asleep, and avoid the use of narcotics. For prophylaxis of severe or frequent migraine attacks, propranolol, amitriptyline, and cyproheptadine are useful. Calcium channel blockers, corticosteroids, and narcotics are rarely necessary for the treatment of childhood migraine.

ACUTE CEREBELLAR ATAXIA OF CHILDHOOD
(Acute Cerebellitis)

The syndrome of acute cerebellar ataxia occurs most commonly in children 2–6 years of age. The onset is abrupt and the evolution of symptoms rapid. In about 50% of cases, there is a prodromal respiratory or gastrointestinal viral-like illness or an exanthematous illness 2–3 weeks before onset. Well-known associated viral infections include varicella, rubeola, mumps, rubella, echovirus, poliovirus, infectious mononucleosis, and influenza. Bacterial infections such as scarlet fever and salmonellosis have also been implicated.

Ataxia of the trunk and extremities may be mild or so severe that the child is unable to stand or sit without support. Intention tremors may impair the child's ability to reach for objects. Hypotonia, tremor, horizontal nystagmus, and dysarthria are frequently present. The child is irritable and vomiting is common. Signs of increased intracranial pressure are absent and the fundi are normal. Sensory and reflex examinations are normal.

Cerebrospinal fluid pressure and protein and glucose concentrations are normal. A mild lymphocytosis (up to 30 lymphocyte/mm) may be present in CSF. Attempts should be made to identify the etiologic infectious agent by appropriate virologic, bacteriologic, and immunologic studies on spinal fluid, blood, stool, throat washings and urine. Head CT and MRI scans are normal. The EEG may show mild, diffuse, generalized background slowing, but these changes are nonspecific and the EEG rapidly returns to normal.

The syndrome of acute, parainfectious cerebellar ataxia must be differentiated from actue cerebellar ataxia due to drugs and toxins, for example, phenytoin, phenobarbital, primidone, and lead. An occult neuroblastoma can produce a paraneoplastic syndrome characterized by ataxia, myoclonus, and opsoclonus, and this neoplasm must be excluded in young children with acute onset ataxia. Posterior fossa tumors must be excluded also. On occasion, acute cerebellar ataxia may be the presenting sign of acute bacterial meningitis, systemic vasculitides, trauma, or an inborn error of metabolism, such as Hartnup's and maple syrup urine disease. Acute disseminated encephalomyelitis and multiple sclerosis can cause acute ataxia in older children and adolescents.

Treatment is supportive. The use of corticosteroids is unnecessary in typical parainfectious, acute cerebellar ataxia. Between 80 and 90% of children with acute cerebellar ataxia recover without permanent sequelae within 6–8 weeks. In the remainder, disorders of behavior and learning, persistent ataxia, abnormal eye movements, and speech impairment may persist for months or years, and recovery may remain incomplete.

NEURODIAGNOSTIC PROCEDURES

Electroencephalography (EEG)

EEG is most useful in evaluation of patients with seizures and patients with unexplained loss of consciousness. Activation procedures such as sleep deprivation, hyperventilation, and photic stimulation help to accentuate and provoke electrocortical, epileptiform abnormalities. Prolonged EEG recordings with or without simultaneous video taping of the patient are valuable in the diagnosis of unusual or difficult to treat seizures as well as sleep apnea, narcolepsy, and other sleep disturbances. An electrically silent EEG supports the diagnosis of death if specific clinical and technical criteria have been met. The limitations of EEG in the evaluation of brain function are considerable, and results should be interpreted with caution and with a good understanding of the clinical context. Most EEGs represent about 45 minutes of recording, and it must be remembered that a routine EEG records electrical events at the surface of the brain. About 15% of normal, nonepileptic people show some paroxysmal activity on routine EEG recordings, and many patients with epilepsy have normal, interictal EEGs.

Evoked Potentials

Cortical auditory, visual, and somatosensory evoked potentials can be recorded from the scalp overlying the temporal, occipital, and frontoparietal cortex after appropriate, repetitive stimulation of the retina, cochlea, or skin. Computer averaging is used to recognize and enhance these cortical responses while eliminating asynchronous background electroencephalographic activity. Abnormalities in the evoked potential waves or their latencies indicate disturbances along sensory pathways in the peripheral or central nervous system. These tests are noninvasive, sensitive, objective, reproducible, and relatively inexpensive extensions of the clinical neurologic examination. When combined with other clinical information, results of these tests may be helpful in localizing neurologic deficits and defining their etiology. Since evoked potentials are largely passive examinations, requiring only that the patient remain still, they are particularly useful in the neurologic evaluation of neonates and small children, as well as patients who are unable to cooperate.

Computed Tomographic (CT) Scans

CT scans consist of a series of cross-sectional, computerized radiographs. The procedure carries minimal risk and can be performed on an outpatient basis. Radiation exposure is approximately the same as that from a skull x-ray with shielded gonads receiving only about 0.1 mrad. CT scans are often done before and after the intravenous injection of iodinated contrast material. The contrast material helps to visualize structures or lesions with a high degree of vascularity. Excessive enhancement is also indicative of cerebral capillary damage and disruption of the blood brain barrier.

Magnetic Resonance Imaging (MRI)

MRI is a noninvasive, risk-free technique that uses the magnetic properties primarily of protons in water molecules within the body to produce signals that are converted by computers into images. MRI can provide information about the histologic, physiologic, and biochemical status of tissues, in addition to anatomic, structural data. MRI can delineate clearly brain tumors, edema, ischemic areas, hemorrhages, hydrocephalus, vascular abnormalities, and inflammatory and infectious lesions. Sequential MRI scans are extremely useful in following the structural changes that occur in the brain and spinal cord in many neurodegenerative and metabolic disorders. Bone produces almost no image on MRI scans, therefore, making this test valuable in evaluating structures within the posterior fossa.

Head Ultrasonography

Head ultrasonography provides an excellent way to rapidly visualize the ventricles and midline brain structures in neonates and young infants with open, anterior fontanelles. Ultrasound studies are used in many nurseries to screen premature neonates for intracranial hemorrhage. This technique is also useful in the diagnosis and follow-up of periventricular ischemic injury and ventriculomegaly.

Cerebral Angiography

Angiography remains a useful procedure in the diagnosis of cerebrovascular disorders, particularly vascular malformations, and is sometimes used to help localize vascular anomalies and tumors or define the vascular supply of cerebral neoplasms. Noninvasive CT and MRI scans together with MR angiography have eliminated the need for invasive angiography in many instances.

Myelography

X-ray and CT scan examinations of the spine following injection of water-soluble contrast material or air into the subarachnoid space may be indicated in selected cases of spinal cord tumors, hematomas, and abscesses or in various forms of spinal dysraphism. In many institutions, MRI and CT scans of the spine without contrast material provide the desired diagnostic information, and these procedures have replaced myelography in the workup of many spinal cord lesions.

Sedation for Neurodiagnostic Procedures

Satisfactory sedation for neuroradiologic and other neurodiagnostic procedures can be achieved with rectally administered chloral hydrate (30–60 mg/kg/dose) or intramuscularly or rectally administered pentobarbital (5 mg/kg/dose). Sedation is given at least 20 minutes before the procedure. If pentobarbital (2–4 mg/kg/dose) or other sedatives are administered intravenously, trained personnel and equipment should be readily available to support blood pressure and respirations in the event of an unexpected adverse reaction. Occasionally, general inhalation anesthesia is necessary to achieve adequate sedation for neuroimaging procedures.

21 | Bones & Joints

Robert E. Eilert, MD

This chapter is organized to be a quick reference for common diseases of the musculoskeletal system as encountered by the house officer or general pediatrician. The presentations are arranged according to pattern of patient complaints, eg, in the newborn nursery, trauma, infection, and pain without trauma as well as common office problems.

ORTHOPEDIC PROBLEMS IN THE NEWBORN

CONGENITAL AMPUTATIONS

Congenital amputations may be due to teratogens (eg, drugs or viruses), amniotic bands, or metabolic diseases (eg, diabetes in the mother) or, in rare cases, may be hereditary defects. Most are spontaneous and not genetically determined. The history of the pregnancy must be carefully reviewed in a search for possible teratogenic factors. According to the currently accepted international classification, amputations are either terminal or longitudinal. In terminal amputation, all parts are missing distal to the level of involvement—eg, absence of the forearm, wrist, and hand in the case of a terminal below-the-elbow amputation. A longitudinal amputation consists of partial absence of structures in the extremity along one side or the other. In radial clubhand, the entire radius is absent, but the thumb may be either hypoplastic or completely absent—ie, the effect on structures distal to the amputation may vary. Complex tissue defects are nearly always associated with longitudinal amputations in that the associated nerves and muscles are usually not completely represented when a bone is absent. Bones within the axial skeleton likewise may be absent. Congenital absence of the sacrum is often associated with diabetes in the mother.

Terminal amputations are treated by means of a prosthesis, eg, to compensate for shortness of one leg. With longitudinal deficiencies, constructive surgery may be feasible with the objective of reducing deformity and stabilizing joints.

Lower extremity prostheses are best fitted at about the time of normal walking (12–15 months of age). Lower extremity prostheses are consistently well accepted, as they are necessary for balancing and walking. Upper extremity prostheses are not as well accepted. Fitting the child with a dummy type prosthesis as early as 6 months of age has the advantage of instilling an accustomed pattern of proper length and bimanual manipulation. Children fitted later than age 2 years nearly always reject upper extremity prostheses.

Children quickly learn how to function with their prostheses and can lead active lives, participating in sports with peers.

METATARSUS VARUS

Metatarsus varus is characterized by adduction of the forefoot on the hindfoot, with the heel in normal position or slightly valgus. The longitudinal arch is often creased vertically when the deformity is more rigid. The lateral border of the foot demonstrates sharp angulation at the level of the base of the fifth metatarsal, and this bone will be especially prominent. The deformity varies from flexible to rigid. Most flexible deformities are secondary to intrauterine posture and usually resolve spontaneously.

If the deformity is rigid and cannot be manipulated past the midline, splinting is appropriate to ensure the resolution of the deformity. The prognosis for this common deformity of the foot is excellent in that 85% correct by age 3–4 years with the remainder having mild problems fitting shoes.

CLUBFOOT

When foot deformity consists of the following 3 elements, the diagnosis of classic talipes equinovarus, or clubfoot, is made: (1) equinus or plantar flexion of the foot at the ankle joint, (2) varus or inversion deformity of the heel, and (3) forefoot varus. The incidence of talipes equinovarus is approximately 1:1000 live births. Any infant with a clubfoot should be examined carefully for associated anomalies, especially of the spine. Clubfoot tends to follow a hereditary pattern in some families or may be part of a generalized neuromuscular syndrome such as arthrogryposis or myelodysplasia.

Treatment consists of massage and manipulation of the foot to stretch the contracted tissues on the medial and posterior aspects, followed by splinting to hold the correction. When this is instituted in the nursery shortly after birth, correction is achieved much more rapidly. When treatment is delayed, the foot tends to become more rigid within a matter of days.

About half of children with clubfoot eventually need an operative procedure to lengthen the tightened structures about the foot.

A supple foot that is easily corrected by strapping and casting has a more favorable prognosis. If the foot is rigid operative correction is indicated for normal function in walking.

DEVELOPMENTAL DYSPLASIA OF THE HIP JOINT

In a child with congenital dysplasia of the hip, the femoral head and the acetabulum may be in partial contact at birth. This condition is termed subluxation of the hip. A more severe defect is complete loss of contact between the femoral head and acetabulum, in which case there is frank dislocation of the hip, with the femoral head nearly always displaced laterally and superiorly due to muscle pull. At birth, there is lack of the development of both the acetabulum and the femur in cases of congenital hip dysplasia. The dysplasia becomes progressive with growth unless the dislocation is corrected. If the dislocation is corrected in the first few days or weeks of life, the dysplasia is completely reversible and a normal hip will develop. As the child becomes older and the dislocation or subluxation persists, the deformity will worsen to the point where it will not be completely reversible, especially after the walking age. It is important to diagnose the deformity in the nursery or, at the latest, the 6-week checkup.

Clinical Findings

The diagnosis of congenital hip dislocation in the newborn depends upon demonstrating instability of the joint by placing the infant on its back and obtaining complete relaxation by feeding with a bottle if necessary. The examiner's long finger is then placed over the greater trochanter and the thumb over the inner side of the thigh. Both hips are flexed 90 degrees and then slowly abducted from the midline. With gentle pressure, an attempt is made to lift the greater trochanter forward. A feeling of slipping as the head goes into the acetabulum is a sign of instability. In other infants, the joint is more stable, and the deformity must be provoked by applying slight pressure with the thumb on the medial side of the thigh as the thigh is adducted, thus slipping the hip posteriorly and eliciting a jerk as the hip dislocates. The signs of instability are the most reliable criteria for diagnosing congenital dislocation of the hip in the newborn. X-rays of the pelvis are notoriously unreliable until about 6 weeks of age.

After the first month of life, the signs of instability become less evident. Contractures begin to develop about the hip joint, causing limitation of abduction. Normally, the hip should abduct fully to 90 degrees on either side during the first few months of life. It is important that the pelvis be held level to detect asymmetry of abduction. When the hips and knees are flexed, the knees are at unequal heights, with the dislocated side lower. After the first few weeks of life, x-ray examination becomes more valuable, with lateral displacement of the femoral head being the most reliable finding. In mild cases, the only abnormality may be increased steepness of acetabular alignment, so that the acetabular angle is greater than 35 degrees.

If congenital dislocation of the hip has not been diagnosed during the first year of life and the child begins to walk, there will be a painless limp and a lurch to the affected side. When the child stands on the affected leg, there is a dip of the pelvis on the opposite side owing to weakness of the gluteus medius muscle. In children with bilateral dislocations, the loss of abduction is almost symmetric and may be deceiving. Abduction, however, is never complete, and x-ray of the pelvis is indicated in children with incomplete abduction in the first few months of life. As a child with bilateral dislocation of the hips begins to walk, the gait is waddling. The perineum is widened as a result of lateral displacement of the hips, and there is flexion contracture as a result of posterior displacement of the hips. This flexion contracture contributes to marked lordosis, and the greater trochanters are easily palpable in their elevated position. Treatment is still possible in the first 2 years of life, but the results are not nearly as effective as in children treated in the nursery.

Treatment

Dislocation or dysplasia diagnosed in the first few weeks or months of life can easily be treated by splinting, with the hip maintained in flexion and abduction. Forced abduction is contraindicated, as this often leads to avascular necrosis of the femoral head. The use of double or triple diapers is never indicated, since diapers are not adequate to obtain proper positioning of the hip. In cases of joint laxity without true dislocation, improvement will be spontaneous and diapers are excessive treatment.

Various splints to maintain flexion and abduction of the hip, such as the ones designed by Pavlik, Ilfeld, or von Rosen, are available. Treatment of children requiring splints is best supervised by an orthopedic surgeon with a special interest in the problem.

In the first 4 months of life, reduction can be obtained by simply flexing and abducting the hip; no other manipulation is usually necessary. If force is used to reduce the hip, the excessive pressure may cause avascular necrosis. In such cases, preoperative traction for 2–3 weeks is important to relax soft tissues about the hip. Following traction in which the femur is brought down opposite the acetabulum, reduction can be easily achieved without force under general anesthesia. It is then necessary to place the child in a plaster cast, which is used for approximately 6 months. If the reduction is not stable within a reasonable range following closed reduction, open reduction may be necessary combined with plication of the lax capsule in order to maintain reduction.

If reduction is done at an older age, operations to correct the deformities of the acetabulum and femur may be necessary during growth.

TORTICOLLIS

Wryneck deformities in infancy may be due either to injury to the sternocleidomastoid muscle during delivery or to disease affecting the cervical spine. In the case of muscular deformity, the chin is rotated to the side opposite to the affected sternocleidomastoid muscle contracture, and the head is tilted toward the side of the contracture. A mass felt in the midportion of the sternocleidomastoid muscle does not represent a true tumor but fibrous transformation within the muscle.

In mild cases, passive stretching is usually effective. If the deformity has not been corrected by passive stretching within the first year of life, surgical division of the muscle will correct it. If the deformity is left untreated, an unsightly facial asymmetry will result.

Torticollis is occasionally associated with congenital deformities of the cervical spine, and x-rays of the spine are indicated in all cases.

Acute torticollis may follow upper respiratory infection or mild trauma in children. Rotatory subluxation of the upper cervical spine should be sought by appropriate x-ray views. Traction or a cervical collar usually results in resolution of the symptoms within 1 or 2 days.

TALIPES CALCANEOVALGUS

Talipes calcaneovalgus is characterized by excessive dorsiflexion at the ankle and eversion of the foot. It is often present at birth and almost always corrects spontaneously. The deformity is the reverse of classic clubfoot (talipes equinovarus) and is due to intrauterine position.

Treatment consists of passive exercises by the parents, stretching the foot into plantar flexion. In rare instances, it may be necessary to use plaster casts to help with manipulation and positioning.

Complete correction is the rule.

MUSCULOSKELETAL TRAUMA
(Basic Principles of Examination & Treatment)

The force involved and the pattern of injury determine the structures which are damaged in musculoskeletal trauma. Spending the time to gain as accurate a history as possible will expedite the examination. After deciding that the rare limb threatening injury has not occurred, the next concern is whether bone and/or soft tissue have been disrupted. Once an initial visual assessment and palpation have been done, a splint should be applied to the injured part to relieve pain and prevent further damage during transportation, even if this move is only to the radiology suite. A fracture causes local tenderness and swelling, if not deformity. It is a rare fracture that cannot be diagnosed by looking and feeling, if the clinician is thorough and suspicious.

SOFT TISSUE TRAUMA
(Sprains, Strains, & Contusions)

General information about soft tissue trauma is presented in Chapter 22. Specific entities will be discussed in greater detail in this section.

1. ANKLE SPRAINS

The history will indicate that the injury was by either forceful inversion or eversion. The more common inversion injury results in tearing or injury to the lateral ligaments, whereas an eversion injury will injure the medial ligaments of the ankle. The injured ligaments may be identified by means of careful palpation for point tenderness around the ankle.

If there is more severe trauma resulting in tearing of a ligament, instability of the joint may be demonstrated by gross examination or by stress testing with x-ray documentation. Such deformity of the joint may cause persistent instability resulting from inaccurate apposition of the ligament ends during healing. If instability is evident, surgical repair of the torn ligament is indicated.

2. KNEE SPRAINS

Sprains of the collateral and cruciate ligaments are uncommon in children. These ligaments are so strong that it is more common to injure the epiphyseal growth plates, which are the weakest structures in the region of the knees of children. In adolescence, however, the joints and growth plates attain adult growth, and a rupture of the anterior cruciate ligament can result from a twisting injury that may avulse the anterior tibial spine. In such instances, the injury is apparent on physical examination and x-ray and requires anatomic reduction and immobilization for 6 weeks. In most instances, this means open operative correction.

3. BACK SPRAINS

Sprains of the ligaments and muscles of the back are unusual in children but may occur as a result of violent trauma from automobile accidents or athletic injuries. A child with back pain should not be presumed to have had trauma to the spine unless the history warrants that conclusion. The reason for back pain should be carefully sought by x-ray and physical examination. Inflammation, infection, and tumors are more common causes of back pain in children than sprains.

4. MYOSITIS OSSIFICANS

Ossification within muscle occurs when there is sufficient trauma to cause a hematoma that later heals in the manner of a fracture. The injury is usually a contusion and occurs most commonly in the quadriceps of the thigh or the triceps of the arm. When such a severe injury with hematoma is recognized, it is important to splint the extremity and avoid activity. If further activity is allowed, ossification may reach spectacular proportions and resemble an osteosarcoma.

Disability is great, with local swelling and heat and extreme pain upon the slightest motion of the adjacent joint. The limb should be rested, with the knee in extension or the elbow in 90 degrees of flexion, until the local reaction has subsided. Once local heat and tenderness have decreased, gentle active exercises may be initiated. Passive stretching exercises are not indicated, because they may stimulate the ossification reaction. It is occasionally necessary to excise excessive bony tissue if it interferes with muscle function once the reaction is mature. Surgery should not be attempted before 9 months to a year after injury, because it may restart the process and lead to an even more severe reaction.

TRAUMATIC SUBLUXATIONS & DISLOCATIONS

Dislocation of a joint is always associated with severe damage to the ligaments and joint capsule. In contrast to fracture treatment, which may be safely postponed, dislocations must be reduced immediately. Dislocations can usually be reduced by gentle sustained traction. It often happens that no anesthetic is necessary for several hours after the injury, because of the protective anesthesia produced by the injury. Following reduction, the joint should be splinted for transportation of the patient.

The dislocated joint should be treated by immobilization for at least 3 weeks, followed by graduated active exercises through a full range of motion. Physical therapy is usually not indicated for children with injuries. As a matter of fact, vigorous manipulation of the joint by a therapist may be harmful. The child should be permitted to perform therapy alone. No stretching should be permitted.

1. SUBLUXATION OF THE RADIAL HEAD
(Nursemaid's Elbow)

Infants frequently sustain subluxation of the radial head as a result of being lifted or pulled by the hand. The child appears with the elbow fully pronated and painful. The usual complaint is that the child's elbow will not bend. X-rays are normal, but there is point tenderness over the radial head. When the elbow is placed in full supination and slowly moved from full flexion to full extension, a click may be palpated at the level of the radial head. The relief of pain is remarkable, as the child usually stops crying immediately. The elbow may be immobilized in a sling for comfort for a day.

Pulled elbow may be a clue to battering. This should be remembered during examination, especially if the problem is recurrent.

2. RECURRENT DISLOCATION OF THE PATELLA

Recurrent dislocation of the patella is more common in loose-jointed individuals, especially adolescent girls. If the patella completely dislocates, it nearly always goes laterally. Pain is severe, and the patient is brought to the doctor with the knee slightly flexed and an obvious bony mass lateral to the knee joint and a flat area over the usual location of the patella anteriorly. X-rays confirm the diagnosis. The patella may be reduced by extending the knee and placing slight pressure on the patella while gentle traction is exerted on the leg. In subluxation of the patella, the symptoms may be more subtle, and the patient may say that the knee "gives out" or "jumps out of place."

In the case of complete dislocation, the knee should be immobilized for 3–4 weeks, followed by a physical therapy program for strengthening the quadriceps muscle. Operation may be necessary to tighten the knee joint capsule if dislocation or subluxation is recurrent. In such instances, if the patella is not stabilized, repeated dislocation produces damage to the articular cartilage of the patellofemoral joint and premature degenerative arthritis.

EPIPHYSEAL SEPARATIONS AND FRACTURES

1. EPIPHYSEAL SEPARATIONS

In children, epiphyseal separations and fractures are more common than ligamentous injuries. This finding is based on the fact that the ligaments of the joints are generally stronger than the associated growth plates. In instances where dislocation is suspected, an x-ray should be taken in order to rule out epiphyseal fracture. Films of the opposite extremity, especially around the elbow, may be valuable for comparison. Reduction of a fractured epiphysis should be done under anesthesia in order to align the growth plate with the least amount of force necessary. Fractures across the growth plate may produce bony bridges that will cause premature cessation of growth or angular deformities in the growth plate. Epiphyseal fractures around the shoulder, wrist, and fingers can usually be treated by closed reduction, but fractures of the epiphyses around the elbow often require open reduction. In the lower extremity, accurate reduction of the epiphyseal plate is necessary to prevent joint deformity if a joint surface is involved. Unfortunately, some of the most severe injuries to the epiphyseal plate occur from compression injuries, where the amount of force is not immediately apparent. If angular deformities result, corrective osteotomy should be necessary.

2. TORUS FRACTURES

Torus fractures consist of "buckling" of the cortex as a result of minimal angular trauma. They usually occur in the distal radius or ulna. Alignment is satisfactory, and simple immobilization for 3–5 weeks is sufficient.

3. GREENSTICK FRACTURES

With greenstick fractures there is frank disruption of the cortex on one side of the bone but no discernible cleavage plane on the opposite side. These fractures are angulated but not displaced, as the bone ends are not separated. Reduction is achieved by straightening the arm into normal alignment, and reduction is maintained by a snugly fitting plaster cast. It is necessary to x-ray children with greenstick fractures again in a week to 10 days to make certain that the reduction has been maintained in plaster. A slight angular deformity will be corrected by remodeling of the bone. The farther the fracture is from the growing end of the bone, the longer the time required for healing. The fracture can be considered healed when there are no findings of tenderness and local swelling or heat and when adequate bony callus is seen on x-ray.

4. FRACTURE OF THE CLAVICLE

Clavicular fractures are very common injuries in infants and children. They can be immobilized by a figure-of-8 dressing that retracts the shoulders and brings the clavicle to normal length. The healing callus will be apparent when the fracture has consolidated, but this unsightly lump will generally resolve over a period of months to a year.

5. SUPRACONDYLAR FRACTURES OF THE HUMERUS

Supracondylar fractures tend to occur in the age group from 3 to 6 years and are potentially dangerous because of the proximity to the brachial artery in the distal arm. They are usually associated with a significant amount of trauma, so that swelling may be severe. Volkmann's ischemic contracture of muscle may occur as a result of vascular embarrassment. When severe swelling is present, the safest course is to place the arm in traction and carefully observe nerve function and the vascular supply to the hand. In these cases, the children should be hospitalized. If the blood supply is compromised, exposure of the brachial artery may be necessary, although this is rarely needed when satisfactory reduction and traction are employed. Complications associated with supracondylar fractures also include a resultant cubitus valgus secondary to poor reduction. It is often difficult to ascertain adequacy of the reduction because a flexed position is necessary to maintain normal alignment. Such a "gunstock" deformity of the elbow may be somewhat unsightly but does not usually interfere with joint function.

6. GENERAL COMMENTS ON OTHER FRACTURES IN CHILDREN

Reduction of fractures in children is usually accomplished by simple traction and manipulation; open reduction is not commonly indicated. Remodeling of the fracture callus will usually produce an almost normal appearance of the bone over a matter of months. The younger the child, the more remodeling is possible. Angular deformities remodel with ease. Rotatory deformities do not remodel, and this produces the cubitus valgus deformity sometimes seen after supracondylar fractures.

The physician should be suspicious of child battering whenever the age of a fracture does not match the history given or when the severity of the injury is more than the alleged accident would have produced. In suspected cases of battering where no fracture is present on the initial x-ray, a repeat film 10 days later is in order. Bleeding beneath the periosteum will be calcified by 7–10 days, and the x-ray appearance is almost diagnostic of severe closed trauma characteristic of a battered child.

INFECTIONS OF THE BONES & JOINTS

OSTEOMYELITIS

Osteomyelitis is an infectious process that usually starts in the spongy or medullary bone and then extends to involve compact or cortical bone. It is more common in boys than in girls or in adults of either sex. The lower extremities are most often affected, and there is commonly a history of trauma. Osteomyelitis may occur as a result of direct invasion from the outside through a penetrating wound (nail) or open fracture, but hematogenous spread of infection (eg, pyoderma or upper respiratory tract infection) from other infected areas is more common. The most common infecting organism is *Staphylococcus aureus*, which seems to have a special tendency to infect the metaphyses of growing bones. Anatomically, circulation in the long bones is such that the arterial supply to the metaphysis just below the growth plate is by end arteries, which turn sharply to end in venous sinusoids, causing a relative stasis. In the infant under 1 year of age, there is direct vascular communication with the epiphysis across the growth plate, so that direct spread may occur from the metaphysis to the epiphysis and subsequently into the joint. In the older child, the growth plate provides an effective barrier and the epiphysis is usually not involved, although the infection spreads retrograde from the metaphysis into the diaphysis and, by rupture through the cortical bone, down along the diaphysis beneath the periosteum.

1. EXOGENOUS OSTEOMYELITIS

In order to avoid osteomyelitis by direct extension, all wounds must be carefully examined and cleansed. Cultures of the wound made at the time of exploration and debridement may be useful if signs of inflammation and infection develop subsequently. In extensive or contaminated wounds, antibiotic coverage is indicated. Contaminated wounds should be left open and secondary closure performed 3–5 days later. If at the time of delayed closure further necrotic tissue is present, it should be excised.

Parenteral administration of antibiotics is satisfactory, and local irrigation is not needed. If the wound is acquired outside the hospital, penicillin is adequate for most wounds. After cultures have been read, an appropriate alternative antibiotic can be chosen if there is lingering inflammation. A tetanus toxoid booster is indicated for any questionable wound.

Once exogenous osteomyelitis has become established, treatment becomes more complicated, requiring extensive surgical debridement and drainage followed by careful antibiotic management (in particular for *Staphylococcus aureus*). Coverage for *Pseudomonas* should be added in cases involving nail puncture wounds. These cases require hospitalization and the use of intravenous antibiotics.

2. HEMATOGENOUS OSTEOMYELITIS

Hematogenous osteomyelitis is usually caused by pyogenic bacteria; 85% of cases are due to staphylococci. Streptococci are rare causes of osteomyelitis today. Children with sickle cell anemia are especially prone to osteomyelitis caused by salmonellae.

Clinical Findings

A. Symptoms and Signs: In infants, the manifestations of osteomyelitis may be quite subtle, presenting as irritability, diarrhea, or failure to feed properly; the temperature may be normal or slightly low; and the white blood count may be normal or only slightly elevated. In older children, the manifestations are more striking, with severe local tenderness and pain, high fever, rapid pulse, and elevated white blood cell count and sedimentation rate. Osteomyelitis of a lower extremity often presents around the knee in a child 7–10 years of age. Tenderness is most marked over the metaphysis of the bone where the process has its origin.

B. Laboratory Findings: Blood cultures are often positive early. The most significant test in infancy is the aspiration of pus when suspicion arises because of lack of movement in a painful extremity. It is useful to insert a needle to the bone in the area of suspected infection and aspirate any fluid present. This fluid can be smeared and stained for organisms as well as cultured. Even edema fluid may be useful for determining the causative organism. The white blood cell count is usually elevated, as is the sedimentation rate.

C. Imaging: The first manifestation to appear on x-ray is nonspecific local swelling. This is followed by elevation of the periosteum, with formation of new bone from the cambium layer of the periosteum occuring after 3–6 days. As the infection becomes chronic, areas of cortical bone are isolated by pus spreading down the medullary canal, causing rarefaction and demineralization of the bone. Such isolated pieces of cortex become ischemic and form sequestra (dead bone fragments). These x-ray findings are late, and osteomyelitis should be diagnosed clinically before significant x-ray findings are present. Bone scan is valuable in suspected cases before x-rays become positive.

Treatment

A. Specific Measures: Antibiotics should be started intravenously as soon as the diagnosis of osteomyelitis is made. Use of methicillin, another semisynthetic penicillin, or a cephalosporin that covers penicillinase-producing *S aureus* is recommended. Gentamicin can also be given to combat gram-negative organisms until the results of cultures are available and Salmonella should be covered in children with Sickle cell. Antibiotics should be continued until swelling, tenderness, and local discharge have ceased and the white blood cell count and erythrocyte sedimentation rate are normal, usually a period of at least 1 month. Serial x-rays can also be used to follow bone healing. Antibiotic therapy by the intravenous route should be continued until all clinical signs are improved, including sedimentation rate. For a reliable family, oral medication may be started at that time (about 10 days), adjusting dosage by serum killing power and continued monitoring of erythrocyte sedimentation rate for at least 1 month after the ESR has returned to normal.

B. General Measures: Splinting of the limb minimizes pain and decreases spread of the infection by lymphatic channels through the soft tissue. The splint should be removed periodically to allow active use of adjacent joints and prevent stiffening and muscle atrophy. In chronic osteomyelitis, splinting may be necessary to guard against fracture of the weakened bone.

C. Surgical Measures: Aspiration of the metaphysis is a useful diagnostic measure in any case of suspected osteomyelitis. Osteomyelitis represents a collection of pus under pressure within the body. In the first 24–72 hours, it may be possible to abort osteomyelitis by the use of antibiotics alone. However, if frank pus is aspirated from the bone, surgical drainage is indicated. If the infection has not shown a dramatic response to antibiotics within 24 hours in questionable cases, surgical drainage is also indicated. It is important that all devitalized soft tissue be removed and adequate exposure of the bone obtained in order to permit free drainage. Excessive amounts of bone should not be removed when draining acute osteomyelitis, since they may not be completely replaced by the normal healing process.

In questionable cases, little damage has been done by surgical drainage, but failure to drain the pus in acute cases may lead to more severe damage.

Prognosis

When osteomyelitis is diagnosed in the early clinical stages and prompt antibiotic therapy is begun, the prognosis is excellent. If the process has been unattended for a week to 10 days, there is almost always some permanent loss of bone structure, as well as the possibility of growth abnormality.

PYOGENIC ARTHRITIS

The source of pyogenic arthritis varies according to the age of the child. In the infant, pyogenic arthritis often develops by spread from adjacent osteomyelitis. In the older child, it presents as an isolated infection, usually without bony involvement. In teenagers with pyogenic arthritis, an underlying systemic disease is usually the cause, eg, an obvious generalized infection or an organism that has an affinity for joints, such as the gonococcus.

In infants, the most common cause of pyogenic arthritis is *S aureus*, although gram-negative organisms may be seen. In children between 4 months and 4 years of age, *Haemophilus influenzae* is a common causative organism.

The initial effusion of the joint rapidly becomes purulent. An effusion of the joint may accompany osteomyelitis in the adjacent bone. A white blood cell count exceeding 100,000/μL in the joint fluid indicates a definite purulent infection. Generally, spread of infection is from the bone into the joint, but unattended pyogenic arthritis may also affect adjacent bone. The sedimentation rate is elevated.

Clinical Findings

   A. Symptoms and Signs: In older children, the signs are striking, with fever, malaise, vomiting, and restriction of motion. In infants, paralysis of the limb due to inflammatory neuritis may be evident. Infection of the hip joint in infants can be diagnosed if suspicion is aroused by decreased abduction of the hip in an infant who is irritable or feeding poorly. A history of umbilical catheter treatment in the newborn nursery should alert the physician to the possibility of pyogenic arthritis of the hip.

   B. Imaging: Early distention of the joint capsule is nonspecific and difficult to measure by x-ray. In the infant with unrecognized pyogenic arthritis, dislocation of the joint may follow within a few days as a result of distention of the capsule by pus. Later changes include destruction of the joint space, resorption of epiphyseal cartilage, and erosion of the adjacent bone of the metaphysis.

Treatment

   Diagnosis may be made by aspiration of the joint. In the hip joint, pyogenic arthritis is most easily treated by surgical drainage because the joint is deep and difficult to aspirate as well as being inaccessible to thorough cleaning through needle aspiration. In more superficial joints, such as the knee, aspiration of the joint at least twice daily may maintain adequate drainage. If fever and clinical symptoms do not subside within 24 hours after treatment is begun, open surgical drainage is indicated. Antibiotics can be specifically selected based on cultures of the aspirated pus. Before the results of cultures are available, treatment by methicillin and gentamicin will cover the usual etiologic organisms. It is not necessary to give intra-articular antibiotics, since good levels are achieved in the synovial fluid.

Prognosis

The prognosis is excellent if the joint is drained early, before damage to the articular cartilage has occurred. If infection is present for more than 24 hours, there is dissolution of the proteoglycans in the articular cartilage, with subsequent arthrosis and fibrosis of the joint. Damage to the growth plate may also occur, especially within the hip joint, where the epiphyseal plate is intracapsular. This damage is usually due to interruption of blood supply producing osteonecrosis.

NONTRAUMATIC HIP PAIN OR LIMP

TRANSIENT ("TOXIC") SYNOVITIS OF THE HIP

The most common cause of limping and pain in the hip of children in the USA is transitory synovitis, an acute inflammatory reaction that often follows an upper respiratory infection and is generally self-limited. In questionable cases, aspiration of the hip yields only yellowish fluid, ruling out pyogenic arthritis. Generally, however, toxic synovitis of the hip is not associated with elevation of the white blood cell count or a temperature above 38.3°C (101°F). It classically affects children 3–10 years of age and is more common in boys. There is limitation of motion of the hip joint, particularly internal rotation, and x-ray changes are nonspecific, with some swelling apparent in the soft tissues around the joint.

Treatment consists of bed rest and the use of traction with slight flexion of the hip. Aspirin may shorten the course of the disease, although even with no treatment the disease usually is self-limited to a matter of days. It is important to maintain x-ray follow-up, since transient synovitis may be the precursor of avascular necrosis of the femoral head (see next section) in a small percentage of patients. X-rays can be obtained at 1 month and 3 months, or earlier if there is persistent limp or pain.

AVASCULAR NECROSIS OF THE PROXIMAL FEMUR
(Legg-Calvé-Perthes Disease)

The vascular supply of bone is generally precarious, and when it is interrupted, necrosis results. In contrast to other body tissues that undergo infarction, bone removes necrotic tissue and replaces it with living bone in a process called "creeping substitution." This replacement of necrotic bone may be so complete and so perfect that a completely normal bone results. Adequacy of replacement depends upon the age of the patient, the presence or absence of associated infection, congruity of the involved joint, and other physiologic and mechanical factors.

Because of their rapid growth in relation to their blood supply, the secondary ossification centers in the epiphyses are subject to avascular necrosis. Even though the pathologic and radiologic features of avascular necrosis of the epiphyses are well known, the cause is not generally agreed upon. Necrosis may follow known causes such as trauma or infection, but idiopathic lesions usually develop during periods of rapid growth of the epiphyses. Thus, the highest incidence of Legg-Calvé-Perthes disease is between 4 and 8 years of age.

Clinical Findings

A. Symptoms and Signs: Persistent pain is the most common symptom, and the patient may present with limp or limitation of motion.

B. Laboratory Findings: Laboratory findings, including studies of joint aspirates, are normal.

C. Imaging: X-ray findings correlate with the progression of the process and the extent of necrosis. The early finding is effusion of the joint associated with slight widening of the joint space and periarticular swelling. Decreased bone density in and around the joint is apparent after a few weeks. The necrotic ossification center appears more dense than the surrounding viable structures, and there is collapse or narrowing of the femoral head.

As replacement of the necrotic ossification center occurs, there is rarefaction of the bone in a patchwork fashion, producing alternating areas of rarefaction and relative density or "fragmentation" of the epiphysis.

In the hip, there may be widening of the femoral head associated with flattening. If infarction has extended across the growth plate, there will be a radiolucent lesion within the metaphysis.

If the growth center of the femoral head has been damaged so that normal growth does not occur, varus deformity of the femoral neck will occur as a result of overgrowth of the greater trochanteric apophysis.

Eventually, complete replacement of the epiphysis will become apparent as new bone replaces necrotic bone. The final shape of the head will depend upon the extent of the necrosis and collapse that has been allowed to occur.

Differential Diagnosis

Differential diagnosis must include inflammatory and infectious lesions of the joints or apophyses. Transient synovitis of the hip may be distinguished from Legg-Calvé-Perthes disease by serial x-rays.

Treatment

Treatment consists simply of protection of the joint. If the joint is deeply seated within the acetabulum and normal joint motion is maintained, a reasonably good result can be expected. The hip is held in abduction and internal rotation in order to fulfill this purpose. Braces are generally used. Surgery may be necessary for an uncooperative patient or one whose social or geographic circumstances do not allow use of a brace.

Prognosis

The prognosis for complete replacement of the necrotic femoral head in a child is excellent, but the functional result will depend upon the amount of deformity that develops during the time the softened structure exists. In Legg-Calvé-Perthes disease, the prognosis depends upon the completeness of involvement of the epiphyseal center. In general, patients with metaphyseal defects, those in whom the disease develops late in childhood, and those who have more complete involvement of the femoral head have a poorer prognosis.

EPIPHYSIOLYSIS
(Slipped Capital Femoral Epiphysis)

Epiphysiolysis is the separation of the proximal femoral epiphysis through the growth plate. The head of the femur is usually displaced medially and posteriorly relative to the neck of the femur. The condition occurs in adolescence and is more common in overweight children. Slightly over 40% of the children so affected are of the obese, hypogenital body type.

Occasionally, the condition occurs as an acute episode resulting from a fall or direct trauma to the hip. This is called a fracture and must be differentiated. Commonly, there are vague symptoms over a protracted period of time in an otherwise healthy child who presents with pain and limp. The pain is often referred into the thigh or the medial side of the knee. It is important to examine the hip joint in any child complaining of knee pain, particularly in adolescents. The consistent finding on physical examination is limitation of internal rotation of the hip. There usually is also an associated hip flexion contracture as well as local tenderness about the hip. X-rays should be taken in both the anteroposterior and lateral planes. These must be carefully examined in early cases in order to show an abnormality where displacement of the femoral head occurs posteriorly, which is usually most easily seen on the lateral view.

Treatment is based on the same principles that govern treatment of fracture of the femoral neck in adults in that the head of the femur is fixed to the neck of the femur and the fracture line allowed to heal. Unfortunately, the severe complication of avascular necrosis occurs in 30% of these patients.

The long-term prognosis is guarded because most of these patients continue to be overweight and overstress their hip joints. Follow-up studies have shown a high incidence of premature degenerative arthritis in this group of patients—even those who do not develop avascular necrosis. The development of avascular necrosis almost guarantees a poor prognosis, since new bone does not replace the femoral head at this late stage of skeletal growth.

About 30% of patients have bilateral involvement, and patients should be followed for slipping of the opposite side, which may occur as long as 1 or 2 years after the primary episode.

NONTRAUMATIC KNEE PAIN

OSTEOCHONDRITIS DISSECANS

In osteochondritis dissecans, there is a pie-shaped necrotic area of bone and cartilage adjacent to the articular surface. The fragment of bone may be broken off from the host bone and displaced into the joint as a loose body. If it remains attached, the necrotic fragment may be completely replaced by creeping substitution.

The pathologic process is precisely the same as that described above for avascular necrosing lesions of ossification centers. However, since these lesions are adjacent to articular cartilage, there may be joint damage.

The most common sites of these lesions are the knee (medial femoral condyle), the elbow joint (capitellum), and the talus (superior lateral dome).

Joint pain is the usual presenting complaint. However, local swelling or locking may be present, particularly if there is a fragment free in the joint. Laboratory studies are normal.

Treatment consists of protection of the involved area from mechanical damage. If there is a fragment free within the joint as a loose body, it must be surgically removed. For some marginal lesions, it may be worthwhile to drill the necrotic fragment in order to encourage more rapid vascular ingrowth and replacement. If large areas of a weight-bearing joint are involved, secondary degenerative arthritis may result.

FIBROUS DYSPLASIA

Dysplastic fibrous tissue replacement of the medullary canal is accompanied by the formation of metaplastic bone in fibrous dysplasia. Three forms of the disease are recognized: monostotic, polyostotic, and polyostotic with endocrine disturbances (precocious puberty in females, hyperthyroidism, and hyperadrenalism, ie, Albright's syndrome).

Clinical Findings

A. Symptoms and Signs: The lesion or lesions may be asymptomatic. Pain, if present, is probably due to pathologic fractures. In females, endocrine disturbances may be present in the polyostotic variety and associated with café au lait spots.

B. Laboratory Findings: Laboratory findings are normal unless endocrine disturbances are present, in which case there may be increased secretion of gonadotropic, thyroid, or adrenal hormones.

C. Imaging: The lesion begins centrally within the medullary canal, usually of a long bone, and expands slowly. Pathologic fracture may occur. If metaplastic bone predominates, the contents of the lesion will be of the density of bone. Marked deformity of the bone may result, and a shepherd's crook deformity of the upper femur is a classic feature of the disease. The disease is often asymmetric, and limb length disturbances may occur as a result of stimulation of epiphyseal cartilage growth.

Differential Diagnosis

The differential diagnosis may include other fibrous lesions of bone as well as destructive lesions such as bone cyst, eosinophilic granuloma, aneurysmal bone cyst, nonossifying fibroma, enchondroma, and chondromyxoid fibroma.

Treatment

If the lesion is small and asymptomatic, no treatment is needed. If the lesion is large and produces or threatens pathologic fracture, curettage and bone grafting are indicated.

Prognosis

Unless the lesions impair epiphyseal growth, the prognosis is good. Lesions tend to enlarge during the growth period but are stable during adult life. Malignant transformation has not been recorded.

UNICAMERAL BONE CYST

Unicameral bone cyst appears in the metaphysis of a long bone, usually in the femur or humerus. It begins within the medullary canal adjacent to the epiphyseal cartilage. It probably results from some fault in enchondral ossification. The cyst is "active" when it abuts onto the metaphyseal side of the epiphyseal cartilage and "inactive" when a border of normal bone exists between the cyst and the epiphyseal cartilage. The lesion is usually identified when a pathologic fracture occurs, producing pain. Laboratory findings are normal. On x-rays, the cyst is identified centrally within the medullary canal, producing expansion of the cortex and thinning over the widest portion of the cyst.

Treatment consists of curettage of the cyst if it is producing pain. The cyst may heal after a fracture and not require treatment. Curettage should be delayed if surgery would risk damage to the adjacent growth plate. In such cases, methylprednisolone injection may be curative.

The prognosis is excellent. Some cysts will heal following pathologic fracture.

ANEURYSMAL BONE CYST

Aneurysmal bone cyst is similar to unicameral bone cyst, but it contains blood rather than clear fluid. It usually occurs in a slightly eccentric position in the long bone, expanding the cortex of the bone but not breaking the cortex, although some extraosseous mass may be produced. On x-rays, the lesion appears somewhat larger than the width of the epiphyseal cartilage, and this feature distinguishes it from unicameral bone cyst.

The aneurysmal bone cyst is filled by large vascular lakes, and the stoma of the cyst contains fibrous tissue and areas of metaplastic ossification.

The lesion may appear quite aggressive histologically, and it is important to differentiate it from osteosarcoma or hemangioma. Treatment is by curettage and bone grafting, and the prognosis is excellent.

BAKER'S CYST

Baker's cyst is a herniation of the synovium in the knee joint into the popliteal region. In children, the diagnosis may be made by aspiration of mucinous fluid, but the cyst nearly always disappears with time. Whereas Baker's cysts may be indicative of intraarticular disease in the adult, they usually are of no clinical significance in children and rarely require excision, usually resolving spontaneously by age 5 years.

FOOT DEFORMITIES

When a child begins to stand and walk, the long arch of the foot is flat with a medial bulge over the inner border of the foot. The forefeet are mildly pronated or rotated inward, with a slight valgus alignment of the knees. As the child grows and muscle power improves, the long arch is better supported and more normal relationships occur in the lower extremities.

FLATFOOT

Flatfoot is a normal condition in infants. Children presenting for examinations should be checked to determine that the heel cord is of normal length when the heel is aligned in the neutral position, allowing complete dorsiflexion and plantar flexion. As long as the foot is supple and the presence of a longitudinal arch is noted when the child is sitting in a non–weight-bearing position, the parents can be assured that a normal arch will probably develop. There is usually a familial incidence of relaxed flatfeet in children who have prolonged malalignment of the foot. In any child with a shortened heel cord or stiffness of the foot, other causes of flatfoot such as tarsal coalition or vertical talus should be ruled out by a complete orthopedic examination and x-ray.

In the child with an ordinary relaxed flatfoot, no active treatment is indicated unless there is calf or leg pain. In children who have leg pains attributable to flatfeet, an orthopedic shoe with Thomas heel may relieve discomfort. An arch insert should not be prescribed unless passive correction of the arch is easily accomplished; otherwise, there will be irritation of the skin over the medial side of the foot.

CAVUS FOOT

In cavus foot, the deformity consists of an unusually high longitudinal arch of the foot. It may be hereditary or associated with neurologic conditions such as poliomyelitis, Charcot-Marie-Tooth disease, Friedreich's ataxia, or diastematomyelia. There is usually an associated contracture of the toe extensor, producing a claw toe deformity in which the metatarsal phalangeal joints are hyperextended and the interphalangeal joints acutely flexed. Any child presenting with cavus feet should have a careful neurologic examination including x-rays of the spine.

In resistant cases that do not respond to shoe adjustments (metatarsal bars and supports), operation may be necessary to lengthen the contracted extensor and flexor tendons. Arthrodesis of the foot may be necessary later. If these feet are left untreated, they are often painful and limit walking.

The overall prognosis is much poorer than with low arch or pes planus.

CLAW TOES

In patients with claw toes, there is a flexion deformity of either or both interphalangeal joints, which results in the "claw." The condition is usually congenital and may be seen in association with disorders of motor weakness, such as Charcot-Marie-Tooth disease or pes cavus. Surgical correction can alleviate symptoms if the toes are painful.

BUNIONS
(Hallux Valgus)

Girls may present in adolescence with lateral deviation of the great toe associated with a prominence over the head of first metatarsal. This deformity is painful only with shoe wear and almost always can be relieved by fitting shoes that are wide enough. Surgery should be avoided in the adolescent age group, as the results are much less successful than in adult patients with the same condition.

OFFICE ORTHOPEDICS

SCOLIOSIS

The term *scoliosis* denotes lateral curvature of the spine, which is always associated with some rotation of the involved vertebrae. Scoliosis is classified by its anatomic location, in either the thoracic or lumbar spine, with rare involvement of the cervical spine. The apex of the curve is designated right or left. Thus, a right thoracic scoliosis would denote a convex leftward curve in the thoracic region, and this is the most common type of idiopathic curve. Posterior curvature of the spine (kyphosis) is normal in the thoracic area, though excessive curvature may become pathologic. Anterior curvature is called lordosis and is normal in the lumbar spine. Idiopathic scoliosis generally begins at about 8 or 10 years of age and progresses during growth. In rare instances, infantile scoliosis may be seen in children 2 years of age or less.

Idiopathic scoliosis is about 4–5 times more common in girls than in boys. The disorder is usually asymptomatic in the adolescent years, but severe curvature may lead to impairment of pulmonary function or low back pain in later years. It is important to examine the back of any adolescent coming in for a physical examination. The examination is performed by having the patient bend forward 90 degrees with the hands joined in the midline. An abnormal finding consists of asymmetry of the height of the ribs or paravertebral muscles on one side, indicating rotation of the trunk associated with lateral curvature.

Diseases that may be associated with scoliosis include neurofibromatosis, Marfan's syndrome, cerebral palsy, muscular dystrophy, and poliomyelitis. Neurologic examination should be performed in all children with scoliosis to determine whether these disorders are present.

Five to 7% of cases of scoliosis are due to congenital vertebral anomalies such as a hemivertebral or unilateral vertebral bridge. These curves are more rigid than the more common idiopathic curve and will often increase with growth, especially during the rapid growth spurt during adolescence.

The most common type of scoliosis is so-called idiopathic scoliosis, which may be due to asymmetry of neuromuscular development. In 30% of cases, other family members are affected.

Postural compensation of the spine may lead to lateral curvature from such causes as unequal length of the lower extremities. Antalgic scoliosis may result from pressure on the spinal cord or roots by infectious processes or herniation of the nucleus pulposus; the underlying cause must be sought. The curvature will resolve as the primary problem is treated.

Clinical Findings

A. Symptoms and Signs: Scoliosis in adolescents is classically asymptomatic. It is imperative to seek the underlying cause in any case where there is pain, since in these instances the scoliosis is almost always secondary to some other disorder such as a bone or spinal cord tumor. Deformity of the rib cage and asymmetry of the waistline are evident with curvatures of 30 degrees or more. A lesser curvature may be detected by the forward bending test as described above, which is designed to detect early abnormalities of rotation that are not apparent when the patient is standing erect.

B. Imaging: The most valuable x-rays are those taken of the entire spine in the standing position in both the anteroposterior and lateral planes. Usually, there is one primary curvature with a compensatory curvature that develops to balance the body. At times there may be 2 primary curvatures, usually in the right thoracic and left lumbar regions. Any left thoracic curvature should be suspected of being secondary to neurologic or muscular disease, prompting a more meticulous neurologic examination.

Treatment

Curvatures of less than 20 degrees usually do not require treatment unless they show progression. Bracing is indicated for curvature of 20–40 degrees in a skeletally immature child. Treatment is indicated for any curvature that demonstrates progression on serial x-ray examination. Curvatures greater than 40 degrees are resistant to treatment by bracing. Thoracic curvatures greater than 60 degrees have been correlated with a poor pulmonary prognosis in adult life. Curvatures of such severity are an indication for surgical correction of the deformity and posterior spinal fusion to maintain the correction. Curvatures between 40 and 60 degrees may also require spinal fusion if they appear to be progressive, are causing decompensation of the spine, or are cosmetically unacceptable.

Prognosis

Compensated small curvatures that do not progress may be well tolerated throughout life, with very little cosmetic concern. The patients should be counseled regarding the genetic transmission of scoliosis and cautioned that their children should be examined at regular intervals during growth. Large thoracic curvatures greater than 60 degrees are associated with shortened life span and may progress even during adult life. Large lumbar curvatures may lead to subluxation of the vertebrae and premature arthritic degeneration of the spine, producing disabling pain in adulthood. Early detection allows for simple brace treatment or surface electrical stimulation. In patients so treated, the long-term prognosis is excellent and surgery is not necessary. For this reason, school screening programs for scoliosis have gained popular support in many sections of the country.

GENU VARUM & GENU VALGUM

Genu varum (bowleg) is normal from infancy through 2 years of life. The alignment then changes to genu valgum (knock-knee) until about 8 years of age, at which time adult alignment is attained. Criteria for referral to an orthopedist include persistent bowing beyond age 2, bowing that is increasing rather than decreasing, bowing of one leg only, and knock-knee associated with short stature.

Bracing may be appropriate, or, rarely, an osteotomy is necessary for a severe problem such as Blount's disease (proximal tibial epiphyseal dysplasia).

TIBIAL TORSION

The physician is often asked about "toeing in" in small children. The disorder is routinely asymptomatic. Tibial torsion is rotation of the leg between the knee and the ankle. Internal rotation amounts to about 20 degrees at birth but decreases to neutral rotation by 1 year of age. The deformity is sometimes accentuated by laxity of the knee ligaments, allowing excessive internal rotation of the leg in small children. In children who have a persistent internal rotation of the tibia beyond 1 year of age, it is often due to sleeping with feet turned in and can be reversed with an external rotation splint worn only at night.

FEMORAL ANTEVERSION

"Toeing in" beyond 2 or 3 years of age is usually based on femoral anteversion, which produces excessive internal rotation of the femur as compared with external rotation. This femoral alignment follows a natural history of progressive decrease toward neutral up to 8 years of age, with slower change to 16 years of age. Studies comparing the results of treatment with shoes or braces to the natural history have shown that little is gained by active treatment. Active external rotation exercises such as ballet, skating, or bicycle riding may be worthwhile. Osteotomy for rotational correction is rarely required. Refer those who have no external rotation of hip in extension.

GANGLION

A ganglion is a smooth, small cystic mass connected by a pedicle to the joint capsule, usually on the dorsum of the wrist.

It may also be seen in the tendon sheath over the flexor surfaces of the fingers. These ganglions can be excised if they interfere with function or cause persistent pain.

INFLAMMATION OF JOINTS

Degenerative arthritis may follow childhood skeletal problems such as infection, slipped capital femoral epiphysis, avascular necrosis, or trauma or may occur in association with hemophilia. Early effective treatment of these disorders will prevent arthritis. Late treatment is often unsatisfactory.

Inflammatory changes in the soft tissues around joints may occur as a result of overuse syndrome in adolescent athletes. Young boys throwing excessive numbers of pitches, especially curve balls, may develop "little leaguer's elbow," consisting of degenerative changes around the humeral condyles associated with pain, swelling, and limitation of motion. In order to enforce the rest necessary for healing, a plaster cast may be necessary. A more reasonable preventive measure is to limit the number of pitches thrown by children.

Acute bursitis is quite uncommon in childhood, and other causes should be ruled out before this diagnosis is accepted.

Tenosynovitis is most common in the region of the knees and feet. Children taking dancing lessons, particularly toe dancing, may have pain around the flexor tendon sheaths in the toes or ankles. Rest is effective treatment. At the knee level, there may be irritation of the patellar ligament, with associated swelling in the infrapatellar fat pad. Synovitis in this area is usually due to overuse and is also treated by rest. Corticosteroid injections are contraindicated.

Sports Medicine | 22

Suzanne M. Tanner, MD

The pediatric sports medicine practitioner aims to prevent injuries and illness in young athletes. Since this goal is not always achievable, a second objective is to provide prompt, appropriate medical care. Practitioners treating young athletes are called upon to perform preparticipation examinations and treat sprains, strains, contusions, and overuse injuries, the most common maladies affecting active youngsters.

THE PREPARTICIPATION EXAMINATION

For many pediatricians, performing sports physical examinations is a principal source of involvement in the realm of sports medicine. The primary goal of the preparticipation evaluation is to enhance the health of athletes. It is not meant to exclude athletes from participation, but to help them participate safely. Although it is not intended as a substitute for an athlete's regular health maintenance examination, 78% of athletes view the preparticipation evaluation as their annual health examination. Careful attention to general health maintenance should therefore be included with the exam, or at another appointment.

The preparticipation examination should ideally be conducted at least 6 weeks prior to the start of practice or competition so that health disorders may be evaluated and previous injuries rehabilitated.

A complete history (Table 22–1) will identify 63–74% of problems affecting athletes. Parents should help the athlete complete the questionnaire since only 39% of histories reported by athletes agree with information given by their parents.

Important entities to detect during the preparticipation examination are listed below. Further evaluation or treatment may be recommended before the athlete is allowed to participate.

Exercise-Induced Asthma (EIA)

EIA is common in children and adolescents. Approximately 10% of the normal population and 80–90% of asthmatics experi-

Table 22-1. Preparticipation physical evaluation form.

	YES	NO
Explain "YES" answers in space below: Sport: _____		
1. Have you ever been hospitalized?	☐	☐
Have you ever had surgery?	☐	☐
2. Are you presently taking any medications or pills?	☐	☐
3. Do you have any allergies (medicine, bees or other stinging insects)?	☐	☐
4. Have you ever passed out during or after exercise?	☐	☐
Have you ever been dizzy during or after exercise?	☐	☐
Have you ever had chest pain during or after exercise?	☐	☐
Do you tire more quickly than your friends during exercise?	☐	☐
Have you ever had high blood pressure?	☐	☐
Have you ever been told you have a heart murmur?	☐	☐
Have you ever had racing of your heart or skipped beats?	☐	☐
Has anyone in your family died of heart problems or a sudden death before age 50?	☐	☐
5. Do you have any skin problems (itching, rashes, acne)?	☐	☐
6. Have you ever had a head injury?	☐	☐
Have you ever been knocked out or unconscious?	☐	☐
Have you ever had a seizure?	☐	☐
Have you ever had a stinger or burner or pinched nerve?	☐	☐
7. Have you ever had heat or muscle cramps?	☐	☐
Have you ever been dizzy or passed out in the heat?	☐	☐
8. Do you have trouble breathing or cough during or after activity?	☐	☐
9. Do you have any special equipment (pads, braces, neck rolls, mouth guard, eye guards, etc.)?	☐	☐
10. Have you had any problems with eyes or vision?	☐	☐
Do you wear glasses or contacts or protective eye wear?	☐	☐
11. Have you ever sprained/strained, dislocated, fractured, broken or had repeated swelling or other athletic injuries of any bones or joints?	☐	☐
12. Have you had any other medical problems (e.g., infectious mononucleosis, diabetes, etc.)?	☐	☐
13. Have you had a medical problem or injury since your last evaluation?	☐	☐
14. When was your last tetanus shot? _____		
When was your last measles immunization? _____		
15. When was your first menstrual period? _____		
Last menstrual period? _____		
What was the longest time between periods last year? _____		

726

ence EIA. Only athletes with severe asthma should be deterred from participating in any sport.

Symptoms include shortness of breath, chest pain, abdominal pain, a feeling of being out of shape, and coughing after activity. Symptoms can be reduced by performing warm-up drills prior to activity and exercise in a warm, humidified environment. Sports well tolerated include swimming (since air is humidified), and wrestling (since bouts are of short duration).

Treatment includes inhaling a β_2-agonist or cromolyn shortly before exercise. More extensive treatment is outlined in Chapter 25.

Cardiovascular Symptoms

Careful attention to the cardiovascular system is crucial since over 95% of sudden deaths in athletes under age 30 involve the cardiovascular system. Syncope, or near syncope, may be a clue to the presence of hypertrophic cardiomyopathy, conduction abnormalities, arrhythmias or valvular problems, such as aortic stenosis or mitral valve prolapse. Exertional chest pain may indicate congenital abnormalities of the coronary arteries or atherosclerotic disease in a child with abnormal lipid metabolism. Lung pathology or valvular problems may cause dyspnea on exertion. Palpitations or skipped beats may signify arrhythmias or conduction abnormalities, such as Wolff–Parkinson–White syndrome.

It is important to determine if family members under 50 years have experienced sudden cardiac death. Causes of sudden cardiac death include hypertrophic cardiomyopathy, Marfan's syndrome and prolonged QT syndrome. These entities may have a familial component.

Repeat measurements of blood pressure, using an appropriate cuff size, should be taken if the pressure is elevated initially. As an easy rule of thumb, blood pressure greater than 125/75 for a child 10 years or younger, or a blood pressure greater than 135/85 for a child over 10 years should be further evaluated.

Children with mild hypertension may compete in all sports. Those with moderate to severe hypertension should be individually evaluated.

Skin Infections

An athlete with herpes simplex, scabies, pubic lice, molluscum contagiosum, furunculosis, carbunculosis, or impetigo may temporarily need to be disqualified from sports such as wrestling, the martial arts, swimming, or gymnastics. Infections may be spread via direct contact, swimming pools, tumbling mats, or shared towels.

Previous Concussions

Brain injuries are the leading cause of athletic death. Football, because it is participated in by more than 1.5 million high school and college athletes, causes more minor head injuries than any other single sport. The incidence is estimated to be 250,000 per year, or approximately 20%.

A concussion is defined as a clinical syndrome characterized by immediate and transient post-traumatic impairment of neural functions, such as alteration of consciousness, disturbance of vision, or equilibrium due to brain stem involvement. The ability to process new information may be reduced after a cerebral concussion, and the severity and duration of functional impairment may be greater with repeated concussions. A grading system for concussions and guidelines for return to play are presented in Table 22–2.

Allergies to Hymenoptera

Allergies to stings by bees, wasps, yellow jackets, and fire ants should be noted so that proper emergency medications (Ana-Kit, EpiPen) are always available on the playing field.

Eating Disorders

Athletes at risk for inadequate nutritional intake while attempting to lose weight include those competing in endurance sports (eg, cross-country running), those sports with weight classes (eg, wrestling) and those in which the body is self-propelled (eg, gymnastics). Girls with a low percentage of body fat may be at risk for amenorrhea, iron-deficiency anemia, and stress fractures.

Previous Injuries

Many sports injuries are reinjuries so the musculoskeletal system should be assessed in detail. The "2-minute orthopedic examination" should be included in all preparticipation examinations (Table 22–3). Complete examination of individual joints should be performed if the athlete has injured a joint or if a joint is painful. Poor range of motion of a joint, ligament laxity, or weakness may signify inadequate rehabilitation of a previous injury.

Table 22–2. Grading concussions in sports and guidelines for return to play.[1,5]

Severity	Signs/Symptoms	Guidelines		
		First Concussion	Second Concussion	Third Concussion
Grade I (Mild)	Confusion without amnesia; No loss of consciousness	May return to play if asymptomatic[4] for at least 20 minutes	Terminate contest/practice May return to play one week after asymptomatic[4]	Terminate season; may return to play in three months if asymptomatic[4]
Grade II (Moderate)	Confusion with amnesia[2]; No loss of consciousness[3]	Terminate contest/practice May return to play one week after asymptomatic[4]	Consider terminating season but may return to play one month after asymptomatic[4]	Terminate season May return to play next season if asymptomatic[4]
Grade III (Severe)	Loss of consciousness[3]	Terminate contest/practice and transport to hospital May return to play one month after two weeks asymptomatic[4] Conditioning allowed after one week asymptomatic[4]	Terminate season May return to play next season if asymptomatic[4]	Strongly discourage return to contact/collision sports

[1] These guidelines are not absolute and therefore should not substitute for the clinical judgement of the examining physician.

[2] Post-traumatic amnesia (amnesia for the events following the impact) or more severe retrograde amnesia (amnesia for events preceding the impact).

[3] Some "brief" loss of consciousness to be included in Grade II and reserve "prolonged" loss of consciousness for Grade III, but the definitions of "brief" and "prolonged" are not universally accepted.

[4] No headache, confusion, dizziness, impaired orientation or concentration, or memory dysfunction during rest or with exertion.

[5] Adapted from Colorado Medical Society. Guidelines for the management of concussion in sports. Sports Medicine Committee, Colorado Medical Society. May 1990.

Table 22–3. The 2-minute orthopedic examination.[1]

Instructions	Observations
Stand facing examiner	Acromioclavicular joints, general habitus
Look at ceiling, floor, over both shoulders; touch ears to shoulders	Cervical spine motion
Shrug shoulders (examiner resists)	Trapezius strength
Abduct shoulders 90° (examiner resists at 90°)	Deltoid strength
Full external rotation of arms	Shoulder motion
Flex and extend elbows	Elbow motion
Arms at sides, elbows 90° flexed; pronate and supinate wrists	Elbow and wrist motion
Spread fingers; make fist	Hand or finger motion and deformities
Tighten (contract) quadriceps; relax quadriceps	Symmetry and knee effusion; ankle effusion
"Duck walk" four steps (away from examiner with buttocks on heels)	Hip, knee and ankle motion
Back to examiner	Shoulder symmetry, scoliosis
Knees straight, touch toes	Scoliosis, hip motion, hamstring tightness
Raise up on toes, raise heels	Calf symmetry, leg strength

[1] Reproduced with permission from *Sports Medicine: Health Care of the Young Athlete*, 2nd ed., 1991, published by The American Academy of Pediatrics, Elk Grove Village, Illinois.

Laboratory Tests

Routine urinalysis, hemoglobin/hematocrit, blood chemistry, sickle cell test, and lipid assay are *not* recommended for screening purposes by the American Academy of Pediatrics (AAP). Athletes with inadequate iron intake, especially girls participating in endurance sports, may be at risk for iron-deficiency anemia and should be screened for this disorder.

Electrocardiogram, echocardiogram, and exercise stress testing are indicated only when history and physical findings identify an individual with increased cardiovascular risks.

Exclusion From Sports

The AAP has classified sports based on strenuousness and probability of collision (Table 22–4). AAP guidelines for participation or exclusion from sports are listed in Table 22–5.

Table 22–4. Classification of sports.[1]

Contact Collision	Limited Contact Impact	Noncontact		
		Strenuous	Moderately Strenuous	Nonstrenuous
Boxing	Baseball	Aerobic dancing	Badminton	Archery
Field hockey	Basketball	Crew	Curling	Golf
Football	Bicycling	Fencing	Table tennis	Riflery
Ice hockey	Diving	Field		
Lacrosse	Field	Discus		
Martial arts	High jump	Javelin		
Rodeo	Pole vault	Shot put		
Soccer	Gymnastics	Running		
Wrestling	Horseback riding	Swimming		
	Skating	Tennis		
	Ice	Track		
	Roller	Weight lifting		
	Skiing			
	Cross-country			
	Downhill			
	Water			
	Softball			
	Squash handball			
	Volleyball			

[1] From American Academy of Pediatrics. Committee on Sports Medicine. Recommendations for participation in competitive sports. *Pediatrics* 1988;**81**:737–739.

Table 22–5. Recommendations for participation in competitive sports.[1]

| | Contact/ Collision | Limited Contact/Impact | Noncontact | | |
			Strenuous	Moderately Strenuous	Nonstrenuous
Atlantoaxial instability	No	No	Yes*	Yes	Yes
* Swimming, no butterfly, breast stroke or diving starts					
Acute illnesses	·	·	·	·	·
* Needs individual assessment eg, contagiousness to others, risk of worsening illness					
Cardiovascular					
Carditis	No	No	No	No	No
Hypertension					
Mild	Yes	Yes	Yes	Yes	Yes
Moderate	·	·	·	·	·
Severe	·	·	·	·	·
Congenital heart disease	†	†	†	†	†
· Needs individual assessment					
† Patients with mild forms can be allowed a full range of physical activities: patients with moderate or severe forms, or who are postoperative, should be evaluated by a cardiologist					
Eyes					
Absence or loss of function of one eye	·	·	·	·	·
Detached retina	†	†	†	†	†
* Availability of American Society for Testing and Materials (ASTM) approved eye guards may allow competitor to participate in most sports, but this must be judged on an individual basis.					
† Consult ophthalmologist					

Inguinal hernia	Yes	Yes	Yes	Yes	Yes
Kidney: Absence of one	No	Yes	Yes	Yes	Yes
Liver: Enlarged	No	No	Yes	Yes	Yes
Musculoskeletal disorders	*	*	*	*	*
*Needs individual assessment					
Neurologic					
History of serious head or spine trauma, repeated concussions or craniotomy	*	*	Yes	Yes	Yes
Convulsive disorder					
Well controlled	Yes	Yes	Yes	Yes	Yes
Poorly controlled	No	No	Yes†	Yes	Yes‡
*Needs individual assessment					
†No swimming or weight lifting					
‡No archery or riflery					
Ovary: Absence of one	Yes	Yes	Yes	Yes	Yes
Respiratory					
Pulmonary insufficiency	*	*	*	*	Yes
Asthma	Yes	Yes	Yes	Yes	Yes
*May be allowed to compete if oxygenation remains satisfactory during a graded stress test					
Sickle cell trait	Yes	Yes	Yes	Yes	Yes
Skin: Boils, herpes, impetigo, scabies	*	*	Yes	Yes	Yes
*No gymnastics with mats, martial arts, wrestling or contact sports until not contagious					
Spleen: Enlarged	No	No	No	Yes	Yes
Testicle: Absence or undescended	Yes*	Yes*	Yes	Yes	Yes
*Certain sports may require protective cup					

1 From American Academy of Pediatrics. Committee on Sports Medicine. Recommendations for participation in competitive sports. *Pediatrics* 1988;**81**:737–739.

The physician should consider the following questions when considering clearing or excluding an athlete from participation:

(1) Does the problem place the athlete at increased risk of injury?

(2) Is any other participant at risk of injury because of the problem?

(3) Can the athlete safely participate with medication, rehabilitation, bracing, or padding?

(4) Can limited participation be allowed while treatment is being initiated?

(5) If clearance is denied only for certain activities, in what activities can the athlete safely participate?

EPIDEMIOLOGY OF SPORTS INJURIES IN THE PEDIATRIC ATHLETE

Injuries by Sport

The yearly injury incidence in all interscholastic high school sports is 27 to 39%. Among popular high school sports, football and wrestling are the most hazardous.

Injuries by Gender

There has been concern that sports are more dangerous for girls than boys. Injury incidence between males and females in high school and college sports, however, is similar.

Injuries by Age

Injury rates tend to increase by age. Teenager and college-age athletes may have a higher rate of injury than youngsters due to increased time at risk. At the high school and college level, games last longer and practices are more frequent, giving the player more opportunity to be injured. In sports such as football, larger size and increased speed make collisions more hazardous.

It is unlikely that any physiologic or anatomic factor associated with aging in children enhances injury risk. In fact, younger children may be at more risk of serious injury since they are skeletally immature.

Methods to prevent injuries are presented in Table 22–6.

SOFT TISSUE TRAUMA

Of injuries in adolescents, soft tissue injures are by far the most common. Sprains, strains, and contusions account for 75%

Table 22–6. Methods of injury prevention.[1]

- Proper conditioning and acclimatization
- Avoidance of training excesses
- A safe environment
- Resolution of previous injuries
- Good supervision
- Enforcement of rules concerned with safety, with continued revision as new risk factors are identified
- Instruction in proper technique
- Appropriate safety equipment
- A careful preparticipation medical assessment
- Matching of competitors by age, weight, and stage of maturation

[1] From Goldberg B, in Dyment PG (ed): *Adolescent Medicine: Sports and the Adolescent.* Hanly and Belfus, Philadelphia, Vol. 2, No. 1, Feb. 1991.

of all high school sport-related injuries. The knee, thigh, and ankle are the sites most commonly injured.

Sprain

A sprain is an injury to a ligament or joint capsule. Ligaments connect adjacent bones at a joint. Common sites of sprains include the lateral ankle, medial collateral ligament of the knee, elbow, and wrist. Sprains are graded according to their severity (Table 22–7). Grading of sprains requires testing ligament integrity through specific tests during which stress is applied across a joint.

Strains

Strains are often referred to as "muscle pulls." The term refers to an injury to a muscle or tendon. Common sites of strains include the shoulder and hamstrings. Grading of strains requires

Table 22–7. Grading of sprains according to severity.[1]

Grade	Fibers Torn	Pain/Swelling	Range of Motion	Laxity
I	Less than 5%	Little	Full	None
II	5–95%	Moderate	Impaired	Noticeable
III	100%	Severe	Poor	Marked

[1] Adapted from Dyment PG (ed): *Adolescent Medicine: Sports and the Adolescent.* Hanly and Belfus, Philadelphia, Vol. 2, No. 1, Feb. 1991.

Table 22–8. Grading of strains by assessing strength.[1]

Grade	Pain on Palpation or Contraction	Loss of Strength	Palpable Defect
I	Little	Little or none	−
II	Moderate	Significant	±
III	Severe	Marked	±

[1] Adapted from Dyment PG (ed): *Adolescent Medicine: Sports and the Adolescent.* Hanley and Belfus, Philadelphia, Vol. 2, No. 1, Feb. 1991.

assessing strength, which is more subjective that grading stability for sprains (Table 22–8).

Contusions

A contusion refers to a crushing of cells and bleeding from a direct blow. A ''Charley Horse'' refers to a contusion of the quadriceps muscles. Since muscles are more vascular than ligaments and tendons, they are prone to hematoma formation after a blow. Repetitive or severe contusions may progress to myositis ossificans, or calcification within the muscle, especially if further activity is not halted.

Treatment of Soft Tissue Injuries

Most grade I and II soft tissue injuries can be managed by the primary care physician. The aim of treatment during the first 48–72 hours following a soft tissue injury is to limit inflammation and bleeding. This promotes healing and speeds up rehabilitation. An acronym, RICE (*r*est, *i*ce, *c*ompression, and *e*levation) should guide initial management.

Rest is accomplished through cessation of activity, immobilization, and eliminating or reducing weight bearing for lower extremity injuries. These steps prevent further injury, relieve pain, and reduce inflammation. Although the length of time a body part requires rest to enhance healing varies according to the injury severity and site, rest should usually be at least 48–72 hours.

Vasoconstriction by application of cold, rather than heat, immediately after an injury decreases bleeding, inflammation, pain and spasm. Applying heat acutely after an injury may have the opposite effect. A plastic bag containing ice cubes or crushed ice can be placed over a towel on the skin. For best results, ice

Table 22–9. Adverse effects of NSAIDS.[1]

Gastritis
Headache
Mental status changes
Hypersensitivity
Impairment of platelet function
Impairment of renal function
Bronchospasm

[1] Adapted from Landry G, in Dyment PG (ed): *Adolescent Medicine: Sports and the Adolescent.* Hanley and Belfus, Philadelphia, Vol. 2, No. 1, Feb. 1991.

may be applied for 10–20 minutes, 2 to 4 times/day for the first 2 to 3 days.

Applying an elastic bandage to the injured part compresses the site and limits swelling.

Elevation is accomplished by raising the injured part on cushions or pillows. Elevation facilitates venous and lymphatic drainage.

Application of the RICE regimen alone usually limits swelling adequately for most soft tissue injuries. The role of anti-inflammatory medications in the management of soft tissue injuries is controversial due to their potential toxicity (Table 22–9).

Management of Soft Tissue Injuries After the Acute Phase

Approximately 72 hours post-injury, when swelling and pain have decreased, rehabilitation may be started. An athletic trainer or physical therapist may help design a rehabilitation program. Range of motion exercises through simple, isolated movement patterns may be performed several times per day. Once range of motion is near normal, strengthening exercises may be added. Strengthening helps the athlete to return to sports sooner and helps prevent a reinjury. Cardiovascular endurance can be maintained during rehabilitation while resting the injured part. For example, a basketball player with a shoulder injury may ride an exercycle. A runner with a sore foot may swim.

Return to Play

Criteria for return to play include:

- Full range of motion
- Full strength

- No swelling
- No joint instability
- No tenderness
- No pain with motion
- Ability to perform the athletic activity without limping or favoring the injured part

OVERUSE INJURIES

Today, millions of children join organized sports teams, train rigorously, and pursue sports at a young age. The reward to a young athlete may be excelling at a sport. Hours of practicing the same movement, however, may produce wear on specific body parts. Overuse, or overload, injuries refer to trauma to a body part due to repetitive microtrauma. Intrinsic and extrinsic factors may lead to overuse injuries (Table 22–10).

Table 22–10. Predisposing factors to overruse injuries.

Intrinsic Factors	Example
Leg-length inequality	May cause low back pain
Weakness	Weak quadriceps may predispose to patellofemoral (kneecap) pain
Inflexibility	Tight Achilles tendons may predispose to Sever's disease (heel pain)
Poor aerobic fitness	Poor general fitness correlates with the presence of low back pain
Growth spurt	Perhaps bones grow faster than muscles, causing inflexibility (unproven)
Extrinsic Factors	**Example**
Training errors	Suddenly increasing running mileage may lead to stress fractures
Improper technique	Deep squats while holding weights may lead to patellofemoral (kneecap) pain
Poor equipment	Shoes with poor support may lead to pain in the arch of the foot
Poor nutrition	Low calcium intake may predispose to the development stress fractures

Examples of overuse injuries in children include the entities listed below. Treatment options are listed in Table 22–11.

Rotator Cuff Tendinitis

The rotator cuff consists of four muscles (SITS muscles = *s*upraspinatus, *i*nfraspinatus, *t*eres minor, and *s*ubscapularis). These muscles form a tendinous cuff around the superior portion of the humerus. Children and teenagers who participate in overhead activities such as throwing, swimming, and playing volleyball may develop pain in the superior aspect of the shoulder due to inflammation of the rotator cuff.

Patellar Tendinitis (Jumper's Knee)

Jumper's knee refers to inflammation of the patellar tendon below the patella. Youngsters involved in running and jumping sports, such as basketball, may develop pain at the area of the patellar tendon during and after activity.

Patellofemoral Pain

Patellofemoral pain refers to discomfort around the patella. Possible sources of pain include irritation of the cartilage posterior to the patella and perhaps synovial inflammation. Predisposing conditions include weakness of the quadriceps, inflexibility of the hamstrings and quadriceps, malalignment of the extensor mechanism of the knee, and increased patellar compressive forces (running, ascending and descending stairs, full squats, and jumping).

Pain usually occurs during and after activity, ascending and descending stairs, while squatting, and after prolonged sitting. The physical examination often reveals that compression on the patella during quadriceps contraction with the knee extended is painful.

Stress Fracture

When a bone is repetitively loaded, such as while running, it may break with a load that would not normally cause it to fail if it were loaded only once. This condition is called a fatigue or stress fracture. Predisposing conditions in children include high training intensity and frequency, and perhaps poor calcium intake and hormonal imbalances associated with athletic amenorrhea.

Common sites include the fibula, metatarsal, tibia, and femoral neck. Localized pain is a presenting symptom of stress frac-

Table 22-11. Treatment options for overuse injuries.

Tissue	Overuse Injury	Rest	Apply Ice	nSAID[1]	Stretching	Strengthening	Shoes	Brace	Injection
Tendon	Rotation cuff tendonitis	+	+	+		Rotator cuff			+ Subacromial – Bursa injection
	Jumper's knee (patella tendonitis)	+	+	+	Quadriceps hamstrings	Quadriceps (straight leg raises)	Proper shoes	± Infrapatella strap	
Cartilage	Patellofemoral pain	+	+	+	Quadriceps hamstrings	Quadriceps (straight leg raises)	Proper shoes	± Sleeve with central patellar hole	
Bone	Stress fracture	+					Proper shoes		
	Spondylolysis	+			Hamstrings	Back and abdomen		+	
Apophysis	Osgood–Schlatter condition	+	+	+	Quadriceps hamstrings			± Infrapatella strap	
	Severe condition	+	+	+	Achilles tendon		Heel lifts Proper shoes		
Epiphyseal growth plate	Little leaguer's elbow (medial humeral epicondylitis)	+	+	+		Wrist flexor		± Elbow sleeve	

[1] nSAID = nonsteroidal anti-inflammatory medication.

tures. Impact, such as heel strike during running, often produces pain. The most important physical examination finding is point tenderness over bone.

Radiographs may not show evidence of a stress fracture, such as a radiolucent line or callous formation, until 7 to 10 days after the onset of pain. Bone scans are more sensitive.

Spondylolysis/Spondylolisthesis

These terms are derived from the Greek. *Spondylo* means vertebra, *-lysis* means crack or fracture, and *-olisthesis* means sliding down an incline. Spondylolysis is a bony defect of the pars interarticularis (a segment of the vertebrae) that usually affects the fifth lumbar vertebra. Spondylolysis may progress to spondylolisthesis, an anterior slippage of a vertebra.

In athletes, the lytic defect is thought to be due to repetitive hyperextension maneuvers, such as performing back walk overs in gymnastics, or while high jumping.

Symptoms include chronic dull aching pain of the lumbosacral spine that is exacerbated by maneuvers requiring hyperextension. Oblique radiographs of the spine are required to view the defect. A bone scan may also confirm the diagnosis.

Progression from spondylolysis to spondylolisthesis is unusual, but when slips do develop, it is often between the ages of 10 and 15 years. Approximately 90% of the slips occur at the fifth lumbar–first sacral level.

Osgood–Schlatter Disease

Osgood–Schlatter's disease is not a disease, but a condition in growing, active children. It refers to traction apophysitis of the tibial tubercle. Sports requiring repetitive flexion and extension of the knee, such as basketball and soccer, are inciting factors. Physical examination reveals tenderness directly over the prominence of the tibial tubercle. Pain resolves once growth is completed, or by decreasing running, but prominence of the tibial tubercle may persist through adulthood.

Sever Disease

Sever disease can be referred to as Osgood–Schlatter disease of the heel. A traction apophysitis at the site of attachment of the Achilles tendon to the calcaneus is the source of pain with this entity.

Little Leaguer's Elbow

The term ''little leaguer's elbow'' refers to all stress changes involved in pitching that occur in the skeletally immature athlete.

The most common cause of elbow pain is due to distraction of the medial side of the elbow during the follow through of a pitch. This may produce tendinitis at the site of insertion of the wrist flexor and pronator muscles to the medial epicondyle of the humerus. More serious causes of little leaguer's elbow include osteochondritis dissecans (bone fragmentation) of the capitellum and radial head due to lateral elbow compression while throwing, or separation of the medial epicondylar epiphyseal growth plate due to medial distraction forces.

Pain, tenderness and loss of extension are common findings. Radiographs may reveal osteochondritis dissecans. Comparison radiographs with the contralateral elbow may show separation of the medial epiphyseal growth plate.

Failure to protect the joint may result in the formation of loose fragments, pain, deformity, and possibly arthritis.

Endocrine & Metabolic Disorders | 23

Ronald W. Gotlin, MD

DISTURBANCES OF GROWTH & DEVELOPMENT

SHORT STATURE

Abnormally short stature in relation to age is a common finding in childhood. In most instances, it is due to a normal variation from the usual pattern of growth. The possible roles of such factors as sex, race, size of parents and other family members, intrauterine factors, nutrition, pubertal maturation, and emotional status must all be evaluated in the total assessment of the child (Table 23–1). The causes of unusually short stature can usually be differentiated on the basis of significant findings in the history, physical examination, and radiographic estimation of skeletal maturation (''bone age'').

1. CONSTITUTIONAL DELAYED GROWTH & ADOLESCENCE

Many normal children have a delay in the onset of skeletal maturation that is considered to be ''constitutional.'' Puberty progresses normally after a delayed onset. In other respects, they appear entirely normal. There is often a history of a similar pattern of growth in one of the parents or other members of the family. These children are usually short throughout childhood but reach normal adult height, although at an age later than average.

2. GROWTH HORMONE DEFICIENCY

The incidence of growth hormone (GH) deficiency is approximately 1:4000. More than 75% of cases are the result of

Table 23–1. Causes of short stature.[1]

Familial, racial, or genetic
Constitutional short stature and delayed adolescence
Endocrine disturbances
Growth hormone deficiency
Hereditary—gene deletion
Idiopathic—deficiency of growth hormone or growth hormone releasing hormone (or both) with and without associated abnormalities of midline structures of the central nervous system
Acquired
Transient—eg, psychosocial short stature
Organic—tumor, irradiation of the central nervous system, infection, or trauma
Hypothyroidism
Adrenal insufficiency
Cushing's disease and Cushing's syndrome (including iatrogenic causes)
Sexual precocity (androgen or estrogen excess)
Diabetes mellitus (poorly controlled)
Diabetes insipidus
Hyperaldosteronism

Inborn errors of metabolism (cont'd)
Sphingolipidoses (eg, Tay-Sachs disease, Niemann-Pick disease, Gaucher's disease)
Miscellaneous (eg, cystinosis)
Aminoacidemias and aminoacidurias
Epithelial transport disorders (eg, renal tubular acidosis, cystic fibrosis, Bartter's syndrome, vasopressin-resistant diabetes insipidus, pseudohypoparathyroidism)
Organic acidemias and acidurias (eg, methylmalonic aciduria, orotic aciduria, maple syrup urine disease, isovaleric acidemia)
Metabolic anemias (eg, sickle cell disease, thalassemia, pyruvate kinase deficiency)
Disorders of mineral metabolism (eg, Wilson's disease, magnesium malabsorption syndrome)
Body defense disorders (eg, Bruton's agammaglobulinemia, thymic aplasia, chronic granulomatous disease)
Constitutional (intrinsic) diseases of bone
Defects of growth of tubular bones or spine (eg, achondroplasia, metatropic dwarfism, diastrophic dwarfism, metaphyseal chondrodysplasia)

Primordial short stature
  Intrauterine growth retardation
    Placental insufficiency
    Intrauterine infection
  Primordial dwarfism with premature aging
    Progeria (Hutchinson-Gilford syndrome)
    Progeroid syndrome
    Werner's syndrome
    Cachectic (Cockayne's syndrome)
  Short stature without dysmorphism
  Short stature with dysmorphism (eg, Seckel's bird-headed dwarfism, leprechaunism, Silver's syndrome, Bloom's syndrome, Cornelia de Lange syndrome, Hallerman-Streiff syndrome)
Inborn errors of metabolism
  Altered metabolism of calcium or phosphorus (eg, hypophosphatemic rickets, hypophosphatasia, infantile hypercalcemia, pseudohypoparathyroidism)
  Storage diseases
    Mucopolysaccharidoses (eg, Hurler's syndrome, Hunter's syndrome)
    Mucolipidoses (eg, generalized gangliosidosis, fucosidosis, mannosidosis)

Disorganized development of cartilage and fibrous components of the skeleton (eg, multiple cartilaginous exostoses, fibrous dysplasia with skin pigmentation, precocious puberty of McCune-Albright)
Abnormalities of density of cortical diaphyseal structure or metaphyseal modeling (eg, osteogenesis imperfecta congenita, osteopetrosis, tubular stenosis)
Short stature associated with chromosomal defects
  Autosomal (eg, Down's syndrome, cri du chat syndrome, trisomy 18)
  Sex chromosomal (eg, Turner's syndrome-XO, penta X, XXXY)
Chronic systemic diseases, congenital defects, and cancers (eg., chronic infection and infestation, inflammatory bowel disease, hepatic disease, cardiovascular disease, hematologic disease, central nervous system disease, pulmonary disease, renal disease, malnutrition, cancers, collagen vascular disease)
Psychosocial short stature (deprivation dwarfism)
Miscellaneous syndromes (eg, arthrogryposis multiplex congenita, cerebrohepatorenal syndrome, Noonan's syndrome, Prader-Willi syndrome, Riley-Day syndrome)

---

[1] From Hathaway WE et al: *Current Pediatric Diagnosis & Treatment*, 10th ed. Appleton & Lange, 1991.

a hypothalamic abnormality affecting GH releasing hormone. Approximately two-thirds of all cases involving the hypothalamus and pituitary are idiopathic (rarely familial), and the remainder are secondary to pituitary, central nervous system, or hypothalamic disease (empty sella syndrome, septooptic dysplasia, craniopharyngioma, infections, tuberculosis, sarcoidosis, toxoplasmosis, syphilis, trauma, reticuloendotheliosis, vascular anomalies, and other tumors such as gliomas). GH deficiency may be an isolated defect or may occur in combination with other pituitary hormone deficiencies.

At birth, affected infants may be small; growth retardation is evident during infancy. There may be infantile fat distribution, youthful facial features, small hands and feet, and delayed sexual maturation. Hypoglycemia and microphallus may occur. Dental development and epiphyseal maturation ("bone age") are delayed to an equal degree or more so than height age (median age for patient's height). Headaches, visual field defects, abnormal skull x-rays, and symptoms of posterior pituitary insufficiency (polyuria and polydipsia) often precede or accompany the GH deficiency in cases resulting from central nervous system disease.

GH deficiency is associated with low levels of IGF, (somatomedin C) and GH in the serum and a failure of the GH level to rise during normal physiologic sleep in response to arginine, oral levodopa, oral clonidine, exercise, or insulin-induced hypoglycemia. Patients with hypothalamic deficiency may have a GH rise in response to growth hormone-releasing hormone.

Laron type dwarfism is a rare condition in which there is an inability to generate somatomedin in response to GH. Rarely children may have an immunoreactive GH with reduced bioactivity.

Treatment is with synthetic human growth hormone (hGH). Growth hormone-releasing hormone may be effective in hypothalamic disease and is expected to be available soon. Protein anabolic agents (testosterone, fluoxymesterone, oxandrolone, etc) may be effective in promoting linear growth, but these drugs may cause acceleration of epiphyseal closure with decrease in eventual height.

Treatment trials employing hGH in conditions with non-hGH-dependent short stature are proceeding and in Turner's syndrome hGH treatment is efficacious. Use of hGH for *normal* short children is controversial.

3. HYPOTHYROIDISM

See section on hypothyroidism later in this chapter under Diseases of the Thyroid.

4. PRIMORDIAL SHORT STATURE
(Intrauterine Growth Retardation)

Primordial short stature may occur in a number of disorders, including craniofacial disproportion (Table 23–1), or may occur in individuals with no accompanying significant physical abnormalities. Children with primordial short stature have birth weight and length below normal for gestational age. Head circumference may be normal or reduced. Thereafter, they grow parallel to but below the third percentile. Plasma GH levels are usually normal but may be elevated. In some instances, somatomedin levels are subnormal. There is an increased incidence of functional fasting hypoglycemia. In most instances, skeletal maturation ("bone age") corresponds to chronologic age or is only mildly delayed, in contrast to the more marked delay often present in children with GH and thyroid deficiency.

There is as yet no satisfactory treatment for primordial short stature, although there may be an increase in growth rate in response to pharmacologic doses of human GH.

5. SHORT STATURE DUE TO EMOTIONAL FACTORS
(Psychosocial Short Stature, Deprivation Dwarfism, Reversible Growth Hormone Deficiency)

Psychologic and emotional deprivation with disturbances in motor and personality development may be associated with short stature. Growth retardation in some of these children is the result of undernutrition; these children may have an increased (often voracious) appetite. In others, undernutrition does not seem to be a factor. There is a delay in skeletal maturation. Plasma GH and somatomedin C levels are reduced. A history of feeding problems during early infancy is common; polydipsia and polyuria are sometimes present. Emotional disturbances in the family are the rule.

Placement in a foster home or a significant change in the psychologic and emotional environment at home usually results in significantly return to normal levels of GH and somatomedin and improved growth, a decrease of appetite and dietary intake to more normal levels, and personality improvement. Treatment with growth-promoting agents is not indicated.

DIFFERENTIAL DIAGNOSIS OF SHORT STATURE

Short stature may accompany or be caused by a large number of conditions (see Table 23–1). When the etiologic diagnosis is not apparent from the history and physical examination, the following laboratory studies, in addition to bone age, are useful in detecting or categorizing the common causes of short stature:

(1) Complete blood count (to detect chronic anemia, infection, cancer).

(2) Erythrocyte sedimentation rate (often elevated in collagen vascular disease, cancer, chronic infection, inflammatory bowel disease).

(3) Urinalysis and microscopic examination (occult pyelonephritis, glomerulonephritis, renal tubular disease, etc).

(4) Stool examination for occult blood, parasites, and parasite ova (inflammatory bowel disease, overwhelming parasitism).

(5) Serum electrolytes and phosphorus levels (mild adrenal insufficiency, renal tubular diseases, parathyroid disease, rickets, etc).

(6) Blood urea nitrogen and creatinine levels (occult renal insufficiency).

(7) Karyotyping (should be performed in all short girls with delayed sexual maturation with or without clinical features of Turner's syndrome).

(8) Thyroid function assessment: serum free thyroxin (FT_4) and thyroid-stimulating hormone (TSH) assay (short stature may be the only sign of hypothyroidism).

(9) GH evaluation. Blood samples for GH determination should be obtained following 20 minutes of exercise, during normal sleep, or after administration of one of the conventional provocative agents (arginine, glucagon, levodopa, clonidine, and insulin-induced hypoglycemia). Random GH samples are of no value.

FAILURE TO THRIVE

Failure to thrive (FTT) is present when there is a perceptible declination of growth from an established pattern or when the patient's height and weight plot consistently below the third percentile. (The term is usually reserved for infants who for various reasons fail to gain weight.) Linear growth and head circumference may also be affected; when this occurs, the underlying condition is generally more severe. There are many reasons for failure to thrive (see below and Table 23–1), although a specific cause often cannot be established. Neglect and nonaccidental trauma may be an important cause of failure to thrive.

Classification & Etiologic Diagnosis

The diagnosis of FTT is usually apparent on the basis of the history and physical examination. In FTT, it is useful to compare the patient's chronologic age with the height age (median age for the patient's height), weight age, and head circumference. On the basis of these measurements, 3 principal patterns can be defined and will provide a starting point in the diagnostic approach.

Group 1: This group is the most common type. The head circumference is normal, and the weight is reduced out of proportion to height. In the majority of cases of FTT, undernutrition is present as a result of deficient caloric intake, malabsorption, or impaired caloric utilization.

Group 2: The head circumference is normal or enlarged for age, and the weight is only moderately reduced, usually in proportion to height. Failure to thrive is due to structural dystrophies, constitutional dwarfism, or endocrinopathies.

Group 3: Although the head circumference is normal, the weight is reduced in proportion to height, owing to a primary central nervous system deficit or intrauterine growth retardation (see Primordial Short Stature, above).

An initial period of observed nutritional rehabilitation, usually in a hospital setting, is often helpful in the diagnosis. The child should be placed on a regular diet for age, and the caloric intake and weight should be carefully plotted for 1–2 weeks. During this period, evidence of lactose intolerance is sought by checking pH and reducing substances in the stool. If stools are abnormal, the child should be placed on a lactose-free diet and further observed. Caloric intake should be increased if weight gain does not occur but intake is well tolerated. The following 3 patterns are often noted during the rehabilitation period. Pattern 1 is by far the most common.

Pattern 1: In this most common type, the intake is adequate and the weight gain is satisfactory, but the feeding technique is at fault. A disturbed infant-mother relationship leads to the decreased caloric intake.

Pattern 2: The intake is adequate, but there is no weight gain. If weight gain is unsatisfactory after increasing the calories to an adequate level (based on the infant's ideal weight for his or her height), malabsorption is a likely diagnosis. If malabsorption is present, it is usually necessary to differentiate pancreatic exocrine insufficiency (cystic fibrosis) from abnormalities of intestinal mucosa (celiac disease). In cystic fibrosis, growth velocity commonly declines from the time of birth, and appetite is good to voracious except during illness (eg, pneumonia). In celiac disease, growth velocity is usually not reduced until 6–12 months of age, and inadequate caloric intake may be a prominent feature.

Pattern 3: The intake is inadequate, owing to the following: (1) Sucking or swallowing difficulties due to central nervous system or neuromuscular disease or to esophageal or oropharyngeal malformations may result in inadequate intake. (2) Inability to eat large amounts is common in patients with cardiopulmonary disease or in anorexic children suffering from chronic infections, inflammatory bowel disease, and endocrine problems (eg, hypothyroidism). Patients with celiac disease often have inadequate caloric intake in addition to malabsorption. (3) Inadequate intake may be due to vomiting, spitting up, or rumination in patients with upper intestinal tract obstruction (eg, pyloric stenosis, hiatal hernia, chalasia), chronic metabolic aberrations and acidosis (eg, renal insufficiency, diabetes mellitus or insipidus, methylmalonic acidemia), adrenogenital syndrome, increased intracranial pressure, or psychosocial abnormalities.

TALL STATURE

Although there are several conditions (Table 23–2) that may produce tall stature, by far the most common cause is a constitutional variation from normal. Tall stature is usually of concern only to adolescent and preadolescent girls.

On the basis of family history, previous pattern of growth, state of physiologic development, assessment of epiphyseal development ("bone age"), and standard growth data, the physician should make a tentative estimate of the patient's eventual height. Hormonal therapy with conjugated estrogenic substances (eg, Premarin), 5–10 mg/d orally (continuously or cyclically),

Table 23-2. Causes of tall stature.

Constitutional (familial, genetic) factors	Genetic causes
Endocrine causes	Klinefelter's syndrome
Androgen deficiency (normal	Syndromes of XYY, XXYY (tall
height as children, tall as	as adults)
adults)	Testicular feminization
Anorchidism (infection,	Miscellaneous syndromes and
trauma, idiopathic)	entities
Klinefelter's syndrome	Cerebral gigantism (Soto's
Androgen excess (tall as	syndrome)
children, short as adults)	Diencephalic syndrome
Pseudosexual precocity	Homocystinuria
True sexual precocity	Marfan's syndrome
Hyperthyroidism	Total lipodystrophy
Somatotropin excess (pituitary	
gigantism)	

has been recommended by some in cases in which the patient's predicted height is considered to be excessive and the physiologic age as determined by stage of sexual maturity and epiphyseal development has not reached the 12-year-old level. Because of known and unknown long-term effects of estrogen administration in children and variable effects of therapy, treatment with estrogen seldom is recommended and should be used with caution.

Testosterone in high doses has been used to decrease final height in excessively tall boys. The results are variable (average reduction in adult height is approximately 5 cm); treatment is probably effective when the bone age is 14 yr or greater. Testicular function may be altered for a variable period after treatment.

DIABETES INSIPIDUS

Diabetes insipidus may result from deficient secretion of vasopressin (ADH), lack of response to the kidney to ADH, or failure of osmoreceptors to respond to elevations of osmolality. Hypofuncion of the posterior lobe of the pituitary with ADH deficiency may be idiopathic or may be associated with lesions of the anterior pituitary or hypothalamus (trauma, infections, suprasellar cysts, tumors, reticuloendotheliosis, or some developmental abnormality). Congenital ADH deficiency may be transmitted as an autosomal dominant trait. In nephrogenic diabetes insipidus, a hereditary X-linked (dominant) disease affecting both sexes but more severe in males, the renal tubules fail to respond normally to ADH, and no lesion of the pituitary or hypothalamus can be demonstrated. See Chapter 18.

Clinical Findings

The onset is often sudden, with polyuria, intense thirst, constipation, and evidence of dehydration. High fever, circulatory collapse, and secondary brain damage may occur in young infants on an ordinary feeding regimen. Serum osmolality may be elevated (above 305 mosm/L), but urine osmolality remains below 280 mosm/L (specific gravity approximately 1.010) even after a 7-hour test period of thirsting. Rate of growth, sexual maturation, and general body metabolism may be impaired, and hydroureter and bladder distention may develop.

Diabetes insipidus may be differentiated from psychogenic polydipsia and polyuria by permitting the normal intake of fluid for several days and then withholding water for 7 hours or until weight loss (3% or more) demonstrates adequate dehydration. With neurogenic or nephrogenic diabetes insipidus, the urine osmolality does not increase above 300 mosm/L even after the period of dehydration. Normal children and those with psychogenic polydipsia will respond to the dehydration with a urinary osmolality above 450 mosm/L. Patients with long-standing psychogenic polydipsia may be unable to concentrate urine initially, and the test may have to be repeated on several successive days. Eventually, dehydration will increase urine osmolality well above plasma osmolality. The ADH and hypertonic saline tests may be employed to distinguish between the various forms of diabetes insipidus.

Treatment

The treatment of choice for central diabetes insipidus is intranasal desmopression acetate (1-desamino-8-D-arginine vasopressin; DDAVP). Individual and temporal variations in degree of deficiency absorbtion and response are the rule.

The cautious use of chlorothiazide and ethacrynic acid may be of value in nephrogenic diabetes insipidus. (Check levels of serum electrolytes, uric acid, and blood glucose periodically.) For nephrogenic diabetes insipidus, also administer abundant quantities of water at short intervals and feedings containing limited electrolytes and minimal (but nutritionally adequate) amounts of protein.

SEXUAL PRECOCITY

In sexual precocity, the onset of secondary sexual development is earlier than anticipated by chronologic age (females less than 8 yrs; males less than 9 yrs of age), body mass, and family history. Sexual precocity is generally divided into 2 *major* types: Gonadotropin releasing hormone dependent (GnRH) or true precocity, and GnRH independent pseudoprecocity. **True (complete) precocity** is the result of premature increases in gonadotropin either from stimulation of the hypothalamic-pituitary mechanism (eg, in children with no abnormality or in those with tumor, infection, trauma, etc) or rarely from gonadotropin-producing tumors (eg, CNS germinoma hepatoma, choriocarcinoma). **Pseudoprecocity** is initiated by nongonadotropin-producing conditions (eg, adrenal, ovarian, and testicular tumors and other lesions) or by administration of sex steroids.

A third type, which resembles true sexual precocity but is not associated with premature elevation of gonadotropin concentrations, has been described and is more common in males and is usually familial.

In the past, true sexual precocity was considered to be idiopathic in approximately 80% of girls and 50% of boys. Currently, through the use of CT and MRI imaging, small abnormalities in the region of the hypothalamus are most commonly recognized.

Sexual precocity has been arbitrarily defined as the development of secondary sex characteristics beginning before age 8 in girls and age 9 in boys. Breast development is usually the first sign in girls, but the pattern of development is variable. Height may be normal initially, but it is often increased; osseous maturation ("bone age") may be even more advanced than height age, particularly in pseudoprecocious patients. Psychologic development tends to correspond to chronologic age. Ovarian luteal cysts may be present in response to gonadotropin stimulation. When sensitive assays are employed, urinary and serum gonadotropin levels are elevated for age, and adrenal androgen levels may be elevated to the pubertal range. Findings on EEG are frequently abnormal, particularly in boys.

Adrenal lesions (see Diseases of the Adrenal Cortex, below) are the most common causes of pseudoprecocity. Gonadal tumors are uncommon causes; the granulosa cell and theca-lutein cell tumors of the ovary are the most common, are generally unilateral and of low malignant potential, and produce excessive amounts of estrogen. In almost all instances, the tumor can be palpated transabdominally or rectally, and is readily visualized by pelvic ultrasonography.

When possible, treatment is directed at the underlying cause. In the GnRH type the treatment of choice is a GnRH agonist. These agents result in gonadotropin suppression through endocrine "down regulation." Treatment with medroxyprogesterone acetate (Depo-Provera) and cyproterone is often unsatisfactory. Psychologic management of the patient and family is important. Children who initially have no definable causative lesion should be examined at periodic intervals for evidence of previously occult abdominal or central nervous system lesions.

Precocious Development of the Breast (Premature Thelarche)

Precocious development of one or both breasts may occur at any age. In most cases, the onset is in the first 2 years of life; in two-thirds of these cases, breast development is obvious in the first year. The condition is not associated with other evidence of sexual maturation (rapid growth, advanced skeletal maturation, and menstruation do not occur). It may represent unusual sensitivity of the breasts to normal amounts of circulating estrogen or a temporarily increased secretion or ingestion of estrogen. Both breasts are usually involved, and enlargement may persist for months or years; the nipples generally do not enlarge. Extensive diagnostic investigation is seldom warranted; no treatment is necessary. Puberty occurs at the normal time.

Premature Adrenarche (Premature Pubarche)

Premature development of sexual hair may occur at any age and in both sexes (more often in females than in males) and must be differentiated from adrenal hyperplasia or neoplasia exogenous androgen intake and gonadal tumors. About a third of cases occur in organically brain-damaged children. Pubic hair usually develops first, but axillary hair is present in about half of cases when these patients are first seen. Children are of normal stature, and osseous development (bone age) is not advanced. The condition results from a premature slight increase in production of adrenal androgens. Premature adrenarche requires no treatment.

Menstruation

The age at menarche ranges from 9 to 16 years; menarche is considered delayed if it has not occurred by age 17 years or within 5 years after development of the breasts. Primary amenorrhea is the result of gonadal lesions (ie, gonadal dysgenesis) in about 60% of patients, and in such cases serum and urine gonadotropin levels are elevated. In the remaining cases of primary amenorrhea, extragonadal abnormalities are present (eg, pituitary-hypothalamic hypogonadotropinism; congenital anomalies of the tubes, uterus, or vagina; androgen excess or other endocrine imbalance; and chronic systemic disease or pelvic inflammatory disease).

Once regular periods are established, amenorrhea (ie, secondary amenorrhea; Table 23–3) during adolescence is often the result of pregnancy, strenuous physical activity, or chronic systemic disease. Secondary amenorrhea should therefore be viewed as a symptom requiring evaluation and, when possible, treatment.

Table 23–3. Causes of secondary amenorrhea.

I. Pregnancy.
II. Decreased ovarian function.
    A. Decreased gonadotropin level (secondary ovarian insufficiency).
        1. Due to organic and idiopathic hypothalamic disease, pituitary disease, or both.[1]
        2. Due to "functional abnormalities of the hypothalamic-pituitary axis" ("psychogenic").
        3. Due to hypothalamic-pituitary disease secondary to chronic systemic illness.
            a. Nutritional disorder (eg, anorexia nervosa).
            b. Chronic infection or systemic disease (eg, cancer, collagen vascular disease, inflammatory bowel disease).
        4. Secondary to endogenous hormones (eg, androgen excess, feminizing or masculinizing ovarian tumor).
        5. Secondary to exogenous drugs (eg, long-term contraceptive drugs, androgens, estrogens, tranquilizers).
        6. Associated with strenuous and prolonged physical activity (eg, ballet dancing, marathon running).
    B. Increased gonadotropin level (primary ovarian insufficiency).
        1. Due to acquired diseases (destruction of ovaries by infection or tumor, "premature menopause," radiation castration, surgical removal of ovaries).
        2. Due to ovarian agenesis and dysgenesis[1] (eg, Turner's syndrome).
III. Congenital and acquired lesions of the uterine tubes and uterus, including cases of chromosomal intersex (eg, adhesions, congenital absence of the uterus, cryptomenorrhea, hysterectomy, synechia of the uterus, testicular feminization syndrome).

[1] Usually or often associated with primary amenorrhea.

GONADAL DISORDERS

Deficiency of gonadal tissue or function may result from a genetic or embryologic defect; from hormone excess affecting the fetus in utero; from inflammation and destruction following infection (eg, mumps, syphilis, tuberculosis); from trauma, irradiation, autoimmune disease, or tumor; or as a consequence of surgical castration. Secondary hypogonadism may result from pituitary insufficiency (eg, destructive lesions in or about the anterior pituitary, irradiation of the pituitary, starvation), diabetes mellitus, androgen excess (eg, adrenogenital syndrome), or insufficiency of either the thyroid or adrenals.

CRYPTORCHIDISM

Cryptorchidism (undescended testes) is a common disorder in children. It may be unilateral or bilateral and may be classified as ectopic, total, or incomplete. About 3% of term male infants and 20% of premature male infants have undescended testes at birth. In over half of these cases, the testes will descend by the second month; by age 1 year, 80% of all undescended testes are in the scrotum. If cryptorchidism persists into adult life, failure of spermatogenesis is the rule, but testicular androgen production usually remains intact. The incidence of cancer (usually seminoma) is appreciably greater in testes that remain in the abdomen after puberty.

Cryptorchidism may merely represent delayed descent of the testes or may be due to prevention of normal descent by some mechanical lesion such as adhesions, short spermatic cord, fibrous bands, or endocrine disorders (ie, decreased gonadotropins). It is probable that many undescended testes are congenitally abnormal and that this abnormality in itself prevents descent.

A causal relationship between failure of spermatogenesis and an abdominal location of testes after puberty is assumed. On occasion, the apparent abnormality of abdominal testes may be reversible (even if the testes are histologically abnormal at the time they are placed in the scrotum).

Clinical Findings

In palpating the scrotum for the testes, the cremasteric reflex may be elicited, with a resultant ascent of the testes into the abdomen (pseudocryptorchidism). To prevent this ascent, the fingers first should be placed across the upper portion of the inguinal canal. Examination in a warm setting or bath is also helpful.

Treatment

The best age for medical or surgical treatment has not been determined, but early childhood is currently recommended. Some recommend surgery before age 5 years; others say during the first year. There appears to be a high incidence of azoospermia in testes operated on after age 10 years; recent evidence indicates that damage to germ and Leydig cells of intraabdominal testes may occur by age 3–4 years, but the relationship of these changes to fertility is unproved. The risk of surgical injury to the testes must be weighed against the possible benefits. Surgical repair is indicated for cryptorchidism persisting beyond puberty, since the incidence of cancer is appreciably greater in glands that remain in the abdomen beyond the second decade of life.

A. Unilateral Cryptorchidism: Most cases are due to local mechanical lesions or a defective testis on the involved side. If pseudocryptorchidism has been ruled out and if descent has not occurred by age 5 years, many investigators recommend surgical exploration, with testicular biopsy and relocation by a surgeon skilled in this procedure.

B. Bilateral Cryptorchidism: The child with bilaterally undescended testes should be evaluated for sex chromosome abnormalities and genetic sex determined by chromosome analysis in the newborn period. Androgen treatment (testosterone enanthate) is indicated only as replacement therapy in the male beyond the normal age of puberty who has been shown to lack functional testes.

C. Pseudocryptorchidism: Retractile testes, ie, those that are sometimes in the scrotum but not at the time of examination, generally require no treatment.

Prognosis

Following surgery, the prognosis is guarded with respect to spermatogenesis in the involved testis.

KLINEFELTER'S SYNDROME

Klinefelter's syndrome is occasionally familial, is typically not diagnosed until the time of puberty, and is characterized by atrophic sclerosis of the seminiferous tubules, normal Leydig cells and virilization. It is often accompanied by bilateral gynecomastia, relatively long extremities, particularly legs, abnormally small testes, and azoospermia or oligospermatogenesis. Gonadotropin levels (particularly luteinizing hormone levels) are usually elevated. Testosterone levels are normal or low. Many patients have mild mental retardation and poor psychosocial skills. There is an extra X chromosome (most commonly an XXY chromosome pattern).

Klinefelter's syndrome must be differentiated from other causes of primary hypogonadism, gonadotropin deficiency, the physiologic gynecomastia that occurs in some boys at puberty, and feminizing tumors of the adrenal cortex or testes.

There is no satisfactory treatment, but depot testosterone, 200–400 mg intramuscularly every 3 weeks, continued for several months, may produce positive physical and behavioral changes and reduce gynecomastia. If not, liposuction or surgical mastectomy for cosmetic purposes is indicated.

DISEASES OF THE THYROID

GOITER

Goiter is not uncommon in children and adolescents and is most commonly due to chronic lymphocytic thyroiditis (see Thyroiditis, below). It may also result from acute inflammation, iodine deficiency, infiltrative processes, neoplasms, ingestion of goitrogens, or an inborn error in thyroid metabolism (familial goiter). With the exception of hyperthyroidism (and possibly pregnancy), thyroid enlargement results from the stimulation of excess thyroid-stimulating hormone (TSH). Regardless of the cause, patients may be clinically and biochemically euthyroid, hypothyroid, or hyperthyroid.

Familial goiter results from enzymatic defects in hormonogenesis, eg, (1) iodide trapping, (2) iodide organification, (3) coupling, (4) deiodination, and (5) production of thyroglobulin and serum carrier protein. Patients with any of these defects display an autosomal recessive mode of inheritance; the organification defect may be associated with severe congenital deafness (Pendred's syndrome). The age at onset of symptoms of hypothyroidism is variable.

Substances implicated in the development of goiter include cabbage, soybeans, turnips, rutabagas, aminosalicylic acid (PAS), resorcinol, phenylbutazone, iodides (particularly in individuals who have also received corticosteroids), and drugs that interfere with iodide trapping (eg, thiocyanates).

Clinical Findings

The clinical features and physical characteristics of patients with goiters vary depending on the cause and are seldom diagnostic.

Nodular goiter may occur during childhood. The likelihood that a nodule is malignant increases when the nodule is single, hard, or associated with paratracheal lymph node enlargement or does not concentrate radioactive iodide (see Carcinoma of the Thyroid, below).

Treatment

Remove or avoid precipitating factors if possible. With the exception of hyperthyroidism and instances where specific causes can be eliminated or corrected (eg, iodide deficiency, goitrogens), treatment is with full replacement of thyroid hormone (see below). Surgery is necessary if cancer is a possibility.

Prophylaxis

Prophylaxis in endemic areas of iodine deficiency consists of the use of bread containing iodides or iodized salt (1 mg of iodine per 100 g of salt) the administration of 1–2 drops of saturated solution of potassium iodide per week or monthly injections of depot iodide preparation. Iodination of the water supply is also a satisfactory preventive measure.

NEONATAL GOITER

Neonatal goiter may result from the transplacental passage, from mother to infant, of iodides, goitrogens, antithyroid drugs, or human-specific thyroid-stimulating immunoglobulin (TSI). The latter may occur in pregnancies in which the mother has or once had Graves' disease. The offspring may temporarily be hyperthyroid, with exophthalmos. Regardless of the cause, the goiter is usually diffuse and relatively soft but may be large and firm enough to compress the trachea, esophagus, and adjacent blood vessels. Treatment varies with the cause; iodides, antithyroid drugs, or thyroid hormone (eg, levothyroxine, 0.05 mg/d) for a few weeks may be indicated. Rarely, surgical division of the thyroid isthmus may be necessary.

HYPOTHYROIDISM

Hypothyroidism may be either congenital or acquired. Congenital hypothyroidism may be due to aplasia, hypoplasia, or maldescent of the thyroid, resulting from an embryonic defect of development; the administration of radioiodide to the mother; or, possibly, an autoimmune disease. It may be cause by defective synthesis of thyroid hormone (familial goiter; see Goiter, above). Other cases of congenital hypothyroidism may result from the maternal ingestion of medications (eg, goitrogens, propylthiouracil, methimazole, iodides), from iodide deficiency (endemic cretinism), or, rarely, from thyroid hormone unresponsiveness. Thyroid tissue in an aberrant location is present in most patients with sporadic "athyreotic" cretinism.

Acquired (juvenile) hypothyroidism is most commonly the result of chronic lymphocytic thyroiditis (see Thyroiditis, below) but may be idiopathic or the result of surgical removal, thyrotropin deficiency (usually associated with other pituitary tropic hormone deficiencies), the ingestion of medications (eg, iodides, cobalt), or a deficiency of iodides. An ectopic thyroid gland, a relatively common cause of hypothyroidism, may maintain normal function for variable periods postnatally. Breast-feeding may mitigate severe hypothyroidism and perhaps diminish impaired neurologic development in the hypothyroid patient.

Clinical Findings

The findings depend on age at onset and the degree of deficiency.

A. Symptoms and Signs:

1. Functional Changes–Findings include decreased appetite; physical and mental sluggishness; pale, dry, coarse cool skin; decreased intestinal activity (constipation); large tongue; poor muscle tone (protuberant abdomen, umbilical hernia, lumbar lordosis); hypothermia; bradycardia; diminished sweating (variable); carotenemia; decreased pulse pressure; hoarse voice or cry; and slow relaxation on eliciting tendon reflexes. Prolonged gestation, large size at birth, nasal obstruction and discharge, large fontanelles, hypoactivity, and persistent jaundice may also be present during the neonatal period. Even with congenital deficiency of thyroid hormone, the first findings may not appear for several days or weeks.

2. Retardation of Growth and Development–Findings include decreased growth velocity with resultant shortness of stature; infantile skeletal proportions, with relatively short extremities; infantile naso-orbital configuration (bridge of nose flat, broad, and undeveloped; eyes seem to be widely spaced); retarded "bone age" and epiphyseal dysgenesis; retarded dental development and enamel hypoplasia; and large fontanelles in the neonate. Slowing of mental responsiveness and retardation of development of the brain may occur. In older children and adolescents, growth failure may be the only manifestation of hypothyroidism.

3. Sexual Precocity–Rarely, isosexual precocity may occur, resulting from elevated gonadotropin levels. Galactorrhea may be present, and menometrorrhagia has been reported in older girls. Testicular enlargement occurs rarely in boys.

4. Other Changes–Myxedema of tissues may occur. The skin may be dry, thick, scaly, and coarse, with a yellowish tinge from excessive deposition of carotene. The hair is dry, coarse, and brittle (variable) and may be excessive. The axillary and supraclavicular pads may be prominent. Muscular hypertrophy (Kocher, Debré-Sémélaigne syndromes) occasionally is present. Psychosis secondary to myxedema has been described. An ectopic thyroid gland may produce a mass at the base of the tongue or in the midline of the neck.

B. Laboratory Findings: Thyroxine (T_4) and thyroid-stimulating hormone (TSH) levels are the most helpful aids in diagnosing hypothyroidism. Levels of T_4 and free T_4 are reduced; TSH levels are increased in primary hypothyroidism. Serum carotene and cholesterol levels are usually elevated in hypothyroid children but may be normal in some hypothyroid infants; a rise to abnormally high levels occurs 6–8 weeks after cessation of therapy. The basal metabolic rate is low (unreliable in children). Serum alkaline phosphatase levels and erythrocyte glucose 6-phosphate dehydrogenase activity are reduced; BUN and creatinine levels may be increased. Sweat electrolyte levels are often increased. Circulating autoantibodies to thyroid constituents may be found. Plasma GH levels and GH response to insulin-induced hypoglycemia and arginine stimulation may be subnormal.

C. Imaging: Epiphyseal development ("bone age") is delayed. The cardiac shadow may be increased. Epiphyseal dysgenesis, coxa vara, coxa plana, and vertebral anomalies may occur. The pituitary fossa may be enlarged.

Treatment

Levothyroxine sodium is a reliable synthetic agent for thyroid replacement therapy. The dose is 100 $\mu g/m^2$ (10–12 $\mu g/kg$ in neonates). Older children, adolescents, and adults require 0.15–0.2 mg daily in one dose. In hypothyroid patients, particularly myxedematous infants, low doses (0.025–0.05 mg) should be used initially and increased weekly in small increments. The therapeutic range is evaluated by clinical response (appearance, growth, development), sleeping pulses, and thyroid function tests. (TSH and free T_4 levels). Improvement usually occurs in 1–3 weeks.

Course & Prognosis

In patients with congenital hypothyroidism, growth and motor development can be returned to normal with adequate replacement therapy. The prognosis for mental development is guarded if treatment is delayed beyond 3 months of life. In patients with acquired hypothyroidism, restoration of physical and mental function to the predisease level is variable following replacement therapy. Overtreatment with thyroid drugs may produce accelerated skeletal maturation and craniosynostosis; osteoporosis is a concern in adults.

HYPERTHYROIDISM

Hyperthyroidism appears to occur in individuals who demonstrate a reduced capacity to remove host-directed thyroid-stimulating immunoglobulins. In addition, psychic trauma, psychologic maladjustments, disturbances in pituitary function, infectious disease, heredity, and imbalance of the endocrine system all have been incriminated in the etiology and pathogenesis of hyperthyroidism. Congenital hyperthyroidism, sometimes persisting or recurring for months or years with or without exophthalmos, may occur in infants of thyrotoxic mothers and be associated with premature cranio synostosis, minimal brain dysfunction, accelerated "bone age," and goiter.

Hyperthyroidism (with normal T_4 levels) may result from

isolated hypersecretion of triiodothyronine (T_3 toxicosis) but is uncommon during childhood except in relapse.

Clinical Findings

A. Symptoms and Signs: The disease usually develops rapidly and is more common in girls, (5:1), with the highest incidence between ages 12 and 14 years. The manifestations may include the following in any combination: "nervousness" (ie, restlessness, mood swings, hand tremors); palpitations and tachycardia, even during sleep, and systolic hypertension with increased pulse pressure; warm and moist skin and flushed face; exophthalmos; diffuse goiter, usually firm, with or without bruit and thrill; weakness and loss of weight in spite of polyphagia; accelerated growth and development; and poor school performance. Amenorrhea is common in adolescent girls.

B. Laboratory Findings: Levels of T_4, free T_4, and T_3 resin uptake are elevated. T_3 levels may be elevated. Serum cholesterol and TSH levels are low. Circulating TSI and other antithyroid antibody levels are usually elevated. There is moderate leukopenia and hyperglycemia. Glycosuria may be present.

Treatment

Antithyroid drugs, radioactive iodide, and surgical methods are equally capable of eliminating the manifestations of hyperthyroidism and yield approximately equal numbers of "cured" patients.

A. General Measures:

1. Restricted Physical Activity–Activity should be restricted in severe cases, in preparation for surgery or during pregnancy.

2. Diet–The diet should be high in calories, proteins, and vitamins.

3. Sedation–Large doses of barbiturates or tranquilizers may be necessary to control nervousness.

4. Sympatholytic Drugs–These drugs (eg, propranolol) decrease the peripheral conversion of T_4 to T_3 and diminish cardiovascular and some neurologic symptoms. They are also helpful in preparation for thyroid surgery.

B. Specific Measures: With medical treatment, clinical response may be noted in about 2–3 weeks, and adequate control may be achieved in 2–3 months. The thyroid gland frequently increases in size after initiation of treatment, but it usually decreases in size after 3 months.

1. Propylthiouracil–This drug blocks the hormonogenesis and release of thyroid hormone as well as the peripheral conversion of T_4 to T_3. It may be used in the initial treatment of the patient with hyperthyroidism, but if the T_4 fails to return to a normal range, surgery or RAI may be necessary, although some patients may be controlled by long-continued (> 5 years) medical therapy. Relapses occur in 25–50% of patients, and severe cases may not respond. Therapy must usually be continued at least 2–3 years with the minimum drug dosage that will produce a euthyroid state.

a. Initial Dosage–Give 100–800 mg/d in 3 or 4 divided doses 6 or 8 hours apart until results of thyroid function tests are normal and all signs and symptoms have subsided. Larger doses may be necessary.

b. Maintenance Dosage–Give 100–150 mg/d in 1–3 divided doses. The drug may be continued at higher doses until hypothyroidism has resulted, and then a supplement of oral thyroid may be added. Thyroid hormone may be necessary if the TSH concentration rises during treatment.

2. Methimazole (Tapazole)–This may be used in $\frac{1}{15}$–$\frac{1}{10}$ the dosage of propylthiouracil. Toxic reactions are slightly more common with this drug than with the thiouracils.

3. Iodide–Elemental iodide is effective only transiently (1–2 weeks) and may be useful in preparation of surgery or RAI and following RAI therapy. Iodide is generally not recommended.

4. Radioactive Iodide–Radioiodide therapy is currently recommended by some either as initial treatment or if medical therapy fails. Regardless of the dose or type of radioactive iodide employed, hypothyroidism generally can be anticipated at variable periods after treatment.

5. Other Drugs–Antithyroid drugs, antibiotics, sedation, propranolol, reserpine, and guanethidine may be of value for the treatment of thyroid storm.

C. Surgical Measures: Subtotal thyroidectomy is considered by some to be the treatment of choice for children, especially if close follow-up is difficult or impossible. The patient should be prepared first with bed rest, diet, propranolol, and sedation (as above) and with propylthiouracil (for 2–4 weeks). Iodide (2–10 drops daily of saturated solution of potassium iodide for 10–21 days) may be of value. Continue for 1 week after surgery.

Course & Prognosis

Medical treatment is usually effective within 2–3 years. With medical treatment alone, prolonged remissions may be expected in about one-third of cases. Hypothyroidism is likely in later life. The risk of developing leukemia or carcinoma of the thyroid after treatment with radioactive iodide has not been determined.

CARCINOMA OF THE THYROID

See also Chapter 29.

Carcinoma of the thyroid is uncommon. It is most likely to occur following irradiation of the neck and chest. Findings include goiter, neck discomfort, dysphagia, and voice changes or a nodule of the thyroid that fails to regress despite therapy with a large dose of thyroid hormones for a period of 1–2 months. Surgical extirpation of the entire gland, with removal of all involved nodes, is the treatment of choice. Radical neck dissection is seldom necessary. Postoperatively, the patient may be allowed to become hypothyroid and a diagnostic scan with radioactive iodide then done; metastases, if present, can be treated with ^{131}I or removed surgically, if feasible. Subsequent thyroid replacement therapy should consist of larger than maintenance doses. Patients with papillary carcinoma have a good prognosis for prolonged (>10 years) survival.

Medullary carcinoma may be familial and associated with multiple endocrine adenomatosis, marfanoid body habitus, mucosal neuromas of the tongue and mucous membranes, and pheochromocytoma or visceral ganglioneuromas. The serum calcitonin level is elevated basally or after stimulation with pentagastrin.

GOITROUS CRETINISM

See Familial Goiter, above.

THYROIDITIS

Acute thyroiditis produces an acute inflammatory goiter and may be due to almost any pathogenic organism (viral or bacterial) or may be nonspecific or idiopathic. Most children are euthyroid and free of symptoms, but hypothyroidism or hyperthyroidism may be present. Specific antibiotic therapy and corticosteroids may be of value.

Subacute thyroiditis (pseudotuberculosis, de Quervain's giant cell thyroiditis) is characterized by mild and transient manifestations of hypermetabolism and an enlarged, very tender, firm thyroid gland. The T_4 concentration is elevated, and ^{131}I uptake by the gland is reduced. Aspirin (mild cases) and corticosteroids and thyroid hormone (severe disease) may be of value.

Chronic thyroiditis (lymphocytic or Hashimoto's struma, autoimmune thyroiditis) is being seen with increasing frequency, particularly in pubertal patients ("adolescent goiter"). It may be associated with other endocrine disorders (eg, Addison's disease, type I diabetes mellitus) resulting from autoimmune damage to the organ. It is characterized by firm, nontender, diffuse or nodular, "pebbly" enlargement of the thyroid with variable activity. Occasionally, there are symptoms of mild tracheal compression. Definitive diagnosis can be made only by histologic examination; thyroid function tests, antithyroid antibody tests, and scanning studies provide varying results. Needle biopsy of the gland is often diagnostic but is not generally indicated. Treatment is with thyroid hormone in full replacement dosage. Hypothyroidism is often an end result, and lifelong treatment may be required.

DISEASES OF THE PARATHYROID GLANDS

HYPOPARATHYROIDISM

Hypoparathyroidism may be idiopathic, may result from parathyroidectomy, or may be one feature of a general autoimmune disorder associated with candidiasis, Addison's disease, pernicious anemia, diabetes mellitus, thyroiditis, ovarian failure, and alopecia. Transient hypoparathyroidism may occur in the neonate as a result of parathyroid gland immaturity; the condition is more common in the offspring of diabetic and of hyperparathyroid mothers.

Clinical Findings

A. Symptoms and Signs:

1. Tetany–Symptoms and signs include numbness, cramps and twitchings of extremities, carpopedal spasm, laryngospasm, a positive Chvostek sign (tapping of the face in front of the ear produces spasm of the facial muscles), a positive peroneal sign (tapping the fibular side of the leg over the peroneal nerve produces abduction and dorsiflexion of the foot), and a positive Trousseau sign (prolonged compression of the upper arm produces carpal spasm).

2. Prolonged Hypocalcemia–In addition to the findings listed above, prolonged hypocalcemia may be associated with growth retardation, blepharospasm and chronic conjunctivitis, cataracts, unexplained bizarre behavior, diarrhea, photophobia, irritability, loss of consciousness, convulsions, poor dentition, skin rashes, ectodermal dysplasias, fungal infections (*Candida*), "idiopathic" epilepsy, symmetric punctate calcifications of basal ganglia, and steatorrhea. Candidiasis, Addison's disease, thyroiditis, and pernicious anemia may precede or follow the hypoparathyroidism in the familial "autoimmune" form.

B. Laboratory Findings: See Table 23–4. Serum parathyroid levels are inappropriately low.

Treatment

The objective of treatment is to maintain serum calcium at a low normal level.

A. Tetany: In patients with acute or severe tetany, immediate correction of hypocalcemia is indicated. Give calcium intravenously and orally. Thiazide diuretics may be used to increase urinary calcium reabsorption.

B. Prolonged Hypocalcemia: For maintenance therapy in patients with hypoparathyroidism and chronic hypocalcemia, use calciferol 1,25 dihydroxycholecalciferol or dihydrotachysterol (see Chapter 38). The diet should be high in calcium, with added calcium lactate or carbonate, and should be adequate in phosphorus.

PSEUDOHYPOPARATHYROIDISM
(Seabright Bantam Syndrome)

Pseudohypoparathyroidism consists of a group of disorders generally having a familial X-linked dominant syndrome in which

Table 23–4. Laboratory findings in rickets and disorders of calcium metabolism.[1]

Condition	Metabolic Features					
	Serum Concentration				Urinary Excretion	
	Ca²⁺	P	Alk P'tase	PTH	Ca²⁺	P
Chronic renal insufficiency	↓ (N)	↑	↑ (N)	↑	↓ (N)	↓
Hypoparathyroid states	↓	↑	N	↓	↓	↓
Malabsorption syndrome	↓ (N)	↓ (N)	↑ (N)	↑ (N)	↓	N (↑↓)
Rickets						
Familial hypophosphatemic vitamin D-resistant	N (↓)	↓	N	N (↑)	N	↑
Hereditary vitamin D-refractory	↓	↓ (N)	↑	↑	↑	↑
Vitamin D-deficient	↓ (N)	↓	↑	↑	↓	↑
Transient tetany of the newborn	↓	N (↑)	N	↓ (N)	↓ (N)	↓ (N)

[1] Tubular reabsorption of phosphate (TRP) normally is 83–98%; the lower values are associated with higher serum levels of phosphorus. In hypoparathyroidism, TRP values vary from 40 to 70%. Low TRP values are also found in some forms of inherited renal tubular disease, eg, vitamin D-resistant rickets.

there is no lack of parathyroid hormone but a failure of response in the end organs (eg, the renal tubule). The symptoms and signs of hypocalcemia are the same as in idiopathic hypoparathyroidism. Patients with pseudohypoparathyroidism have round, full faces, stubby fingers (shortening of the first, fourth, and fifth metacarpals), mental subnormality, shortness of stature, delayed and defective dentition, and early closure of the epiphyses. X-rays may show dyschondroplastic changes in the bones of the hands, demineralization of the bones, thickening of the cortices, exostoses, and ectopic calcification of the basal ganglia and subcutaneous tissues. Corneal and lenticular opacities may be present.

Treatment is with vitamin D and supplementary oral calcium lactate or carbonate.

Pseudohypoparathyroidism type II is the result of a cellular defect in which neither cAMP nor parathyroid hormone produces a phosphaturic effect.

HYPERPARATHYROIDISM

Hyperparathyroidism may be primary (occasionally familial) or secondary. Primary hyperparathyroidism may be due to adenoma or diffuse parathyroid hyperplasia. The most common causes of the secondary form are chronic renal disease (glomerulonephritis, pyelonephritis), congenital anomalies of the genitourinary tract, pseudohypoparathyroidism, and vitamin D-refractory rickets. Rarely, it may be found in osteogenesis imperfecta, cancer with bony metastases, and vitamin D-resistant rickets.

Clinical Findings

A. Symptoms and Signs:

1. Due to Hypercalcemia*–Findings include hypotonicity and weakness of muscles; nausea, vomiting, and poor tone of the gastrointestinal tract, with constipation; loss of weight; hyperextensibility of joints; bradycardia; and shortening of the QT interval.

---

* Hypercalcemia may also be secondary to immobilization, excess intake of vitamin D, sarcoidosis, milk-alkali syndrome, extensive fat necrosis of the newborn, or certain types of cancer, or it may occur as a familial disease.

2. Due to Increased Calcium and Phosphorus Excretion–Polyuria, hyposthenuria, polydipsia, and precipitation of calcium phosphate in the renal parenchyma or as urinary calculi (ie, sand or gravel) may occur.

3. Related to Changes in the Skeleton–Findings include osteitis fibrosa, absence of lamina dura around the teeth, spontaneous fractures, and a "moth-eaten" appearance of the skull.

B. Laboratory Findings: Serum calcium and parathyroid hormone, urinary phosphorus, cAMP, and hydroxyproline excretion are increased (Table 23–5).

C. Imaging: Bone changes usually do not occur in children with an adequate calcium intake. When bone changes occur, there is a generalized demineralization with a predilection for the subperiosteal cortical bone. The distal clavicle and phalanges are usually first affected. Nephrocalcinosis is an important additional x-ray finding.

Treatment

Complete removal of tumor or subtotal removal of hyperplastic parathyroid glands is indicated. Preoperatively, fluids should be forced and the intake of calcium restricted. Postoperatively, the diet should be high in calcium, phosphorus, and vitamin D.

Treatment of secondary hyperparathyroidism (viz renal disease) is directed at the underlying disease. Decrease the intake of phosphate by use of aluminum hydroxide orally and by reduction of milk consumption.

Course & Prognosis

Although the condition may recur (particularly in patients with familial forms of hyperparathyroidism), the prognosis following subtotal parathyroidectomy or removal of an adenoma is usually quite good. The prognosis in the secondary forms depends on correcting the underlying defect. Renal function may remain abnormal.

IDIOPATHIC HYPERCALCEMIA

Idiopathic hypercalcemia (Williams's syndrome) is an uncommon disorder probably related to either excessive intake or increased sensitivity to vitamin D. The disease is characterized in its severe form by peculiar facies (receding mandible, de-

Table 23-5. Laboratory findings in hypercalcemia.

| | Metabolic Features | | | | | |
| | Serum Concentration | | | Urinary Excretion | | Bone Pathology |
Condition	Ca^{2+}	P	P'tase	Ca^{2+}	P	
Excessive vitamin D	↑	↑	N	↑	N (↑)	
Hyperparathyroidism	↑	↓	N (↑)	↑	↑	Generalized osteitis fibrosa
Hyperparathyroidism with impaired renal function	↑	N (↑)	↑	↑	↑	Generalized osteitis fibrosa
Hyperproteinemia	↑ (total) N (ionized)	N	N	N	N	
Idiopathic hypercalcemia	↑	N	N	↑	N	See text
Neoplasms of bone	N (↑)	N	N (↑)	↑	N (↑)	Bone destruction

pressed bridge of nose, relatively large mouth, prominent lips, hanging jowls, large low-set ears, "elfin" appearance), failure to thrive, mental and motor retardation, irritability, purposeless movements, constipation, hypotonia, polyuria, polydipsia, hypertension, and heart disease (especially supravalvular aortic stenosis). Generalized osteosclerosis is common, and there may be premature craniosynostosis and nephrocalcinosis with evidence of urinary tract disease. Hypercholesterolemia, azotemia, and serum vitamin A elevations may be present. Familial benign hypercalcemia has been reported.

Clinical manifestations may not appear for several months. Severe disease may end in death. Mild disease may occur without the typical facies and other findings and has a good prognosis.

Treatment is by rigid restriction of dietary calcium and vitamin D and, in severely involved children, the administration of corticosteroids in high doses.

HYPOPHOSPHATASIA

Hypophosphatasia is an uncommon heritable condition characterized by rickets and a deficiency of alkaline phosphatase. The earlier the age at onset, the more severe the condition. Failure to thrive, premature loss of teeth, widening of the sutures, bulging fontanelles, convulsions, bony deformities, dwarfing, and renal lesions have been reported. Premature closure of cranial sutures may occur. Late features include osteoporosis, pseudofractures, and rachitic deformities. Signs and symptoms may be similar to those of idiopathic hypercalcemia. The serum calcium level is frequently high. The urinary hydroxyproline level is low during infancy. The plasma and urine contain phosphoethanolamine in excessive amounts. No specific treatment is available; corticosteroids may be of value.

DISEASES OF THE ADRENAL CORTEX

ADRENOCORTICAL HYPOFUNCTION
(Adrenal Crisis, Addison's Disease)

Adrenocortical hypofunction may be due to atrophy; autoimmune disease; destruction of the gland by a tumor, hemorrhage (Waterhouse-Friderichsen syndrome), or infection (eg, tuberculosis); congenital absence of the adrenal cortex; or congenital hyperplasia of the cortex associated with glucocorticoid insufficiency with or without androgen excess. It may occur as a consequence of inadequate secretion of corticotropin (ACTH) due to anterior pituitary or hypothalamic disease. Any acute illness, surgery, trauma, or exposure to excessive heat may precipitate an adrenal crisis. A temporary salt-losing disorder (possibly due to hypoaldosteronism) may occur during infancy.

Adrenogenital syndrome and associated adrenal insufficiency, congenital adrenocortical insufficiency, autoimmune adrenal insufficiency, and neoplasms are the most common causes of chronic adrenocortical insufficiency. Autoimmune Addison's disease may be associated with hypoparathyroidism, lymphocytic thyroiditis, candidiasis, pernicious anemia, ovarian failure, alopecia, and diabetes mellitus. Antiadrenal antibodies may be present.

Clinical Findings
A. Symptoms and Signs:
1. Acute Form (adrenal crisis)–Signs and symptoms include nausea and vomiting; diarrhea; dehydration; fever, which may be followed by hypothermia; circulatory collapse; and confusion or coma.

2. Chronic Form (Addison's disease)–Signs and symptoms include vomiting (which becomes forceful and sometimes projectile), diarrhea, weakness, fatigue, weight loss or failure to gain weight, increased appetite for salt, dehydration, increased pigmentation (both generalized and over pressure points and scars and on mucous membranes), hypotension, and small heart size.

B. Laboratory Findings:
1. Adrenal Insufficiency–Findings suggestive of adrenal insufficiency include the following:

a. Serum sodium, chloride, and carbon dioxide levels are decreased.

b. Serum potassium and blood urea nitrogen levels are increased.

c. Urinary sodium levels are increased despite low serum sodium levels.

d. Eosinophilia and moderate neutropenia occur.

e. Fasting blood glucose levels are generally normal but may be low in crisis.

f. There is inability to excrete a water load.

2. Adrenal Cortex Function–Results of confirmatory tests to measure the functional capacity of the adrenal cortex include the following:

a. Blood cortisol and urinary 17-hydroxycorticosteroid levels and ketogenic steroid excretion levels are decreased. ACTH levels are increased in primary adrenal insufficiency.

b. Blood Androstenedione and DHEA concentrations and urinary 17-ketosteroid levels are decreased except in cases due to congenital hyperplasia or tumor of the cortex.

c. Circulating eosinophil counts are elevated.

d. Corticotropin and metyrapone administration are associated with subnormal responses.

e. In the prolonged corticotropin (ACTH) test, blood and urine levels of cortisol on the day before and on the day of ACTH infusion are compared. A rise of 50–100% or more in cortisol excludes primary adrenal insufficiency.

Treatment

A. Acute Form (Adrenal Crisis):

1. Treat infections with large doses of the appropriate antibiotics or other antimicrobial agents.

2. Treat hypovolemia with adequate fluid and electrolyte therapy (Normal saline). Infusion of a solution of human albumin may be necessary in severe cases.

3. In Waterhouse-Friderichsen syndrome with fulminant infections, adrenocorticosteroids and isoproterenol should be used.

4. For replacement therapy, use the following:

a. Initially, hydrocortisone sodium succinate (Solu-Cortef), 2 mg/kg diluted in 2–10 mL of water intravenously, is given over 2–5 minutes. Follow this with an infusion of normal saline and 5–10% glucose, 100 mL/kg/24 h intravenously.

b. Hydrocortisone sodium succinate, 1.5 mg/kg (12.5 mg/m^2), is given intravenously every 4–6 hours until stabilization is achieved and oral therapy tolerated.

c. Ten percent glucose in normal saline, 20 mL/kg intravenously in the first 2 hours, may be of value, particularly in infants with adrenal crisis who have congenital adrenal hyperplasia. Avoid overtreatment.

5. Fruit juices, ginger ale, milk, and soft foods should be started as soon as possible.

B. Chronic Form (Addison's Disease): There may be variable response to different glucocorticoids in some patients. (See

Table 23–6. Corticosteroids.

Generic and Chemical Name	Potency per Milligram Compared with Hydrocortisone[1]	
	Glucocorticoid Effect	Mineralocorticoid Effect
Glucocorticoids		
Hydrocortisone	1	1
Betamethasone	33	
Dexamethasone	30	Minimal
Fluprednisolone	13	
Methylprednisolone	5	Minimal
Paramethasone	10–12	
Prednisolone	4	Minimal
Prednisone	4	Minimal
Triamcinolone	5	Minimal
Mineralocorticoids		
Aldosterone	30	500
Fludrocortisone		15–20

[1] To convert hydrocortisone dosage to equivalent dosage in any of the other preparations listed in this table, divide by the potency factors shown.

Table 23–6 for conversion of other corticosteroids to hydrocortisone equivalents.) Maintenance therapy following initial stabilization generally requires the use of a corticosteroid together with a liberal intake of salt and a fluorinated steroid. Children requiring prolonged adrenocorticosteroid administration should have periodic determinations of height, weight, and blood pressure (taken in the recumbent position) and assay of blood glucose, ACTH, sodium, and potassium.

1. Hydrocortisone–Dosages are as follows:

a. Physiologic replacement–

(1) Intramuscularly–0.44 mg/kg or 13–20 mg/m^2 once daily.

(2) Orally*–0.66 mg/kg in infants or 10–15 mg/m^2/d.

b. Therapeutic use–

(1) Intramuscularly–4.4 mg/kg or 130 mg/m^2 once daily.

(2) Orally*–6.6 mg/kg or 200 mg/m^2/d.

* In 4 doses 6 hours apart (preferred) or 3 doses every 8 hours, providing approximately 50% of the total dose in the early morning.

c. Therapeutic maintenance–

(1) Intramuscularly–1.3–2.2 mg/kg or 40–65 mg/m² once daily.

(2) Orally*–2–3.3 mg/kg or 60–100 mg/m²/d.

d. Development of infection–If infection occurs while the patient is receiving a large dose of glucocorticoid, give about 2–3 times the physiologic maintenance dose for 3 or 4 days and then resume the larger dose.

e. Long-term maintenance–Except when used for replacement therapy (ie, in the treatment of Addison's disease and the adrenogenital syndrome) and in the treatment of certain malignant states, the total 2-day dose of glucocorticoid for long-term maintenance therapy may be administered as a single dose once every 48 hours. This will not diminish the therapeutic efficacy but will diminish the side effects; there may be normal growth and decreased tendency to cushingoid appearance.

2. Fludrocortisone–Give fludrocortisone, 0.05–0.2 mg daily in 2 divided doses.

3. Sodium Chloride–Give 1–3 g/d (as enteric-coated salt pills if they can be taken). Reduce the dose if edema appears.

4. Increased Dosages–Additonal glucocorticoids (2–3 times the maintenance dose) may be necessary with moderate to severe acute illness, surgery, trauma, or other stress reactions after optimal glucocorticoid stabilization has been achieved.

C. Other Recommendations:

1. If corticosteroids have been administered for more than 1 month, terminate their use gradually. Abrupt withdrawal may cause a severe "rebound" of the disease or rarely produce symptoms of adrenal insufficiency.

2. Give corticosteroids to any child undergoing surgery, severe infection, or other significant stress who has received prolonged therapy with corticosteroids in the past.

3. If a child receiving maintenance doses of corticosteroids develops chickenpox, the dosage of glucocorticoids should be increased to pharmacologic levels (eg, 3 times maintenance). Corticosteroid withdrawal in these circumstances may have a fatal outcome.

4. Use of topical corticosteroids for the treatment of inflammatory skin conditions may result in absorption of significantly large amounts of corticosteroid.

---

* In 4 doses 6 hours apart (preferred) or 3 doses every 8 hours, providing approximately 50% of the total dose in the early morning.

D. Corticosteroids in Patients Requiring Surgery: In patients with current or previous adrenocortical insufficiency who undergo surgery, corticosteroids are given as follows:

1. Preoperatively–Give oral glucocorticoids in twice the maintenance dose 24 hours before surgery.

2. During Operation–Give hydrocortisone sodium succinate (Solu-Cortef), 1–2 mg/kg by intravenous infusion over a 6- to 12-hour period.

3. Postoperatively–Continue intravenous delivery until oral intake is resumed. Begin oral preparation as soon as possible, and give full maintenance doses daily. If the maintenance dose is unknown, give 1.25 mg/kg intramuscularly as follows: 100% of total dose at 8:00 AM and 50% of dose at 2:00 PM and at 10:00 PM. If significant stress occurs postoperatively, give 3–5 times the maintenance dose.

ADRENOCORTICAL HYPERFUNCTION

1. CUSHING'S SYNDROME

The principal findings in Cushing's syndrome in children result from excessive secretion of glucocorticoid and androgenic hormones, leading to varying degrees of abnormal carbohydrate, protein, and fat metabolism and virilization. In noniatrogenic disease there may also be overproduction of mineralocorticoids and adrenal androgens.

Cushing's syndrome is more common in females; in children under 12 years of age, noniatrogenic disease is usually due to adrenal tumor. Hemihypertrophy may be present. Cushing's syndrome is a common result of therapy with one of the corticosteroids. Rarely, it may be associated with an apparently primary adrenocortical hyperplasia or hyperplasia secondary either to basophilic adenoma of the pituitary gland or to an ectopic ACTH-producing tumor. Spontaneous remission has been reported.

Clinical Findings

A. Symptoms and Signs:

1. Due to Excessive Secretion of the Carbohydrate-regulating Hormones–"Buffalo type" adiposity, most marked on the face, neck, and trunk, may occur; a fat pad in the interscapular area is characteristic. Other findings include easy fatigability and muscle weakness, striae, plethoric facies, easy bruisability, osteoporosis, increased appetite, growth failure, hyperglycemia, psychologic disturbances, and pain in the back.

2. Due to Excessive Secretion of Androgens–Findings include hirsutism, acne, varying degrees of clitoral or penile enlargement, advanced skeletal maturation, and deepening of the voice. Menstrual irregularities occur in older girls.

3. Due to Excessive Production of Mineralocorticoids–Sodium retention with hypertension (rarely edema) occurs.

B. Laboratory Findings:

1. Serum chloride and potassium levels may be low.

2. Serum sodium, pH, and carbon dioxide content may be elevated.

3. Plasma and urine cortisol levels are increased, and plasma diurnal variation may not occur.

4. Excretions of urinary 17-ketosteroids, 17-hydroxycorticosteroids, 17-ketogenic steroids, and free cortisol are generally increased; the test for free cortisol is the assay of choice. Increased secretion of ACTH occurs in patients with adrenal hyperplasia and with ACTH-secreting nonendocrine tumors but not with other adrenal tumors. Suppression of blood cortisol and 17-hydroxycorticosteroids by high doses of dexamethasone occurs with adrenal hyperplasia but not with adrenal tumors.

5. Eosinophil counts are below 50/μL.

6. Glycosuria alone or with carbohydrate intolerance and hyperglycemia may be present ("diabetic" type of glucose tolerance curve).

7. Abdominal ultrasonography, CT or MRI scanning, and radioactive cholesterol uptake studies may be helpful in localizing a tumor.

Treatment

Since almost all cases of primary adrenal hyperfunction in childhood are due to tumor, surgical removal (if possible) is indicated. Corticotropin has been recommended for pre- and postoperative use to stimulate the nontumorous adrenal cortex, which is generally atrophied. Corticosteroids should be administered for 1 or 2 days before surgery and continued during and after operation. Supplemental potassium, normal saline solution, and fludrocortisone may be necessary.

Pituitary surgery, irradiation, or cyproheptadine may be of value to control Cushing's disease resulting from adrenal hyperplasia. If these measures are ineffective, bilateral adrenalectomy and hypophysectomy may be tried.

Prognosis

If the tumor is malignant, the prognosis is poor. If it is benign, cure should result following proper preparation and surgery. Following total bilateral adrenalectomy, pituitary tumors may appear in Cushing's disease.

2. ADRENOGENITAL SYNDROME

Adrenogenital syndrome is most commonly the result of tumor or congenital adrenal hyperplasia; maternal androgens from endogenous and exogenous sources and tumor may also be causative.

The congenital form of adrenogenital syndrome (due to adrenal hyperplasia) is an autosomal recessive disease due to an inborn error of metabolism with a deficiency of an adrenocortical enzyme. Various types are recognized, including the following:

(1) Deficiency of 21-hydroxylase (approximately 90% of cases), resulting in inability to convert 17-hydroxyprogesterone into 11-deoxycortisol. Mild forms result in androgenic changes (virilization) alone, but severe cases are associated with salt loss and electrolyte imbalance.

(2) Deficiency in 11β-hydroxylation and a failure to convert 11-deoxycortisol to cortisol. This is associated with virilization and usually with hypertension.

(3) A defect in 17-hydroxylase, with the enzyme deficiency in both the adrenals and the gonads. Hypertension, virilization, amenorrhea, and eunuchoidism may be present.

(4) A partial or complete defect in 3β-hydroxysteroid dehydrogenase activity and a failure to convert Δ^5-pregnenolone to progesterone. This is associated with incomplete masculinization, hypospadias, and cryptorchidism in the male. Some degree of masculinization may occur in the female. Severe sodium loss occurs, and the infant mortality rate is high in the complete form.

(5) Cholesterol desmolase deficiency with congenital lipoid adrenal hyperplasia. Clinical features are similar to those of 3β-hydroxysteroid dehydrogenase deficiency (above).

Adrenogenital Syndrome in Females (Pseudohermaphroditism)

In congenital bilateral hyperplasia of the adrenal cortex (pseudohermaphroditism), abnormalities of the external genitalia include an enlarged clitoris with partial to complete labial fusion and a common urogenital sinus. Growth in height is excessive and "bone age" advanced, and patients may have excessive muscularity and sexual development. Pubic hair appears early; acne may be excessive; and the voice may deepen.

Pseudohermaphroditism in the female may also be produced as a result of the administration of androgens, progestins, diethylstilbestrol, and related hormones to the mother during the first trimester of pregnancy or as a result of virilizing maternal tumors. In these cases, the condition regresses after birth.

Adrenogenital Syndrome in Males (Macrogenitosomia Praecox)

In males, precocious sexual development is along isosexual lines. With congenital bilateral hyperplasia of the adrenal cortex, the infant may appear normal at birth; however, during the first few months of life, the penis enlarges, the scrotum darkens, the rugae become more prominent, and acne and pubic and axillary hair appear. The testicles generally remain small, and spermatogenesis does not occur. Other symptoms and signs are similar to those of the congenital form in females. If an adrenal or testicular tumor is the cause, the tumor may be palpable or readily appreciated with ultrasound, CT or MRI imaging. Rarely, an adrenal tumor in either sex produces feminization, with gynecomastia resulting in males.

Laboratory Findings

A. 21-Hydroxylase Deficiency–Blood and urine adrenal androgens and testosterone are elevated and the 17 OH progesterone level is elevated to diagnostic levels in cord and newborn blood. Aldosterone may be reduced, and excessive sodium loss occurs in salt-losing forms.

B. 11β-Hydroxylase Deficiency–11-Deoxycortisol (and its tetrahydro derivative), 17-hydroxycorticoid, deoxycorticosterone, 17-ketosteroid, and testosterone levels are increased.

C. 17-Hydroxylase Deficiency–17-Ketosteroid and 17-hydroxycorticoid levels are decreased; aldosterone, corticosterone, and deoxycorticosterone levels are increased.

D. 3β-Hydroxysteroid Dehydrogenase Deficiency–With the exception of Δ^5 compounds all adrenal steroid levels in the blood and urine are low.

E. Cholesterol Desmolase Deficiency–All steroid excretion is markedly decreased.

F. Tumor–Excretion of dehydroepiandrosterone may be greatly elevated.

G. Other Findings–Urinary excretion of gonadotropins may be elevated for age.

Dexamethasone Suppression Test

If the administration of dexamethasone, 2–4 mg/d orally in 4 doses for 7 days, reduces serum and urine metabolite levels, hyperplasia rather than adenoma is the probable diagnosis.

Imaging

Genitograms using contrast material may indicate the presence of a urogenital sinus. Displacement of the kidney and calcification in the area of the adrenal may be seen on urograms or plain films of patients with tumors. "Bone age" is typically advanced with 21- and 11β-hydroxylase defects after the first year of life in the untreated child.

Treatment

A. Congenital Hyperplasia of the Adrenal Cortex:

1. Hydrocortisone–Approximately 20–25 mg/m^2/d orally will produce adrenal suppression and normal linear growth. Dosages of 10–25 mg/d for infants and 25–100 mg/d for older children initially are usually necessary. The drug should be given orally in divided doses several times a day, two-fifths of the total dose given as the first morning dose and two-fifths as the last dose at night. After suppression is achieved, the maintenance doses necessary to sustain control are generally 10–15 mg/m^2/day.

2. Mineralocorticoids–For patients with salt-losing forms of adrenogenital syndrome, therapy with fludrocortisone and sodium chloride is necessary (see pp 885–887).

3. Glucocorticoids–Glucocorticoids should be increased (by 3–4 times) during acute severe stress, surgery or moderate infectious illnesses.

4. Surgical Measures–Recession or partial clitoridectomy is occasionally indicated in a girl with an abnormally large or sensitive clitoris but may be delayed for 1 or 2 years until the effect of therapy is determined. Surgical correction of the labial fusion and urogenital sinus may require several operations.

B. Tumor: Because the malignant lesions cannot be distinguished clinically from the benign ones, surgical removal is indicated whenever a tumor has been diagnosed. Preoperative and postoperative treatment are as for Cushing's syndrome due to a tumor (see Cushing's Syndrome, above).

Course & Prognosis

Untreated patients with congenital adrenal hyperplasia will show precocious virilization throughout childhood. Because of accelerated skeletal maturation, these individuals will be tall as children but short as adults. Adequate corticosteroid treatment permits normal growth and sexual maturation.

Female pseudohermaphrodites mistakenly raised as males for more than 3 years may have serious psychologic disturbances if their sex role is changed after that time.

When the adrenogenital syndrome is caused by a tumor, progression of signs and symptoms will cease after successful surgical removal; pubic hair, pigmentation, and deepening of the voice may regress or persist.

3. PRIMARY ALDOSTERONISM

Primary hyperaldosteronism may be caused by an adrenal tumor or by adrenal hyperplasia. It is characterized by paresthesias, tetany, weakness, periodic "paralysis," low serum potassium levels, hypertension, alkaline urine, proteinuria, metabolic alkalosis, carbohydrate intolerance, suppressed plasma renin activity, polyuria, and hyposthenuria that does not respond to vasopressin. The urinary aldosterone level is increased, but other steroid levels are variable. Adrenal tumors may be visualized with CT scanning ultrasonography or MRI. Treatment of the tumor is by surgical removal. With hyperplasia, subtotal or total adrenalectomy is recommended if pharmacologic doses of glucocorticoid are ineffective after 2 months.

A form of secondary hyperaldosteronism, possibly due to increased prostagladins, occurs in which both renin and aldosterone levels are elevated in the absence of hypertension (Barter's syndrome). There is associated renovascular disease, with hyperplasia of the juxtaglomerular apparatus and renal electrolyte wasting.

DISEASES OF THE ADRENAL MEDULLA

PHEOCHROMOCYTOMA
(Chromaffinoma)

Pheochromocytoma is an uncommon tumor that may be located wherever there is any chromaffin tissue (eg, adrenal medulla, sympathetic ganglia, carotid body). The condition may be familial (eg, multiple endocrine adenomatosis type II), and in children the tumors are often multiple and bilateral.

Clinical Findings

Clinical manifestations of pheochromocytoma are due to excessive secretion of epinephrine or norepinephrine (or both). Attacks of anxiety and headaches should arouse suspicion. Other findings are palpitation, dizziness, weakness, nausea, vomiting, diarrhea, dilated pupils with blurring of vision, abdominal and precordial pain, rapid pulse, hypertension (usually persistent), and discomfort from heat. The symptoms may be sustained, producing all of the above findings plus papilledema, retinopathy, and cardiac enlargement.

Urine and serum catecholamine levels are increased. The 24-hour urine collection shows markedly increased urinary excretion of total catecholamines, metanephrine, and vanilmandelic acid. *Caution:* Attacks may be provoked by mechanical stimulation of the tumor or by histamine or tyramine. Results of the phentolamine (Regitine) test are positive, but the test is not specific for pheochromocytoma and may not be necessary for diagnosis. Displacement of the kidney may be shown by routine x-ray. The tumor may be defined by ultrasonography or by CT scanning or MRI of the abdomen.

Treatment

Surgical removal of the tumor is the treatment of choice, but a sudden paroxysm and death during surgery are not uncommon. The oral administration of propranolol and phentolamine preoperatively has been recommended to prevent the extreme fluctuations of blood pressure that sometimes occur during surgery. Medical treatment includes phenoxybenzamine to reduce hypertension and propranolol to lessen tachycardia and ventricular dysrhythmias.

Prognosis

Complete relief of symptoms, except those due to longstanding vascular or renal changes, is the rule after recovery. If no treatment is given, severe cardiac, renal, and cerebral damage may result.

DIABETES MELLITUS*

Insulin dependent diabetes mellitus (IDDM) or Type I diabetes (previously referred to as juvenile diabetes) is the main type

---

* This section authored by H. Peter Chase, MD.

of diabetes occurring in people under age 40 years and is characterized by a gradual loss of insulin production. Although the majority of children in the US no longer present in acidosis (due to the earlier diagnosis by lay and professional people), if untreated long enough acidosis will ensue.

Noninsulin-dependent diabetes mellitus (NIDDM) or Type II diabetes occurs primarily in people over 40 years of age who are overweight, but can occur in overweight teenagers and is then referred to as maturity-onset diabetes in youth (MODY). Insulin production is often elevated in NIDDM (and MODY) and the etiology is related to ineffective insulin activity. Treatment is with weight loss, exercise, oral hypoglycemic agents, and a high-fiber diet. Insulin is not initially required and acidosis is usually not a problem.

Transient diabetes may occur in the newborn and may not require insulin treatment. Similarly, the stress of illness may result in hyperglycemia and glucosuria (and even mild acetonuria) in some children. Treatment with insulin is usually not necessary. However, up to 25% of these children will have islet cell antibodies (see below) and may eventually develop Type I diabetes.

Etiology

The etiology of Type I diabetes is now believed to involve a genetic predisposition, environmental factors (such as viruses or chemicals) and an immunologic component. The genetic component is associated with the HLA groups DR3 and DR4 (present in 95% of Caucasian children with diabetes and 53% have DR3/DR4). In addition, the presence of aspartic acid on position 57 of the DQ beta chain of the HLA complex is considered protective of diabetes and its absence provides a marker for susceptibility. In spite of these genetic associations, there is no close family member with Type I diabetes in 75% of newly diagnosed children.

It is now recognized that Type I diabetes has a gradual onset and that immunologic markers (islet cell antibodies [ICA], insulin autoantibodies [IAA], and other antibodies) may be present in the sera of prediabetic children for years prior to developing insulin dependence.

Clinical Findings

A. Symptoms and Signs:

1. Early Manifestations–The 3 main symptoms are thirst (polydipsia), frequent urination (polyuria) which may include nocturia or enuresis, and weight loss (or a failure to gain weight). A loss of energy is common. The presence of ketones may result in nausea and/or vomiting and, eventually, ketonemia and acidosis and a sweet-smelling breath and deep respirations (Kussmal) and, eventually, coma.

2. Chronic Complications–One-third of children with diabetes develop joint contractures, particularly of the fifth fingers. However, these are not usually disabling. Severe diabetic retinopathy and early nephropathy develop in one-third of pubertal adolescents and young adults who have had diabetes for 10–20 years. Mild retinal changes, such as microaneurysms, are much more common. The severe renal and retinal complications are more likely in patients with longitudinal poor glucose control or higher blood pressures. Thyroid gland enlargement is present in 20% of adolescents with diabetes and 5% have elevated TSH levels (subclinical thyroiditis). Psychological problems also seem to be more common among adolescents with IDDM. Fortunately, stunting of growth and hepatomegaly (Mauriac's syndrome) due to chronic poor glucose control is now quite rare. Also, since it has been realized that recurrent ketoacidosis is almost always due to missed insulin shots, the incidence of this problem has been reduced greatly.

B. Laboratory Findings: Findings include glycosuria, fasting hyperglycemia ($>$ 120 mg/dL or 6.7 mmol/L), and hyperglycemia 2 hours after a meal ($>$ 200 mg/dL or 11.1 mmol/L). Similarly, a random blood glucose above 300 mg/dL (16.6 mmol/L) is usually indicative of diabetes. A glucose tolerance test is usually not necessary, but if done should involve giving 1.75 g/kg body weight (up to a maximum of 75 g) of glucose orally. Antibody levels (see Etiology, above) may be helpful in the borderline patient. Other findings may include ketonuria, hyperlipidemia, hemoconcentration, and ketoacidemia. The venous pH is the best test to detect the degree of acidemia. Hemoglobin A1c levels may be elevated in new, long-standing, or poorly controlled patients. Insulin levels are usually not measured, but may be elevated (as with C-peptide levels) in obese adolescents with MODY.

Treatment

A. Education: Good initial education is important in making the family feel secure and competent to handle the insulin injections, blood glucose testing, urine ketone testing, hypoglycemia, and other management that they must do. This usually requires that both parents be present for approximately 3 days (but depends on the rate of learning).

B. Insulin: Most children with moderate or large ketonuria who are not acidotic and who are not dehydrated so as to require intravenous fluid therapy are initially treated (usually as outpatients) with regular insulin IM (every 1 hour) or SQ (every 2–3 hours) at a dose of 0.1 to 0.2 Units per kg body weight. When ketonuria diminishes, a mixture of regular insulin and long-acting insulin (usually NPH; see Table 23–7) is started at 0.5 to 1.0 units per kg (total dose) per 24 hours. If ketonuria is not present at onset, usually signifying greater endogenous insulin production, the usual starting dose is 0.25 to 0.5 units per kg body weight per 24 hours. Two-thirds of the total dose is usually given in the morning and one-third in the evening, preferably 30 to 60 minutes before meals. Children under age 4 years usually need only ½ to 2 Units of regular insulin, children between 4 and 12 years need 1 to 5 Units of regular insulin, and pubertal children need 5 to 10 Units of regular insulin. The remainder of the dose is given as long-acting insulin. Dosages are usually closely monitored by phone in the first week and are titrated to home blood glucose monitoring. At puberty, the insulin dose generally increases and can reach up to 1.5 units per Kg body weight per 24 hours.

C. Diet: Five-year data are now available to show that glucose control is similar for children receiving a ''sugar-restricted'' diet with freedom to eat other foods to appetite, versus a specified American Diabetes Association exchange diet (originally de-

Table 23–7. Summary of bioavailability characteristics of the insulins.

	Insulin Type	Onset	Peak Action	Duration
Short-acting	Regular, Actrapid, Velosulin	15–30 min	1–3 h	5–7 h
	Semilente, Semitard	30–60 min	4–6 h	12–16 h
Intermediate-acting	Lente, Lentard, Monotard	2–4 h	8–10 h	18–24 h
	NPH, Insulatard, Protaphane	2–4 h	8–10 h	18–24 h
Long-acting	Ultralente, Ultratard, PZI	4–5 h	8–14 h	25–36 h

veloped for weight control and still useful if weight is a problem). If an exchange diet is used, the 24-hour caloric intake is calculated as 1000 Kcal plus an additional 100 Kcal per year of age up to 2500 Kcal. Calories are usually divided with 55% from carbohydrate, 20% from protein, and 25% from fat. Snacks are used at peak times of insulin activity or before exercise to prevent hypoglycemia (usually at 3–4 PM and sometimes at 10–11 AM) and a solid snack containing protein and fat should consistently be consumed prior to bedtime to help prevent noctural hypoglycemia.

D. Outpatient Management: In most children and adolescents, blood should be tested 3 times each day (in the morning, before supper, and/or at bedtime). This can be done with diagnostic paper strips (eg, Chemstrip bG Strips), which permit visual estimation of the glucose concentration when compared to a color chart, or by use of a meter (eg, The One-Touch meter manufactured by LifeScan). If the blood glucose concentration is above 240 mg/dL (13.30 mmol/L) or if the patient feels ill, urine ketone levels must also be checked. Physical examination every 3 months with particular attention to the retinas, thyroid, liver, injection sites, fingers (for blood test pricks and for contractures), and neurologic examination is recommended. The patient's understanding of the disease should be reviewed. After puberty, hemoglobin A1c (glycosylated hemoglobin) levels should be determined every 3 months. In the young child hemoglobin A1c levels may be determined only twice yearly if in a good range (<1.3 times the upper limit of normal). Poor control of blood glucose levels is most commonly due to inadequate insulin dosage, missed insulin injections, frequent infections, or non-compliance with diet or timing of injections.

E. Other Factors Influencing the Regulation of Diabetes:

1. Activity–Strenuous exercise tends to lower the insulin requirement. Exercise in moderation (and without significant day to day variations) is beneficial. However, patients should be cautioned against strenuous exercise unless they take extra carbohydrates beforehand or reduce the insulin dosage.

2. Infection–Any infection is serious in a diabetic patient; it completely upsets the equilibrium established by therapy, usually increasing the need for insulin. Infection may precipitate ketoacidosis. During severe infections, it is often necessary to add small doses of supplemental regular insulin every 2–4 hours until acetonuria clears. Supplements of approximately 10 to 20% of the total daily insulin dose are given every 3 hours as regular insulin if the patient has moderate or large ketonuria and a blood glucose level above 150 mg/dL (8.30 mmol/L). When vomiting is present without ketoacidosis, it is often best to reduce the daily insulin dose by half; regular insulin may be supplemented later if high glucose and ketone levels develop. It may also be necessary to give beverages containing sugar (eg, soda pop) to keep the blood glucose level normal if vomiting is a problem.

3. Surgery–Prior to elective surgery, the patient should be given half the usual dose of long-acting insulin in the morning; following this, 5 or 10% dextrose in water should be administered slowly intravenously before, during and after surgery to cover the insulin. Blood glucose levels should be monitored during surgery and the early postoperative period. If blood glucose levels exceed 300 mg/dL (16.65 mmol/L) or if moderate or large levels of urine ketones appear, regular insulin may be administered as a continuous intravenous solution at the rate of 0.05 Unit/kg/hour. If the patient is unable to return to oral food intake promptly, intravenous glucose and electrolytes are continued and intravenous insulin may be continued as necessary. On the day after surgery, if the patient is able to resume eating, the usual amount of long-acting insulin should be administered. As soon as possible, feedings by mouth and the usual insulin regime should be reinstituted.

4. Prevention of Hypoglycemia–Prevention of hypoglycemia is particularly important in the child under age 4 years when the brain is still developing. Hypoglycemia and posthypoglycemic hyperglycemia (Somogyi's syndrome) may be due to overdosage with insulin. This should be suspected in children receiving an insulin dosage that exceeds 1.5 Units/kg/day, although the relative insulin resistence of adolescence may result in insulin doses of 1.5 units/kg/day or more during the adolescent growth spurt. All families should receive thorough education about hypoglycemia and how to handle it. Most physicians recommend the family keep glucagon (1.0-mg vials) available for emergencies (0.3 mg for children under 10 years old or 0.5 mg [SQ or IM] for older children).

DIABETIC ACIDOSIS
(Diabetic Coma)

Clinical Findings

A. Symptoms and Signs: Diabetic acidosis is characterized by marked thirst and polyuria, followed by nausea and vomiting, abdominal pain, and general malaise. Dehydration and acidosis (pH < 7.3) develop rapidly. Respirations then become long, deep, and labored; headache, irritability, drowsiness, stupor, and (finally) coma may develop. On physical examination, the patient is irritable, drowsy, or unconscious, and there is marked dehydration. The skin and mucous membranes are usually dry, lips cherry-red, eyeballs soft, blood pressure low, pulse usually rapid and thready, hyperventilation present, temperature low, and a sweetish (''fruity'') acetone breath may be detected. The abdomen may show diffuse spasm and tenderness suggestive of an acute abdominal disorder. The signs and symptoms of the precipitating cause (infection, trauma, missed injection, emotional upset, etc) will usually be found.

A syndrome of hyperosmolar nonketotic diabetic coma in children has been described. It is characterized by the presence of severe hyperglycemia, severe dehydration, and metabolic acidosis and may occur secondary to hypernatremia. The duration of illness is short. There is little or no polydipsia and polyuria, and these children are frequently insulin-resistant. In treatment, sufficient insulin (and isotonic parenteral fluid initially) should be used to normalize glucose metabolism; insulin may not be necessary when the disorder follows hypernatremia.

B. Laboratory Findings: Findings include glycosuria, ketonemia, ketonuria, and hyperglycemia. Acidosis results, and the pH may be below 7.1 (severe ketoacidosis), between 7.1 and 7.2 (moderate ketoacidosis), or between 7.2 and 7.3 (mild ketoacidosis). Serum sodium and chloride levels and the plasma carbon dioxide content are low. Serum potassium and inorganic phosphorus levels may be increased initially, but there is a major total body depletion of these elements, and levels usually decline rapidly with correction of acidosis. Total protein, hemoglobin, and blood urea nitrogen levels may be increased. Leukocytosis and increased hematocrit are often present.

Treatment

A. Objectives: Objectives are the restoration of circulation, correction of fluid and electrolyte deficit, reestablishment of normal carbohydrate metabolism, and eradication of the cause of acidosis and the hyperosmolar state.

B. Emergency Measures:

1. Hospitalize the patient if diabetic acidosis is severe. Patients with mild acidosis can be treated without hospitalization. Keep the patient warm, but avoid excessive warmth. Do not give narcotics or barbiturates.

2. Treat shock, if present, with albumin and other antishock measures (see Chapter 28).

3. Evaluate the degree of dehydration and shock by physical examination and by close inquiry to determine if there is a history of recent weight loss.

4. Obtain urine for estimation of glucose and ketone levels, specific gravity, and evidence of infection.

5. Take venous blood for measurement of pH and determination of levels of carbon dioxide, sodium chloride, potassium, glucose, inorganic phosphorus, urea nitrogen, and ketone bodies. Measurement of the blood lactic acid level may also be of value in the acidotic nonketotic patient.

6. Insulin is given as follows:

a. Intravenous insulin should not be given until the blood glucose level is known, particularly if subcutaneous injections were given previously.

b. A constant intravenous infusion of regular insulin, 0.1–0.2 unit/kg/h, is given by use of a constant infusion pump if that method of delivery is available. One method to prepare an insulin infusion is to add regular insulin, 30 units, to 150 mL of 0.9% sodium chloride to give a dilution of 1 unit/5 mL. If 50 mL of this solution is run through the tubing prior to use, the insulin binding sites on the tubing will be saturated. A similar dose of insulin may be given intramuscularly instead of intravenously but will then need to be repeated every hour. With either route of administration, blood glucose levels should be determined hourly. Insulin may be given subcutaneously every 2–4 hours in less severely involved patients, except in markedly dehydrated patients who may have varied absorption of the drug.

7. Gastric lavage may rarely be necessary to relieve distention of the stomach and to reduce vomiting.

8. Fluids and electrolytes are given as follows:

a. First correct extracellular dehydration, shock, anoxia, and impaired renal function with normal saline solution or, if acidosis is severe (pH < 7.0), a solution containing the following: sodium, 150 meq/L; chloride, 100 meq/L; and bicarbonate, 50 meq/L. Give 20–40 mL/kg over the first 1 or 2 hours of therapy. If shock is present, the use of albumin or other volume expander is essential.

b. Then give 50% physiologic solution (usually without bicarbonate) at a rate calculated to restore deficits, supply maintenance amounts, and replace intercurrent losses.

c. When urine flow and circulatory efficiency are satisfactory, the blood pH level is above 7.1, and signs of hyperpnea have begun to subside (generally in 1–2 hours), replace intracellular electrolytes (potassium and phosphorus). Although serum potassium and phosphorus concentrations are usually normal or high early in acidosis, they may fall to low levels following correction of acidosis.

d. Replace the remainder of the water deficit, and when the blood glucose level falls below 250 mg/dL, 5% glucose should be added to the intravenous fluids.

C. General Measures:

1. Ascertain the precipitating cause of the acidosis, and initiate appropriate treatment.

2. Use an indwelling catheter if spontaneous voidings are not possible (rarely necessary).

3. Measure urinary glucose and acetone, blood glucose and carbon dioxide, venous pH, and serum electrolytes at frequent intervals.

4. Continuous or intermittent monitoring of the ECG is helpful to follow the effect of potassium therapy.

5. After 12–18 hours, if there is no vomiting, the remainder of the day's fluid and electrolyte requirements may be given orally in a suitable vehicle (orange juice, ginger ale, or milk). Vomiting generally subsides after ketosis has been corrected.

6. For continued fluid and electrolyte therapy, see Chapter 5.

Prognosis

With prompt and adequate therapy, the prognosis is good. The largest number of serious side effects and sequelae result from central nervous system complications. The risk of these may be minimized by attention to correction of fluid and electrolyte losses and avoidance of overzealous correction of the hyperglycemia, dehydration, or acidosis. Recurrent episodes of acidosis are due to failure to take the proper insulin or diet, to emotional problems, to omitting insulin altogether, or to chronic or repeated infections.

HYPOGLYCEMIA
(See also Neonatal Hypoglycemia, Chapter 7.)

Low blood glucose levels can occur when a patient with diabetes receives excessive insulin, fails to eat, or exercises too strenuously. In children who do not have diabetes, the diagnosis of hypoglycemia *should not be made* unless the blood glucose level is below 40 mg/dL; in a newborn, below 30 mg/dL. The diagnosis is unfortunately assigned frequently to children with behavioral or other problems who have never had a documented low blood glucose level.

The most common known cause of severe hypoglycemia in infants during the first year of life is inappropriate insulin secretion. During episodes of hypoglycemia, insulin levels are inappropriately elevated. When the pancreas is examined histologically, the islet cells may be hypertrophied in some cases; in other cases, there may be excessive numbers of islet cells, which may be arising from pancreatic ductules (nesidioblastoma). Treatment consists of avoidance of insulin stimuli (simple carbohydrates and certain amino acids viz leucine arginine). A trial of diazoxide, 10–20 mg/kg, to inhibit insulin release should be attempted. If this is unsuccessful, 80–90% pancreatomy may be indicated.

The most frequent known cause of hypoglycemia in children between 1 and 5 years of age is functional fasting ("ketotic") hypoglycemia. Functional fasting hypoglycemia is more common in males and in children who had birth weights below 2500 g, who were small for gestational age, or who have minor neurologic or behavioral disorders. There is often a history of vomiting or of decreased appetite or failure to eat during the previous 24 hours. Early morning seizures with the concurrent appearance of ketones in the urine are common in the young child. Treatment should consist of preventing excessive fasting and monitoring the urine for ketones whenever the child is ill or appears to be deviating from normal behavior patterns. If ketones are present, foods high in simple sugars should be encouraged. If the child is vomiting, parenteral glucose and fluids to prevent dehydration may be necessary.

Islet cell adenoma is the most frequent known cause of severe hypoglycemia in patients over 6 years of age. Inappropriate insulin secretion occurs and a tumor can sometimes be detected by means of ultrasonography or arteriography. Treatment is surgical removal.

There are some cases in which a cause for hypoglycemia cannot be found (group IV, idiopathic spontaneous hypoglycemia; Table 23–8). Genetic metabolic disorders (group VI) should be considered in the differential particularly when the hypoglycemia occurs in association with vomiting, seizures, feeding disorders and physical signs of increased intracranial pressure and hepatomegaly history or the physical examination (eg, large liver).

Clinical Findings

A. Symptoms and Signs: Findings include weakness, hunger, irritability, faintness, sweating, changes in mood, epigastric pain, vomiting, nervousness, tachycardia, hypothermia, unsteadiness of gait, semiconsciousness, tremors, and convulsions. Symptoms are relieved by administration of glucose. If left untreated, hypoglycemia may lead to extensive central nervous system damage; symptomatic hypoglycemia is more commonly associated with mental deterioration, disintegration of the personality, and death, but the course and prognosis are variable.

B. Laboratory Findings: (See Table 23–8.)

1. Blood glucose levels are low during an attack. There is no sharp dividing line below which a level can be regarded as abnormal, but consistent or repeated levels below 40 mg/dL, associated with signs and symptoms should be investigated.

2. Serum insulin levels may be inappropriately elevated in hyperinsulinemic states when compared with the simultaneous glucose level.

3. No single test of blood glucose regulation reliably confirms the diagnosis of hypoglycemia, and no combination of tests reliably establishes the mechanism of hypoglycemia in all children.

Treatment

Long-term treatment for specific types of hypoglycemia is outlined in Table 23–8. Acute treatment is usually necessary prior to definitive diagnosis and includes the following:

A. Glucose:

1. Infuse 10–20% dextrose via peripheral vein, at a constant rate, maintaining a blood glucose level that controls central nervous system symptoms (eg, 30 mg/dL in newborns and 40–50 mg/dL in children). If hyperinsulinemia is suspected or is a possibility, avoid bolus (''push'') infusions of concentrated dextrose solutions are frequently associated with hyperinsulinemic rebound. (Fifty percent dextrose solutions are not indicated during infancy and childhood.)

2. Instruct the patient's family to give glucose as follows if the patient is unconscious and a physician is not available: Place Insta-Glucose between the child's cheek and gums or under the

Table 23–8. Hypoglycemia.

Classification	Clinical and Laboratory Findings	Treatment
I. Antenatal period disorders (1) Fetal malnutrition (placental insufficiency) (2) Sepsis Offspring of diabetic mothers Erythroblastosis fetalis (3) Neonatal cold injury (4) Hypoglycemia, cardiomegaly, and pulmonary edema	Offspring of diabetic mothers and infants with erythroblastosis fetalis may have hyperinsulinemia with rebound hypoglycemia to insulinogenic stimuli; blood ratios of insulin to glucose are elevated. The other conditions listed have in common depleted hepatic glycogen and fat stores and fasting hypoglycemia.	Infusion of 10–20% glucose by peripheral vein. Frequent oral feedings. Avoidance or cautious administration of insulinogenic agents (eg, arginine, 50% dextrose) in hyperinsulinism states.
II. Hyperinsulin states (1) Islet cell hyperplasia (2) Islet cell adenoma or adenocarcinoma (3) Islet cell nesidioblastosis (4) Leucine sensitivity (5) Beckwith-Wiedemann syndrome	As a whole, this group is prone to fasting hypoglycemia and rebound hypoglycemia to insulinogenic stimuli. Diagnosis is dependent on finding of abnormally elevated insulin or proinsulin levels during the fasting state or following insulin provocation with glucose, amino acids (ie, leucine, arginine), glucagon, or tolbutamide (1–5); or finding of clinical characteristics of the EMG triad, ie, exomphalos, macroglossia, and gigantism with abdominal organomegaly (5).	(1) Avoidance of insulinogenic stimuli. (2) Catecholamines or diazoxide (or both). (3) A diet low in simple sugars and, sometimes, low in leucine. (4) Pancreatectomy.
III. Functional fasting hypoglycemia ("Ketotic hypoglycemia")	Findings include a history of low birth weight for gestational age; onset between ages 1 and 6 yr; and triad of hypoglycemia, ketosis, and blunted glycemic response to glucagon. Patients may have abnormalities in gluconeogenesis with abnormalities in hepatic handling of alanine during a fast.	Frequent feedings with diet high in carbohydrates and protein. Avoid periods of prolonged fasting.

IV. Primary neurologic disorders ("central")	Hypoglycemia is frequently observed in children with neurologic disorders of various types. No definite pattern or consistent metabolic abnormality has been demonstrated, although hyperinsulinemia has not been a feature.	Frequent feedings. Anticonvulsants when indicated.
VI. Metabolic disorders (1) Liver glycogen storage disease (2) Liver glycogen synthase deficiency (3) Fructose intolerance (4) Maple syrup urine disease (5) Deficiency of liver 1,6-diphosphatase activity	Definitive diagnosis is dependent on enzyme determination. Blunted hyperglycemia response to glucagon (1, 2, and 5), history of hypoglycemia after fructose ingestion (3), and a characteristic odor (4) are helpful for diagnosis.	(1 and 2) Frequent feedings with diet high in carbohydrates. Hyperalimentation. Portacaval diversion in severe type 1 glycogen storage disease may be indicated. (3 and 4) Rigid avoidance of offending substrate.
VII. Endocrine insufficiency syndromes (1) Hypopituitarism (2) Hypopituitarism and hyperinsulinemia (3) Adrenocortical insufficiency (4) Adrenomedullary insufficiency (Broberger-Zetterström syndrome) (5) Congenital hypothyroidism (6) Glucagon deficiency	Definitive diagnosis is dependent on biochemical establishment of hormone deficiency. History of failure to thrive, growth retardation, and features of hypopituitarism (1 and 2), excessive tanning (3), and abnormal weight for gestational age (4) are helpful for diagnosis.	Replacement of deficient hormone or hormones.
VIII. Severe malnutrition states (1) Chronic diarrhea (2) Liver disease	Characteristics include fasting hypoglycemia and depleted glycogen and fat stores.	Nutritional rehabilitation.

tongue. If there is no response in 10 minutes, give an initial deep intramuscular injection of glucagon, usually 0.5 mL (0.5 mg). If there is no response, wait 10 more minutes and inject an additional 0.5 mL of glucagon.

3. If a diagnosis of hypoglycemia not due to hyperinsulinism or an inborn error of metabolism has been established, carbohydrates can be safely administered via any route without risk of hypoglycemic rebound.

4. If a diabetic patient is unconscious and a diagnosis of coma or insulin reaction is possible, infuse glucose (20–25%) solution, give intravenously, up to 1 mL/kg. This will overcome the insulin reaction.

B. Drugs:

1. In general, drug therapy should be employed only after a definite diagnosis (see Table 23–8) is established.

2. If the cardiorespiratory status permits, catecholamines (eg, acqueous epinephrine or subcutaneous epinephrine in oil [Sus-Phrine]) may be useful and have the unique advantage in the undiagnosed case of avoiding insulin stimulation.

3. Corticosteroids, corticotropin, and glucagon may be helpful in controlling hypoglycemia, but they may stimulate insulin production, and the action of glucagon in neonates is unpredictable. Glucagon is useful in hyperinsulin states; corticotropin and corticosteroids are occasionally successful over acute short intervals.

4. In severe chronic hyperinsulinism states, an oral preparation of diazoxide is useful. Diazoxide, a nondiuretic benzothiadiazine, may be of value in controlling chronic idiopathic hypoglycemia and certain cases of hyperinsulinism. The dosage has varied from 5 to 20 mg/kg/d. Side effects include hypertrichosis, advancement of epiphyseal maturation, hyperuricemia, fluid retention, neutropenia, and depression of immunoglobulin G. Failure of adequate response to therapy with diazoxide should prompt consideration of subtotal pancreatectomy.

5. Recent experience suggests that somatostatin analogs may be useful and safe in children with hyperinsulinism. Somatostatin inhibits insulin secretion.

6. Sedatives and anticonvulsant therapy may be helpful to reduce convulsions and neuromuscular irritability. (Phenytoin has the added effect of reducing insulin stimulation.)

C. Diet: In patients with functional fasting "ketotic" hypoglycemia, provide a liberal carbohydrate diet and place a moderate restriction on ketogenic foods.

1. In hyperinsulinemic states avoid simple sugars and foods high in leucine and arginine. Employ long chain slowly metabolized carbohydrates.

2. Give small frequent feedings (6 or more meals a day). It may be necessary to feed the patient at regular intervals throughout the 24 hours and to give small carbohydrate feedings 30–45 minutes after regular meals.

D. Surgical Measures: Surgical removal of a portion of the pancreas (or of a tumor if present) should be undertaken for any individual with hyperinsulinemia who cannot be controlled by the above measures.

Prognosis

With prompt corrective treatment and normalization of glucose concentrations, the prognosis is good.

GALACTOSEMIA

Galactosemia is an autosomal recessive disease with an incidence of 1:40,000 live births; the condition is due to congenital absence of the activity of the enzyme galactose-1-phosphate uridyl transferase, which is necessary to convert galactose-1-phosphate. There is decreased activity of the enzyme in heterozygous individuals. Galactosemia is characterized by vomiting, feeding difficulties, hepatomegaly, cataracts, mental retardation (not universal), and jaundice during the neonatal period. Untreated *E coli* sepsis and death is frequent. Other findings include renal Fanconi syndrome, ovarian failure and increased levels of galactose in the blood and galactose-1-phosphate in erythrocytes. A screening test is available to diagnose the condition during the newborn period.

A second form of galactosemia is due to galactokinase deficiency and does not affect the liver, kidneys, or central nervous system; cataracts may develop in patients during the first few months of life.

Treatment consists of excluding galactose (especially milk and its derivatives) from the diet. This prevents development of the signs and symptoms of the disease or may result in improvement after they have developed. A more normal diet may be tolerated later in childhood.

The mother of a known galactosemic child should be on a restricted galactose diet during subsequent pregnancies.

GLYCOGEN STORAGE DISEASE

Numerous disorders affecting the biosynthesis and degradation of glycogen have been described, including:

Type I, Von Gierke's Disease: Type I, the most common glycogen storage disease, is an autosomal recessive disorder that involves the liver and kidneys. It starts at birth or in early infancy and is characterized by anorexia, weight loss, vomiting, convulsions, and coma. Organomegaly of the liver and kidneys, growth retardation, obesity with a "doll-like" appearance, and bleeding tendencies may be noted. Laboratory findings include a deficiency in glucose 6-phosphatase, flat epinephrine and glucagon tolerance curves, elevated blood lipid lactic and pyruvic acid levels, and abnormal glycogen deposition in the liver. Treatment includes frequent high-carbohydrate feedings, sometimes including nighttime intragastric tube feedings.

Type II, Pompe's Disease (Maltase Deficiency): Findings include muscle weakness, cardiomegaly, macroglossia, hepatomegaly, normal mental development, and deficiency of the lysosomal enzyme α1,4-glucosidase.

Type III, Cori's Disease: Type III involves the liver, striated muscle, and red blood cells. The clinical features are similar to those of type I but less severe. A defect in debranching enzymes (amylo-1,6-glucosidase or oligo-1,4-glucantransferase) and hepatomegaly are typical findings.

Type IV, Andersen's Disease (Amylopectinosis): Findings include abnormal levels of glycogen in the liver and reticuloendothelial system, diminished response to glucagon and epinephrine, a defect in the branching enzyme (amylo-1,4 → 1,6-transglucosidase), hepatosplenomegaly, severe cirrhosis, ascites, and normal mental development.

Type V, McArdle's Syndrome: Type V (muscle phosphorylase deficiency) involves the skeletal muscle with clinical muscle weakness, stiffness and easy fatigability. There is a defect in muscle phosphorylase.

Type VI, Hers' Disease: Type VI is clinically similar to type I but less severe. There is a deficiency in liver phosphorylase.

Type VII: Other types involve reduced activity of phosphoglucomutase, phosphofructokinase, or phosphohexoisomerase.

Findings include weak muscles, partial defect of other glycolytic enzymes, and elevated levels of AST (SGOT), serum aldolase, and phosphocreatine kinase.

PHENYLKETONURIA
(Phenylpyruvic Oligophrenia)

Phenylketonuria is an autosomal recessive condition that affects 1:10,000 live Caucasion births. The classic form is due to a deficiency of phenylalanine hydroxylase.

Clinical Findings

Affected children (most often blond and blue-eyed) appear normal at birth but soon develop vomiting, irritability, a "mouse like" odor, patchy eczematous lesions of the skin, convulsions, schizoid personality, and abnormal findings on EEG. If untreated, mentality is retarded. (An occasional patient may have normal intelligence without treatment.) Affected children are hyperactive, with erratic behavior. Perspiration is excessive. Serum and urinary phenylalanine levels are markedly high as determined by ferric chloride test, Phenistix Reagent Strips, or Guthrie bacterial inhibition assay (of particular value in young infants). Some normal infants, particularly those with physiologic jaundice of the newborn, may have transiently elevated (> 6 mg/dL) blood levels of phenylalanine. Orthohydroxyphenylacetic acid is usually present in the urine.

Treatment

A diet low in phenylalanine (58 ± 18 mg/kg) should be instituted to keep plasma phenylalanine levels between 5 and 10 mg/dL; when started in patients during the first weeks of life, this diet prevents severe retardation. It has also been shown that it is possible to breast-feed an infant in combination with giving a milk substitute that is deficient in phenylalanine. The diet should be titrated against the nutritional status of the child and the serum phenylalanine levels to ensure that the diet is restricted enough to prevent manifestations of the disease but liberal enough to prevent hypophenylalaninemia with resultant malnutrition, retarded growth and development and cerebral damage. It is now generally recommended that weekly serum phenylalanine assays be done during the first year of life. In established cases, proper diet may arrest the condition and produce improvement in personality and in symptoms other than the mental deficiency. It may be discontinued after several years.

The blood phenylalanine levels of phenylketonuric females should be maintained in the normal range during the childbearing years to decrease the risk of abnormalities (eg, growth and mental retardation, microcephaly) in their offspring who may be non-phenylketonuric.

Hyperphenylalaninemia may be a transient phenomenon in some newborns who have normal urinary metabolites and do not require treatment.

Genetics & Inborn Errors | 24

Eva Svjansky, MD

The identification of genetic disorders often has important implications for the prognosis and management of affected children. A correct diagnosis is also important for establishment of an accurate recurrence risk and allows the parents to make informed reproductive decisions. Traditionally, genetic disorders included **chromosomal abnormalities, single gene defects,** and **multifactorial conditions.** The recent progress in molecular genetics allowed the identification of additional causes of genetic disorders collectively called **nontraditional modes of inheritance.** These include **gonadal mosaicism, uniparental disomy, imprinting, contiguous gene syndromes,** and **mitochondrial inheritance.**

CHROMOSOME ABNORMALITIES

Normal humans have 46 chromosomes (23 of maternal and 23 of paternal origin) in every cell except gonads, which have 23 chromosomes. Errors during cell division will result in chromosome abnormalities. Uneven division of chromosomes into two daughter cells (non-disjunction) is responsible for numerical abnormalities; breaks in chromosomes, which rejoin randomly and form new combinations are responsible for structural aberrations. While only a handful of numerical abnormalities are compatible with livebirth, the number of possible structural abnormalities is infinite. Collectively, chromosome abnormalities can be found in approximately .5% of all newborns.

The **numerical** chromosome abnormalities (any deviation from the normal 46 chromosomes per cell) are most frequently **trisomy** or **monosomy.** Abnormalities of chromosome **structure** include **deletion** (a chromosome segment missing), **duplication** (presence of an additional chromosome segment), and **translocation** (a segment of one chromosome is attached to another chromosome). Translocation is **balanced** if the total amount of chromosome material per cell is normal, or **unbalanced** if translocation resulted in a partial monosomy or duplication of chromosome material. Less common structural abnormalities include **inversion** (the middle portion of a chromosome is inverted, turned "upside-down") and **ring** chromosome (both ends of a chromosome are lost, deleted, and the new ends are reconnected to form a ring).

Mosaicism denotes the presence of 2 different chromosome constitutions in different cells of an individual. For example, a child with Down's syndrome mosaicism has some cells with the normal number of chromosomes, others show trisomy 21.

Chromosome Nomenclature

The results of chromosome analysis are routinely reported in a cytogenetic "shorthand," using standard symbols. See examples below:

46,XX: normal female.

46,XY: normal male.

47,XY, + 21: male with trisomy 21 (note: trisomy is depicted by " + " symbol before the chromosome number).

46,XX,4p −: deletion of a short arm (p) of chromosome 4 (note: the symbol " − ", indicating deletion, is after the chromosome).

46,XX,5q +: duplication of a long arm (q) of chromosome 5.

45,XX, − 14, − 21, + t(14;21): 45 chromosomes with one copy of the normal chromosomes 14 and 21 missing and having one translocation chromosome consisting of 14 and 21.

46,XY,t(1;8)(q32:p22): translocation between the long arm of chromosome 1, at the band 32 and the short arm of chromosome 8, at the band 22.

CLINICAL SIGNIFICANCE

Chromosome abnormality should be suspected in children with any of the following: dysmorphic features, congenital malformations, developmental delay, mental retardation, prenatal and/or postnatal growth retardation, and/or abnormal sexual characteristics. The identification of other potentially etiologic factors in such children, such as fetal exposure to alcohol, parental consanguinity or perinatal hypoxia, does not rule out the presence of a chromosome abnormality. Fragile X syndrome, XXY, and XYY often are associated with excessive growth. In general, abnormalities of the autosomes (chromosomes number 1 through 22) have more severe consequences for morbidity and mortality than abnormalities of the sex chromosomes (X and Y), some of which may cause only learning and behavioral problems; trisomy or monosomy of a whole chromosome is more deleterious than duplication or deletion of a small segment and deletion is more damaging than duplication. Table 24–1 describes examples of characteristic physical findings associated with some chromosome abnormalities.

DIAGNOSIS

Tissues Used for Chromosome Analysis

(1) Peripheral blood lymphocytes, obtained from a few milliliters of sterile heparinized blood (green top tube) are the most accessible and most frequently used. A 3-day culture is done routinely; 2-day culture can be requested for preliminary results, if needed.

(2) **Skin** or other tissue (gonads, thymus) is obtained post mortem or to look for mosaicism. A sterile piece of tissue is placed into tissue culture media or sterile saline (never into formalin!) and immediately sent to the cytogenetic laboratory. The tissue culture takes 1 to 2 weeks before chromosome study can be performed.

(3) **Bone marrow** is the only tissue with sufficient number of mitoses present to allow an immediate chromosome analysis. Since it is not as readily available as a blood sample, bone marrow is used only if immediate results (within 6–12 hours) are needed for appropriate management (eg, a newborn with complex congenital heart disease requiring immediate intervention is suspicious for having trisomy 13).

(4) **Amniocytes** obtained by amniocentesis or **chorionic villi** obtained by chorionic villi sampling are used for prenatal diagnosis.

Techniques of Chromosome Analysis

(1) **Routine,** conventional chromosome analysis results in production of a **karyotype** (a layout of paired chromosomes, arranged from number 1 through 22 and sex chromosomes) in which all chromosomes demonstrate a light and dark stained

Table 24-1. Phenotypic features of selected chromosomal syndromes.

Syndromes	Signs
Trisomy 21 Down's syndrome	Mongoloid slant of eyes, brushfield spots of iris, protruding tongue, 3rd fontanelle, low set auricles, excess nuchal skin, Simian lines, single flexion crease and incurving (clinodactyly) of 5th fingers, increased distance between 1st and 2nd toes, mottling of skin, hypotonia, CHD (endocardial cushion defect, VSD, other).
Trisomy 13	IUGR in all 3 parameters, coloboma of iris (pupil of keyhole shape), capillary hemangioma, skin defect of skull, hyperconvex nails, polydactyly, rocker bottom feet, arrhinencephaly, cleft lip and palate, CHD, urinary tract abnormalities.
Trisomy 18	IUGR, anti-mongoloid slant of eyes, short palpebral fissure, small mouth, micrognathia, low set, abnormal auricles, prominent occiput, short sternum, abnormal position of fingers (2nd overlapping 3rd and 5th overlapping 4th), hypoplastic finger nails, rocker bottom feet, CHD, spasticity, feeding problems.
Turner syndrome 45,X	Triangular face, antimongoloid slant of eyes, abnormal shape of ears, webbed or wide neck, broad "shield" chest, wide set nipples, edema of hands and feet, shortened 4th and 5th metacarpals and metatarsals, cubitus valgus; short stature, primary amenorrhea, CHD especially coarctation of aorta. Mostly normal I.Q., infertility.
Klinefelter syndrome 47,XXY	Tall stature, postpubertally small testicles, gynecomastia, eunuchoid build. Increased risk for mild MR, learning and behavior problems, infertility.
47,XYY	No characteristic physical findings, except tall stature. Increased risk for behavior problem, mild MR.
Wolf-Hirschhorn 4p-	IUGR, prominent nasal bridge ("roman warrior profile") V-shaped glabella with abnormally arched eyebrows, beaked nose, carp shaped mouth, feeding problems.
13 q-	IUGR, radial ray defects, if involving q 14 segment: retinoblastoma.
Recombinant 8 syndrome Dup 8q 22→qter Del 8p 23→pter	Hispanic ancestry, AGA, postnatal FTT; broad forehead, upturned nares, long philtrum, thin upper lip, thick lower lip, low set ears, brachycephaly, deep plantar furrow, CHD, especially conotruncal abnormalities.
18q-	Deep set eyes, atretic ear canals, abnormal auricles.

banding pattern, characteristic for each chromosome pair. This technique is appropriate to detect numerical abnormalities and those structural abnormalities which involve a chromosome segment large enough to be visualized as a missing or additional chromosome band.

(2) **High resolution** chromosome analysis is a technique by which the chromosome division is stopped earlier in the mitosis, while the chromosomes are more elongated, and therefore, the resolution of chromosome bands is much better. Thus, smaller structural abnormalities can be detected. This method is very time consuming and therefore it is not used when numerical abnormalities are suspected. During the first 6 months of infants' life, the resolution is not as good as later; therefore, it is advisable to postpone the request for this study until at least 6 months of age.

(3) **Fragile X study** is a special technique aimed at the detection of a fragile site at the distal end of the long arm of the X chromosome (Xq27.3) associated with a specific type of X-linked mental retardation, called Fragile X syndrome. The study involves utilization of culture media deficient in folate or thymidine, which enhances fragile sites. The fragile site can be detected by this method in 80% of males and 60% of females with the gene. Recently, molecular analysis established that while normal individuals have less than 200 base pairs of cytosine phosphate guanosine dinucleotides repeats, carriers of the gene have as many as 500 base pairs (premutatin) and affected individuals with Fragile X syndrome have over 600 base pairs repeats (full mutation). The molecular analysis has a much lower frequency of false negative test results than the cytogenetic analysis and is less labor intensive.

(4) **Detection of excessive chromosome fragility.** Excessive chromosome breaks and rearrangements and sister chromatid exchanges, found in some well defined single gene syndromes such as Bloom syndrome, Fanconi anemia, ataxia-telangiectasia, etc can be detected easier, if the laboratory is informed ahead of time of the clinical suspicion of one of these disorders; techniques known to enhance the abnormality are used in such instances.

(5) **Fluorescent in-situ hybridization** (FISH) is a new technique for the detection of structural chromosome abnormalities, based on molecular methods. It utilizes fluorescent DNA probes for specific chromosome segments which allow the detection of cryptic rearrangements, invisible by high resolution chromosome analysis. FISH can be used if there is a strong clinical

suspicion for a particular chromosome abnormality (example: 4p- or trisomy 21), but the karyotype is normal. In addition, it can be useful for identification of the origin of abnormal additional chromosome material which is either attached to other chromosomes or standing separately as a marker chromosome.

(6) **Chromosome painting** is another molecular technique, similar in principle to FISH, but identifies a whole chromosome utilizing different color DNA probes for individual chromosomes; ie, the whole chromosome is "painted." This technique is not yet available routinely in most cytogenetic laboratories.

Useful Principle

The cytogenetic laboratory needs to be informed about the reason for requesting chromosome analysis. The more information (description of dysmorphic features, malformations, etc) the laboratory has about the clinical suspicion of a chromosome abnormality, the better they can choose the most appropriate technique(s).

RECURRENCE RISKS

(1) Numerical abnormalities are most frequently sporadic; however, some families have shown hereditary predisposition to a non-disjunction; therefore, the empirical recurrence risk after the first affected child is 1–2%.

(2) Structural chromosome abnormalities: De novo abnormalities (both parents have normal chromosomes) have a very low recurrence risk because gonadal mosaicism can not be excluded. If one parent has a balanced chromosome rearrangement, the recurrence risk is significantly increased. The specific risk varies according to the chromosome involved and the type of rearrangements.

PREVENTION

(1) **Identification of families with an increased recurrence risk,** which include: previous child with chromosome abnormality, parent with balanced translocation, or a history of multiple fetal losses.

(2) **Prenatal diagnosis.** Amniocentesis at 14–16 weeks of pregnancy or chorionic villi sampling at 9–10 weeks of gestation.

SINGLE GENE DEFECTS

Disorders caused by a mutation of a single gene are responsible for a large number of genetic disorders. Some of these diseases are very rare, but collectively single gene disorders affect approximately 1% of the general population. A complete listing of all known single gene disorders can be found in Victor A. McKusick's text *Mendelian Inheritance in Man*.

All genes are paired (allele). Allele are located in corresponding places (loci) of chromosome pairs; thus, one allele of each pair is of maternal, the other of paternal origin. On the basis of gene location and modes of inheritance, we can recognize **dominant** genes (one copy of abnormal gene, ie, **heterozygous** state causes morbidity) and **recessive** genes (both alleles have to be abnormal, ie, **homozygous** state causes a disease); **autosomal** genes are located on autosomal chromosomes 1 through 22 and **sex-linked** genes are located on X chromosome (majority) and Y chromosome (very few). Thus, single-gene disorders include those caused by autosomal dominant, autosomal recessive, X-linked dominant and X-linked recessive genes.

AUTOSOMAL DOMINANT INHERITANCE

Principles of Inheritance
(1) Vertical transmission: multiple generations can be affected.

(2) Both sexes equally affected; male to male transmission possible: either parent, if affected, can pass the disorder to male or female offspring.

(3) Each offspring of affected has 50% recurrence risk: the affected parent passes the normal or the abnormal allele to each child.

(4) Variable clinical expressivity of the disorder: the inter- and intra-familial severity of the disorder varies.

(5) Nonpenetrance-skipped generation: some individuals with the abnormal gene do not show any clinical symptoms of the disorder.

Reasons for Negative Family History
(1) New germinal mutation.
(2) Non-penetrance.

(3) Non-paternity.

(4) Phenocopy: clinically similar disorder of different etiology.

Clinical Significance

Autosomal dominant disorders may demonstrate clinical signs and symptoms at birth or later in life, sometimes in the 3rd or 4th decade. Thus, in some disorders, asymptomatic child of an affected parent might have inherited the abnormal gene. Presymptomatic DNA testing, if available, may be used for clarification of the child's genotype.

Examples of autosomal dominant disorders include: neurofibromatosis, Marfan syndrome, osteogenesis imperfecta, Huntington's disease, and adult-type polycystic kidney disease.

AUTOSOMAL RECESSIVE INHERITANCE

Principles of Inheritance

(1) Both parents are heterozygous carriers, ie, they have one normal and one abnormal allele of the gene. Carriers are usually clinically normal, but they might show abnormal laboratory findings, which is the basis for carrier testing (sickle cell, Tay Sachs, etc.)

(2) Increased frequency of consanguinity: consanguinity between the parents increases the chance for both of them to be carriers of the same gene.

(3) Each offspring of 2 carrier parents has 25% risk to inherit both abnormal alleles and to be affected, 50% chance to inherit the abnormal allele from one parent and the normal from the other and to be carrier and 25% chance to inherit both normal alleles.

(4) Horizontal transmission—affected sibs, clinically normal parents.

(5) All offspring of an affected parent are carriers: a parent with 2 abnormal alleles has to pass 1 copy to each offspring.

Clinical Significance

Autosomal recessive disorders are usually more severe than autosomal dominant disorders. If a correct diagnosis of the first affected child is not made, multiple affected siblings may be born before the genetic nature of the disorder is appreciated. Examples of autosomal recessive disorders are infantile polycystic kidney disease, hemoglobinopathies, cystic fibrosis, oculo-cutaneous albinism, Meckel syndrome and other dysmorphic syndromes and most inborn errors of metabolism.

X-LINKED RECESSIVE INHERITANCE

Principles of Inheritance

(1) Mostly males affected: A mutated gene on the only X chromosome of a male will be expressed, as there is not the same allele on his Y to compensate for the effect of the abnormal gene.

(2) Affected males are related to each other through usually unaffected females who have two X chromosomes, one of which is randomly inactivated in each cell. Consequently, in females, the mutated gene is active in approximately 50% of cells, and the normal gene, active in 50% of cells is sufficient for a normal function.

(3) Less severe symptoms in occasionally affected females: females show symptoms if the X inactivation is not random and the abnormal gene is active more frequently.

(4) No male to male transmission: a son inherits a Y and not an X chromosome from his father.

(5) Affected male passes the gene to *all* daughters who inherit the X chromosome and are then carriers.

(6) Carrier female has 50% chance of passing the gene to each offspring—the daughters who inherit the gene are carriers, the sons with the gene are affected.

Clinical Significance

Although X-linked disorders are much more common in males, they have to be considered in females with a compatible clinical presentation.

Affected females usually have milder symptoms, caused by the presence of active abnormal and inactive normal X in more than expected 50% of cells. In rare instances, females may be as severely affected as males. In those cases, chromosome analysis, aimed at ruling out monosomy or a structural abnormality of X, is indicated.

Examples of X-linked recessive disorders include hemophilia, Duchenne muscular dystrophy, ocular albinism, and numerous X-linked mental retardation syndromes including fragile X syndrome. However, although the gene is X-linked, the inheritance of the fragile X syndrome does not strictly follow the general principles of X-linked inheritance: Both males and females with the premutation (see under chromosome techniques) are asymptomatic carriers and individuals of both sexes with a full mutation are affected. In addition, genomic imprinting plays a role in the clinical expression of the gene: The premutation has to be passed through a female to change into a full mutation.

X-LINKED DOMINANT INHERITANCE

(1) **Principles** are similar to the X-linked recessive inheritance with the exception that heterozygous females are also affected.

(2) **Clinical Significance.** This is a rare form of inheritance. Examples include incontinentia pigmenti and vitamin D resistant rickets.

DIAGNOSIS OF SINGLE GENE DISORDERS

(1) **Physical examination** leading to the detection of characteristic physical findings. For example, the presence of multiple café-au-lait spots, neurofibromas, and lisch nodules of irises is diagnostic for neurofibromatosis 1.

(2) **Family history.** For example, finding of members of multiple generations of both sexes affected with a neurodegenerative disorder is compatible with autosomal dominant inheritance even in the absence of a specific diagnosis.

(3) **Diagnostic tests,** specific for the given disorder, ie, detection of enzyme defects in inborn errors of metabolism, abnormal sweat test in cystic fibrosis, abnormal amount of dystrophin in muscle biopsy in Duchenne muscular dystrophy, etc.

Molecular Testing

(1) **Direct Detection** of the mutation.

Prerequisites: The specific mutation is known and the mutation is responsible for either adding or abolishing a restriction enzyme recognition site, thus the size of the fragment and its movement on the gel is different from a normal gene. Advantage of this technique is 100% reliability and the ability to make the diagnosis on patients with a negative family history. Examples of disorders with a detectable mutation include Duchenne muscular dystrophy, retinoblastoma, neurofibromatosis, 21-hydroxylase deficiency, hemophilia, myotonic dystrophy and fragile X syndrome.

(2) **Indirect detection** through utilizing linkage analysis is to be considered, if the specific mutation is unknown, but the chromosome location of the gene is known.

Prerequisites: Multiple family members affected with the disease and the availability of polymorphic DNA markers so closely linked to the disease gene, that they are unlikely to segregate independently from the disease gene. The closer the linkage between the markers and the gene in question and the more DNA markers are utilized, the higher the probability that the linkage study is accurate. The disadvantages of linkage study include the necessity of multiple affected and unaffected family members to participate in the study and the possibility of crossing over between the markers and the gene, which results in inaccurate diagnosis. Disorders with available linkage analysis include Huntington disease, neurofibromatosis, tuberous sclerosis, retinoblastoma, Duchenne muscular dystrophy without detectable deletion, spinal muscular atrophy, etc.

DNA testing was greatly advanced by the development of the polymerase chain reaction (PCR) technique which decreased significantly the sample size and the time required for the test, making it less expensive and more accessible. Molecular testing can be helpful for presymptomatic and prenatal diagnosis and for confirmation of a diagnosis in mildly affected patients.

PREVENTION OF SINGLE GENE DISORDERS

The following options are available for couples concerned about having an affected offspring:

(1) **Artificial insemination by donor** if the father is affected with X-linked or autosomal dominant disease, or if both parents are carriers of an autosomal recessive gene.

(2) **Donor egg** and in vitro fertilization if the mother does not wish to pass her abnormal autosomal dominant or X-linked gene.

(3) **Prenatal diagnosis** of disorders with available molecular testing (direct or linkage analysis).

(4) **Pre-implantation testing** of a polar body or an early zygote is being developed.

MULTIFACTORIAL INHERITANCE

The inheritance of many frequently familial disorders does not fit the single gene model. Traditionally, the additive effect of multiple common genes with a threshold effect, in combination with further unidentified environmental factors, have been implicated as the cause of these disorders. However, it has been suggested recently on the basis of statistical evidence, that single major loci are important in at least 2 traditionally multifactorial defects: cleft lip and palate and congenital heart defects. This information is somehow tentative, and at the present, the principles of empirical recurrence risk of multifactorial models are still valid.

CLINICAL SIGNIFICANCE

Disorders with multifactorial inheritance include the majority of isolated congenital malformations such as congenital heart disease, cleft lip and/or palate, congenital dislocation of hip, pyloric stenosis, celiac disease, Hirschsprung disease, neural tube defects and club foot; the majority of mental retardation; common, later onset diseases such as hyperlipidemia, hypertension and allergies; and normal traits such as height, pigmentation and intelligence. Sporadic cases, or multiple family members, scattered throughout the kindred can be affected with multifactorial disorder. The recurrence risk of relatives of affected person is increased and empirical recurrence risk tables are available for different disorders.

The recurrence risk is not constant, as in single gene defects (ie, each offspring of a parent with autosomal dominant disorder has 50% recurrence risk, regardless of how many siblings have been already affected), but it is directly related to the number of affected family members, how closely they are related, if they are of the less commonly affected sex, and how severely they are affected. In general after one first degree affected relative (parent, child, or sib) the recurrence risk for most multifactorial disorders is 3–5%; after two affected first degree relatives, the risk is approximately 10%.

PREVENTION

(1) Parents of affected children need to be informed about the increased recurrence risk.

(2) Prenatal diagnosis (ultrasound, alpha fetoprotein) can be utilized for the detection of congenital malformations.

(3) Children at increased risk for a multifactorial disorder must be closely monitored for a recurrence as early intervention may prevent complications.

NON-TRADITIONAL INHERITANCE

GONADAL MOSAICISM

A new gene mutation affecting not one, but a cluster of gametes, will result in gonadal mosaicism. Thus, two clinically normal parents may have two or more affected offspring, mimicking autosomal recessive inheritance. An example is osteogenesis imperfecta, type 2 (lethal), which was previously thought to be caused by an autosomal recessive disorder, but molecular analyses confirmed gonadal mosaicism. The recurrence risk in cases of gonadal mosaicism is unknown, but is estimated to be 5–10%.

UNIPARENTAL DISOMY

Under normal circumstances, one chromosome of each chromosome pair is of maternal, the other of paternal origin. In uniparental disomy, both alleles originated from the same parent and none from the other. Uniparental disomy cannot be detected by chromosome analysis, which is normal. Only molecular analysis, using specific polymorphic markers can identify the parental origin of the chromosomes. Uniparental trisomy has been documented for human chromosomes 7, 11, 15 and X. Uniparental disomy is responsible for Beckwith-Wiedemann, Prader-Willi and Angelmann syndromes in some patients. It has been found to be responsible for passing homozygosity for cystic fibrosis from a mother to her child; it has been documented that both X and Y chromosomes have been past from a father with hemophilia to his affected son. In addition, uniparental disomy has been implicated in some cases of prenatal and postnatal growth retardation (Russell-Silver syndrome) and in fetal demise.

IMPRINTING

Imprinting is a process by which the expression of a gene depends on its parental origin. For example, a uniparental disomy of chromosomes 15 of maternal origin will result in Prader–Willi syndrome, whereas a paternal uniparental disomy of the same chromosome pair will cause Angelmann syndrome.

CONTIGUOUS GENE SYNDROMES

Some well-defined dysmorphic syndromes, previously of unknown etiology, have been found to be caused by a sub-microscopic or visible chromosome deletion. Thus, they are believed to be caused by a number of genes located in linear arrangement on the chromosome, i.e. contiguous genes. Currently recognized contiguous gene syndromes include DiGeorge syndrome (deletion 22q11), Miller-Dieker syndrome (del 17p13), WAGR syndrome (Wilm's tumor, aniridia, genitourinary abnormalities and retardation) on chromosome 11p13 and retinoblastoma—mental retardation (13q14).

MITOCHONDRIAL INHERITANCE

In addition to mutation of genes found in nuclei of cells, human disorders may be caused by mutation of mitochondrial genes, located in the cytoplasm of cells. The normal function of mitochondrial genes is very important for normal energy metabolism, through oxidative phosphorylation and formation of ATP. This generates energy especially important for a normal function of the central nervous system and cardiac and peripheral muscles. Thus, the mutations of mitochondrial genes have adverse effects predominantly on these organs. Since cytoplasmic mitochondria are inherited through the egg (the sperm contains a minimal amount of cytoplasm), mitochondrial diseases are inherited through the maternal lineage; affected males usually do not pass the mutation to their offspring. Mitochondrial inheritance is implicated in Leber optic atrophy and a variety of neuromuscular degenerative disorders.

PRINCIPLES OF PEDIGREE ANALYSIS

(1) **Negative family history** does not exclude the presence of single gene disorder. Explanations include a new mutation,

or decreased penetrance of a dominant gene, autosomal recessive or multifactorial inheritance.

(2) **Multiple generations affected** are compatible with autosomal or X-linked dominant disorders.

(3) **Mostly males are affected** and they are related to each other through unaffected or mildly affected females: X-linked recessive (can be passed through affected males) or mitochondrial (not passed through affected males) inheritance.

(4) **Only sibs affected:** Compatible with autosomal recessive inheritance, gonadal mosaicism or multifactorial.

(5) **Affected individuals are scattered** in irregular fashion through the kindred: multifactorial.

INBORN ERRORS OF METABOLISM

Inborn errors of metabolism (IEM) are disorders caused by blocks in metabolic pathways. The clinical symptoms of these disorders are caused either by the accumulation of a substrate behind the block or by the deficiency of the product of a normal metabolic reaction. The recognition of an IEM, most of which are inherited as autosomal recessive disorders, is extremely important. Inborn errors of metabolism frequently present as a medical emergency, and because many of them can be successfully treated, early diagnosis is paramount to the prevention of significant morbidity and mortality. Although infants with IEM are best managed in centers with expertise in treatment of metabolic diseases, the primary care physicians have to be the ones to suspect the diagnosis of IEM and to initiate an appropriate laboratory workup.

WHEN SHOULD IEM BE CONSIDERED?

(1) Acutely ill newborn with symptoms of neonatal sepsis: vomiting, poor feeding, jaundice, lethargy, seizures, or jitteriness, especially if the alteration of the mental status is out of the proportion to systemic findings or if there is a peculiar body odor, or history of unexplained neonatal death in a sib or maternal uncle.

(2) Typical Reye or Reye-like syndrome: encephalopathy, vomiting, hepatomegaly.

(3) Vomiting, especially cyclic, or associated with acidosis.

(4) Acutely altered neurologic/mental status, ataxia, seizures, hypertonia in neonate or hypotonia in a child.

(5) Mental retardation, especially if there is slowing or regression of development.

(6) Unexplained metabolic imbalance: acidosis, hyperammonemia or hyperglycemia.

(7) Unusual body odor—smell of sweaty feet or mouse-like smell.

(8) Coarse facial features and other physical findings compatible with storage disorders (see below).

(9) Sudden, unexplained death after rapid deterioration of a previously well infant.

The suspicion of inborn errors is heightened by a history of consanguinity, unexplained infant deaths in siblings or maternal male relatives, aversion to certain food and appearance of symptoms with changes in diet.

Suspicious physical findings include abnormal hair, retinal changes (cherry red spot or retinitis pigmentosa), corneal clouding, coarse facial features, hepatomegaly, skeletal changes, microcephaly or macrocephaly, abnormal muscle tone and failure to thrive. The presence of another specific cause which can explain the symptoms, such as intercurrent infection, does not exclude IEM as some disorders become symptomatic during infection; others like galactosemia, increase the risk of gram-negative septicemia. The presence of facial dysmorphism and/or congenital malformations does not rule out IEM (Table 24–2).

CLASSIFICATION OF IEM'S

- Disorders of carbohydrate metabolism (eg, galactosemia, glycogen storage diseases, fructose intolerance, primary lactic acidemias).
- Defects of amino acid metabolism (eg, phenylketonuria, tyrosinemia, maple syrup urine disease, homocystinuria, nonketotic hyperglycinemia, urea cycle disorders such as transcarbamoylase deficiency).
- Organic acidurias (eg, glutaric acidemia, type I and II, methylmalonic acidemia, primary lactic acidemia, isovaleric acidemia).
- Defects of fatty acid oxidation (eg, deficiencies of long chain and medium chain acyl-CoA dehydrogenase: LCAD, MCAD).

- Disorders of purine metabolism (eg, Lesch–Nyhan syndrome).
- Lysosomal storage disorders (eg, mucopolysaccharidoses such as Hurler syndrome, mucolipidosis such as Mannosidoses or I-cell disease, lipidoses such as Niemann–Pick diseases).
- Peroxisomal disorders (eg, Zellweger syndrome).

The clinical and laboratory features of these categories are listed in Table 24–2.

DIAGNOSTIC EVALUATION

(1) Acutely ill infant or child: *Blood*: CBC, ammonia, glucose, acid-base status, amino acids, carnitine total and free. *Urine*: pH, reducing substances, ketones, organic acids, amino acids. Other studies such as CSF glycine, plasma lactate and pyruvate depending upon age and specific presentations.

(2) Stable child with mental retardation/developmental delay: *Blood*: CBC, acid-base status, amino acids. *Urine*: amino acids, organic acids, mucopolysaccharides, ketones, pH, reducing substances. Consider on the basis of above tests results and clinical findings: urine oligosaccharides, blood lactate and pyruvate, or other studies. Instructions on handling the samples for metabolic evaluations are in Table 24–3.

MANAGEMENT OF ACUTELY ILL INFANT OR CHILD WITH IEM

(1) Treatment must be prompt and vigorous. Treatment has to be started as soon as hyperammonemia or acid-base imbalance are diagnosed, while waiting for the results of other tests.

(2) Stop oral intake (stop intake of all protein, all sugars, except glucose).

(3) Give glucose IV in amounts **sufficient** to stop catabolic process.

(4) Treat hyperammonemia with dialysis or pharmacologically.

(5) Treat acidosis with bicarbonate.

(6) More specific treatment may be instituted after establishment of diagnosis.

Table 24–2. Clinical and laboratory features of inborn errors.[1–4]

	Defects of Carbohydrate Metabolism	Defects of Amino Acid Metabolism[2]	Organic Acid Disorders[3]	Defects of Fatty Acid Oxidation	Defects of Purine Metabolism	Lysosomal Storage Diseases	Disorders of Peroxisomes
Neurodevelopmental							
Mental/developmental retardation	—	+++	+++	—	++	+++	+++
Developmental regression	+++	—	+	—	—	+++	++
Acute encephalopathy	+++	+++	+++	+++	—	—	++
Seizures	++	+++	+++	+	—	+++	+
Ataxia/movement disorder	—	+	++	—	+++	—	+++
Hypotonia	++	++	++	+++	—	+	+++
Hypertonia	—	++	+++	—	++	+	—
Abnormal behavior	—	++	++	—	++	+++	—
Growth							
Failure to thrive	+++	+++	+++	—	—	+	—
Short stature	++	—	+	—	—	++	—
Macrocephaly	—	—	+	—	—	+++	++
Microcephaly	+	++	+++	—	—	+	—
General							
Vomiting/anorexia	++	+++	+++	+++	—	—	++
Food aversion or craving	++	+++	+++	+++	—	—	—
Odor	—	++	++	—	—	—	—
Dysmorphic features	—	+	+	—	—	++	++
Congenital malformations	—	++	++	—	—	—	++
Organ specific							
Hepatomegaly	+++	—	++	+++	—	+++	+++

Clinical/Laboratory feature	[1]	[2]	[3]					
Liver disease/cirrhosis	++	+	—	—	—	—	—	+
Splenomegaly	—	—	—	—	—	++	++	+
Skeletal dysplasia	—	—	—	+++	—	++	++	++
Cardiomyopathy	++	—	+	++	+++	++	++	—
Tachypnea/hyperpnea	++	++	++	++	++	—	—	—
Rash	—	+	++	—	—	—	—	—
Alopecia or abnormal hair	++	+	—	—	—	—	—	+
Cataracts or corneal opacity	++	—	—	—	—	++	++	++
Retinal abnormality	—	+	++	+	—	++	++	—
Frequent infections	++	—	++	—	++	—	—	—
Deafness	—	—	+	—	—	++	—	—
Laboratory–general								
Hypoglycemia	+++	+	++	++	—	—	—	—
Hyperammonemia	—	++	++	++	—	—	—	—
Metabolic acidosis	++	++	+++	+++	—	—	—	—
Respiratory alkalosis	—	++	—	—	—	—	—	—
Elevated lactate/pyruvate	++	—	+++	++	—	—	—	—
Elevated liver enzymes	++	++	++	+++	—	+	+	+
Neutropenia or thrombocytopenia	+	—	+	—	++	—	++	—
Ketosis	+++	++	+++	—	—	—	—	—
Hypoketosis	—	—	+++	+++	—	—	—	—

[1] +++, most conditions in group; ++, some; +, one or few; —, not found.
[2] Includes disorders of urea cycle but not maple syrup urine disease.
[3] Includes maple syrup urine disease and disorders of pyruvate oxidation.
[4] From Goodman SI, Greene CL: Inborn errors of metabolism. In: Hathaway WE et al (editors) *Current Pediatric Diagnosis & Treatment*, 11th ed. Appleton & Lange, 1993.

Table 24–3. Obtaining and handling samples to diagnose inborn errors.[1]

Test	Comments
Acid-base status	Accurate estimation of anion gap must be possible. Samples for blood gases should be kept on ice and analyzed immediately.
Blood ammonia	Sample should be collected without a tourniquet, kept on ice, and analyzed immediately.
Blood lactic acid and pyruvic acid	Sample should be collected without a tourniquet, kept on ice, and analyzed immediately. Reduction of pyruvic acid to lactic acid must be prevented. Normal literature values are for the fasting, rested state.
Amino acids	Blood and urine should be examined. CSF glycine should be measured if nonketotic hyperglycinemia is to be ruled out. Normal literature values are for the fasting state. Growth of bacteria in urine should be prevented. At autopsy: liver, kidney, or vitreous may be analyzed if urine is not available.
Organic acids	Urine preferred for analysis. At autopsy: liver, kidney, or vitreous may be analyzed if urine is not available.
Urine mucopolysaccharides	Variations in urine concentration may cause errors in screening tests. Diagnosis requires knowing which mucopolysaccharides are increased. Some patients with Morquio's disease do not have abnormal mucopolysacchariduria.
Enzyme assays	Specific assays must be requested. Exposure to heat may cause loss of enzyme activity. Enzyme activity in whole blood may become normal after transfusion or vitamin therapy. Leukocyte or fibroblast pellets should be kept frozen prior to assays. Fibroblasts may be grown from skin biopsies taken up to 72 hours after death. Tissues such as liver and kidney should be taken as soon as possible after death, frozen immediately, and kept at $-70°C$ until assayed.

[1] From Goodman SI, Greene CL: Inborn errors of metabolism. In: Hathaway WE et al (editors): *Current Pediatric Diagnosis & Treatment,* 11th ed. Appleton & Lange, 1993.

SPECIFIC TREATMENT FOR IEM

The goal of the treatment is to compensate the metabolic imbalance caused by the block in the pathway. This can be accomplished by supplementing a deficient metabolite (eg, arginine in disorders of urea cycle), eliminating a harmful substrate from the diet (eg, phenylalanine in phenylketonuria), providing coenzyme (eg, vitamin B_{12} therapy in some types of methylmalonic acidemia), pharmacologically removing accumulated substrate (isovaleric acidemia), or replacing the missing enzyme (by infusion or transplant). Ideally, a permanent solution would be gene replacement and research trials are underway.

THE EVALUATION OF A DYSMORPHIC CHILD

Disruption of normal morphogenesis during intrauterine life is responsible for the presence of major malformations and dysmorphic features such as single flexion creases of the palms (Simian lines), hypoplastic finger nails, upslant or downslant eyes, epicanthic folds, abnormal shape of auricles, etc.

ETIOLOGY

Dysmorphogenesis can be caused by chromosome abnormalities, single gene defects, adverse environmental factors—teratogens or by a combination of multiple factors. In approximately 50% of dysmorphic children, specific etiology cannot be identified.

PATHOGENESIS

On the basis of pathogenesis, dysmorphic features can be classified as **malformations,** ie, true primarily abnormal development caused by intrinsic factors such as a chromosome abnormality; **deformations,** caused by external mechanical forces acting upon a normally developing fetus, such as uterine constraint; and **disruptions,** the result of extrinsic interruption of normal development such as amniotic bands interfering with normal closure of body cavities or of separation of fingers.

THE VALUE OF RECOGNITION OF
DYSMORPHIC FEATURES

(1) Pattern of dysmorphic features allows diagnosis of specific syndromes, thus establishing correct prognosis and recurrence risk (eg, Down's syndrome). This is especially valuable in newborns as the correct diagnosis of a specific syndrome might influence the management (eg, Trisomy 13 or 18).

(2) Presence of dysmorphic features in children with developmental delay or mental retardation helps to establish timing of the harmful insult to prenatal versus perinatal or postnatal periods and aid in the identification of the etiology.

(3) Multiple dysmorphic features are known to be associated with an increased frequency of major malformations, thus, their presence alerts the professionals to look for major malformations. In addition, there are some more consistent associations, eg, abnormally formed auricles are associated with higher frequency of hearing loss, etc. Alternatively, the presence of dysmorphic features in a child with a known major malformation helps to differentiate a child with an isolated multifactorial defect such as CHD from a child with a more complex syndrome, eg, Noonan syndrome with CHD.

PRINCIPLES OF SYNDROME IDENTIFICATION

(1) Recognition of dysmorphic features. These have to be differentiated from familial features found in normal relatives and normal variations frequent in the general population, such as mongolian spots.

(2) Familiarity with a large number of syndromes and their clinical variability. The clinician with limited knowledge of syndromes is at danger of misdiagnosing the patient. Excellent extensive reviews of specific syndromes can be found in *Smith's Recognizable Pattern of Human Malformations* edited by Dr. Ken Jones and Dr. Gorlin's book: *Syndromes of the Head and Neck*.

(3) Establishment of a differential diagnosis starting with the patient's abnormality which has the lowest incidence in the general population, i.e. use radial ray defect rather than more common VSD if both present. Comparison of the patient's other findings with known syndromes with radial ray defect, helps to find the syndrome most compatible with the patient's diagnosis.

(4) **Do not over-diagnose.** If a specific syndrome cannot be confidently identified, diagnosis has to be deferred. The child needs to be periodically re-evaluated (the younger the child, the more frequently). A diagnosis may become apparent later either because (a) the child developed new signs, which aid the diagnosis (eg, a child with severe prenatal and postnatal growth retardation, originally seen at 2 months of age, developed facial erythema upon a sun exposure at 9 months of age allowing the diagnosis of Bloom syndrome, confirmed by chromosome analysis) or (b) the diagnostic techniques improve (eg, a retarded child, reminiscent of 4p deletion, was reported to have a normal karyotype; recently developed FISH technique detected 4p deletion).

THE ROLE OF TERATOGENS IN DYSMORPHOGENESIS

The exposure of a genetically susceptible fetus to a potential teratogen increases the chance of malformations. Although many environmental agents are potentially teratogenic, very few are proven teratogens. These include the following:

- Infectious agents (rubella virus, cytomegalic virus, toxoplasma, herpes virus, varicella virus).
- Drugs and medications (including alcohol, cocaine, anticonvulsants, vitamin A derivatives).
- Maternal diseases (such as diabetes mellitus, phenylketonuria).
- Uterine conditions (malformed uterus, twinning).

Prerequisites for Teratogenic Action

(1) **Teratogenicity of agents:** Documentation of teratogenicity in humans is important. Information can be obtained from the Teratogen Information Service available in many states or from clinical genetics centers.

(2) **Genetic predisposition of the fetus:** All fetuses exposed to known teratogens are not affected adversely; the genetic makeup may influence the absorption, metabolism, excretion, etc, of a teratogen.

(3) Exposure during vulnerable stages of fetal development. Exposures during the organogenesis may be responsible for major congenital malformations; later exposures may contribute to a neuro-developmental dysfunction.

(4) *Caution*: The history of teratogenic exposure does not rule out the contribution of other etiologies to the patient's dysm-

orphogenesis; a chromosome abnormality or single gene syndrome may need to be considered, if clinically warranted.

MENTAL RETARDATION

The American Association of Mental Deficiency defines mental retardation (MR) as a concurrent presence of intellectual functioning more than 2 standard deviations below the mean (ie, IQ < 70) and a deficit in adaptive behavior. The purpose of this changed definition is to prevent overlabeling with mental retardation children who in fact have learning disability or undetected sensory deficit. While over-diagnosis of MR in a child with normal intellectual potential may be detrimental for the future, lack of detection of MR is also harmful. There are a number of mandated services for MR children, which are unavailable without the diagnosis. In everyday practice, the diagnosis of MR is still mostly based on IQ < 70. The incidence of MR is approximately 2–4%.

ETIOLOGY OF MENTAL RETARDATION

Multifactorial mental retardation (physiological, familial MR) comprises 90% of all MR. This group of MR represents the lowest tail of normal Gaussian distribution of IQ of general population. The MR is mild (IQ 70–50), is not associated with minor or major malformations, is more common in lower socioeconomic classes and frequently there is positive family history for mildly MR family members. One parent with multifactorial MR has approximately 20%, both parents with MR 40% chance for affected offspring. Normal parents with one affected child have approximately 5% recurrence risk.

The remaining categories of MR collectively represent 10% of all MR children and .3% of the general population. Most of the children in these categories have severe MR (IQ 50–30), although some are only mildly retarded. The etiologies include **chromosome abnormality:** Down's syndrome is most common and fragile X is the second most common genetic cause of MR. Other chromosome anomalies are present in 1–4% of severely MR children surviving past 1 year. **Single gene defects** include inborn errors of metabolism (3–7% of severe MR), neurocutaneous and other disorders, and syndromes such as Smith–Lemli–Opitz and Rett syndrome. **Teratogenic exposures** include fetal alcohol syndrome and fetal hydantoin syndrome, congenital rubella, and CMV. **Infections** cause 2.8–8.5% of severe MR. **Environmental factors** such as Rh incompatibility, lead-poisoning, and accidental or non-accidental trauma account for approximately 1% of MR. **Syndromes of unknown etiology** such as Cornelia de Lange are associated with MR.

MR associated with **other CNS dysfunction** of heterogeneous etiology includes MR associated with **cerebral palsy** (over 50% has documented prenatal etiology); MR with **multiple congenital malformations** (chromosomal, single gene defect or teratogenic); and MR with **CNS malformations** such as hydrocephalus, neural tube defects, midline brain defects etc.

Recurrence risk in these categories corresponds with the genetic mechanisms involved, as discussed under those headings.

Diagnostic evaluation of MR children includes detailed family, pregnancy, medical and developmental histories; physical examination aimed at detection of dysmorphic features and signs of single gene disorders such as depigmented ash-leaf spots of tuberous sclerosis; laboratory testing is based on the clinical suspicion of an etiology and may include chromosome analysis, studies for inborn errors of metabolism, brain imaging, etc.

GENETIC EVALUATION AND COUNSELING

Purpose of Referrals to Genetics Clinic

The genetics clinic can assist the primary care provider with any of the following:

    (1) Establishment of correct **diagnosis.**
    (2) Explanation of **natural history** of the disorder.
    (3) **Management** issues.
    (4) Establishment of **recurrence risk.**
    (5) Identification of available **reproductive options.**
    (6) Help families to **adjust** to having an affected child.

Correct diagnosis is of utmost importance, before further information listed below can be provided. Detailed history (prenatal, developmental, medical, family), and review of the results of previous tests in combination with physical examination and select laboratory studies aid the dysmorphologist/geneticist in establishment of diagnoses.

While the diagnostic features of most genetic disease and various syndromes are well known, the specific information about the natural history and about the impact of various management approaches on the course of many disorders is often inadequate.

The recurrence risk for individual family members is established according to the principles of inheritance of different disorders. In cases with unknown etiology, where a specific diagnosis cannot be established, the genetic evaluation may be reassuring because the absence of a known genetic disorder indicates probable low recurrence risk.

Available reproductive options may include any of the following: (a) taking chances; (b) no reproduction; (c) artificial insemination by donor (paternal chromosomal, autosomal dominant or X-linked disease, both parents are carriers of autosomal recessive disorder); (d) donor egg and in vitro fertilization (to avoid passing an abnormal maternal gene or chromosome); (e) prenatal diagnosis (ultrasound, amniocentesis, chorionic villi sampling, maternal serum alpha fetoprotein); and (f) pre-implantation genetic evaluation is in a developmental stage.

Genetic counseling should be **nondirective.** It should provide all available information about all aspects of the disorder. The counselors should support the family in any decision they deem appropriate for their family's goals and moral values.

Indications for Referral to a Genetic Clinic

(1) Child with birth defects and/or developmental delay/mental retardation.

(2) Dysmorphic child.

(3) Parent or child affected with known or suspected genetic disorder (chromosomal or single gene or multifactorial).

(4) Positive family history of birth defects or retardation in aunts, uncles, grandparents or other relatives, especially if multiple members are affected.

(5) Possible teratogenic exposure or other abnormalities of pregnancy.

(6) Advanced maternal age (over 35 years) or other indications for prenatal diagnosis.

The **advantages of a genetic evaluation** include (1) the establishment of a diagnosis which in turn may clarify the child's prognosis and indicate the appropriateness of supportive therapies (OT, PT, etc); (2) the clarification of the etiology helps to identify recurrence risk and the appropriate reproductive options; and (3) provision of extensive information may help to alleviate parental guilt for producing an abnormal child and help the parents to accept the situation.

25 | Neoplastic Diseases

Linda C. Stork, MD

Cancer in children differs biologically from cancer in adults (Fig. 25–1). Neoplastic disease is the second leading cause of death in the pediatric age group in the USA. Solid tumors represent 70% of cases and acute leukemia the remaining 30%.

For solid tumors in general, the less the tumor burden and the more localized the tumor at diagnosis, the better the chance of cure. For the leukemias, various clinical and laboratory features present at diagnosis correlate with ultimate prognosis. Present-day treatment of pediatric cancers is complex, multimodal, and multidisciplinary and should be carried out under the direction of centers specializing in the care of children with neoplastic diseases.

BRAIN TUMORS

Brain tumors represent the second most common type of childhood cancer, with leukemia being the most common. About 50% of these arise in the posterior fossa. Cerebellar tumors include medulloblastomas or primitive neuroectodermal tumors (PNET), astrocytomas, and ependymomas. Supratentorial tumors include astrocytomas (high and low grade), optic gliomas, craniopharyngiomas, choroid plexus tumors, teratomas and germinomas. Gliomas and astrocytomas occur in the brainstem.

The entire symptom complex of an intracranial space-consuming lesion, including vomiting, increase in intracranial pressure, and papilledema, can be caused by lesions that are not neoplastic. The principal ones are abscess, hemorrhage, CNS infections, and venous sinus thrombosis. CT scan and MRI can help differentiate among these lesions. Some brain tumors grow slowly over years before diagnosis and others develop quickly over months.

Clinical Findings

A. Symptoms and Signs: Evidence of increased intracranial pressure includes headache, vomiting (often without nausea and

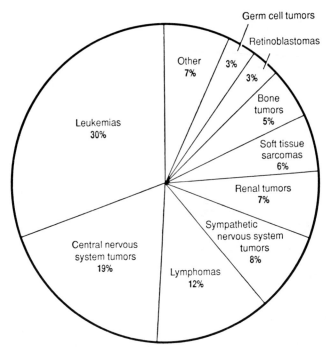

Figure 25–1. Approximate incidence of the principal cancers in children less than 15 years old (SEER program, 1973–1982).

before breakfast), diplopia, blurred vision, and papilledema. Personality changes, including irritability, apathy, disturbances in sleep and eating patterns, are frequent. Sudden enlargement of the head, if head circumferences have been plotted, is detectable when sutures are still open, or after sutures have split. Alterations of consciousness and stiff neck with tonsillar herniation may be seen.

1. Cerebellar and 4th Ventricle Tumors–Evidence of increased intracranial pressure is often present along with cerebellar signs, including ataxia, dysmetria and nystagmus. Pressure on adjacent structures may cause head tilt, cranial nerve signs, pyramidal tract signs and stiff neck.

2. Supratentorial Tumors–Evidence of increased intracranial pressure is usually present, along with seizures (generalized, psychomotor, focal) in about 40% of cases. Hemiparesis, visual field defects, and personality changes often develop. Tumors of the diencephalon (like optic gliomas) are often associated with emaciation despite good oral intake (diencephalic syndrome). Tumors of the suprasellar region are often associated with visual disorders, diabetes insipidus, and pituitary insufficiency.

3. Brainstem Tumors–Cranial nerve palsies are especially common in these tumors along with hemiparesis and ataxia. Signs of increased intracranial pressure are uncommon.

B. Imaging: CT scan with contrast usually identifies the mass, hydrocephalus, midline shift, and edema. MRI is often better than CT scan at identifying intracranial spread beyond the primary mass. Brainstem gliomas are best imaged with MRI. The presence of calcification and cysts correlate with specific tumor types. Spinal MRI and/or myelograms are necessary to diagnose "drop mets" in patients with medulloblastoma, ependymomas and germinomas.

Treatment

Complete surgical resection should be attempted whenever the tumor location permits this. Ventriculoperitoneal shunts may be necessary to correct hydrocephalus. Many tumors are not resectable, including those of the brainstem and diencephalon. In these cases stereotactic biopsy is usually recommended to establish histologic diagnosis. Until the 1980s, radiation therapy was the mainstay of treatment for brain tumors. Unfortunately, severe learning disabilities and endocrine dysfunction often developed in survivors. Chemotherapy along with radiation therapy has been shown to increase survival in incompletely resected medulloblastomas, high-grade astrocytomas, and ependymomas. In addition to radiation therapy to the posterior fossa, radiation therapy to the entire craniospinal axis is necessary to prevent recurrence and "drop mets" in medulloblastomas (PNET). Cooperative clinical trials are currently evaluating the role of intensive chemotherapy in the treatment of many types of brain tumors. Trials are also evaluating whether radiation can be delayed or omitted in young children.

Prognosis

The prognosis depends on tumor location, histology, and grade (low versus high) and extent of surgical resection. At least

50% of patients with medulloblastoma (PNET) survive 5 years; fewer than 25% of patients with brainstem gliomas survive 5 years; and over 75% of patients with completely resected low-grade astrocytomas survive 5 years.

HODGKIN'S DISEASE

Hodgkin's disease occurs twice as frequently in men as in women, with its peak incidence in the third decade. It has been reported in children as young as 3 years of age. The cause is not known. The clinical and surgical staging system is shown in Table 25–1.

Clinical Findings

A. Symptoms and Signs: Painless lymph node enlargement, variable degrees of anorexia, weight loss, fatigue, weakness, fever, malaise, pruritus, and night sweats (Table 25–1). The most common site of nodal involvement is the cervical region, but Hodgkin's disease can arise in any lymph node. Involved nodes

Table 25–1. Staging classification for Hodgkin's disease.[1]
(Ann Arbor classification.)

Stage[2]	Distinctive Features
I	Involvement of a single lymph node region (I) or a single extra-lymphatic organ or site (I_E).
II	Involvement of 2 or more lymph node regions on the same side of the diaphragm (II) or localized involvement of an extralym-phatic organ or site and of one or more lymph node regions on the same side of the diaphragm (II_E).
III	Involvement of lymph node regions on both sides of the dia-phragm (III), which may be accompanied by localized involve-ment of an extralymphatic organ or site (III_E) or of spleen (III_S) or both (III_{SE}).
IV	Diffuse or disseminated involvement of one or more extralym-phatic organs with or without associated lymph node involve-ment. The organs involved should be identified by a symbol.

[1] Modified and reproduced, with permission, from Kempe CH, Silver HK, O'Brien D (editors): *Current Pediatric Diagnosis & Treatment,* 8th ed. Lange, 1984.
[2] Stages are also classified as IA, IB, IIA, IIB, etc. on the basis of symptoms and signs: A = asymptomatic; B = fever, night sweats, or weight loss > 10% of body weight in the 6 months prior to diagnosis.

are usually firm and nontender and may produce pressure symptoms depending upon their location. Hepatosplenomegaly and extranodal disease, particularly in lung and bone marrow, may be present. Splenomegaly does not necessarily imply splenic involvement with Hodgkin's disease, however. Other infections and inflammatory causes of lymphadenopathy are in the differential diagnosis, including infectious mononucleosis and atypical mycobacterial infections.

B. Laboratory Findings: Hematologic findings may be normal or may show anemia, leukocytosis, leukopenia, thrombocytosis, thrombocytopenia, eosinophilia, or elevated sedimentation rate. Acute phase reactant proteins, including fibrinogen, ceruloplasmin, C-reactive protein, and ferritin, may be elevated in serum and can serve as sensitive markers of response to therapy and of early recurrent disease. Kidney and liver function tests may reflect abnormalities if these organs are involved with disease. Cell-mediated immunity is often impaired in patients with Hodgkin's Disease. Hemolytic anemia and abnormal levels of immunoglobulins may also occur. The diagnosis of Hodgkin's disease is made by biopsy of the involved node. Clinical staging should include bilateral bone marrow aspirates and biopsies. General anesthesia may be contraindicated if a large mediastinal mass is present.

C. Imaging: Clinical staging includes a number of x-ray modalities. Chest x-rays or chest CT scan may show parenchymal or mediastinal nodal disease. Lymphangiography may reveal a "foamy" enlarged node, which implies tumor filling the node. Abdominal CT scan may show enlarged periaortic nodes or spleen and liver abnormalities. Gallium scan may help identify areas of occult disease.

D. Staging: Surgical staging by laparotomy, with splenectomy, liver biopsy, and lymph node sampling is still recommended in fully grown patients who may be successfully treated with radiation therapy alone. However, pediatric oncologists prefer to treat growing children with chemotherapy and limited radiation, thus eliminating the need for laparotomy and the risk of postsplenectomy sepsis.

Treatment

Fully grown patients with surgical stages I and II disease can be successfully treated with extended field irradiation alone. Therapy for growing children with low-stage disease remains controversial, but chemotherapy with or without low-dose radiation to involved areas is becoming widely used. Chemotherapy is the primary treatment modality for stages III and IV disease. Chemotherapeutic agents commonly employed in combination are vincristine, mechlorethamine or cyclophosphamide, procarbazine, prednisone, vinblastine, bleomycin, doxorubicin, and dacarbazine (Table 25–2).

Prognosis

In adequately treated patients, 5-year survival rates have improved greatly. In stages I and II disease, rates range from 85 to 90%. In stages III and IV disease, rates range from about 50 to 80%. Late side effects of treatment with radiation and chemotherapy include infertility, impaired bony growth, hypothyroidism, and second cancers.

NON-HODGKIN'S LYMPHOMA

Non-Hodgkin's lymphomas encompass a more diverse group of lymphomas in adults than in children. Histologic classification into 2 main groups, lymphoblastic and nonplymphoblastic, is important in childhood lymphomas for determining appropriate therapy and prognosis.

Burkitt's tumor (African lymphoma) is a special type of childhood lymphoma found principally in Africa. This tumor is responsible for half of all cancer deaths in children in Uganda and Central Africa. A viral cause has been assumed and the role of Epstein-Barr virus in this disease is under scrutiny. The tumor is characterized by (1) predilection for the facial bones and mandible *or* (2) primary involvement of abdominal nodes and viscera and (3) massive proliferation of primitive lymphoid cells. When Burkitt's tumor is seen in patients outside of Africa, it generally presents as an abdominal tumor.

Clinical Findings

A. Symptoms and Signs: Non-Hodgkin's lymphoma of childhood tends to grow rapidly. The gastrointestinal tract in the region of the terminal ileum, cecum, appendix, ascending colon, and mesenteric nodes is the most common site of nonlymphoblastic lymphoma (aside from African Burkitt's). Acute abdominal pain, intussusception, gastrointestinal tract perforation, and hemorrhage may occur. Lymphoblastic lymphoma presents most commonly with a mediastinal mass, with or without pleural

Table 25–2. Antineoplastic agents.[1]

Agent	Indications	Toxicity
Asparaginase (Elspar)	Acute lymphoblastic leukemia.	Nausea, vomiting, fever, hypersensitivity, pancreatitis, hyperglycemia thromboses.
Bleomycin (Blenoxane)	Hodgkin's disease, non-Hodgkin's lymphoma, testicular tumors.	Nausea, vomiting, stomatitis, fever, chills, pulmonary fibrosis, hyperpigmentation, alopecia.
Carmustine (BCNU)	Malignant gliomas, medulloblastoma, advanced Hodgkin's disease and other sarcomas, neuroblastoma, malignant melanoma.	Nausea, vomiting, hepatotoxicity, chemical dermatitis. Bone marrow depression (3- to 4-wk delay).
Cisplatin (Platinol, CDDP)	Germ cell tumors, osteogenic sarcoma, brain tumors, neuroblastoma.	Nausea, vomiting, anorexia, alopecia, bone marrow depression, renal failure, magnesium and calcium wasting hearing impairment.
Cyclophosphamide (Cytoxan)	Leukemia, Hodgkin's disease, neuroblastoma, sarcomas, retinoblastoma, hepatoma, rhabdomyosarcoma, Ewing's sarcoma.	Nausea, vomiting, anorexia, alopecia, bone marrow depression, hemorrhagic cystitis.
Cytarabine (cytosine arabinoside; Cytosar-U)	Acute myeloblastic and acute lymphocytic leukemia.	Nausea, vomiting, anorexia, bone marrow depression, hepatotoxicity.
Dacarbazine (DTIC)	Hodgkin's disease, neuroblastoma, sarcomas.	Bone marrow depression, flulike syndrome, rash, liver failure, pain at IV infusion site.

(Continued)

Table 25–2. Antineoplastic agents (continued)

Agent	Indications	Toxicity
Dactinomycin (Cosmegan)	Wilms's tumor, sarcomas, rhabdomyosarcoma.	Nausea, vomiting, anorexia, bone marrow depression, alopecia. Chemical dermatitis if leakage at intravenous site. Tanning of skin if used with radiation therapy.
Daunorubicin (daunomycin)	Acute myelogenous, monomyelogenous, and monoblastic leukemias.	Same as for doxorubicin (below).
Doxorubicin (Adriamycin)	Acute lymphoblastic and myelocytic leukemia, lymphoma, Hodgkin's disease, Wilms's tumor neuroblastoma, ovarian or thyroid carcinoma, Ewing's sarcoma, osteogenic sarcoma, rhabdomyosarcoma, other soft tissue sarcomas.	Alopecia, stomatitis, esophagitis, nausea, vomiting. Severe chemical cellulitis and necrosis if extravasated. Bone marrow depression, irreversible myocardial damage (rare if cumulative dose less 350 mg/m^2).
Etoposide (VP-16)	Leukemias, germ cell tumors, neuroblastoma, brain tumors, sarcomas.	Allergic reactions, bone marrow depression, nausea and vomiting, neurotoxicity.
Fluorouracil (Adrucil)	Hepatoma, gastrointestinal carcinoma.	Nausea, vomiting, oral ulceration, bone marrow depression, gastroenteritis, alopecia, anorexia.
Ifosfamide	Sarcomas, recurrent solid tumors.	Bone marrow depression, hemorrhagic cystitis, nausea and vomiting, renal failure, alopecia, neurotoxicity.

(continued)

Table 25–2. Antineoplastic agents (continued)

Agent	Indications	Toxicity
Lomustine (CCNU; CeeNu)	Brain tumors, Hodgkin's disease.	Nausea, vomiting, alopecia, stomatitis, hepatotoxicity. Bone marrow depression (4- to 6-wk delay).
Mechlorethamine (nitrogen mustard)	Hodgkin's disease, non-Hodgkin's lymphoma.	Nausea, vomiting, bone marrow depression, strong vesicating effect on skin and veins.
Mercaptopurine (Purinethol)	Acute myeloblastic and acute lymphocytic leukemia.	Nausea, vomiting, rare oral ulcerations, bone marrow depression.
Methotrexate	Acute lymphocytic leukemia, central nervous system leukemia, lymphoma, choriocarcinoma, brain tumors, Hodgkin's disease.	Oral ulcers, gastrointestinal irritation, bone marrow depression, hepatotoxicity. Do not use in presence of impaired renal function.
Prednisone	Acute myeloblastic and lymphocytic leukemia, lymphoma, Hodgkin's disease, bone pain from metastatic disease, central nervous system tumors.	Increased appetite, sodium retention, hypertension, osteoporosis, provocation of latent diabetes or tuberculosis.
Procarbazine (Matulane)	Hodgkin's disease, lymphoma.	Nausea, vomiting, anorexia. Bone marrow depression (3-wk delay). Do not give with narcotics or sedatives; has "disulfiram effect." Monitor liver and renal function.
Vinblastine	Histiocytosis, Hodgkin's disease, germ cell tumors.	Bone marrow depression, alopecia, mucositis, neurotoxicity, chemical dermatitis.

(continued)

Table 25–2. Antineoplastic agents (continued)

Agent	Indications	Toxicity
Vincristine (Oncovin)	Acute lymphocytic and myeloblastic leukemia, lymphoma, Hodgkin's disease, rhabdomyosarcoma, Wilms's tumor, neuroblastoma, Ewing's sarcoma, retinoblastoma, hepatoma, sarcomas, osteogenic sarcoma, brain tumors.	Alopecia, constipation, abdominal cramps, jaw pain, paresthesia, myalgia, muscle weakness, neurotoxicity, decrease in deep tendon reflexes, chemical dermatitis. Do not use in presence of severe liver impairment.

[1] Since the dosage of these agents varies widely depending on number of drugs used simultaneously, type of tumor being treated, bone marrow reserve, and previous toxicities and therapies (eg, irradiation), the dosages are not given in this handbook.

effusion. Chronic cough, dyspnea, and orthopnea are often associated. Involvement of the tonsillar region, cervical nodes, and nasopharynx may be diagnosed by the presence of a mass or compression symptoms. Other less common sites of primary disease include bone, ovaries, skin, and CNS.

B. Laboratory Findings: Spread to the bone marrow and CNS often occurs with lymphoblastic or disseminated nonlymphoblastic lymphoma. Thus, bone marrow aspirates and biopsies and spinal fluid cytology need to be obtained. The CBC is usually normal in non-Hodgkin's lymphoma unless widespread disease and marrow infiltration is present. Serum uric acid and LDH are often very elevated in patients with Burkitt's lymphoma and moderately elevated in patients with lymphoblastic lymphoma.

C. Imaging: These patients should be evaluated radiographically as is done for Hodgkin's lymphoma, with the exception of lymphangiogram and the addition of bone scan.

Treatment

Staging laporatomy is not performed in non-Hodgkin's lymphoma. Complete surgical resection of nodal, extranodal, or gastrointestinal disease, when possible, is advocated. However, debulking of widespread abdominal disease or mediastinal mass is not advised. General anesthesia may be contraindicated in patients with large mediastinal masses. Multiple-drug chemotherapy should be started as soon as possible after diagnosis. Severe tumor lysis syndrome may develop following the initiation of treatment. Hyperuricemia, hyperphosphatemia, hypocalcemia with tetany, and renal failure may develop (see below, Leukemia, Supportive Measures). Duration of therapy depends on location, type of lymphoma, and extent of disease, and currently ranges from 6 to 18 months. The drugs most commonly employed are vincristine, cyclophosphamide, doxorubicin, prednisone, methotrexate, and cytarabine (Table 25–2). In patients at high risk for CNS involvement, prophylactic intrathecal therapy should be given. Radiation therapy is no longer recommended in children.

Prognosis

The prognosis in children with non-Hodgkin's lymphoma depends primarily on histology and extent of disease. Overall, at least 70% of children with non-Hodgkin's lymphoma can be cured.

NEUROBLASTOMA

Neuroblastoma is a tumor arising from cells in the sympathetic ganglia and adrenal medulla. It is the third most frequent pediatric neoplasm seen in children less than 5 years old. This tumor may be seen in the newborn period; the highest incidence is at 2 years of age. The tumors may regress spontaneously in infants less than 1 year old. Presentation in the abdominal area is most commonly associated with distant metastases and carries a poor prognosis.

Clinical Findings

A. Symptoms and Signs: General symptoms include failure to thrive, anorexia, fatigue, periorbital ecchymoses, chronic diarrhea, hypertension, pallor, irritability, bone pain, limp, and bluish skin nodules. Opsoclonus and myoclonus ("dancing eyes and dancing feet") have been associated with neuroblastoma.

1. Cervical Tumors–Involvement of the cervicothoracic ganglion may be associated with Horner's syndrome.

2. Posterior Thoracic Tumors–Tumors may present with respiratory symptoms such as cough, croup, dysphagia, and fatigue, or with symptoms of spinal cord compression.

3. Abdominal Tumors–Tumors may cause abdominal swelling from adrenal or paraspinal tumor. They may be very large and cross the midline or may be deep and difficult to palpate. Other findings include abdominal pain, change in bowel habits, delay in walking, paraplegia, or shock if a large tumor has ruptured.

B. Laboratory Findings: Anemia is common at diagnosis and results from chronic disease, hemorrhage into tumor, or marrow invasion. Thrombocytosis is common. Bone marrow is a common site of metastases and may reveal classic rosettes or sheets of anaplastic neuroblasts. Urine levels of catecholamines (vanillylmandelic acid [VMA] and homovanillic acid [HVA]) are elevated in nearly 90% of patients. An elevated VMA or HVA and evidence of metastatic disease in bone marrow is sufficient for the diagnosis of neuroblastoma and can obviate the need to biopsy the primary mass. Uric acid, lactate dehydrogenase, and liver and renal function should be evaluated as baseline studies. Elevated levels of serum ferritin (> 150 ng/mL), serum neuron-specific enolase (> 100 ng/mL), and amplification of the n-*myc* oncogene in the tumor itself are indicators of poor prognosis.

C. Imaging: Multiple destructive lesions of bone with a "moth-eaten" appearance may be seen in all bones. Pathologic fracture may also occur. Both skeletal survey and bone scan are necessary to determine extent of bony metastases.

1. Thoracic Tumors–Chest x-ray often shows soft tissue areas with clear borders and scattered calcifications close to the spine and in the upper chest. There may be erosion and separation of posterior ribs. CT scan or MRI should be obtained to define the tumor mass and its involvement with adjacent vital structures and spinal canal.

2. Abdominal Tumors–Abdominal x-ray may reveal a soft tissue mass in the region of the adrenal gland or along the spine. Many tumors show calcification. CT scan should be obtained to delineate the tumor and to look for hepatic metastases. Spinal MRI may be necessary to evaluate for intercanalicular disease.

Treatment

Current therapeutic recommendations include surgery alone with close follow-up for patients with stage I disease. (See Table 25–3 for staging). Patients with stage II disease and small or microscopic residua after surgery can also be safely treated with surgery alone and close follow-up. Improved treatments for advanced disease continue to be evaluated. Agents shown to be

Table 25–3. International staging system for neuroblastoma.

Stage I:	Localized tumor confined to the area of origin; complete gross excision, with or without microscopic residual disease; identifiable lymph nodes negative microscopically.
Stage IIA:	Unilateral tumor with incomplete gross excision; identifiable lymph nodes negative microscopically.
Stage IIB:	Unilateral tumor with complete or incomplete gross excision; with positive ipsilateral regional lymph nodes; identifiable contralateral lymph nodes negative microscopically.
Stage III:	Tumor infiltrating across the midline with or without regional lymph node involvement; or unilateral tumor with contralateral regional lymph node involvement; or midline tumor with bilateral regional lymph node involvement.
Stage IV:	Dissemination of tumor to distant lymph nodes, bone, bone marrow, liver and/or other organs (except as defined in stage IV).
Stage IVS:	Localized primary tumor as defined for stage 1 or 2 with dissemination limited to liver, skin, and/or bone marrow.

effective in neuroblastoma include vincristine, cytoxan, dacarbazine, etoposide, doxorubicin, cisplatin, and melphalan (Table 25–2). Neuroblastoma is very radiosensitive. Very-high-dose chemotherapy with total body irradiation, followed by autologous bone marrow transplant, is currently being evaluated in treatment of advanced disease. Retinoic acid may help differentiate neuroblastoma cells into ganglion cells, and this drug is currently being studied in clinical trials.

Prognosis

The most important variables for predicting prognosis are age and stage. Children diagnosed at less than 1 year of age have about an 80% survival rate, while survival of children diagnosed at older than 2 years (of whom two-thirds present with metastatic disease) is about 25%. Patients with stage I disease have a survival rate of about 80%, whereas survival in stage IV disease treated with conventional chemotherapy may be as poor as 10%.

WILMS'S TUMOR
(Nephroblastoma)

The most common abdominal masses encountered in early childhood are hydronephrosis, neuroblastoma, and Wilms's tumor. Wilms's tumor is believed to be embryonal in origin. It develops within renal parenchyma and enlarges with distortion and invasion of adjacent renal tissue. It occurs most commonly in children between 2 and 5 years old. Bilateral Wilms's tumors occur in up to 5% of patients. This tumor may be associated with congenital anomalies such as hemihypertrophy, aniridia, ambiguous genitalia, hypospadias, undescended testes, duplications of ureters or kidneys, horseshoe kidney, multiple nevi, and Beckwith's syndrome.

Clinical Findings

A. Symptoms and Signs: Ninety percent of patients present with an abdominal mass, but only about 30% complain of abdominal discomfort. Anemia is observed at diagnosis in about 24% of patients, hypertension in 20%, and hematuria in 15%.

B. Laboratory Findings: Results of urinalysis are usually normal, but hematuria or pyuria may be found. Blood urea nitrogen levels are usually normal; uric acid may be increased. A normochromic, normocytic anemia may be present.

C. Imaging: A soft tissue mass may be seen on a plain film of the abdomen and calcification may occur in a marginal concentric fashion. Hepatomegaly may be present if the liver has extensive metastases. Abdominal ultrasound and CT scan can define the mass, which usually appears well encapsulated. Ultrasound may demonstrate tumor thrombus in the renal vein or inferior vena cava. CT scan of chest or 4-view chest x-ray may reveal metastases.

Treatment

Surgical excision of the entire mass, without prior biopsy, is the standard surgical procedure in the USA. A transabdominal approach is essential to allow adequate mobilization, prevent excess manipulation of the tumor, and allow examination of abdominal viscera, nodes, and the opposite kidney. Conservative surgery is appropriate when bilateral disease is present at diagnosis.

Treatment of Wilms's tumor depends on surgical staging and histology (Table 25–4). Improvement in survival has resulted from cooperative clinical trials in the USA and Europe. Chemotherapy agents used to treat Wilms's tumor include dactinomycin and vincristine for the lower stages, with the addition of doxorubicin and occasionally cytoxan for the higher stages or unfavorable histology. Radiotherapy to the tumor bed is no longer recom-

Table 25–4. Wilms's tumor stages.

Stage	Findings
I	Tumor *limited* to kidney; intact capsule; completely resected
II	Tumor extension *beyond capsule* into perirenal soft tissues or renal vessels but *no* residua beyond margin of resection; surgical rupture: *flank* only
III	*Residual* tumor in abdomen: 1) + lymph nodes 2) massive rupture 3) peritoneal implants 4) not fully resected secondary to local infiltration into vital structures
IV	Hematogenous metastases
V	Bilateral; each side staged as above

mended in stages I and II disease, but appears to be of benefit in stages III and IV disease.

Prognosis

The survival rate is best in children with localized disease and favorable histology. Survival rates have significantly improved over the past 30 years, and the overall 5-year survival rate is now about 80%.

TUMORS OF SOFT TISSUE

The most common malignant soft tissue tumor seen in children is rhabdomyosarcoma. Rhabdomyosarcoma is one of the tumors associated with neurofibromatosis. The most common primary site of occurrence is the head and neck, followed in decreasing frequency by genitourinary, extremity, trunk, and retroperitoneal sites. Pathologic evaluation of a biopsy specimen or of the completely removed tumor (depending on size and location) is necessary to distinguish rhabdomyosarcoma from other soft tissue sarcomas, lymphomas, and neuroblastoma.

Clinical Findings

A. Symptoms and Signs: The child usually presents with a firm mass in the region of tumor. Orbital rhabdomyosarcoma often presents with proptosis. Middle ear and parameningeal tumors may present with chronic otitis media, cranial nerve palsies, and headaches.

B. Laboratory Findings: CBC and serum chemistries are usually normal, although LDH may be elevated. Bone marrow aspirates and biopsies need to be performed to evaluate for metastatic disease.

C. Imaging: CT scan or MRI of the primary mass is necessary to determine extent of disease and resectability. Evaluation for metastatic disease should include skeletal survey and bone scan, CT of the abdomen and lungs.

Treatment and Prognosis

Treatment depends on location of the tumor, histologic type, and extent of disease. Treatment modalities include surgery, chemotherapy, and radiation therapy. Effective chemotherapy includes vincristine, dactinomycin, cytoxan, ifosfamide, etoposide, and doxarubicin (Table 25–2).

The overall disease-free survival is about 70%. Orbital tumors have the best prognosis.

Fibrosarcomas and liposarcomas are rare lesions and should be surgically excised when possible. In certain circumstances, electron beam therapy (4000–6000 rads) may be of benefit. The role of adjuvant chemotherapy is unclear.

Benign tumors are generally slow-growing and nontender. Most commonly seen are the fibromas and lipomas. These may be excised if they are symptomatic.

TUMORS OF BONE

Malignant bone tumors are more common in children over 10 than in younger age groups. Osteogenic sarcoma and Ewing's sarcoma are the most common types of bone tumors; rare tumors include chondrosarcoma, fibrosarcoma, and synovial sarcoma. Osteogenic sarcoma typically arises in the metaphyses of long bones. The distal femur is the most common site, followed by the proximal tibia and proximal humerus. Ewing's sarcoma arises in long and flat bones, including the pelvis.

Clinical Findings

A. Symptoms and Signs: Bone tumors may present with bone pain, with or without associated mass, limitation of motion, and x-ray changes in the involved bones.

B. Laboratory Findings: CBC may show anemia of chronic disease if widespread metastatic disease is present. LDH and sedimentation rate are often elevated in Ewing's sarcoma and alkaline phosphatase and sedimentation rate may be elevated in osteogenic sarcoma. Uric acid may transiently increase following initial treatment of osteogenic sarcoma.

Imaging

Plain x-rays of osteogenic sarcoma typically display a "sunburst" appearance with lytic and blastic elements within the lesion. X-rays of Ewing's sarcoma typically show a moth-eaten and lytic appearance with elevation of the periosteum ("onion-skinning"). CT or MRI scan of the lesion allows assessment of extent of disease and involvement of the neurovascular bundle. Metastatic disease to lungs and other bones is not uncommon at diagnosis and should be sought with chest CT scan and bone scan prior to planning therapy.

Treatment and Prognosis

Survival rate for patients with osteosarcoma was less than 20% with surgical amputation alone, but significant improvement has resulted from the combination of aggressive surgery (amputation or complex limb-preservation surgery) and multiple drug chemotherapy. A few courses of chemotherapy is usually given prior to definitive surgery. Effective chemotherapeutic agents for osteogenic sarcoma include high-dose methotrexate with leucovorin rescue, doxorubicin, cisplatin, and ifosfamide (Table 25–2). Radiation therapy is not effective in osteogenic sarcoma. Local high-dose radiation therapy (5000–6000 rads) has traditionally been used along with chemotherapy for Ewing's sarcoma. However, many centers now advocate full surgical resection, when possible, as for osteogenic sarcoma. Effective chemotherapy for Ewing's sarcoma includes cytoxan, adriamycin, vincristine, actinomycin, ifosfamide, and etoposide (Table 25–2). The 5-year disease-free survival for osteogenic sarcoma is about 60%, and for Ewing's sarcoma about 50%. Newer chemotherapy regimens may improve these survival rates. Patients who present with metastatic disease have a very poor prognosis. Ewing's sarcoma can recur many years after completion of treatment.

There are a number of fibrous, cartilaginous, and osseous benign tumors. Some have classic x-ray findings. In general, they should be biopsied or excised to rule out the possibility of a malignant tumor. Osteoid osteoma is a relatively common benign tumor of bone in adolescents and young adults. It is characterized by pain, limp (if the lower extremity is involved), atrophy of muscle, normal laboratory findings, and prompt and dramatic relief of pain in response to aspirin.

RETINOBLASTOMA

Retinoblastoma is a malignant ocular tumor that occurs before the age of 5 in over 90% of cases. The tumor may arise sporadically or be inherited. Patients with inherited retinoblastoma often have bilateral disease, while those with the sporadic form have unilateral disease.

Clinical Findings

A. Symptoms and Signs: The most common presenting complaint is leukocoria (white "cat's eye reflex") noted by parents. Strabismus, signs of orbital inflammation, and retinal detachment may be associated. The diagnosis is usually made by inspection of the globe under anesthesia by an ophthalmologist experienced with these tumors. The differential diagnosis includes lesions of *Toxocara canis*, toxoplasmosis, and retrolental fibroplasia. The tumor is typically confined to the globe but is extraocular in about 15% of cases.

B. Laboratory Findings: Metastatic evaluation should include cerebrospinal fluid cytology and bone marrow aspirate and biopsy. It is very rare for retinoblastoma to spread to the spinal fluid or bone marrow without extra-ocular spread, however.

C. Imaging: Metastatic evaluation should include orbital CT scan to define extraocular extension and ocular nerve involvement. Head CT or MRI should be obtained in bilateral cases to look for retinoblastoma involving the pineal gland (trilateral retinoblastoma).

Treatment

Eradication of the tumor by enucleation depends on the potential for useful vision. Since the majority of unilateral tumors involve over one-half the retina by the time of diagnosis, enucleation is most commonly advised. For smaller lesions where vision may be saved, cryotherapy, photocoagulation, or radiotherapy have been successful treatments. Combination chemotherapy should be given to patients with regional or distant extraocular spread. Ophthalmologic evaluation of the uninvolved eye should be performed at regular intervals for several years in order to detect early bilateral disease.

Prognosis

Survival of retinoblastoma is greater than 90%. Patients with the inherited form have a high risk of second cancers throughout their lives, the most common being osteogenic sarcoma. Genetic counseling is important for families of patients with retinoblastoma. The risk of a subsequent sibling developing retinoblastoma varies from 1 to 50%, depending on the presence of other affected family members. Siblings should be carefully examined and followed by an ophthalmologist.

GERM CELL TUMORS

Germ cell tumors are derived from primordial germ cells and can be benign or malignant, gonadal or extragonadal. Extragonadal midline sites are involved in about two-thirds of cases, including the sacrococcygeal area, mediastinum, retroperitoneum, and CNS. Patients with gonadal dysgenesis (as in Turner's syndrome) and those with undescended testes are at increased risk of developing germ cell tumors, particularly gonadoblastomas and germinomas. Teratomas can be benign or malignant, depending on the degree of maturity of the tissue elements involved. Since therapy is different for benign and malignant teratomas, very careful pathologic evaluation of the tumor is necessary. Malignant germ cell tumors characteristically secrete alpha-fetoprotein (AFP) or beta-subunit human chorionic gonadotropin (β-hCG), which are valuable serum markers of disease activity.

Sacrococcygeal teratomas are found more often in neonates than in older infants and children. The majority of these tumors have an external component, allowing for rapid diagnosis. Most of these tumors are benign at the time of diagnosis. However, since benign teratomas have the capacity to become malignant, full surgical excision is necessary. The coccyx should be removed as well since the chance of recurrence in that area is high.

Tumors of the Ovary

Tumors of the ovary are characterized by an enlarging palpable mass in the lower abdomen or pelvis. Severe abdominal pain may occur due to a twisted pedicle. The majority of ovarian tumors in children are benign teratomas; about 25% are malignant germ cell tumors. Sexual precocity, uterine bleeding, and advanced bone age as a result of excessive estrogen production occur only in patients with granulosa cell tumors (which are almost always large enough to palpate). These tumors arise from stromal rather than germ cell elements and may be malignant or benign.

Treatment of ovarian tumors is by complete surgical removal for localized disease. Postoperative chemotherapy is used to treat malignant germ cell tumors, whether completely or incompletely excised. The best treatment results so far have been obtained with cisplatin, vinblastine or etoposide, and bleomycin. Prognosis is generally very good.

Tumors of the Testis

Testicular tumors vary from highly malignant (embryonal carcinoma, germinoma, or malignant teratoma) to relatively benign (Leydig cell tumor or benign teratoma). They are rare in boys under 15 years of age. Paratesticular rhabdomyosarcoma may also present as a scrotal mass in the male child. Tumors are characterized by painless, solid swelling of the testicle, which does not transilluminate and appears to have a purplish discoloration. Hydrocele may be associated.

Orchiectomy with high ligation of the cord is indicated in all testicular tumors. Radiographic staging with abdominal and chest CT scan, bone scan, and skeletal survey is necessary prior to treatment of malignant tumors. Metastases may occur in lungs, mediastinum, bones, and regional and abdominal lymph nodes. For boys without radiographic evidence of lymphatic or hematologic spread, orchiectomy without chemotherapy but with close serial follow-up of serum AFP levels appears to be adequate initial treatment. The most successful chemotherapy for malignant testicular germ cell tumors is as described for ovarian primaries. The prognosis is very good.

LANGERHANS CELL HISTIOCYTOSIS
(Histiocytosis X)

The diseases discussed under this heading comprise a heterogeneous group of proliferative disorders of the reticuloendothelial system. The disorders are of unknown cause, but immune system dysfunction may be involved in their pathogenesis. They differ in behavior from true neoplasms. Eosinophilic granuloma of bone, Hand-Schüller-Christian disease, and Letterer-Siwe disease constitute a complex of diseases previously grouped

under the term **histiocytosis X.** Langerhans histiocytes—phago-
cytes normally found in skin—are the proliferating cells in these
disorders. Whether these cells are immature, normal, or malignant is unclear. Various immunologic abnormalities have been
observed in patients with these diseases.

Clinical Findings

Certain patients present primarily with signs and symptoms
of lytic lesions limited to the bones—especially the skull, ribs,
clavicles, and vertebrae. These lesions are well demarcated on
x-ray and occasionally are painful with overlying soft tissue
swelling. Biopsy reveals eosinophilic granuloma, which may be
the only lesion the patient will develop, although further bone
and even visceral lesions may occur.

Another group of patients present with otitis media, seborrheic skin rash, and evidence of bone lesions, usually in the
mastoid or skull area. They frequently also have visceral involvement, which may be indicated by lymphadenopathy and hepatosplenomegaly. This chronic disseminated form is usually known
as Hand-Schüller-Christian disease. The classic triad of Hand-
Schüller-Christian disease (bony involvement, exophthalmos,
and diabetes insipidus) is rarely seen; however, diabetes insipidus may develop over time.

A third group of patients present early in life primarily with
visceral involvement. They often have a petechial or macular
skin rash, generalized lymphadenopathy, enlarged liver and
spleen, pulmonary involvement, and hematologic abnormalities
such as anemia and thrombocytopenia. Bone lesions can occur.
This acute visceral form, Letterer-Siwe disease, is often fatal.

The principal diseases to be differentiated from histiocytosis
X are infections with histiocyte proliferation (eg, toxoplasmosis,
tularemia), bone tumors (primary or metastatic), lymphomas or
leukemias, immune deficiency states, and storage diseases. The
diagnosis is established by biopsy of abnormal areas of bone,
skin, bone marrow, lymph node, or liver. Complete immunologic
evaluation is essential to distinguish Letterer-Siwe disease from
severe combined immune deficiency.

Treatment

Isolated bony lesions, if progressive or symptomatic (or
both), are best treated by curettage and local radiotherapy. Multiple bony involvement and visceral involvement often respond
well to prednisone, vinblastine, cyclophosphamide, methotrex-

ate, and etoposide (Table 25–2). Combination chemotherapy does not appear to offer significant advantage over single- or double-agent chemotherapy. Immunotherapy may also play a role in the treatment of these disorders. If diabetes insipidus occurs, treatment with vasopressin gives good control.

Prognosis

In patients with Langerhans histiocytosis, the prognosis is often unpredictable. Many patients with considerable bony and visceral involvement have shown apparent complete recovery. The disease can also smolder for years, causing significant morbidity without mortality. In general, the younger the patient and the more extensive the visceral involvement, the worse the prognosis.

LEUKEMIAS IN CHILDHOOD

Most leukemias (97.5%) in childhood are acute. The most common type is acute lymphoblastic leukemia (ALL), which accounts for about 80% of cases (Table 25–5). The highest incidence of leukemia occurs in patients between 2 and 5 years of age. There is an increased risk of leukemia in patients with chromosomal abnormalities or immune deficiency states.

Clinical Findings

A. Symptoms and Signs: Initial signs and symptoms, in order of decreasing frequency, include fever, pallor, petechiae and purpura, lymphadenopathy, hepatosplenomegaly, anorexia, fatigue, bone and joint pain, abdominal pain, and weight loss. Nonmalignant conditions in the differential diagnosis include juvenile rheumatoid arthritis, immune thrombocytopenic purpura, Epstein-Barr viral disease, and aplastic anemia. CNS infiltration may cause manifestations simulating meningitis, with increased intracranial pressure and cranial nerve palsies. Septicemia may occur during the course of the disease due to neutropenia.

B. Laboratory Findings:

1. Blood–Red blood cell counts and hemoglobin levels are usually low. The white blood cell count may be elevated, normal, or reduced, but neutropenia is often present. In some cases, large numbers of abnormal cells (blasts) are seen on smear; in others, no peripheral blasts are noted. Thrombocytopenia is very frequent.

Table 25-5. Acute leukemias of childhood.

Type	Approximate Frequency	Morphology	Immunophenotype (Histochemical Staining)
Lymphoblastic (ALL)	80%	Typically small blasts (≤2 RBC diameters), scant cytoplasm, indistinct nucleoli.[2]	
B-Cell Precursor ALL	84%[1]		Majority are CALLA (+)
T-Cell ALL	15%		E-rosette or T-cell surface antigen (+)
B-Cell ALL	1%	Blasts with deeply basophilic cytoplasm and vacuolization.	Surface immunoglobulin (+)
Nonlymphoblastic (ANLL)	20%		
Myeloblastic	45%[3]	Blasts with few or many cytoplasmic granules; may have Auer rods.	Myeloperoxidase (MP) (+)
Promyelocytic	4%	Promyelocytes with numerous cytoplasmic granules.	MP(+)
Myelomonocytic	26%	Myeloblasts with cytoplasmic granules and monoblasts.	MP (+) and nonspecific esterase (NSE) (+)
Monocytic	21%	Monoblasts with smooth or irregular, folded nuclear contour.	NSE (+)
Erythroid	2%	Erythroblasts amid dyserythropoiesis.	
Megakaryocytic	2%[4]	Blasts look like lymphoblasts or undifferentiated myeloblasts.	Platelet peroxidase (+) endoplasmic reticulum on electron microscopy

[1] % of ALL.

[2] Some lymphoblasts are larger, with more cytoplasm and more prominent nucleoli; similar morphologically to undifferentiated myeloblasts.

[3] % of ANLL.

[4] Frequency may be underestimated since megakaryocytic leukemia has only recently been recognized.

2. Bone Marrow–By definition, leukemia is present when more than 25% of cells in a bone marrow aspirate are malignant blasts. In almost all cases, 50–98% of nucleated cells are blast forms with marked reduction in the normal erythroid, myeloid, and platelet precursors. Blasts from the majority of cases of childhood ALL have an antigen present on the cell surface called the common ALL-antigen (CALLA). These blasts are derived from B-cell precursors early in their development. Less commonly, lymphoblasts are of T-cell origin or of mature B-cell origin.

3. Chromosomes–A variety of chromosome abnormalities have been reported in the blasts of all forms of acute leukemia. Certain abnormalities, including reciprocal translocations [eg, t(4;11) and t(9;22)] or monosomy 7 are associated with a very poor prognosis.

4. Serum–Levels of uric acid and lactate dehydrogenase are often elevated.

5. Cerebrospinal Fluid–Pleocytosis (consisting of blast forms), elevated levels of protein, and decreased levels of glucose may be seen.

Treatment of Leukemias

A. Acute Lymphoblastic Leukemia:

1. Remission Induction–Most patients (95%) achieve complete remission following 4 weeks of treatment with vincristine, prednisone, asparaginase, and intrathecal methotrexate (Table 25–2).

2. Central Nervous System Leukemia–Because of the risk of CNS leukemia, patients should be treated prophylactically with intrathecal chemotherapy and sometimes CNS irradiation as well. Treatment of frank CNS leukemia requires whole brain and spinal irradiation along with intrathecal drugs.

3. Maintenance–Commonly used maintenance therapy lasts 2–3 years, with daily oral mercaptopurine and weekly methotrexate as mainstays of treatment, along with monthly vincristine and prednisone.

4. Relapse–If the disease recurs, another remission may be induced with selected combinations of the above drugs or other antineoplastic agents. Ultimate prognosis for patients who relapse depends on when relapse occurs in relation to completion of initial therapy. Allogeneic bone marrow transplant may allow the only chance of cure for patients who relapse.

B. Acute Nonlymphocytic Leukemia (ANLL): ANLL of childhood is more difficult to cure than ALL. Remission induction has been successful with a number of agents; the most commonly used are cytarabine and daunorubicin (Table 25–2). CNS prophylaxis with intrathecal cytarabine (but without cranial irradiation) is necessary. Questions that remain to be answered include the optimal length of maintenance therapy and the advantages of bone marrow transplantation over conventional chemotherapy for long-term cure in patients who achieve remission.

C. Supportive Measures: Transfusions of packed red blood cells and platelets should be given as needed. Fevers in the face of neutropenia should be treated with broad-spectrum antibiotics. Hyperuricemia due to the degradation of nucleic acids may occur following the initiation of antileukemic therapy (tumor lysis syndrome). Allopurinol taken orally is effective in reducing the hyperuricemia. Intravenous hydration and alkalinization (to decrease uric acid precipitation in kidneys) is also of value. Hyperphosphatemia and hypocalcemia can occur during initial treatment as well. Hyperkalemia, severe hyperphosphatemia, tetany, or oliguria may require temporary hemodialysis.

Prognosis

Aggressive combination chemotherapy and supportive therapy with blood products and antibiotics have contributed to improved survival. As many as 95% of children with ALL will achieve remission within 1 month of starting therapy, and long-term "cure" rates are between 50 and 85%, depending on various prognostic features (including age and white blood cell count) present at diagnosis. In general, children diagnosed with ALL between the ages of 2 and 10 with a white blood cell count of less than 50,000/µL at diagnosis have the best chance of cure. Children with ANLL have a poorer prognosis, with long-term cure rates between 25 and 40%.

INFECTIONS IN THE ONCOLOGY PATIENT

Immunodeficiency may be congenital in cancer patients but more often is due to suppression of the immune system by the cancer or drugs. Deficiencies of neutrophils, T lymphocytes, or B lymphocytes tend to predispose the host to infection with different agents. Neutropenia caused by chemotherapy predisposes to infection with gram-negative or gram-positive bacteria and fungi. B lymphocyte deficiency can develop from repeated exposure to steroids, cyclophosphamide, and methotrexate, and predisposes to infection with extracellular bacteria such as pneumococci and staphylococci. T lymphocyte deficiency caused especially by exposure to steroids and radiation predisposes to infection with intracellular bacteria (mycobacteria, *Listeria*, etc), fungi (*Candida*, *Aspergillus*, etc), protozoa (*Pneumocystis*, etc), and viruses (herpes simplex, etc). Patients receiving intensive chemotherapy or steroids require TMP/SMZ prophylaxis against pneumocystis.

Many opportunistic organisms do not produce disease except in the immunodeficient host. Such hosts are often infected with a number of pathogens simultaneously. Infections caused by common organisms may present uncommon clinical manifestations. Determination of the specific infecting agents is essential for effective treatment.

Approach to Treatment of Febrile Neutropenia

For patients with absolute neutropenia [WBC × (% bands + segs) < 500/μL] and temperature > 38.5°C (oral), broad-spectrum antibiotics should be initiated immediately after blood, throat, and urine cultures are obtained even if the patient appears clinically well. This practice is necessary because signs of infection (ie, exudate, fluctuance, swelling, erythema, pain) are decreased or absent when neutrophil counts are very low. Thorough physical exam should include close inspection of skin for septic emboli and perirectal area for signs of cellulitis. No digital rectal exams or rectal temperatures should be performed in neutropenic patients.

Central venous catheters may have to be removed if bacteremia persists despite antibiotics. If disseminated varicella or herpes zoster is suspected, IV acyclovir should be started immediately, prior to culture confirmation. Fungal infection should be suspected in a patient who remains febrile after a number of days on broad-spectrum antibiotics. Granulocyte transfusions may be able to tide the patient over a period of profound neutropenia when appropriate antibiotics have failed to eradicate bacteremia. Serum immunoglobulin levels should be measured and IV IgG replacement given if IgG levels are low. Once an infectious agent is identified, antimicrobial drug therapy should be specific and lethal for it. Combinations of antibiotics may be necessary, since multiple infectious agents may be involved in some cases.

The hemotopoietic growth factor called G-CSF, or Neupogen, has been available since 1991 for use in patients receiving chemotherapy. This agent stimulates proliferation and maturation of neutrophil precursors in bone marrow and accelerates neutrophil recovery follow chemotherapy. G-CSF has decreased the incidence of febrile neutropenia following chemotherapy by as much as 40% in both adults and children.

Allergic Diseases | 26

David S. Pearlman, MD

Allergic reactivity, that is, the specific ability to reject foreign substances, is normal. Some forms of allergy, however, occur only in certain individuals in whom a presumably hereditary predisposition is important. These disorders—allergic rhinitis, asthma, and atopic dermatitis—are called "atopic disorders." In most instances allergic reactivity based on IgE antibody to innocuous inhaled or ingested materials is an important cause of the disorder. The most important of these materials are animal allergens, house dust mite and insect allergens, spores from indoor and outdoor molds, and tree, grass, and weed pollen. Inhalants generally induce symptoms in the upper and/or lower respiratory tract. Sensitivity to foods, drugs and stinging insects, and other ingested materials contribute to perennial, seasonal, or episodic problems, some of which can be life-threatening.

PRINCIPLES OF DIAGNOSIS

Diagnosis is based first on the history and physical findings. Identification of the allergic antibody that may be involved is helpful and sometimes essential for determining the nature of the reaction and the environmental culprit. **These tests are not diagnostic in themselves, and their interpretation requires knowing the child,** including his or her environmental exposures. Atopic disorders tend to occur in families, and multiple disorders often occur in the same child. A history of time and place (eg, at school or at home) where a reaction occurs is helpful in determining environmental culprits. Some reactions occur within minutes ("early reaction"), but others can develop hours after allergen exposure.

Laboratory Tests

The principal allergic antibody identified belongs to the IgE class, also called skin sensitizing antibody. There are two basic kinds of tests for IgE antibody: skin tests and serologic tests.

A. Skin Tests: These are very sensitive "biologic" tests and measure allergic antibody as a manifestation of the local release of mediators from sensitized cells on which the allergic reaction takes place. Sensitized mediator cells are found throughout the body, including the skin, which provides an extremely convenient site for testing. Prick tests generally are done first, since they are relatively painless, a large number of allergens can be applied conveniently, and they are safer in highly sensitive children than are intradermal tests. Intradermal tests are significantly more sensitive than are prick tests but are reserved for allergens that do not elicit a positive prick test but are still considered to be likely culprits of the disorder. The end point of these tests is a wheal and erythema reaction (hive), which occurs rapidly and peaks within 15–20 minutes. Skin testing is potentially dangerous in highly sensitive individuals. Most test materials are impure and in high concentration can produce an irritant reaction easily misinterpreted as positive for antibody ("false-positive test"). Positive tests may or may not be of significant clinical relevance, hence it is important to interpret test results strictly within the context of the clinical circumstances of the patient.

B. Serologic Tests: These tests measure serum IgE antibody per se. The best known is the radioallergosorbent test (RAST), a radioimmunoassay, but various enzymatic immunoassay variations are commonly available (ELISAs). Serologic tests correlate best with skin tests when high levels of antibody are present, but are less sensitive than skin tests. Theoretically, these tests should be especially useful for testing severe drug and stinging insect hypersensitivity. However, particularly with drug sensitivity, the important drug metabolites responsible for drug sensitivity rarely are available for serologic or skin testing and the lesser sensitivity of serologic tests make these tests less valuable for determining potentially life-threatening sensitivity.

C. Immunoglobulin Levels: IgE levels are measured by radioimmunosorbent or ELISA tests. Elevated IgE levels do occur in some allergic disorders, but the frequency of this occurrence and correlation with the presence or absence of allergy is so imperfect that this is not generally a useful screening procedure. Greatly elevated IgE levels in infancy are highly predictive of an atopic diathesis but a normal or low IgE level does not rule out either an atopic disorder or specific allergic sensitization.

D. Provocative Testing: Challenging the patient with a suspected allergen and observing the response also is useful, particularly with possible food sensitivity. It should not be used when life-threatening sensitivity is suspected, however. A positive response can establish a cause-and-effect relationship but not necessarily the mechanism involved (eg, a positive challenge to milk may be due to allergy or to lactase deficiency).

Eosinophils are a component of allergic inflammation, and the presence of a large number in secretions or in blood often is seen in atopic disorders. Large numbers are suggestive but not diagnostic of an allergic reaction, and their absence does not rule out allergy. Nasal eosinophilia is especially helpful in diagnosing allergic rhinitis, but nasal eosinophilia in infants up to 3 months of age can be normal.

Controversial Techniques for Diagnosis and Treatment

Intracutaneous end-point titration (sometimes called the "Rinkel test"), sublingual and serial intracutaneous provocation titration tests, and sublingual desensitization—all used for diagnosing or treating "allergy"—are not scientifically validated. They are rarely used by trained allergists certified by the American Board of Allergy and Immunology.

GENERAL PRINCIPLES OF TREATMENT

Controlling the Environment

Avoiding the offending allergen is the most effective treatment of all allergic disorders. Although complete avoidance may be impossible, often it is feasible to reduce the degree of exposure to the point that reactions are trivial. The avoidance of nonallergic add-on irritants such as smoke also is important. The single most important area of exposure is a child's bedroom. Here the greatest effort is made to control house dust (the most allergenic ingredients of which are house dust mites or insects and animal saliva or dander). Overnight exposure to pollens and molds can be diminished by keeping the bedroom window closed overnight or employing an air conditioner as a partial filter in the bedroom or centrally. Animals should not be allowed in the bedroom if there is any question of animal sensitivity and should be kept out of the house or eliminated from the environment altogether depending upon the degree of the child's sensitivity. Frequent bathing (eg, once a week) of indoor animals can reduce allergen levels. The remainder of the house is the second most

important environmental area, but exposures at babysitters',
preschools or schools, or at friends' houses can be problematic
and may require alternative arrangements.

Hyposensitization
(Immunotherapy)

Specific hyposensitization is attempted if the allergen is not
sufficiently avoidable and is considered a significant problem.
Its value is documented both for upper respiratory tract inhalant
allergy and for allergic asthma, and it is effective for Hymenoptera insect sting allergy. Evidence for effectiveness is greatest
for pollens, house dust mites, and Hymenoptera venom. It also
may be efficacious for mold sensitivity. Injection therapy to
foods is experimental and may be dangerous. The use of bacterial
extracts is of little value.

The procedure involves injecting extremely small amounts
of allergen subcutaneously in gradually increasing dosage at frequent intervals (generally once or twice a week) until a top or
maintenance dose is reached. This is usually the highest tolerated
dose, or the amount that induces a state of clinical hyporeactivity
to the allergen as demonstrated after natural contact. The top
dose is used as the maintenance dose with carefully regulated
lengthening of intervals, eventually to perhaps every 4 weeks if
tolerated. Injection therapy is given for a minimum of 2 years,
often 3–5 years, and occasionally for longer periods.

Drug Therapy

The following are principal groups of therapeutic agents
used for the treatment of allergic disorders:

A. Adrenergic Agents: Epinephrine is the single most important agent for treating acute severe allergic reactions. It is
used to decrease bronchospasm in acute severe asthma, although
more selective beta-2 adrenergic agents such as terbutaline by
injection are available. Moreover, selective beta-2 adrenergic
drugs used by inhalation are generally as effective as injectable
adrenergic agents in relieving asthma and are associated with
fewer side effects. Orally active beta-2 agents also can be effective. The vasoconstrictive properties of certain adrenergic agents
such as phenylephrine and pseudoephedrine also are useful in
decongestion of allergic and nonallergic rhinitis. They can be
used topically in the nose for short (5 days or less) periods, or
orally, alone or in conjunction with antihistamines.

B. Antihistamines: Antihistamines are specific antagonists of histamine and are useful therefore when histamine is an important mediator of the reaction. Since histamine is only one of the numerous mediators involved, however, antihistamines rarely are completely therapeutic. There are at least two major classes of antihistamines: H_1-receptor inhibitors, which are the classic antihistamines used for many years in allergic disorders, and H_2-receptor inhibitors, marketed for inhibiting gastric acid secretion but which also have vascular properties. H_1 antihistamines are particularly useful for allergic rhinitis and urticaria and as a part of the treatment of anaphylaxis. The addition of H_2 antihistamines (eg, cimetidine and ranitidine) to an H_1 antihistamine can help control urticaria not controlled by H_1 antihistamines alone, and both classes are sometimes recommended for the treatment of anaphylaxis. Antihistamines are *not* the drugs of first choice in allergic emergencies—epinephrine is—but they may be administered after epinephrine has been given. Since antihistamines are competitive antagonists, they are best used in advance of histamine liberation and of anticipated symptoms. Most antihistamines are potentially soporific and they should be used cautiously during school hours. Antihistamines are most effective in reducing symptoms of rhinorrhea, nasal itching and sneezing, eye tearing, itching, and hives. In contrast to general warnings in the *PDR*, antihistamines can be used when asthma is present (and may even have some beneficial effects in asthma!).

C. Theophylline and Aminophylline: Theophylline and its ethylene diamine derivative aminophylline are effective but potentially toxic bronchodilators, the improper use of which has been associated with severe reactions and in some instances even death. Periodic monitoring of blood theophylline levels is important in patients on long-term theophylline therapy. Theophylline can be therapeutic over a wide range of blood concentrations, but levels between 10 and 20 µg/mL have been considered "optimal" for severe asthma since *major* toxicity rarely occurs with peak blood levels below 20 µg/mL. Since levels can vary significantly owing to viral infections, diet, the use of erythromycin and other drugs, peak levels higher than 15 µg/mL on a long-term basis are discouraged. In early to mid-infancy, metabolism is markedly diminished and these drugs rarely should be employed at these ages.

D. Expectorants: Glyceryl guaiacolate (guaifenesin) is used mainly to thin mucus in asthma and upper respiratory tract disorders but it is not clear how effective it is. Iodides appear to be more effective but, especially with prolonged use, goiter, salivary gland inflammation, gastric irritation, and skin eruptions such as acne can occur.

E. Corticosteroids: These are extremely potent antiallergic drugs but side effects associated with prolonged therapy limit their use mainly to those conditions that are refractory to other measures or are life-threatening. Topically active corticosteroids which are inactivated rapidly upon absorption have been developed, giving them a high local therapeutic potency with low systemic effects. Intranasal topical steroids, and inhalant topical steroids for chronic asthma, have been shown to be relatively safe and effective in these conditions, as have topical steroids for eczema. In the latter case, however, significant absorption of active drug occurs with extensive use over inflamed skin or with occlusive dressings, especially with the halogenated preparations. Systemic corticosteroids should be considered for short-term use for acute severe asthma not immediately responsive to nonsteroid therapy, for severe contact dermatitis, and for medical emergencies due to allergic reactions as a second- or third-line medication after adrenergic agents and antihistamines have been given. Long-term use of systemic steroids should be considered when nonsteroid agents or topical steroids cannot control symptoms sufficiently. When long-term use is necessary, alternate-day therapy with a short-acting preparation such as prednisone in the early morning should be attempted, using the least amount necessary to control symptoms.

F. Sedatives: Sedatives have little place in the treatment of allergic disorders and are contraindicated in asthma since they can depress the respiratory center. Anxiety associated with extreme asthma is more a reflection of the severity of asthma than its cause.

G. Oxygen: Oxygen is extremely important in the treatment of severe asthma since hypoxemia virtually always is present with severe obstruction.

H. Antibiotics: There are no special indications for antibiotics in allergic disorders. In most instances viral infections precipitate respiratory problems such as asthma.

I. Cromolyn Sodium (Intal, Nasalcrom, and Opticrom): Cromolyn sodium is a topically active agent useful in treatment of asthma, allergic rhinitis, and conjunctivitis. In asthma it is effective particularly as a preventive when used 15–20 minutes prior to contact with an asthmogenic agent such as an allergen or exercise. It can be used alone or in conjunction with adrenergic or other agents. If used routinely on a long-term basis, it is best given 3–4 times a day, although twice a day usage may be effective. It is a relatively safe and nonirritating drug.

PROPYHLAXIS OF ATOPIC ALLERGIC DISORDERS

There is evidence that avoidance of certain foods in the first few months of life, specifically cow products, eggs, wheat, and chicken, with or without concomitant dust and animal control, can lessen development of food sensitivity, allergic rhinitis, asthma, or eczema in the first year or so of life. Although some studies show no benefit from these procedures, it seems prudent to institute dietary and environmental restrictions in the first few months of life in children with a strong family history of atopy.

MEDICAL EMERGENCIES DUE TO ALLERGIC REACTIONS

Anaphylactic shock, angioedema particularly of the airway, and bronchial obstruction, alone or in combination, are the principal life-threatening manifestations of severe allergic reactions. Sweating, flushing, palpitations, lightheadedness, paresthesias, and urticaria may precede or accompany severe reactions.

Treatment
A. Immediate:
1. Epinephrine, aqueous, 1/1000, 0.2–0.4 mL should be injected intramuscularly without delay, and may be repeated at intervals of 15–20 minutes as necessary. If the reaction is due to the injection of a drug, serum, or sting on an extremity, a tourniquet should be applied proximal to the site to delay absorption and 0.1 mL of adrenaline injected into the site to delay absorption.

2. Antihistamines should be given intramuscularly, or **slowly** intravenously. An H_1 antihistamine such as diphenhydramine should be used initially; the addition of an H_2 antihistamine (eg, cimetidine) is recommended.

3. An asthmatic component should be treated with aminophylline and inhaled adrenergics, with other treatment appropriate for asthma as indicated.

4. Tracheostomy can be life-saving in cases of profound laryngeal edema.

5. Hypovolemia secondary to massive transudation of intravascular fluid can be a part of the reaction; maintenance of proper fluid volume by IV replacement may be necessary.

B. Subsequent Measures: Adrenocorticosteroids should be given only after epinephrine and antihistamines have been administered. The patient should be watched for 24 hours since a recurrence (''delayed anaphylaxis'') can occur many hours after the initial reaction and treatment.

Insect Sting Sensitivity

Life-threatening insect allergy is due mostly to the venom of stinging insects of the class Hymenoptera (bees, wasps, hornets, and fire ants). Venom immunotherapy in children is reserved mainly for those instances in which a life-threatening reaction—for example, involving the cardiovascular or respiratory tract—has occurred. A large local reaction or generalized urticaria without respiratory or cardiovascular compromise probably is not an indication for hyposensitization. Venom antigens for diagnosis and treatment are more efficacious than whole-body extracts although the latter may be useful for fire ant allergy. Treatment kits for anaphylactic reactions (ANA-KKIT) or spring-loaded epinephrine injectables (Epi-Pen or Epi-Pen, Jr.) should be made available for immediate use for children with extreme insect sensitivity and should be kept in the home or taken along by a responsible person in times of travel. The single most important item in such a kit is epinephrine.

ALLERGIC RHINITIS

Major symptoms include chronic or recurrent nasal congestion generally with nasal itching and sneezing, with serous to mucoid discharge. Itching of the eyes with or without tearing also occurs, particularly in the seasonal or episodic variety. The appearance of the nasal mucosa can vary from somewhat hyperemic to very edematous with purplish pallor. Rhinitis may be perennial owing to exposure to perennially present allergens, seasonal owing to pollens or seasonal molds, episodic owing to occasional encounter with allergens such as animals, or any combination of these. The disease can occur even in infancy, but becomes more frequent and intense with age due to increased exposure to environmental allergens. ''Allergic facies'' can include allergic shiners, suborbital edema that takes on a bluish discoloration secondary to nasal congestion, flattened malar eminences, and a transverse crease across the nose from pushing the nose upward in an attempt to relieve nasal itching ("allergic salute"). Differential diagnosis includes chronic sinusitis and nonallergic ("vasomotor") rhinitis. Other conditions to be considered in chronic nasal "congestion" include adenoid hypertrophy, foreign bodies (usually unilateral), choanal stenosis or atresia, nasopharyngeal neoplasms, and palatal malformations. Helpful laboratory findings include nasal eosinophilia; this is not a universal finding, however, nor does its presence establish an allergic etiology. Allergy tests reveal IgE antibody to offending allergens.

Associated Conditions

Allergic rhinitis is a risk factor for chronic or recurrent otitis media with effusion. Nasal polyps are unusual in children and even though they often contain eosinophils, generally they are not caused by allergy. They can be associated with cystic fibrosis. Sinusitis may accompany allergic rhinitis.

Treatment

Known or suspected allergens need to be avoided. When symptoms are severe or other symptomatic measures have failed, or when associated with complications, immunotherapy should be considered.

A. Drug Therapy: Table 26–1 lists various drugs useful in treating rhinitis and the symptoms and signs most relieved by each. Chronic rhinitis is more of a congestive problem, whereas acute or seasonal rhinitis tends to involve more itching, sneezing, and rhinorrhea. Antihistamines, with or without decongestants, and nasal and ocular cromolyn are first-line drugs, whereas topical corticosteroids are reserved for more resistant cases.

Table 26–1. Drugs useful in treating rhinitis.

	Decon-gestant	Anti-histamine	Cromolyn	Anti-cholinergic	Steroid
Sneezing	(x)	x	(x)		x
Itching	(x)	x	(x)		x
Rhinorrhea	(x)	(x)	(x)	x	x
Congestion	x	±			x

BRONCHIAL ASTHMA

Asthma is an obstructive disorder of the tracheal bronchial tree, in which the obstruction is variable and largely reversible. The major symptoms of asthma are cough and wheezing, a high-pitched squeaky sound from the partially obstructed large airways, shortness of breath, and chest tightness. **Wheezing is not an invariable symptom or sign;** asthma may present with chronic cough ("cough variant asthma"). Obstruction is due to mucosal edema, bronchospasm, increased and unusually viscid secretions, and chronic inflammation of mucosal walls often with sloughing of epithelium. Asthma is a chronic disorder, the symptoms of which may be only episodic. It can be mild, severe, infrequent, or constant. Because of great pulmonary reserve, obstruction can be profound without causing death, but deaths from asthma do occur. The adolescent age group is at special risk. It is a very common disorder, grossly underdiagnosed; its severity often is underestimated and generally undertreated, and it may be diagnosed as recurrent bronchitis or pneumonia. A large proportion of childhood asthma begins before age 3. Approximately twice as many males are affected as females before adolescence, after which there is not a major difference between the sexes.

Most children with asthma eventually demonstrate evidence of allergy, which can play a minor to major role in asthma. Especially early in life viral respiratory infection is a frequent precipitating event; precipitants most often are multifactorial and can include irritants, exercise, some medications (aspirin infrequently), and sometimes emotional factors (mainly indirectly, through maladaptive behaviors with asthma). Asthma can occur alone or with allergic rhinitis and/or atopic dermatitis. Inhalants are most important in causing symptoms, but occasionally foods, especially early in life, may be causative. The prognosis of asthma is variable; the likelihood that asthma will be "outgrown" increases with the milder form of the disorder **but probably no more than half of even milder asthmatics outgrow the disorder.** Moderate or severe asthma generally is not outgrown. If symptoms *are* lost, the most common time is around puberty.

An important feature of at least chronic symptomatic asthma is an extraordinary generalized hyperreactivity of the tracheobronchial tree to various chemical inflammatory mediators and in turn to numerous insulting environmental agents or events. Because of this feature, asthma sometimes is called "reactive airways disorder.'' Reactions to allergens and irritants may be immediate, occurring within minutes of exposure, but with sufficient sensitization and strong allergen exposure, a second kind of reaction occurs 4–12 hours after allergen exposure and can be prolonged. There is a large inflammatory component to chronic asthma. Beta-2 adrenergic drugs, and cromolyn as a preventive, are most effective for immediate responses, whereas corticosteroids and cromolyn are the most effective for late inflammatory responses. Signs and symptoms of asthma are only a crude reflection of the obstructive process, and in many patients, neither the child's nor the physician's assessment of the asthma are very accurate. *The most accurate indicator of the degree of obstruction is measurement of airflow with a pulmonary function device.* A reliable simple peak flowmeter such as a Wright Peak Flow Meter, *used properly* (by patient and medical personnel), is important to the diagnosis and treatment of children with asthma.

In infancy, predominant symptoms may be dyspnea, excessive secretions, noisy and rattly breathing, cough, and intercostal or suprasternal retractions rather than the typical pronounced expiratory wheezes that occur in older children. Physical findings depend upon the degree of obstruction. Between episodes, findings can be normal. With progressive obstruction, air exchange diminishes, expiration becomes prolonged, and wheezing generally occurs and increases in intensity; with greater obstruction, wheezing will decrease due to poor air exchange, hyperinflation may be apparent, and in later stages retractions and use of accessory respiratory muscles increases. Pulsus paradoxicus may be present. There may be pallor; **cyanosis is a very late sign.** Tachycardia may occur and ultimately there can be respiratory failure. The hallmark of asthma is responsiveness to bronchodilators, both a therapeutic and diagnostic point. In the later stages of an asthmatic paroxysm or simply with severe asthma, response to bronchodilators is poor, a condition sometimes called ''status asthmaticus.''

Eosinophil accumulations in bronchial secretions and blood are common. The hematocrit can be elevated with dehydration or in severe chronic obstructive disease. In severe asthma, the first blood gas abnormality is hypoxemia without CO_2 retention. Since hyperpnea is usual in an attack, $Paco_2$ tends to be low with the hypoxemia so that ''normal'' Pco_2 in an attack should be taken as CO_2 retention. Particularly in young children, some metabolic acidosis is not unusual. Early in asthmatic paroxysms, the pH tends to be alkaline from hyperventilation. If obstruction is severe, there can be CO_2 retention with a respiratory acidosis, often with a metabolic component. X-ray may show bilateral hyperinflation, bronchial thickening, peribronchial infiltration, and areas of density that may represent patchy atelectasis (common) or associated bronchopneumonia. The former is often confused with the latter. In uncomplicated asthma, a chest x-ray is not always necessary. Lung functions reveal a decrease in flow rates, particularly FEV_1. There is hyperinflation of the chest with increased residual volume and functional residual capacity. During asymptomatic intervals, all of the above may be normal, but there frequently is residual hyperinflation on a chronic basis even in asthmatic children asymptomatic for prolonged periods. Allergy tests may reveal IgE antibodies to potentially causative allergens.

Bronchial asthma may be confused with acute bronchiolitis, laryngotracheobronchitis, bronchopneumonia, or pertussis, especially in the very young. Some children with immunodeficiency disease, particularly in the first 3 years of life, have associated cough and wheezing due to chronic lower respiratory tract infection. Nasal wheezes can be transmitted to the chest especially in infants, and other forms of upper airway obstruction such as adenoidal hypertrophy and foreign body may cause wheezing sounds. The predominant wheeze from lower airway obstruction is expiratory, although inspiratory wheezing along with expiratory wheezing can occur. Wheezing that is predominantly inspiratory more often than not is laryngeal or higher in origin. In tracheal or bronchial foreign body obstruction, dyspnea and wheezing is usually of sudden onset and often unilateral, although it may be bilateral. Characteristic x-ray findings are not always present. The differentiation between bronchial asthma and cystic fibrosis is made on the basis of high sweat chloride in the latter, and a history often present in cystic fibrosis of serious pulmonary infections since birth, along with a personal and family history of associated intestinal disturbances with profuse, bulky stools and pancreatic enzyme deficiency. In asthma, chronic inflammatory changes generally are not seen on chest x-ray, in contrast to that seen in cystic fibrosis and other chronic infectious lower pulmonary disorders. Cystic fibrosis and asthma can and frequently do coexist. Tracheal or bronchial compression by extramural forces may be due to the presence of a foreign body in the esophagus, anomalous vessels, or neoplastic of inflammatory lymphadenopathy.

Treatment

A. General: Identify and avoid known or suspected allergens and irritants!

Hyposensitization should be considered for allergens that cannot be avoided and that play a substantial role in the disorder. Educate the parents and the child, if old enough, to understand asthma, the importance of avoidance or other therapy, and the proper use of medications. The major pharmacotherapeutic agents are bronchodilators of the adrenergic and methylxanthine (theophylline or aminophylline) classes, preventives (cromolyn sodium), and anti-inflammatory drugs (corticosteroids).

Adrenergic aerosols are extremely useful but must not be abused. Overreliance on these drugs can lead to delays in obtaining other therapy needed and possibly may make asthma worse. Adrenergic inhalants can be as effective as injected drugs in reversing acute severe asthma and are attended with fewer side effects. Cromolyn sodium is used on an around-the-clock basis 3–4 times daily for chronic symptoms, or acutely to prevent asthmatic insults from allergenic or irritant agents, or before exercise; it is used alone or in conjunction with inhaled adrenergic drugs. Encourage exercise in children with asthma, as in all children. The use of a peak flowmeter at home to assist in assessment of airflow can be useful and even lifesaving. Children with frequent overt asthma attacks (eg, 1 or 2 per week other than from exercise alone) and evidence of more or less constant pulmonary obstruction should be on constant pharmacologic therapy.

Cromolyn sodium or theophylline can be considered firstline drugs for chronic symptomatic asthma. Adrenergic drugs by inhalation, with or without additional oral adrenergic agents, are adjuncts. In patients who do not require constant bronchodilator therapy, adrenergic agents by inhalation are first-line drugs. Systemic corticosteroids are used acutely (days) for the treatment of acute severe asthma not responsive to nonsteroidal bronchodilators; they also are employed chronically (weeks to months) and occasionally even longer, mainly on an alternate-day early morning dosage regimen when all other measures are not sufficient to keep the asthma under control. Inhalant corticosteroids also can be considered firstline drugs for long-term therapy and are used in addition or in place of theophylline, and as a substitute for long-term alternate-day systemic steroid therapy.

Table 26–2. Adrenergic drugs.

Drug	Route[1]	Dose	Frequency
Terbutaline mg/mL (1:1000)	SC	0.01 mg/kg up to 0.30 mL	q 20 min × 2
Epinephrine aqueous 1:1000	SC	0.01 mg/kg up to 0.30 mL	q 20 min × 3
Epinephrine suspension 1:200 (Sus-Phrine)	SC	0.005 mL/kg up to 0.15 mL	single dose
Albuterol 0.5%[2]	NA	0.25–0.5 mL in 2 mL saline	q 30 min
Metaproterenol 5%[2]	NA	0.10–0.20 mL in 2 mL saline	q 30 min
Isoetharine 1%[2]	NA	0.25–0.50 mL in 2mL saline	q 30 min

[1] SC = subcutaneous; NA = nebulized aerosol.
[2] Each of these is also available as a metered dose inhaler and can be used, 2 inhalations per dose. For mild to moderate asthma, use every 4 hours.

TREATMENT OF ACUTE SEVERE ASTHMA
(Status Asthmaticus)

This is a medical emergency and requires prompt and aggressive treatment. Injectable adrenergic agents, or if the child is sufficiently cooperative, aerosolized adrenergic drugs given by a compressed air device or preferably by oxygen are the drugs of first choice (Table 26–2). Sensitivity to adrenergic drugs may improve after initiation of other therapy, particularly corticosteroids, and responsiveness may occur even as early as 1–2 hours after their administration.

Hospital or Emergency Room Care

(1) Give moisturized oxygen by face mask or nasal prong, at a flow rate of approximately 4 L/min.

(2) Give 5% dextrose solution with 0.2% saline IV with poor responsiveness to initial therapy, poor fluid intake, vomiting, or dehydration. *Do not overhydrate.* Particularly if corticosteroids are used, add potassium (approximately 10–20 mEq/L of intravenous fluids) after urination is established.

(3) Give aminophylline,* 4–6 g/kg in intravenous tubing over a 10–20 minute period if not used in the previous 3 hours, and either repeat in 4–6 hours or give as a constant infusion using a rate of 0.6–1 mg/kg/hr. The rate should be determined, however,

---

* The effectiveness of aminophylline for acute severe asthma when inhalant beta-adrenergic agents are maximized is debated, for children and adults.

by measurement of theophylline blood levels, aiming for a level of 15 ± 3 µg/mL on a constant basis. Average total daily dosages of theophylline to achieve levels between 10–20 µg/mL are listed below, but there is much individual variation in requirements. Also, viral infections, diet, and medications can alter metabolism (eg, erythromycin impedes metabolism).

Age	Average Total Daily Dose ± SD
1–8 yr	25 ± 5 mg/kg
8–16 yr	20 ± 5 mg/kg
>16 yr	12 ± 3 mg/kg

(4) Take an arterial blood sample for pH, P_{CO_2}, and P_{O_2}, or use oximetry for P_{O_2} determination (but this does *not* tell you the Pa_{CO_2}). Repeated monitoring of gases and pH may be necessary.

(5) Correct acidosis of pH of ≤ 7.3 with sodium bicarbonate. The appropriate bicarbonate dose can be calculated with the following formula:

mEq bicarbonate needed = negative base excess × 0.3 × body weight in kg

(6) Give albuterol 0.5% by inhalation every 30 minutes to 1 hour until there is a response. Interval can be extended to every 4 hours as tolerated.

(7) If the patient is already receiving corticosteroids, increase the dose temporarily. Patients requiring hospitalization or who have severe asthma not responsive to other therapy within the first 2 hours should receive corticosteroids promptly. Give the equivalent of 2 mg/kg of prednisone every 4–6 hours until a therapeutic response is obtained, following which taper the dosage as rapidly as possible over a 3–7 day period.

(8) Give antibiotics if specifically indicated.

(9) Consider intravenous isoproterenol therapy in younger children with respiratory failure unresponsive to the above therapy. This is not recommended for older adolescents or adults, however, because of the increased risk of inducing cardiac arrest in these age groups. Such an infusion should be undertaken in an intensive care unit where continuous cardiac and blood pressure monitoring facilities are available. Alternatively, mechanical

ventilation using a volume respirator capable of producing high expiratory pressures can be used, by personnel expert in such use. Failure to respond adequately to the previously defined measures can be considered as CO_2 retention above 45 mm Hg (arbitrary) or increasing arterial Pa_{CO_2}.

(10) Obtain a chest x-ray if there is a question of pneumothorax, massive atelectasis, or other *significant* intrathoracic complication.

Do Not's

(1) Do not use narcotics or barbiturates (they depress the respiratory center).

(2) Do not use epinephrine excessively; inhaled beta-2 adrenergic agents are preferred.

(3) Do not treat acute severe paroxysm as purely an acute problem. Follow-up therapy including eventually adequate fluid intake with shifting from IV to oral medications and the continued use of pharmacotherapy out of hospital is important until pulmonary functions reverse to essential normality. Treatment in hospital generally is not required for more than 2 or 3 days for acute severe asthmatic paroxysms but aggressive therapy on an outpatient basis must be continued for many days thereafter.

ATOPIC DERMATITIS
(Infantile Eczema)

This ordinarily begins in early infancy after age 2 months. It is a condition of itchy skin in which the threshold for itching is abnormally low, and it usually is associated with skin dryness and sometimes ichthyosis. The majority of children exhibit evidence of IgE antibody to a variety of allergens, but the role of IgE antibody in the disease process often is unclear. Food allergens by ingestion, and inhalant allergens (mites, pollens, molds, animal allergens) particularly by direct contact can play an important role in some children. Foods most often implicated are milk, egg white, peanuts, and, to a lesser extent, peas, wheat, pork, beef, and corn.

Lesions generally begin as erythematous papules, sometimes secondary to scratching, which can result in variable degrees of scaling, vesicular oozing lesions, and, in the more chronic forms, lichenification. In infants, there is predilection for the cheeks and extensor areas; in older children and adolescents, the flexural creases are most commonly affected. Pruritus is characteristic and frequently intense. Scratching plays a major role in the pathogenesis and predisposes to secondary infection. Skin dryness, sweating, and contact with rough materials and detergents all can aggravate itching. Psychologic factors also can intensify itching.

Differential Diagnosis

Seborrheic dermatitis, contact dermatitis, and scabies with a secondary eczematoid reaction may be confused with atopic dermatitis. Disorders in which skin eruptions can resemble atopic dermatitis include Wiscott-Aldrich syndrome, x-linked agammaglobulinemia, ataxia-telangiectasia, phenylketonuria, severe combined immunodeficiency. Hurler's and Hartnup syndromes, and ahistidinemia. Although this disorder may be lost by age 3, it persists into later childhood and adulthood more often than is generally appreciated. Various immune abnormalities have been identified but there are no laboratory findings that are pathognomonic. IgE antibody is found in approximately 80% of patients and IgE immunoglobulin levels are elevated in many cases as well. Secondary bacterial infections, especially with staphylococci and streptococci, occur frequently. Viral infections, mainly with herpes virus, may produce extensive viral lesions (Kaposi's varicelliform eruption).

Treatment

Good skin care, vigorous specific skin treatment, and identification and elimination of any allergens or irritants that may aggravate the disease are the mainstays of treatment. Hyposensitization is of uncertain value.

Adequate hydration is important, particularly in dry climates. There are basically two approaches, "wet" and "dry." The dry approach (Scholtz regimen) avoids bathing with water completely; instead, Cetaphil Lotion is applied liberally as a cleansing agent and wiped from the skin after foaming, leaving a thin film of lotion on the skin. In drier climates, daily baths without soap or with the occasional use of mild soaps (eg, Dove, Basis, Nutragena) are used to hydrate the skin, and the skin then is patted partly dry and covered with a bland cream or one that contains hydrocortisone if there is active inflammation. Topical corticosteroids are the mainstay of control of inflammation by both methods. A strong (eg, fluorinated) corticosteroid is used 2–3 times a day initially to control intense inflammation, but with more chronic use, the weakest corticosteroid needed is used. This generally is 1% hydrocortisone in a variety of available bases.

For acute severe dermatitis with weeping, Burow's solution (aluminum subacetate) soaks made up to $\frac{1}{20}$ solution is used for 20 minutes at a time, with gauze or cloth thoroughly moistened with solution applied 4 times a day or more for up to 3 days. Systemic antibiotics are used for secondary infections. Antihistamines can be used as antipruritic agents, but are of secondary effectiveness in controlling pruritus compared with topical corticosteroids. The use of potent topical corticosteroids frequently and extensively over inflamed skin can lead to significant systemic absorption. There is a high likelihood that a child with atopic dermatitis will develop allergic rhinitis, asthma, or both.

ADVERSE REACTIONS TO FOODS

Serious allergic reactions to foods include anaphylaxis, hives, angioedema of the upper airway, and severe asthma; however, a wide variety of signs and symptoms can be encountered. The more severe the reaction, the faster it is likely to occur; the majority of severe reactions occur within minutes to a couple of hours after ingestion of the food. Many (and probably most) reactions to foods, however, are caused by nonallergic mechanisms and include pharmacologic or metabolic, toxic, or idiosyncratic reactions. Reactions occur most frequently in infancy. Evidence of IgE antibody to a food allergen can be obtained by skin prick testing (intradermal tests are too nonspecific), serologic tests, or both. The apparent presence of IgE antibody does not in itself establish the diagnosis, nor does the apparent absence rule it out. A reaction may depend upon the amount of food ingested, rate of absorption, and other concurrent factors such as the presence of an enteric infection, which alters the intestinal permeability.

Good evidence for a reaction to a suspected food is improvement of symptoms on avoidance of the food (elimination diet), and aggravation of symptoms on adding back the food (challenge). Food challenges should not be done, however, in cases of life-threatening sensitivity.

Syndromes sometimes associated with food sensitivity include angioedema and urticaria; anaphylaxis; gastrointestinal intolerance; and allergic rhinitis, asthma, and eczema (see previous sections). In addition, "tension-fatigue syndrome"—a syndrome of symptoms ranging from irritability, disturbed behavior, sleeplessness, fatigue, lassitude, and disinterest, associated with allergic shiners, sometimes with headache and vague abdominal complaints—has been blamed on food allergy. When it occurs, however, it is not clear that allergic mechanisms are involved. There are numerous claims that various foodstuffs including sugar, food dyes, various specific foods, and natural salicylates in foods, can produce hyperactivity or other behavioral changes in children with attention deficit disorder. If these substances do contribute, it would appear to occur in an extremely small subpopulation of children. Various foods contain vasoactive material that can intensify vascular (migraine) headaches on a nonallergic basis; the most common foods implicated are chocolate, cheeses, liver, and some wines and beers. Allergic reactions to foods also may intensify vascular headaches. Eosinophilic enterocolitis, pulmonary hemosiderosis related to milk sensitivity, and villous atrophy with malabsorption also can be caused by foods. The diagnosis is based upon a suspicion that a particular food may be causing a problem, elimination of the food and then challenge to determine whether symptoms abate and then reappear. Children tend to have sensitivity only to one food at a time, occasionally two; multiple food allergies are rarely documented. A high level of IgE antibody to a food is more likely to be of clinical significance than a low level. The most common allergens implicated in young children are milk, peanut, egg, soy, and wheat. In older children, shellfish, fish, and nuts also are involved with some frequency.

Other disorders from which "food allergy" should be differentiated include those producing gastrointestinal intolerance—carbohydrate enzyme deficiency (eg, lactase), irritable bowel syndrome, gastrointestinal malformations, acute or chronic intestinal infections, celiac disease, pyloric stenosis, and cystic fibrosis.

Treatment

Treatment is based primarily on avoiding the food, although in less sensitive children, small amounts can be tolerable. *It is important to ensure nutritional adequacy when eliminating foods from the diet.* Food allergies can be outgrown—most likely to milk and soy—but when severe allergy exists, especially to peanuts, other nuts, fish, and shellfish, it is not likely. Loss of sensitivity to eggs is highly variable. In children with potential life-threatening sensitivity, an emergency medical kit with epineph-rine should be available for use by the older child or a responsible adult.

DRUG SENSITIVITY

Reactions to drugs can be due to toxicity; an idiosyncratic or peculiar response to the usual action of the drug; anaphylactoid (pseudoallergic), in which the mediators associated with allergic reactants occur by nonallergic mechanisms (eg, some reactions to radiocontrast dyes); or allergic, in which IgE and perhaps other immune reactions play an important role. Manifestations of drug allergy are extremely varied. Most commonly, skin erup-tions occur. A prolonged syndrome of serum sickness, previ-ously due mostly to foreign serum, can occur particularly with penicillins and sulfonamides. Some drugs given in repository forms or by mouth may linger in the body for weeks and continue to induce symptoms during this period of time. Any drug is a potential sensitizer, but the penicillins and sulfonamides are at the top of the list. Sulfonamides and tetracyclines can be photo-sensitizing.

It is often difficult to know whether a rash that develops when a drug is administered is in fact due to the agent. In many instances, the eruption is unrelated, and there is no drug sensitiv-ity. Unfortunately, diagnostic tests for drugs are highly imperfect and particularly with antibiotics it usually is wisest to make a tentative presumption of drug sensitivity and substitute a struc-turally different drug. In most instances, drug reactions are due to sensitivity to by-products of the drug, and in only a few in-stances have these been identified. Penicillin is the best stud-ied—reagents available for testing are useful, but tests are not foolproof.

Treatment

Treatment consists of discontinuing the drug and supportive therapy depending upon the symptoms involved (see other sec-tions). Pretreatment with antihistamines and corticosteroids in cases in which contrast dyes that previously induced reactions must be used has been successful but *is not foolproof.* Reactions to such dyes generally are "pseudoallergic" and tests of the dye, including use of small test doses, are not accurate or advised.

URTICARIA

Urticaria, or "hives," are multiple, although occasionally single, pruritic erythematous wheals of varying sizes, consisting of localized edema and surrounding erythema. Hives can be allergic or nonallergic. Emotional tension may aggravate hives but rarely is the only cause. Angioedema, essentially urticaria of the deeper skin, results in more diffuse edema, and resolves more slowly than hives. It is a problem mainly if it affects the respiratory tract. The most common classes of allergens inducing urticaria are foods and medications. **"Physical" urticarias** include a cold-induced form in which exposure to cold air, cold water, or other cold objects induces localized urticaria or angioedema. In severe forms, death from sudden massive mediator release can occur—for example, from swimming in cold water. **"Cholinergic" urticaria** is a form relating to overheating, characterized by intense itching and small wheals with much erythema. Exercise or fever are precipitants of this form. There is a form of exercise-anaphylaxis phenomena in which urticaria and angioedema can occur with exercise, to an extent that it may be part of a more generalized anaphylactic syndrome, but generally without pulmonary involvement; it can be life-threatening. **Papular urticaria** is a term given to multiple papules induced by insect bites, found especially on the extremities. Papules secondary to infection from scratching and scabies also occurs. **Dermographism** is a familial or acquired form of "skin sensitivity" in which the threshold of the vascular response to stroking of the skin is lowered. Stroking the skin may produce erythema with or without a wheal; it is not necessarily related to allergy. **Hereditary angioedema** is a rare, nonallergic genetic disorder, characterized by periodic bouts of angioedema that are nonpruritic and can be life-threatening.

Diagnosis depends mainly upon a thorough historical review with implication of possible causative agents, and, if necessary, elimination and challenge. Allergy tests to causative agents can be useful sometimes. Inhalant or contact allergens occasionally can induce hives, the former particularly on a seasonal basis. Treatment consists of avoiding the causative factors and use of H_1 antihistamines such as diphenhydramine or hydroxyzine. With more chronic forms, the addition of an H_2 antihistamine such as cimetidine can be helpful. With severe acute urticaria and angioedema, epinephrine may be necessary. Occasionally, short courses of corticosteroids are necessary.

27 | Collagen Diseases

Elaine Van Gundy, MD

"Collagen diseases" are not limited pathologically to alterations of collagen but also involve changes in the connective tissue, and therefore, they are often called connective tissue diseases. However, although many diseases involve the connective tissue, 7 disorders with similar characteristics can accurately be called collagen diseases: rheumatic fever, rheumatoid arthritis, Lyme disease, polyarteritis (periarteritis) nodosa, systemic lupus erythematosus, scleroderma, and dermatomyositis. The similarities can be summarized as follows: (1) frequently overlapping clinical features, (2) chronicity with relapses, (3) changes in immunologic state, (4) common pathologic features (fibrinoid degeneration, granulomatous reaction with fibrosis, vasculitis with proliferation of plasma cells), and (5) improvement with use of corticosteroids (often only symptomatic).

Arthritis is a common feature seen in the collagen diseases. Therefore, a brief discussion regarding evaluation of childhood arthritis will precede the discussion of the specific collagen diseases.

EVALUATION OF THE CHILD PRESENTING WITH ARTHRITIS

The differential diagnosis for arthritis may be categorized as Orthopedic, Rheumatic, Infectious, Neoplastic and Systemic. Please refer to Table 27–1 for a partial list of conditions that may present with arthritis.

The evaluation of the child presenting with arthritis requires an accurate history and physical emphasizing character of presenting symptoms. Historical clues supporting an organic condition include signs of systemic illness (weight loss, fever, night sweats, rash, diarrhea). Initial laboratory evaluation may include CBC, sedimentation rate and ANA titer. Table 27–2 summarizes

Table 27–1. Conditions that may present with arthritis.

Orthopedic	Infectious Disease
Musculoskeletal trauma	Osteomyelitis
Chondromalacia patella	Septic arthritis
Hypermobility	Viral arthritis
Rheumatic	Lyme disease
JRA	Neoplastic
SLE	Leukemia
Juvenile dermatomyositis	Neuroblastoma
Henoch-Schönlein purpura	Systemic Conditions
Rheumatic fever	Inflammatory bowel disease
Spondyloarthropathy	Sickel cell anemia
	Hemophilia

laboratory and clinical clues seen with conditions presenting with arthritis.

In summary, the differential diagnosis that one considers in evaluating a child with arthritis is broad. Characteristics on history and physical examination will help to guide in further evaluation. Laboratory screening tests are often abnormal with organic conditions, although they can be normal (early JRA, early leukemia, toxic synovitis). In orthopedic conditions laboratory screening tests will be normal. Chronic arthritis of undetermined etiology requires repeat examination, stepwise laboratory and possible radiographic evaluation.

RHEUMATIC FEVER

Rheumatic fever is the most common cause of symptomatic acquired heart disease in childhood. The incidence of rheumatic fever had been decreasing in the USA and other developed countries until the mid 1980s. Since then, there has been an increase in the incidence of rheumatic fever, with carditis being the dominant feature. It is clear that group A β-hemolytic streptococci are implicated in the etiology of rheumatic fever, but the pathogenetic mechanism remains obscure. This relation to a specific bacterial component sets rheumatic fever apart from the other collagen diseases.

A β-hemolytic streptococcal infection invariably precedes by 1–3 weeks the initial attack and subsequent relapses of rheumatic fever, although not all of these infections are clinically manifest. Since rheumatic heart disease represents a hypersensi-

Table 27-2. Childhood arthritis and associated laboratory and clinical characteristics.

Condition	CBC	ESR	ANA	Other Characteristics
Orthopedic conditions	Normal	Normal	Normal	History of precipitating events
Rheumatic disease	WBC = nl, ↑ or ↓ H/H = nl or ↓	nl or ↑	nl or positive	Arthritis persistent
Leukemia	WBC = nl, ↑ or ↓ H/H = nl or ↓ Abnormal smear	nl or ↑	nl or mildly positive	Systemically ill
Inflammatory bowel disease	Anemia	nl or ↑	negative	Diarrhea, wt. loss, monoarthritis
Sickle cell disease	Anemia	nl or ↑	negative	Abnormal hemoglobin, electrophoresis
Septic arthritis	↑ WBC	↑ ESR	negative	Child toxic appearing, joints warm, ↑ WBC, synovial fluid: purulent with >50,000 WBC
Viral arthritis	Usually normal	Normal or sl ↑	negative	Usually hip involved (sometimes knee), child appears well
Lyme disease	Normal	Normal or sl ↑	negative	Tick exposure; rash; positive serology

tivity reaction, it is reasonable to assume that several infections with group A β-hemolytic streptococci are necessary to trigger the first episode of rheumatic fever.

Predisposing Factors

Lower socioeconomic status (overcrowding), a familial predisposition, and reinfection with β-hemolytic streptococci place an individual at increased risk.

Clinical Findings

The diagnosis is usually certain if the child has either (a) 2 major manifestations or (b) one major and 2 minor manifestations (modified after Jones), along with supportive evidence of recent streptococcal infection.

A. Major Manifestations:

1. Signs of active carditis.

2. Polyarthritis. Inflammation of the large joints (ankles, knees, hips, wrists, elbows, and shoulders) is usually in a migratory fashion.

3. Subcutaneous nodules.

4. Erythema marginatum.

5. Chorea.

B. Minor Manifestations:

1. Fever.

2. Arthralgia.

3. Previous rheumatic fever.

4. Electrocardiographic changes, particularly prolonged PR intervals.

5. Abnormal blood test results. Increased ESR, C-reactive protein, white blood cell count, anemia.

C. Supportive Evidence:

1. Recent scarlet fever.

2. Throat culture positive for Group A streptococci.

3. Increased ASO or other streptococcal antibodies.

Diagnosis

There is no specific laboratory test for rheumatic fever. Combined use of clinical and laboratory findings may aid in diagnosis and subsequent evaluation of the degree of rheumatic activity. Echocardiography is helpful in diagnosis by showing that the posterior mitral valve leaflet thickens and separates from the anterior leaflet.

Treatment

A. Specific Measures:

1. Corticosteroids–Corticosteroids should be administered for management of acute-onset congestive heart failure associated with carditis. However, long-term controlled studies show no benefit from corticosteroid therapy in preventing chronic rheumatic heart disease. Thus, corticosteroids are not recommended for patients with carditis who are not in congestive heart failure.

2. Salicylates–The salicylates markedly reduce fever, alleviate joint pain, and reduce joint swelling. The rapid response of rheumatic fever to salicylates is usually quite dramatic and is a useful diagnostic test in differentiation from rheumatoid arthritis, which responds much more slowly. Salicylates should be continued as long as necessary for the relief of symptoms. If the withdrawal of salicylates results in a recurrence, they should immediately be reinstituted. The average dose of aspirin is 80–120 mg/kg/day every 4–6 hours. The highest dosage is recommended for the first 48 hours.

3. Penicillin–Penicillin in full dosage should be used in all cases for 10 days; followed by daily prophylaxis to prevent recurrences (see below).

B. General Measures:

Resumption of full activity should be gradual and related to the severity of the attack, particularly if a significant degree of carditis is present.

Prophylaxis

The main principle of prophylaxis is the prevention of recurrent infection with β-hemolytic streptococci.

A. Penicillin: The unequivocal treatment of choice is benzathine penicillin G, given intramuscularly every 28 days; 1.2 million units is sufficient for school-age children. In day-care settings or other extreme situations of exposure, the interval should be every 21 days. Oral penicillin G, 200,000 units twice daily may be used but because of possible poor compliance is a poor second choice. Therapeutic doses of penicillin are recommended before tooth extraction or other surgery if valvular involvement is present.

B. Erythromycin: Use of erythromycin, 125–250 mg/day orally, is of value in children who cannot tolerate penicillin.

Course & Prognosis

The course varies markedly from patient to patient. It may be fulminating, leading to death early in the course of the acute rheumatic episode, or it may be entirely asymptomatic, the diagnosis being made in retrospect on the basis of pathologic findings. With adequate penicillin prophylaxis, recurrences are virtually eliminated. The prognosis for life largely depends on the intensity of the initial cardiac insult and the prevention of repeated rheumatic recurrences.

RHEUMATOID ARTHRITIS

Rheumatoid arthritis in childhood, commonly known as juvenile rheumatoid arthritis (JRA), is an inflammatory disease of unknown etiology. Although familial clustering of arthritis occurs, no definite genetic pattern exists. It is the most common collagen vascular disease seen in childhood.

There are three subgroups of JRA, distinguished by their clinical manifestations, disease course and prognosis, and serologic findings. The three types—systemic, polyarticular, and pauciarticular—are summarized in Table 27–3.

Rheumatoid arthritis should be distinguished from ankylosing spondylitis. Ankylosing spondylitis is 10 times more frequent in males. It is sometimes familial and affects the spine (particularly the sacroiliac joints). Transient and nondeforming periph-

Table 27–3. Types and clinical presentation of JRA.

Type	Peak Age of Onset	Sex	Clinical Manifestation
Systemic	no peak	F = M	Fever, rash, hepatosplenomegaly, arthritis, pericarditis, no uveitis
Polyarticular	1–3 yr & 9 yr	F > M	≥5 joints, symmetrical, infrequent systemic features, chronic uveitis in 5%
Pauciarticular	1–3 yr	F > M	<5 joints, asymmetrical, no systemic features, chronic uveitis in 20%

eral arthritis, usually confined to a few large joints—especially in the lower extremities—occurs in about half of patients; it may occur before back complaints appear. Acute iritis and aortitis are characteristic extra-articular manifestations. Spondylitis has also been associated with psoriasis, inflammatory bowel disease (eg, ulcerative colitis, regional enteritis), and Reiter's syndrome. Autoantibodies are not present, but 90% of affected individuals will carry the HLA-B27 histocompatibility antigen. Treatment with phenylbutazone and indomethacin may be of value.

Clinical Findings

All three types of JRA share the common feature of arthritis (which by criteria, must be present ≥6 weeks) but clinically present very differently.

A. Symptoms and Signs:

1. Systemic–This onset accounts for 10% of cases of JRA. It is hallmarked by high spiking fever (usually to 39°C or higher) once or twice a day, rapidly returning to baseline or even to a subnormal temperature. The fever may be associated with a characteristic evanescent morbilliform rash most commonly found on the trunk and proximal extremities. Arthritis may occur at any time during the course of the disease. Other features include hepatosplenomegaly, pleuritis, pericarditis, and abdominal pain. The children are characteristically quite ill-appearing while febrile but appear surprisingly well the rest of the time.

2. Polyarticular–This onset accounts for 50% of cases of JRA. This subgroup is characterized by arthritis in 5 or more joints. Joint involvement usually consists of symmetrical involvement of fingers, toes, knees, ankles, wrists, hips, and mandibular joints. Cervical spondylitis may be present. Joints are slightly swollen and tender and motion is limited. The finger joints become characteristically spindle-shaped with shiny smooth skin over them. Rheumatoid nodules are infrequent but if they occur are most common in the older female who is RF positive. Systemic features are uncommon. Uveitis occurs in a small percentage of patients (5%), although the patients that are antinuclear antibody (ANA) positive are at increased risk for eye disease.

3. Pauciarticular–This subgroup accounts for 40% of cases of JRA and its onset is characterized by involvement of 4 or fewer joints. The knees and ankles are most commonly involved, and the process is usually asymmetrical. These children do not have any systemic symptoms and appear well. Chronic uveitis is most common in this group (20%), with the majority of patients with uveitis (90%) being ANA positive.

B. Laboratory Findings: Findings include polymorphonuclear leukocytosis and accelerated sedimentation rates, especially in active disease. Moderate anemia is present. HLA-B27 antigen is frequently present in ankylosing spondylitis but is not common in juvenile rheumatoid arthritis. The rheumatoid factor is rarely positive in juvenile rheumatoid arthritis. The ANA is commonly positive in the polyarticular and pauciarticular forms of the disease. Synovial fluid may show an inflammatory reaction. Synovial biopsy demonstrates chronic inflammation, although it is not specific for rheumatoid arthritis.

C. Imaging: Findings in the early phase of disease usually include swelling of periarticular soft structures, synovial effusion, and slight widening of the joint spaces. Accelerated epiphyseal maturation, increase in size of ossification centers, and disproportionate longitudinal bone growth may occur. Later findings include obliteration of the joint space, erosions of bone, and generalized osteoporosis of all bones of the involved areas.

D. Other Findings: Electrocardiographic findings are usually normal unless cardiac involvement is present. Echocardiography may show pericarditis.

Treatment

A. Specific Measures:

1. Nonsteroidal Anti-inflammatory Drugs (NSAIDs)–Aspirin is the most satisfactory anti-inflammatory agent. Its recommended anti-inflammatory dose is 80–120 mg/kg/day in divided doses. Levels of 20–30 mg/dL are therapeutic. The response of rheumatoid arthritis to salicylates occurs within 3–4 days and is usually not as dramatic as in rheumatic fever. In patients who cannot tolerate aspirin, use of tolmetin (Tolectin), 20–30 mg/kg/day, Naproxen (Naprosyn) 10–15 mg/kg/day, or other NSAIDs should be tried. Both aspirin and NSAIDs have potential deleterious effects. Some patients receiving aspirin have developed Reye's syndrome, and renal papillary necrosis has been noted after use of NSAIDs.

2. Gold Salts and Penicillamine–These are being used with increasing frequency in patients who do not respond to salicylates.

3. Methotrexate–Studies of low-dose (10.0 mg/m^2/week) methotrexate use in children show a therapeutic benefit in JRA. Whether or not this drug can induce long term remission of the disease has not been answered. Use in children should be restricted to those who have failed conventional therapy.

4. Corticosteroids–Corticosteroids do not alter the natural remission rate, or the length of the illness. However, there is a place for them (eg, prednisone, 1–2 mg/kg/day) in cases of myocarditis and in any case where the disease appears to be life-threatening. They are used topically for the treatment of uveitis and systemically in low doses (5–10 mg/day) if the uveitis is unresponsive to topical therapy. Low-dose therapy is also used in patients with severe debilitating morning stiffness, and those beginning on slow-acting anti-inflammatory drugs. Intra-articular corticosteroids have a place in the management of JRA when there is a monarticular involvement or when one or 2 joints appear to retard rehabilitation.

B. General Measures:

1. Physical Therapy–The overall goal is to prevent deformities and maintain muscle strength and function. The type of therapy prescribed depends on the disease activity. Acutely inflamed joints should not be subjected to weight-bearing exercise, but range-of-motion exercises should be prescribed. Later, stretching and strengthening should be added. Heat and hydrotherapy may be a useful adjunct to a well-planned exercise program.

2. Orthopedic Care–The wearing of splints during the night will ensure proper alignment of joints. Cylinder casts are to be avoided.

3. Ophthalmic Care–Periodic slit lamp examination is the only means for early diagnosis of iridocyclitis, which may otherwise continue undiagnosed until vision fails.

4. Rest–As fatigue is a frequent symptom, periods of rest should be alternated with periods of activity. However, complete bed rest should be discouraged, since it can lead to osteoporosis, renal calculi, muscle atrophy, or joint deformities.

5. Psychologic Care–In view of the long duration of this disease, the family should understand the necessity of fulfilling the patient's social, educational, and psychologic needs.

6. Diet–There is no special diet. Ferrous sulfate should be given if iron deficiency is present.

Course & Prognosis

Rheumatoid arthritis is a chronic disease with waxing and waning of inflammatory activity. The systemic features (fever, rash, pericarditis, etc) remit more often than the joint manifestations.

With good medical management, one can expect that more than 70% of patients will have complete functional recovery and less than 10% will be severely disabled. Deaths are reported in the pediatric age group, but they are rare.

LYME DISEASE
(Lyme Arthritis)

Lyme disease is a form of arthritis that is often chronic. The first case was reported in Connecticut in 1975, and is known to be due to a spirochete transmitted by a tick (*Ixodes dammini*).

The onset is usually in summer and early symptoms are commonly characterized by influenzalike symptoms (fever, malaise, headache, stiff neck). A target-shaped skin rash (erythema chronicum migrans) develops (usually within 30 days of exposure to the tick vector) and may be confused with ringworm. Later, disseminated disease often involves the heart (myocarditis, AV block), the nervous system (aseptic meningitis, neuropathies), and the joints (arthritis). Later manifestations usually occur within three months of tick exposure. All of these symptoms can recur, and the arthritis can be chronic.

Diagnosis is based on clinically supporting evidence of Lyme Disease, and laboratory confirmation. An enzyme linked immunosorbent assay (ELISA) should be performed. If this is positive, a Western Blot (WB) analysis, which is more specific, more sensitive yet more expensive than the ELISA test, should be done. The combination of a positive ELISA and WB supports the diagnosis of Lyme disease, especially with a history of typical symptoms or rash of Lyme disease.

The treatment is by use of either Amoxicillin, Doxycycline (>9 years of age) or Erythromycin (penicillin allergic child <9). Intravenous antibiotics (ceftriaxone, cefotoxime) are indicated for CNS disease or arthritis failing oral treatment, and early treatment may avoid later complications.

POLYARTERITIS NODOSA

Polyarteritis (periarteritis) nodosa is a rare systemic disease characterized by inflammatory damage to blood vessels, with resulting injury to involved organs. Pathologically, there is segmental inflammation of small- and medium-sized arteries, with fibrinoid changes and (more rarely) necrosis in the vessel wall. Mucocutaneous lymph node syndrome (Kawasaki disease) and infantile polyarterits nodosa bear many pathologic similarities to polyarteritis nodosa.

Clinical Findings

Clinical manifestations vary, depending on the location of the involved arterioles.

A. Symptoms: Symptoms are generally those of a rapidly progressive, wasting disease: fever, lassitude, weight loss, and generalized pains in the extremities or abdomen (or both).

B. Signs: Skin eruptions of the urticarial, purpuric, or macular type occur. Subcutaneous nodules are frequently present along the course of the blood vessels. Involvement of the kidneys, gastrointestinal tract, heart, and nervous system often occur. Features include hypertension, myocardial infarction, seizures, and peripheral neuropathy.

C. Laboratory Findings: Abnormalities reflect the organ involved. These include anemia, with moderate leukocytosis and eosinophilia; accelerated sedimentation rate; proteinuria; intermittent microscopic hematuria and showers of casts; elevated levels of nonprotein nitrogen; sterile blood cultures; and cardiomegaly on x-ray. Muscle, skin, or testicular biopsy may show vasculitis and aid in diagnosis.

Treatment

Treatment with corticosteroids usually produces symptomatic improvement and suppressive doses may prolong life, but the response is unpredictable and quite variable.

Prognosis

Prognosis is poor for patients with renal, cardiac, or central nervous system involvement, although spontaneous and corticosteroid-induced remissions are seen.

SYSTEMIC LUPUS ERYTHEMATOSUS

Systemic lupus erythematosus (SLE) is a multisystem progressive disease whose protean symptomatology and relentless course present a diagnostic and therapeutic challenge. Pathologically, immune complex vasculitis, extensive fibrinoid degeneration, and necrosis are found. The disease is 9 times more common in females than in males. In the pediatric population, the disease onset peaks during the adolescent years. The cause is unknown. It is believed that multiple factors (viral, immunologic, and genetic) play a role. A lupuslike syndrome (including positive findings in LE cell preparations and ANA tests) may occur during procainamide or anticonvulsant therapy.

Clinical Findings

A. Symptoms and Signs: Children often present with fever, rash, arthralgia, and arthritis. Myalgia, fatigue, weakness, and weight loss frequently occur. Table 27–4 summaries typical clinical presentations.

B. Laboratory Findings: Antinuclear antibodies are present in 100% of active cases; the antinuclear antibody test has replaced the LE cell preparation as the most sensitive diagnostic test. Table 27–5 summarizes common laboratory findings.

Diagnosis & Treatment

The diagnosis of SLE is based on clinical findings and presentation, although specific laboratory abnormalities aid in the diagnosis. Consistent features include the episodic nature of the disease, multisystem involvement, and positive ANA.

Nonsteroidal anti-inflammatory drugs should be given for joint symptoms. Prednisone, given in doses of at least 60 mg/m^2/day, not only suppresses the acute inflammatory manifestations but, in many cases, also modifies or halts progressive glo-

Table 27–4. Clinical manifestations pf SLE.

System	Presentation
Cutaneous	Butterfly rash, mucocutaneous ulcers, alopecia, photosensitivity, digital ulcerations, Raynaud's phenomenon.
Cardiac	Pericarditis (most common), endocarditis and myocarditis (less common)
Pulmonary	Pleuritis, basilar pneumonitis.
Gastrointestinal	Abdominal pain, diarrhea, esophageal dysmotility.
Renal	Nephritis, hypertension, uremia, nephrotic syndrome.
Musculoskeletal	Arthralgia, arthritis, myalgia.
Nervous system	Seizures, organic brain syndrome.
Lymphoreticular	Splenomegaly, hepatomegaly, lymphadenopathy.

Table 27–5. Laboratory findings in SLE.

Autoantibodies
Anemia
Thrombocytopenia
Hypocomplementemia
Leukopenia
Hematuria, proteinuria
Elevated ESR
Positive Coombs'
False (+) VDRL

merular involvement. Antibiotics should be used at the first sign of an infection. Hydroxychloroquine may be of value for skin and joint symptoms.

Azathioprine (Imuran) and cyclophosphamide (Cytoxan) are effective in controlling renal and systemic manifestations of the disease in some children who are resistant to corticosteroids alone. Recent evidence suggests that long-term survival in cases of lupus nephritis has improved when cytoxan and prednisone are used together.

Intravenous pulse therapy with methylprednisolone sodium succinate (Solu-Medrol) may be tried in critically ill patients.

Because of their well-known photosensitivity, patients should use sunscreens when exposed to the sun.

Course & Prognosis

Renal complications and central nervous system involvement are the most frequent causes of death. With good medical management, the 5-year survival rate increased from 51% at 5 years in 1954 to 71% at 10 years in 1979, and later data are even more encouraging.

SCLERODERMA

Scleroderma is a collagen disease chiefly involving the skin, but any organ may be involved. In local benign scleroderma (morphea), there is a linear distribution of lesions that first show erythema and edema and subsequently scarring and shrinking. In the progressive generalized form (sclerodactyly), there is more extensive thickening and induration of the skin, followed by contractures. Interstitial and perivascular fibrosis may occur in the viscera.

Table 27–6. Diagnostic features
of dermatomyositis.

Proximal muscle weakness
Muscle enzyme elevation
Characteristic skin rash
Electromyogram findings
Muscle biopsy histology

Trophic ulcers, calcific deposits, and Raynaud's phenomenon are common. Raynaud's phenomenon is often the initial presenting symptom and may precede other manifestations by years. Disturbances in esophageal motility lead to dysphagia, and small bowel involvement leads to malabsorption. Antinuclear antibodies are frequently observed.

There is no specific therapy. Physiotherapy given early may minimize contractures. Corticosteroids are of little value. Phenoxybenzamine (Dibenzyline) has been used to relieve peripheral vasospasm. Bethanechol, cimetidine, and antacids have been used for dysphagia. Colchicine and D-penicillamine therapy have produced inconsistent results.

The prognosis is excellent for patients with local scleroderma but only fair for those with the severe generalized form, in which death may occur within a year. Some deformity may occur with the former and is the rule with the latter. Renal or cardiac involvement implies a poor prognosis.

DERMATOMYOSITIS

Juvenile dermatomyositis is a multisystem inflammatory disease of unknown cause, involving primarily the muscles, skin, and subcutaneous tissues. It may be an autoimmune disorder. The pathologic process can and sometimes does involve the gastrointestinal tract and the central nervous system. Theoretically, since dermatomyositis in childhood appears to be a vascular process leading to arteritis and phlebitis, any organ could be involved. Muscles show segmental or focal necrosis, inflammation, fibrinoid changes in capillaries of blood vessels, and, finally, atrophy.

Clinical Findings

Diagnostic features of juvenile dermatomyositis are listed in Table 27–6.

A. Symptoms: Symptoms include symmetrical proximal muscle weakness; fever; muscle tenderness and pain; malaise and weight loss; arthralgia and arthritis; dyspnea; and dysphagia.

B. Signs: The pathognomonic rash of this disease is a violaceous (heliotrope) discoloration of the eyelids.

C. Laboratory Findings: Elevation of muscle enzymes (SGOT, CPK, aldolase) is a useful laboratory tool. Anemia, increased sedimentation rate, and increased levels of serum globulin may be present. Myopathy on electromyogram, and inflammation on muscle biopsy will aid in the diagnosis.

Treatment

Corticosteroid therapy is indicated in all patients with acute or active disease. Prednisone (1–2 mg/kg/day in divided doses) during the first month after diagnosis is usually required. Treatment should be vigorous and be modulated to produce normal muscle enzymes. The immunosuppressive drugs methotrexate and azathioprine may be of value in life-threatening disease and in children whose disease is not adequately controlled with corticosteroid therapy alone.

Physiotherapy is a very important part of the treatment; the principles outlined in the section on rheumatoid arthritis should be followed.

Course & Prognosis

The clinical course of juvenile dermatomyositis varies considerably. The prognosis is favorable in most cases with early treatment. A small percentage of children will experience a relapsing course. The majority of patients can be returned to functional normality. Calcinosis, contractures, and atrophy produce long-term residua. Intractable muscle weakness, sepsis, and gastrointestinal vasculitis can be responsible for death in a small number of patients. Unlike adults, the juvenile form of this disease is not associated with cancer.

Pediatric Emergencies | 28

F. Keith Battan, MD, FAAP

The primary mission of a Pediatric Emergency Department (PED) is *resuscitation and stabilization* of the life-threatened child. A large amount of definitive care for less serious illnesses and injuries is provided as well. The complete spectrum of illnesses and injuries is seen, from minor acute illnesses to life- or limb-threatening injuries or illnesses. Care provided by the PED to critically ill patients overlaps with that provided in pediatric intensive care units; therefore many of the topics discussed in this chapter relate only to initial stabilization and treatment; more comprehensive treatments are described elsewhere in this book.

Most emergency pediatricians feel that care of the severely injured child is an essential part of their mission. Trauma causes more deaths after the first year of life than any other diagnosis.

APPROACH TO THE VERY ILL OR INJURED CHILD

Children, unlike adults, rarely exhibit sudden death from cardiac etiologies. Rather, pediatric cardiopulmonary arrests are usually due to respiratory causes, and are the result of a prolonged period of deterioration, during which significant insults to brain, heart, liver, kidneys and other vital organs have occurred. By the time cardiopulmonary arrest occurs, the attendant hypoxia and acidosis that have occurred lead to a very dismal outcome. Very few children suffering total arrest survive or are left without significant neurologic impairments. Therefore the key to good outcomes is early recognition and intervention *before* an arrest occurs. *Recognition of the child who is at risk for cardiopulmonary arrest, and early intervention, is essential.*

When the arrival of a very sick child is anticipated or occurs abruptly, adequate nursing and physician staff must be assembled. Subspecialists are included as indicated, eg, neurosurgeons or general surgeons. Team roles are assigned, ensuring that the team leader is clearly designated. Radiology, the blood bank, OR, and the lab are notified, as appropriate.

History

A brief problem-oriented history should be obtained from the parents soon after immediate resuscitation begins and without interrupting the resuscitation. A physician not involved with the resuscitation can obtain a history and counsel the parents on the current status of their child. Essential elements of the history are included in the mnemonic "AMPLE":

A: Allergies and immunizations. Injuries breaking the skin will require determining the status of tetanus immunization.

M: Medications, including over-the-counter and prescription drugs. Many of these agents can produce toxic effects such as altered mental status and cardiorespiratory symptoms.

P: Past illnesses. Determine chronic illnesses, especially bleeding disorders or immunodeficiencies; previous surgeries or hospitalizations; and developmental disabilities.

L: Last meal. Children can be presumed to have a full stomach unless quantity and timing of the last oral intake can be determined. This information has implications for airway management given the risk for vomiting and aspiration.

E: Events preceding the injury or illness. Include timing, duration of symptoms, fever, and treatment. For injured children, determine supervision, witnesses to the event, mechanism of injury, secondary impacts, and pre-hospital course and care.

EXAMINATION; THE ABCS
(Rapid Assessment and Intervention)

Systematic use of the "*Airway, Breathing, Circulation*" method of examination (ABCs) allows rapid assessment of the degree of the child's physiologic derangement, and indicates the immediate interventions necessary to prevent further deterioration. In this system, the patency of the airway is assessed, and if there is obstruction, measures to correct the obstruction are initiated immediately. Once airway patency is assured, the presence and adequacy of breathing is assessed. Again, if respiratory efforts are inadequate, interventions such as bag-valve-mask ventilation are begun to normalize oxygenation and ventilation. Once airway and breathing have been determined to be adequate or have been stabilized, then assessment of and intervention in circulation are done. The ABCs are detailed below. Basic life support measures will not be reviewed here.

Airway

   A. Assessment: Assess airway patency by *look, listen, and feel: Look* for chest wall movement, signs of upper airway obstruction such as increased work of inspiration, and level of consciousness. *Listen* for abnormal breath sounds such as stridor or gurgling. *Feel* for air movement at the mouth and nose by lowering your face to the child's mouth and nose.

   B. Intervention: If airway obstruction is present, begin airway maneuvers in order of increasing invasiveness. If neck injury is possible, immobilize the cervical spine and maintain normal alignment.

   (1) Perform head tilt with chin lift or jaw thrust: Gently extend the head on the neck, and lift the chin (Fig. 28–1) with fingers on the mandible or by exerting upward traction on the angle of the jaw. If airway obstruction persists, reposition the head before proceeding.

   (2) Suction the mouth of secretions or foreign materials.

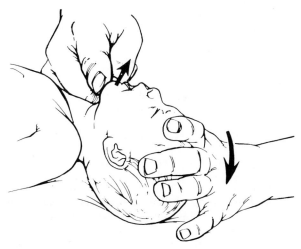

Figure 28 1–1. Head tilt with chin lift. (Used, with permission, from *Textbook of Pediatric Advanced Life Support,* American Heart Association/American Academy of Pediatrics, 1988.)

Table 28–1. Estimation formulas.

Estimated body weight (kg) = (age in yrs × 2) + 8
Median blood pressure (systolic) = (age in years × 2) + 90
5th percentile systolic BP (hypotension) = (age in years × 2) + 70
Endotracheal tube size = (age + 16)/4

(3) Attempt to visualize foreign bodies, with a laryngoscope if necessary, and remove with fingers or Magill forceps. Blind finger sweeps for foreign bodies are contraindicated.

(4) Insert an oropharyngeal airway. This eliminates obstruction due to posterior prolapse of the tongue into the posterior pharynx, which is the most common cause of upper airway obstruction in the unconscious child. In a conscious child, a nasopharyngeal airway may be used to avoid vomiting and possible aspiration.

(5) Consider performing foreign body maneuvers if the airway remains obstructed at this point.

(6) Place an endotracheal tube (see Table 28–1 for sizes) if obstruction persists, or if the child needs assisted ventilation for other reasons.

(7) Needle cricothyroidotomy may be necessary in the rare patient when endotracheal intubation is not possible.

Breathing

A. Assessment: *Look* for apnea, hypoventilation, or signs of respiratory distress. Signs include:

(1) Abnormal respiratory rate for age. Tachypnea is common and frequently non-specific, but its cause must be sought. In a sick or injured child, *an abnormally low heart or respiratory rate with or without respiratory distress is a pre-arrest sign and requires aggressive immediate intervention.*

(2) Increased work of breathing, manifested by retractions, flaring of the alae nasae, or grunting. Retractions can be intercostal, supraclavicular, or substernal. An increased reliance on the diaphragm for breathing in children leads to abdominal or "see-saw" respirations, as the stomach protrudes during inspiration and vice-versa.

(3) Adequate and symmetric chest rise and fall (tidal volume).

(4) Altered mental status. Hypercarbia results in lethargy, while early hypoxia is manifested by agitation or restlessness.

(5) Skin color change. Cyanosis is a late finding due to the relative anemia of children and signifies profound hypoxia, whereas less severe alterations in Pao_2 may result in mottled, gray, or pale skin.

Listen for adventitious breath sounds such as wheezing. Auscultate for rales, wheezing, and symmetry of breath sounds. The smaller the chest, the more transmitted breath sounds may impair your ability to localize auscultatory findings.

Feel for subcutaneous crepitus or tracheal deviation, eg, from pneumothorax. The majority of the respiratory assessment comes from inspection; as Yogi Berra said, "You can see a lot by just looking!"

Intervention

(1) Oxygen should be immediately given to any patient exhibiting respiratory distress.

(2) For spontaneously breathing patients with minimal distress, a nasal cannula can be used. Non-rebreather masks deliver a higher F_1O_2 and are appropriate for more seriously ill patients.

(3) If there is inadequate or absent breathing, begin positive-pressure ventilation with an appropriate size bag-valve-mask device (Table 28–2). Ensure that there is adequate chest rise and fall, and auscultate for air entry bilaterally. If there is resistance to bagging, repeat the interventions in "Airway" above.

(4) Consider needle thoracostomy to alleviate pneumothorax for patients in severe distress or arrest who have asymmetric breath sounds, jugular venous distension, or subcutaneous crepitus.

(5) Endotracheal intubation should be performed for children in severe distress, those unresponsive to bag-mask ventilation, those in coma or who otherwise require airway protection, and in children who will require prolonged mechanical ventilation.

(6) Intravenous access is second in priority to the above interventions but should be established in children with severe distress or respiratory failure (see below). Advanced airway techniques are described in standard texts of pediatric emergency or critical care medicine. Further discussion follows under "respiratory failure," below.

Circulation

Assessment: Unlike respiratory assessment, the assessment of circulatory status is largely by hands-on examination. The

Table 28-2. Equipment sizes and estimated weight by age.

Age (yr)	Weight (kg)	ETT[1] Size	Laryngoscope Blade	Chest Tube (fr.)	Foley (fr.)
Premature newborn	1–2.5	2.5 uncuffed	0	8	5
Term newborn	3.0	3.0	0–1	10	8
1	10	3.5–4.0	1	18	8
2	12	4.5	1	18	10
3	14	4.5	1	20	10
4	16	5.0	2	22	10
5	18	5.0–5.5	2	24	10
6	20	5.5	2	26	12
7	22	5.5–6.0	2	26	12
8	24	6.0 cuffed	2	28	14
10	32	6.0–6.5	2–3	30	14
Adolescent	50	7.0	3	36	14
Adult	70	8.0	3	40	14

[1] ETT = endotracheal tube; NB, cuffed ETTs used about age 8.

diagnosis of shock can be made by the following clinical signs without a blood pressure determination. Assess for:

(1) Tachycardia or bradycardia. As mentioned above, bradycardia is ominous and requires aggressive intervention.

(2) Capillary fill time: This is a very useful index of circulatory integrity. CFT > 2 seconds is abnormal.

(3) Warmth of the extremities: Palpate hands or feet. If they are cool, determine the point at which the extremities become warm; the more proximal coolness begins, the more profound the shock.

(4) Pulses: Pulses should be assessed as normal, bounding (as in early phases of warm shock), thready, or absent. If peripheral pulses are absent, more proximal pulses should be sought.

(5) Skin color: Mottling, cyanosis, or grayness reflect hypoxia/ischemia.

(6) Altered mental status: Ischemia or hypoxemia will be reflected in altered levels of consciousness.

(7) Blood pressure: Because of the ability of children to respond to hypovolemia with marked increases in systemic vas-

cular resistance, blood pressure doesn't fall until very late in the course of shock, making BP an insensitive indicator of shock. It is not necessary to know BP to determine perfusion status: If the patient has an abnormal heart rate and one of the other signs described above, he is in shock and should be treated accordingly. Poor perfusion as determined by CFT and the other clinical signs above with a normal BP is *compensated shock,* when the blood pressure also falls it is *uncompensated shock. Shock* from which the patient cannot be resuscitated has been termed *irreversible shock.* When time permits, BP should be determined with the appropriate-sized cuff. Standard charts of BP for age can be consulted or the following estimation formula used: Systolic BP should be greater than $(2 \times \text{age in years}) + 70$ for children over one year of age, newborns to one-month-olds should have a SBP > 60. See discussion of treatment under "Shock," below. *Hypotension is a late finding in shock. The diagnosis of shock can be made by physical examination.*

Interventions

Hypoperfusion or circulatory failure necessitates IV access, volume replacement, and, at times, pressors. Establishing access can be problematic in patients in shock. Lack of pulses or frank arrest, of course, requires CPR (external cardiac massage).

To summarize, rapidly assess the ABCs, taking care to sequentially assess each system and intervene appropriately before moving to the next step.

RESPIRATORY FAILURE

Respiratory failure is characterized by the inability of the body to maintain normal partial pressures of oxygen and/or CO_2 in the blood. It can be caused by conditions intrinsic (eg, asthma, pneumonia) or extrinsic (head injury, trauma) to the lungs. Respiratory failure can result from either upper, or more commonly, lower airway obstruction. In the acute care setting, early recognition and timely intervention are again key.

Respiratory distress is characterized by increased work of breathing. It can be further subdivided into early or late respiratory distress. Minute ventilation is equal to tidal volume times respiratory rate, therefore respiratory failure can occur with a high respiratory rate but inadequate tidal volume, and vice versa. Signs of respiratory distress are listed above in the assessment of breathing. As early respiratory distress progresses into late respiratory distress or *respiratory failure,* the increased work of breathing will eventually decrease, accompanied by a decrease in mentation. With increasing hypercarbia there will be lethargy; with hypoxia, initial agitation will give way to increasing obtundation. As the patient tires, or as in the case of insufficient central respiratory drive, there will be decreasing or no respiratory distress. Thus, a child with a history of breathing difficulty may exhibit no respiratory distress and yet be in respiratory failure. *Respiratory failure is characterized by a depressed level of consciousness with or without signs of respiratory distress.*

The vast majority of cardiopulmonary arrests in children are caused by respiratory etiologies, and severe illness or injury of any type almost invariably has associated respiratory failure; therefore, ensuring the patency of the airway and normalizing respiration are essential in any resuscitation. Failure to manage the airway successfully is the leading cause of preventable mortality. *Stabilization of airway and breathing are the keys to successful pediatric resuscitations.*

Assessment

(1) History. A knowledge of duration of symptoms, history of choking or gagging episode, cough, the presence or absence of fever, past respiratory symptoms or diagnoses, or prematurity may help in localizing the site of disease.

(2) Physical examination as above is generally sufficient to make the diagnosis of respiratory failure. Frequent reassessment is critical for the child in respiratory distress to ensure that no progression to respiratory failure is occurring.

(3) Labs: Pulse oximetry is mandatory in any child with respiratory distress. Arterial blood gases if necessary will confirm hypoxia and determine acid-base status and P_{CO_2}. Radiographs of the neck in cases of upper airway obstruction, and of the chest in lower airway obstruction may be helpful. Radiographs to rule out foreign-body aspiration should include the entire airway, stomach, and include an assisted expiration view to assess air trapping.

Upper vs. lower airway obstruction causes of respiratory distress. Table 28–3 lists common causes. The upper airway extends from nasopharynx to carina, the lower airway from carina to the most distal gas exchange unit. Upper airway obstruction is characterized by increased work of breathing during inspiration and signs of upper airway narrowing such as stridor. This

Table 28–3. Common causes of upper and lower airway obstruction.

Upper Airway	
Common	**Uncommon**
Croup	Epiglottitis
Foreign body	Bacterial tracheitis
	Retropharyngeal abscess/cellulitis
	Peritonsillar abscess
	Congenital defects
Lower Airway	
Common	**Uncommon**
Reactive airway disease	Pulmonary edema
Pneumonia	Acidosis, any cause
Foreign body	Pulmonary contusion
	Congestive heart failure
	Severe anemia

inspiratory work leads to an increase in the ratio of inspiration to expiration, which is normally roughly 1:1. Conversely, lower airway obstruction will lead to expiratory work and an I:E ratio of 1:2 or more. Stridor will be absent, but wheezing, rales, or other adventitious breath sounds may be heard.

SHOCK

Shock is defined as inadequate tissue perfusion. It is a clinical diagnosis, not relying on BP determination or lab values. The diagnosis of shock can and should be made by examination.

Assessment
Assessment is described above under "Circulation." See Table 28–4 for differentiation and initial therapy for shock states.

Treatment
(1) Institute ALS care as described above. Maintain a patent airway and support breathing if necessary. Hypotensive or severely acidotic patients should be intubated and ventilated.

(2) Administer 100% oxygen.

(3) Place patient in Trendelenburg position unless respiratory distress is present.

(4) Establish IV access. Two large-bore IV catheters are

Table 28-4. Differentiation of shock states and initial therapy.

	Hypovolemic	Distributive	Cardiogenic
Etiologies	Vomiting/ diarrhea, blood loss	Anaphylaxis, sepsis, neurogenic	Dysrhythmias, congenital heart disease, myocarditis
Pathophysiology	Inadequate intravascular volume	Vasogenic maldistribution of vascular volume	Pump failure, inadequate cardiac output or increase afterload
Diagnosis	History, normal cardiac exam	History (allergic or infectious etc), toxic appearance with septic shock, normal cardiac exam	Exam: poor perfusion, rales, hepatomegaly, abnormal heart sounds
Initial treatment	Crystalloid infusion	Crystalloid infusion, pressors if refractory	Fluid restriction, pressors, diuretics, ± afterload reducers

required for hypotensive patients. Consider intraosseous access. Follow access guidelines described below.

(5) Rapidly infuse isotonic crystalloid (LR or NS). Use 20 mL/kg boluses, with reassessment of perfusion between boluses. Colloid infusion, (eg, albumin) can be considered after 3 boluses or if signs of increased capillary permeability are present.

(6) Consider vasopressor support (Table 28-5) if there is inadequate response to volume infusion.

(7) CVP determination will guide therapy in refractory shock states.

(8) Place foley catheter and maintain urine output of > 1 mL/kg/h.

(9) Send blood for indicated lab determinations.

MONITORING

All very sick or injured children should have a minimum level of monitoring, lines, and tubes: (1) 100% oxygen; (2) continuous cardiorespiratory monitoring; (3) pulse oximetry; (4) intra-

Table 28–5. Emergency pediatric drugs and pressors.[1]

Atropine

Indications: 1) Bradycardia, due to cardiac etiologies
2) Vagal tone excess, eg, during laryngoscopy and intubation
3) Anticholinesterase poisoning
4) Asystole, after epinephrine use.
5) Epinephrine first-line for hypoxic/ischemic induced bradycardia

Dose: 0.01–0.02 mg/kg
maximum 1–2 mg

Route: IV, IO, ET

Note: Atropine may be useful in hemodyanically significant primary cardiac-based bradycardias. Because of paradoxical bradycardia somtimes seen in infants, a minimum 0.1 mg dose is recommended by the American Heart Association.

Sodium Bicarbonate

Indications: 1) Documented metabolic acidosis
2) Empiric treatment for presumed acidosis
3) Hyperkalemia

Dose: 1–2 meq/kg empirically, or by ABG

Route: IV, IO

Note: Sodium bicarbonate will be effective only if the patient is adequately oxygenated, ventilated, and perfused. Has some adverse side effects.

Calcium chloride

Indications: 1) Documented hypocalcemia
2) Calcium-channel blocker overdose
3) Hyperkalemia, hypermagnesemia

Dose: 10–30 mg/kg slowly

Route: IV, preferably centrally; IO

Note: Calcium is no longer indicated for asystole or EMD. Potent tissue necrosis if infiltration occurs. Use with caution.

Epinephrine

Indications: 1) Bradycardia, especially hypoxic–ischemic
2) Hypotension (by infusion)
3) Asystole
4) Fine ventricular fibrillation refractory to initial defibrillation
5) Electromechanical dissociation
6) Anaphylaxis

Dose/route: IV/IO: 0.01 mg/kg of 1:10,000 solution. Repeat at no more than five minute intervals. If initial dose unsuccessful, use at least twice the initial dose for subsequent doses.
ET: .02–.03 mg/kg
IO: as IV
SC: (anaphylactic shock): 0.01 mg/kg 1:1000 solution = .01 mL/kg max dose 0.3–0.5 mL.
Infusion: 0.1–1.0 μg/kg/min

Note: Epinphrine is the single most important drug in pediatric resuscitation. Evidence from animal studies and small series of human subjects indicates that the present recommended dose may be insufficient and that doses of 0.2–0.3 mg/kg may be a more optimal dose. A randomized controlled trial has not been done.

(continued)

Table 28–5. Emergency pediatric drugs and pressors.[1] *(continued)*

Glucose

Indications: 1) Hypoglycemia
              2) Altered mental status, empirically
              3) With insulin, for hyperkalemia
Dose: 0.5–1.0 g/kg
Route: IV, IO
Note: Neonates—2 mL/kg D_{10}
              Older child—2–4 mL/kg D_{25}
              6–10 mL/kg D_{10}

Naloxone (Narcan)

Indications: 1) Opiate overdose
              2) Altered mental status—empiric
Dose: 0.1 mg/kg <10 kg
              .01 mg/kg >10 kg
Route: IV, IO, ETT
Note: Side effects are few. A dose of 2.0 mg may be given in young children, 4.0 mg in adolescents. Repeat as necessary, or as constant infusion in narcotic overdoses.

Dopamine: Usually first line inotrope. Stimulates beta and dopaminergic receptors. At higher doses alpha effects predominate. Dose 5–20 μg/kg/minute. Renal and splanchnic vasodilation at low doses. Central access recommended for all pressors.

Dobutamine: Increases stroke volume without increasing myocardial oxygen consumption. Safer than epinephrine or isoproterenol infusions. Beta-adrenergic. Dose 1–10 μg/kg/minute.

Amrinone: Phosphodiesterase inhibitor. Provides inotropy and afterload reduction. May cause dysrhythmias. Dose; initial bolus 0.75 mg/kg over 3 minutes, then infusion 5–10 μg/kg/minute.

Epinephrine: Very potent inotrope and chronotrope. Increases SVR markedly. Alpha-adrenergic . Significant potential toxicities, eg, dysrhythmias, ischemia. Dose: 0.05–1.0 μg/kg/minute.

Isoproterenol: Pure beta agonist. Useful for resistant heart block. May drop SVR and cause peripheral vasodilation, therefore ensure normal volume status when initiating. Increases myocardial oxygen consumption and may cause tachdysrhythmias. Dose: 0.05–1.0 μg/kg/minute.

[1] ET = endotracheal; IO = intraosseous; IV = intravenous; SC = subcutaneous.

venous access of at least one and preferably two short, large-bore peripheral IVs. If peripheral IV access is not established within ninety seconds, initiate attempts at more central access, including intraosseous lines, percutaneous catheterization of the femoral, internal or external jugular, or subclavian veins, or cutdown of the antecubital, saphenous, or femoral veins, depending on the expertise of the providers available. Central access is preferred for infusion of vasopressors or CVP monitoring. Consider arterial monitoring for beat-to-beat BP monitoring or for frequent lab draws. (5) blood pressure determinations every five to ten minutes; (6) nasogastric tube placement for any patients receiving positive-pressure ventilation or with ileus or surgical abdomens; (7) foley catheter placement for children in shock or receiving prolonged ventilation, if no contraindications exist (see Trauma); (8) cervical spine immobilization and placement on a backboard if spinal injury is possible.

Empiric Treatment

Patients with altered mental status should receive 100% oxygen, naloxone 1 mg IV in a younger child, 2 mg IV in an older child, and dextrose 0.5–1.0 g/kg (2–4 mL/kg D_{25}). Patients presenting with cardiorespiratory failure, particularly if there is a history suggestive of infection or the patient is immunosuppressed, (eg, oncology, transplant, sickle-cell anemia patients), should receive empiric broad-spectrum IV antibiotics such as cefotaxime or ceftriaxone, and ampicillin in infants < 3 mos. Cultures can be obtained after stabilization occurs.

Additional Physical Examination

Following assessment and stabilization of the ABC's, perform a more detailed examination, including: (1) general state, including Level of Consciousness (LOC), hydration status, and tone; (2) head and neck, ruling out trauma; (3) cardiovascular exam; (4) abdominal exam, looking for masses, tenderness, or organomegaly; (5) genitourinary exam; (6) musculoskeletal exam, ruling out injuries; (7) complete neurologic exam including pupil size and reactivity and funduscopic exam; (8) the skin, for signs of injury or infection. Keep in mind the possibility of ingestions or exposures for patients without clear etiologies for their deterioration.

Labs & Radiographs

(1) Obtain a bedside glucose determination. Particularly in infants and small children, serious illness is often accompanied by hypoglycemia.

(2) For children presenting with cardiorespiratory collapse, obtain complete blood count, electrolytes, serum glucose, creatinine, BUN, arterial blood gas, and blood culture.

(3) Consider liver function tests and serum ammonia, particularly if there is altered mental status or hypoglycemia.

(4) Do urinalysis and toxicology screen.

(5) Consider calcium, magnesium and phosphorus determinations if the patient may be postictal or is actively seizing.

Diagnostic imaging is directed by history or exam findings. Consider cranial CT for children with altered mental status if there is a possibility of trauma, if there are lateralizing neurologic findings, or signs of intracranial hypertension.

Summary

Care of the critically ill or injured child is a team effort. An organized approach with strict attention to the stabilization of Airway, Breathing, and Circulation will ensure an optimal outcome. *Frequent reassessment* is mandatory to detect deterioration.

EMERGENCY DRUGS

Maintenance of breathing and circulation remain the mainstays of pediatric resuscitations. Oxygen and epinephrine are the principal drugs of use in pediatrics, although the full complement of ALS medications are used. Principles of use include:

(1) Use the appropriate pediatric dose based on weight in kilograms.

(2) Be aware of different delivery modalities, eg, any drug that can be given intravenously can be given IO, and some drugs can be given via endotracheal tube (naloxone, epinephrine, atropine, and lidocaine).

(3) Administer medications close to the IV catheter and flush in with saline,

(4) Use code cards or sheets with preprinted drug dosages and equipment sizes whenever possible to minimize dosing errors. A resuscitation tape is available that uses the child's height to estimate weight, determined by placing the patient directly on the tape, to directly give drug doses and equipment sizes.

Table 28–5 contains a list of the most commonly used drugs and vasopressors.

TRAUMA

Background

Death due to injuries is the leading cause of death for children. Previously, trauma care was solely the domain of surgeons.

It is now clear that optimal outcomes for this very important subset of the pediatric population come from a multidisciplinary approach utilizing emergency pediatricians, pediatric surgeons, pediatric intensivists, and other essential support services such as neurosurgery and orthopedics. This impressive array of resources can be found at designated pediatric trauma centers. However, the majority of injured children are not taken care of in these centers; therefore, pediatricians must be able to participate in initial assessment and stabilization before transport to a referral facility. Pediatricians need to be aware of trauma's sobering statistics and become actively involved in the entire spectrum of care of the traumatized child, from injury prevention to pre-hospital, hospital-based care, and rehabilitation. The federal Emergency Medical Services for Children grants have helped to upgrade the pediatric capability of existing EMS services nationwide.

Epidemiology

Common mechanisms of injury include motor vehicle accidents, either as occupants or pedestrians, falls, sporting injuries, and drownings. Blunt injuries predominate over penetrating injuries from gunshot wounds or stabbings by 9:1. Toddlers and teenagers are most at risk, and males are more frequently injured than females. Head injury is common in major injuries and is usually the cause of death. Abdominal injuries are common and frequently difficult to diagnose. Injury prevention efforts at every level of the health-care system are essential.

Approach

(1) Organize a trauma receiving team with appropriate composition and a designated team leader.

(2) Assign roles for the resuscitation, including airway management, establishment of IV access, lab drawing, and so on.

(3) Assemble subspecialists, eg, neurosurgeons, as indicated by prehospital communications, and technologists, eg, radiology technicians.

(4) Assign a pediatric trauma score to assist in prognosis.

(5) Document interventions with times.

(6) A calm atmosphere in the trauma receiving unit will enhance thoughtful care.

(7) Compile a problem list as pathology is identified to assist in determining priorities for care.

(8) Never neglect a child's pain and fear. Strongly consider

analgesia and sedation in appropriate patients. Constant reassurance is helpful. Enlist the aid of social workers or Child Life workers whenever possible.

Primary Survey

The assessment of the trauma patient is divided into the primary and secondary surveys. This system is useful in the approach to the child with multi-system, life-threatening injuries, or life- or limb-threatening single-system injuries, as well as to apparently less severely injured children. The primary survey is the rapid initial assessment which attempts to identify and immediately treat life-threatening problems. It ascertains physiologic derangements, eg, respiratory failure or shock, and does not include anatomic diagnoses such as fractured pelvis. The primary survey is the *resuscitation* phase, while the secondary survey represents steps toward diagnosis and definitive care for each injury. The primary survey is comprised of:

A: Airway, with cervical spine control.
B: Breathing.
C: Circulation, with hemorrhage control.
D: Disability, a rapid neurologic assessment.
E: Expose and examine.

The approach to the trauma ABCDEs is exactly like the ABCs above, ie, each system is assessed sequentially, and the integrity of that system assured before moving to the next system. Small children are notorious for having significant internal injuries with an initially normal appearance and no cutaneous signs of significant injury. Assessment and initial interventions in the primary survey are described below.

A. Airway With Cervical Spine Control: Considerations are similar to airway assessment and management as discussed above, with the addition of in-line cervical immobilization. (1) Initially, maintain in-line immobilization of the head in neutral position with gentle axial manual traction. (2) Then provide a rigid collar and tape across the forehead and chin. These precautions should be left in place until appropriate radiologic and clinical exams have been conducted. (3) The head should be padded with towel rolls across the top and sides of the head. (4) The entire child should be strapped tightly to a backboard. If the child vomits, the backboard can then be log-rolled while maintaining the entire spine in-line. (5) Suction the mouth and nose of blood and secretions. (6) Remove foreign bodies in the mouth and loose teeth. (7) Every patient should receive 100% oxygen while the assessment proceeds. (8) Intubate the trachea of severely injured patients who have airway obstruction or who are unconscious. Consider rapid-sequence neuroinduction for non-flaccid patients. Oral intubation is generally possible even while maintaining cervical spine precautions and is the route of choice. Nasotracheal intubation is an alternative in teens with spontaneous respirations, if cribriform plate fracture is unlikely. (9) Consider needle cricothyroidotomy if severe midface trauma is present or if endotracheal intubation cannot be achieved.

B. Breathing Assessment: Assessment proceeds just as detailed in the first section. (1) Determine respiratory effort, rate, adequacy and symmetry of chest rise and fall, increased work of breathing, and focal decreases in breath sounds. (2) In the trauma setting, always consider hemo- and/or pneumothorax. Signs include tracheal shift, decreased breath sounds on the side of the pneumothorax, and subcutaneous crepitus. Cyanosis, bradycardia, jugular venous distension, and hypotension may be present. Suspicion of pneumothorax or hemothorax calls for immediate tube thoracostomy placement of sufficient diameter to drain blood. Placement is in the fifth intercostal space in the midaxillary line. (3) Quickly examine the chest for wounds sufficient to cause open pneumothorax (sucking chest wound). Occlude these on three sides with vaseline-impregnated gauze and ensure positive-pressure ventilation.

C. Circulation Assessment With Hemorrhage Control: Circulation is again assessed in an identical fashion to that described above. (1) Bleeding wounds are controlled quickly by direct pressure with a gauze bandage. (2) Remember to detect the early signs of shock in the child with tachycardia and delayed CFT. (3) Insert two large-bore, short peripheral IV catheters. Alternatives for access are discussed above in circulation. If it is necessary to place IO lines, obtain additional personnel to then place a more secure central line. (4) When placing lines, obtain blood for lab work as below. (5) *Shock management of trauma patients:* Begin rapid intravascular replacement with boluses of crystalloid (Lactated Ringer's solution or normal saline), at a rate of 20 mL/kg of body weight, with reassessment of perfusion after each bolus. If hypoperfusion or hypotension persist after three crystalloid boluses, begin blood infusions of 10 cc/kg. Use cross-matched blood, or type-specific if unavailable. Patients in extremis may receive O⁻ blood. Use a fluid warmer for all administered fluids. (6) Muffled heart sounds, poor pulses, nar-

Table 28–6. AVPU system for evaluation of level of consciousness.

A—Alert
V—responsive to Voice
P—responsive to Pain
U—Unresponsive

rowed pulse pressure, and hypotension suggest cardiac tamponade and mandate immediate pericardiocentesis.

D. Disability: A brief neurologic examination is performed to exclude conditions requiring immediate treatment. (1) Characterize the LOC by the AVPU system (Table 28–6). (2) Determine pupil size and reactivity. If one or both pupils are dilated and unreactive or sluggishly reactive to light, begin treating for presumed intracranial hypertension. (3) Briefly check for spinal cord integrity by looking for spontaneous movement of the extremities or localization of painful stimulus in the legs. (4) Suspected *ICP elevation* is treated by elevating the head to 30°, hyperventilation to a PCO_2 of 24–28, maintaining the head in the midline to avoid impedance to venous return from the head, and avoidance of painful stimuli, and administering mannitol 0.5–1.0 g/kg IV. Obtain immediate neurosurgical consultation.

E. Expose & Examine: The child should be completely undressed and examined, and logrolling used to examine the back. During this time it is important to maintain temperature with warming lights and/or warmed blankets applied to previously inspected areas.

Secondary Survey

After the resuscitative or primary phase has been completed, a detailed head-to-toe exam is done. Ensure that all appropriate tubes have been placed. Space permits only a brief description below.

A. Skin: Look for abrasions, lacerations, and contusions. Cutaneous findings may signify underlying pathology, eg, a contusion on the thorax may overlie a pulmonary contusion. Careful cleaning and selective debridement is important. Ensure immunization status is made current.

B. Head & Neck: Perform a detailed exam. Palpate for bony defects. Look for signs of CSF leak (clear or serosanguinous drainage from ears or nose) or basilar skull fracture (hemotympanum, raccoon eyes, or Battle's sign). Rule out broken or misaligned teeth, nasal septal displacement, tracheal deviation, jugular venous distension, limitation of extraocular movements, and cranial nerve palsies.

C. Chest: Tamponade and hemopneumothoraces will have been decompressed in the primary survey. Chest x-ray or chest CT may reveal pulmonary contusions. Myocardial contusions are rare but should be considered with blunt direct anterior thorax injury, as should dissecting aortic injuries. Paradoxic chest wall movements suggest flail chest segments.

D. Abdomen: Penetrating injuries violating the peritoneum require operative exploration. Blunt injuries to liver, spleen, kidneys, and hollow viscera represent a diagnostic challenge. Diagnosis depends on: (1) serial examinations for bowel sounds, tenderness, and organ size; (2) plain films to rule out free intra-abdominal air and CT with double contrast; (3) liver functions tests, which have fair sensitivity but good specificity for liver injuries, and amylase testing for traumatic pancreatitis. (4) in selected unstable patients, diagnostic peritoneal lavage (DPL) to look for blood or intestinal contamination.

E. Pelvis & Genitourinary: Palpate for pelvic instability, pain with direct pressure, or crepitus. Blood at the urinary meatus or in the scrotum, an abnormal prostate, or pelvic fracture suggest the possibility of urethral disruption. Urethrogram should be done before foley catheter placement when these signs are present. Examine the vagina for injuries. Rectal examination is always done to assess tone and to hemetest.

F. Musculoskeletal: Inspect for bony swelling, pain, tenderness, and neurovascular status. Examine the back by logrolling. Assess pulses, perfusion, and neurologic function distal to fractures. Delayed diagnoses of long-bone fractures are unfortunately not uncommon in unconscious children.

G. Neurologic: Perform a detailed examination of mental status, speech, cranial nerves, tone, strength, sensation, cerebellar signs, and reflexes. Perform serial AVPU assessments or employ pediatric Glasgow coma scales (Table 28–7). Consider high-dose methylprednisolone therapy for acute spinal cord injuries.

Discussion of closed head injury follows.

Labs & Radiographs

(1) Laboratory determinations: Routine tests include complete blood count, electrolytes, amylase, and liver function tests,

TAble 28–7. Glasgow Coma Scale.

Eye opening response	
Spontaneous	4
To speech	3
To pain	2
None	1
Verbal response	
Oriented	5
Confused conversation	4
Inappropriate words	3
Incomprehensible sounds	2
None	1
Best upper limb motor response	
Obeys	6
Localizes	5
Withdraws	4
Abnormal flexion	3
Extensor response	2
None	1

type and crossmatch for one unit of PRBC's for each 10 kg of body weight, and urinalysis for hematuria. Consider coagulation studies, creatinine, and toxicology screens.

(2) Radiographs: Routine films include lateral, anterior-posterior, and odontoid view of the cervical spine, chest, and pelvis. Abdominal and long bone films are performed as indicated.

CT of the head and abdomen have become very common. Special studies such as urethrograms and aortograms are obtained in consultation with subspecialty members of the trauma team.

CLOSED HEAD INJURY (CHI)

CHI is one of the most common injuries seen in a pediatric ED. Complications include subdural, epidural, and parenchymal hemorrhage, cerebral edema, and CSF leak and subsequent infection. A clinical classification system (Table 28–8) allows one to determine which patients deserve observation, cranial CT, neurosurgical consultation, admission, or emergent neuroresuscitation.

Assessment

Apply the ABCDEs of trauma resuscitation. *Historical points* to be determined:

Table 28–8. Clinical classification of head-inhjured patients.[1]

Mild:	No LOC[2] or amnesia; alert, oriented; asymptomatic or slight headache with dizziness only
Moderate:	Possible findings: History of LOC,[2] amnesia; posttraumatic seizure; vomiting; more than slight headache; listlessness, lethargy
Severe:	Possible findings: Disoriented, unable to follow commands; decreasing level of consciousness; focal neurologic signs; penetrating skull injury or depressed skull fracture

[1] From Rosenthal BW, Bergman I: Intracranial injury after moderate head trauma in children. *J Pediatr* 1989;**115**:346–350. By permission.
[2] LOC = loss of consciousness.

(1) Mechanism of injury: How significant was the decelerative force? Shear stresses result from the shaken baby syndrome.

(2) Mental status immediately following the injury: Was there loss of consciousness or subsequent confusion or amnesia?

(3) Behavior since the injury: Has there been vomiting, headache, altered vision, or abnormal mental status?

Examination should center on:

(1) General level of consciousness and trend: Is the child becoming more obtunded, remaining stable, or gradually lightening?

(2) Rule out associated injuries, eg, mandibular fractures, scalp or skull injuries, CSF leak, signs of basilar skull fracture, or cervical spine injuries.

(3) Complete neurologic examination, including serial mental status assessments and evidence of antero- or retrograde amnesia.

(4) Complete vital signs, paying attention to signs of Cushing's triad (bradycardia, hypertension, irregular respirations).

(5) Consider non-accidental trauma if the injuries observed are inconsistent with the history given.

Diagnostic Imaging

Plain films of the skull are of little therapeutic significance unless there is concern for depressed skull fracture or penetrating injury. Fractures across the distribution of the middle meningeal artery are no longer thought to deserve CT for the perception of increased risk for intracranial bleeding. The morbidity from CHI stems from intracranial processes, not skull fractures *per se*. Obtain CT of the head for patients with persistent vomiting, an abnormal neurologic exam, or deteriorating level of consciousness.

Concussion

A brief loss or alteration of consciousness followed by a return to the normal state is defined as a concussion. Patients may present with amnesia, pallor, or several episodes of vomiting. The examination is normal and there is no anatomic damage to brain tissue.

Contusion

A bruise of the brain tissue constitutes a cerebral contusion. Level of consciousness is depressed, and focal neurologic findings correspond to the contused area of the brain.

Acute Intracranial Pressure Elevation

Acute ICP elevation occurs not only in the setting of CHI, but also with CNS infections, metabolic derangements (eg, DKA or Reye's syndrome), hydrocephalus, ventriculoperitoneal shunt obstruction, cerebrovascular accident, and tumor. Herniation syndromes may or may not be associated. Early recognition and immediate treatment are essential to avoid disastrous outcomes.

Diagnosis

Symptoms include: (1) increasing headache; (2) decreasing level of consciousness, usually listlessness progressing to lethargy and obtundation; (3) visual changes, eg, diplopia or loss of visual acuity; and (4) vomiting.

Examination findings may include: (1) decreased level of consciousness; (2) stiff neck; (3) cranial nerve palsies; and the late findings of (4) sluggish or frankly unreactive, dilated pupils; (5) Cushing's triad; (6) papilledema.

Management

Measures to control ICP must be immediately instituted. Strict attention to the ABCs is paramount.

(1) Intubate the trachea and hyperventilate to a P_{CO_2} of approximately 25. Use a neuroinductive rapid sequence technique to avoid the elevation in ICP that comes with laryngoscopy and intubation.

(2) Elevate the head of the bed to 30°.

(3) Keep the head in the midline to avoid impedance of venous flow from the head.

(4) Administer mannitol 0.5–1.0 g/kg IV.

(5) Infuse fluids at no more than two-thirds of maintenance rates while maintaining a normal intravascular volume with intermittent boluses as needed.

(6) Avoid painful stimuli.

(7) Treat fever.

(8) Obtain neurosurgical consultation.

(9) Admit to a PICU or operating room.

A common problem is a child who is hypotensive but who appears to have increased ICP. In this case restoration of circulating volume takes precedence over restriction of fluids in consideration of ICP. Remember that cerebral perfusion pressure is the ICP minus the mean arterial pressure, therefore MAP needs to be maintained to have adequate CPP. Once normal intravascular volume has been restored, fluids can be reduced to two-thirds of the maintenance rates. Invasive monitoring will guide further therapy. Never perform lumbar puncture acutely if there is concern for elevated ICP.

Disposition

(1) Mild injuries: Children with no history of loss of consciousness and no vomiting who have a normal general and neurologic exam on presentation have a very low risk of serious intracranial injuries and can be discharged after a brief period of observation with detailed discharge instructions.

(2) Moderate injuries: Patients with the above risk factors of vomiting or LOC and who may not have a normal mental status on admission to the ED require serial neurologic examinations. If the child's mental status is becoming more normal with time and there are no lateralizing signs, the patient may be observed for a period of hours until normal, then discharged with instructions. Advise the parents that intracranial hemorrhages can slowly accumulate, such that they may not present for several days after the injury. If the child isn't responsive to voice commands, has lateralizing signs, or has progressive decrease in level of consciousness, obtain a cranial CT. If CT is normal, the child can be observed further in the ED or in-hospital and discharged when completely normal. Abnormal CT's mandate consultation by a neurosurgeon.

(3) Severe injuries: As detailed above, these children deserve cerebral resuscitation, neurosurgical consultation, and admission to PICU.

BURNS

Thermal injury has a horrible morbidity and mortality to children. The nature, extent and thickness of the burn, as well as associated injuries, should be ascertained in the initial evaluation.

Classification

The depth of thermal injury through epidermis and dermis determines classification. *Superficial* burns (formerly first-degree), as typified by sunburn, are dry, warm, painful, and hypersensitive. They heal without specific treatment. *Partial-thickness* (formerly second-degree) burns affect epidermis and variable but not complete elements of the dermis. Partial thickness burns can be superficial, resulting in burns that are red, painful, and potentially blistered; or deep, resulting in dry, white, and hyposensitive burns. Treatment depends on depth of damage. *Full-thickness* (formerly third-degree) burns affect all epidermal and dermal elements, and are anesthetic, white, avascular, dry, and leathery-appearing. Skin grafting helps ameliorate the uneven and hard fibrotic scar formation as healing proceeds.

Management

A. Superficial Burns: cool compresses and analgesia.

B. Partial-Thickness Burns: These should be aseptically debrided, washed with 1% dilute povidone-iodine solution, copiously irrigated with normal saline, and dressed with topical antibiotic, commonly silver sulfadiazine, although Polysporin or Neosporin can be used in smaller areas. Open blisters should be debrided. The wounds should be covered with a bulky dressing and serially examined, starting within 24 hours. Burns of the hands, feet, face, perineum, or other sensitive areas with the potential for contractions or disfiguration should be referred to a burn surgeon. Always provide appropriate analgesia.

C. Full-Thickness Burns & Extensive or Deep Partial-Thickness Burns: These injuries place particular importance on the ABC's of trauma management, as the pediatric airway may become obstructed by thermal injury, there may be hypoxic or smoke inhalation injury to the lungs, and there are substantial fluid management problems associated with major burns. Be aware of the possibility of toxic byproducts of combustion such as cyanide and carbon monoxide. A burn surgeon should be promptly consulted. See the burn resuscitation protocol.

MAJOR BURN RESUSCITATION PROTOCOL

- Secure the airway.
- Administer 100% oxygen.
- Assist ventilation if needed.
- Obtain IV access.
- Normalize perfusion.
- Remove all clothing.
- Stop the burning process (irrigate).
- Perform complete examination.

Fluid Management for Major Burns

Substantial fluid loss occurs through burned skin, and there is increased capillary permeability. It is essential to maintain normal intravascular volume. Fig 28–2 shows percentage of BSA by body part for infants and children. The Parkland formula for fluid replacement is 4 mL/kg/percent BSA burned for the first 24 hours, with half in the first 8 hours, in addition to maintenance rates.

Disposition

Minor superficial burns and superficial partial-thickness burns can be treated as outpatients if appropriate follow-up and analgesia can be provided. Admission will be necessary for major burns, defined as > 10% BSA for superficial and partial-thickness burns, or > 2% if full thickness, or burns involving eyes, ears, face, perineum, hands or feet, or associated with fractures.

ELECTRICAL INJURIES

Complications of electrical injuries include

(1) Burns: even brief contact with a high voltage source will cause thermal damage. Search for exit wounds. Care is the same as that for other burns.

(2) Dysrhythmia: Current traversing the heart from lightning or household/industrial sources can cause non-perfusing ventricular dysrhythmia.

(3) Neurologic injuries: Early signs include disorientation and peripheral nerve injury; late injuries are neuropsychiatric in nature, eg, concentration or memory defects.

(4) Internal injuries: Passage of current through the body can cause an arc of thermal injury with extensive damage to deep tissues.

Name_____ Age_____ Ward_____

First-degree erythema not to be included. 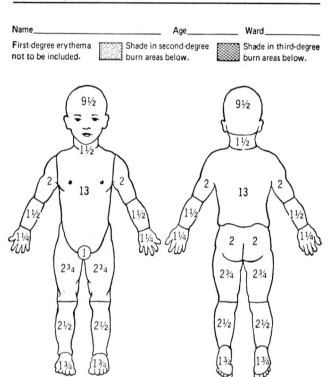 Shade in second-degree burn areas below. Shade in third-degree burn areas below.

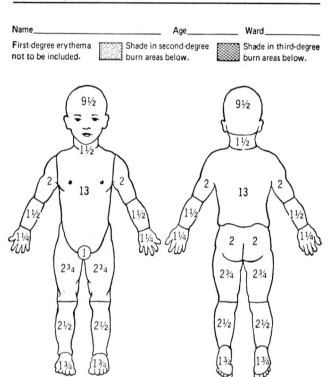

(Above: Infant < 1 yr of age)

Area*	Age (yr)					
	0	1	5	10	15	Adult
Head area	19%	17%	13%	11%	9%	7%
Trunk area	26%	26%	26%	26%	26%	26%
Arm area	7%	7%	7%	7%	7%	7%
Thigh area	5½%	6½%	8½%	8½%	9½%	9½%
Leg area	5%	5%	5%	6%	6%	7%

Total third-degree burns_____ %
Total second-degree burns_____ %   TOTAL BURNS _____ %

*The neck, hands, buttocks, genitalia, and feet are not included in this chart.

Figure 28–2. Lund and Browder modification of Berkow's scale for estimating extent of burns.

Electric cord injuries deserve special mention. Commonly a young child will bite an electric cord, sustaining burns to the oral commissure. Initially the burns appear gray and necrotic. Delayed coagulation around the mouth may occur. Sloughing of the eschar as the wound heals days later may lead to brisk bleeding.

Disposition

All but the most superficial injuries will require hospital admission. Surgical revision of burns may be necessary.

BITES AND STINGS

Bites

Many ED visits are due to bites, generally from domestic animals. Most fatalities are from dog bites, infectious complications can result from cat and human bites.

General Care

All wounds require that tetanus immunization be current, administer tetanus immune globulin if unimmunized. The occurrence of rabies is unusual, except in feral animals. Follow local reporting rules. Suture bite wounds, especially cat and human bites, only if necessary for cosmetic reasons. If a bite involves a joint capsule, periosteum, or neurovascular bundle, consult an orthopedic surgeon. All wounds should receive high-pressure, high-volume irrigation with judicious debridement of ragged or devitalized edges, and removal of foreign material.

Dog Bites

Wounds are generally laceration/puncture. Infecting organisms include *Pasteurella multocida,* streptococci, staphylococci, and anaerobes. Prophylactic antibiotics have not been shown to improve outcome in uncomplicated dog bites not involving hands or feet. Dog bites that have become infected can be treated with penicillin for coverage against *P multocida,* or broader spectrum coverage can be provided by cefalexin or amoxicillin and clavulanic acid, if parenteral therapy is not made necessary by toxicity, bony involvement, or extensive cellulitis. Complications of dog bites include CNS infections, osteomyelitis, septic arthritis, sepsis, and endocarditis.

Cat Bites

Because a cat bite creates a puncture-wound inoculum, there should be even greater reluctance to suture, and prophylactic antibiotics are recommended. *P multocida* is the most common infecting organism, and antibiotic coverage is as recommended for dog bites. Complications include cat scratch disease, cellulitis, tenosynovitis, osteomyelitis, and septic arthritis.

Human Bites

Most human bites stem from assaults, particularly the "fight bite," where the clenched fist strikes teeth, exposing the metacarpophalangeal joint to infection. These wounds should receive operative debridement by a hand surgeon and intravenous antibiotics. Infected human bites commonly grow from culture streptococci, anaerobes, staphylococci, and *Eikenella corrodens*. Coverage against these organisms is recommended.

Insect Stings & Arthropod Bites

Stings are common and generally not serious. Biting arthropods such as spiders, millipedes, scorpions, ticks, and mites abound, but rarely cause serious injury or mortality. Anaphylaxis is the most important sequela.

A. Insect Stings: Bee and wasp stings cause immediate pain, swelling, pruritus, and redness. Myriad home remedies such as meat tenderizer have been advocated but never proven to be effective. Presentation and treatment of anaphylaxis is described below.

B. Spider Bites: Only a few species, such as black widows, tarantulas, and brown recluse spiders commonly cause serious envenomations. Black widow bites may pass unnoticed by the child. Local erythema and edema may progress to significant symptoms such as excruciating pain within one hour. Classically, severe abdominal pain and/or thorax and back pain are present.

Treatment

A. Anaphylaxis: Anaphylaxis accounts for many deaths per year and requires aggressive therapy. Symptoms include chest or neck tightness, faintness, dizziness, syncope, or disorientation. Signs may include face and neck swelling, upper airway obstruction, wheezing, urticaria, and hypotension. Immediate treatment consists of: (1) 100% oxygen; (2) subcutaneous epinephrine 0.01 mL/kg of 1:1000 solution, up to 0.5 mL maximum dose; (3) endotracheal intubation if upper airway obstruction is evolving; (4) IV access; (5) volume support, and vasopressors if unresponsive to crystalloid infusion; and (6) treat bronchospasm with albuterol or other inhaled beta-adrenergic agents. Children experiencing systemic symptoms should be referred to an allergist for consideration of desensitization and provision of an epinephrine auto-injection pen.

B. General Treatment: (1) Apply cool compresses and elevate the sting or bite site. (2) Cleanse the wound site. (3) Ensure tetanus immunization status is current. (4) Administer oral antihistamines, eg, diphenhydramine or hydroxyzine, for pruritus. (5) Admit children with moderate or severe symptoms to the hospital.

Black widow antivenom is available but has significant side effects. Calcium and benzodiazepines have been used for severe black widow bite symptoms.

HYPOTHERMIA

Hypothermia is defined as a core temperature less than 35°C. Most often in pediatrics it is associated with cold-water submersion accidents. Other associations include sepsis, static encephalopathy, ingestions, and metabolic disorders. Hypothermia represents a failure of the normally closely-regulated physiologic mechanisms to maintain a normal body temperature. As core temperature falls, peripheral vasoconstriction gives way to hypothalamic-mediated increases in muscle tone, metabolism, and shivering.

Clinical Findings

Signs depend on depth of temperature depression. Severe cases (<28°C.) mimic death: pupils are fixed and dilated, there is no discernable pulse or respirations, and muscles are rigid. If these changes are a *primary* result of hypothermia and are not simply post-mortem changes, then death cannot be declared until the patient has been rewarmed and resuscitative efforts are unsuccessful. Hence the ED saying: "They're not dead until they're warm and dead." Children have survived core temperatures as low as 19 °C neurologically intact.

Treatment

(1) Handle the patient gently, as the hypothermic myocardium is prone to ventricular fibrillation. (2) Document rewarming

with an indwelling low-reading rectal thermometer. (3) Treat ventricular fibrillation and asystole per PALS protocols including chest compressions. Spontaneous reversion to sinus rhythm may occur at 28–30°C degrees as rewarming proceeds. (4) If peripheral pulses are present, even as low as 6 per minute, withhold chest compressions, as even that low rate may be sufficient to satisfy the metabolic demands of the hypothermic child. (5) Correct hypoxemia and hypercapnia, clotting disturbances, acidemia, and glucose or electrolyte disturbances.

Rewarming

Rewarming interventions are passive or active, and the latter external or core.

Passive rewarming, such as by blankets, is appropriate only for mild cases (>33°C).

Active external rewarming: use warming lights, hot water bottles, heating pads, and warmed bags of IV fluid. Immersion in warm baths can be used only if monitoring is not necessary. Be aware of the potential for the ''core temperature afterdrop'' phenomenon as warmed cool acidemic blood is shunted to the core and rewarming proceeds.

Active core rewarming: This is the most effective method, and should be employed in any case of serious hypothermia. Techniques include: warmed humidified oxygen, IV fluids warmed (to 40°C) for gastric, bladder, and mediastinal lavage. Controlled core rewarming, and volume and electrolyte disturbances can be managed most effectively with hemodialysis and extracorporeal blood rewarming, and should be used whenever available.

HEAT ILLNESS

Heat injury and illness can be life-threatening, as in heat stroke, or mildly disabling, as in heat cramps. Most mild to moderate forms of heat illness can be avoided by acclimization and liberal salt and water intake during exercise.

Heat Stroke

A true emergency, representing a failure of thermoregulation. Diagnosis is based on a rectal temperature greater than 40°C, with associated neurologic findings. An exposure history must be present. Lack of sweating is *not* a necessary criterion.

CNS dysfunction is prominent, along with the symptoms of heat exhaustion, described below. Combativeness and disorientation are common, and in more severe cases, coma, nuchal rigidity, seizures and posturing are present. Cardiac output can be low, normal, or high. Complications are protean, and include rhabdomyolysis, DIC, myocardial and renal tubular necrosis, hepatic degeneration, ARDS, renal failure, electrolyte derangements, and hepatic degeneration. *After* rapid cooling is begun, consider other differential diagnoses: malignant hyperthermia, infection, neuroleptic malignant syndrome.

A. **Management:**

(1) Remove the patient from the heat source.

(2) Stabilize the ABCs.

(3) Immediately begin cooling the patient with ice, cooling fans, cool water mist, etc.

(4) Administer crystalloid: LR or NS for hypotension, 20 mL/kg initially, and D_5NS for maintenance fluid. Consider CVP determination.

(5) Initiate monitoring and tubes as detailed above, page 17.

(6) Laboratory tests: Electrolytes, liver function tests, glucose, BUN and creatinine, blood culture, PT/PTT, creatine kinase, serum magnesium, phosphate, calcium, arterial blood gases, and urinalysis.

(7) Admit to a PICU.

Heat Cramps

Heat cramps are brief and self-limited, albeit quite painful. Core temperature is normal or only slightly elevated. Cramping occurs in skeletal or abdominal muscles, but there is no muscle rigidity. Treat mild cases with oral salt-containing fluids; severe cases may require isotonic IV fluid.

Heat Exhaustion

Core temperature is normal or slightly elevated. Constitutional symptoms of weakness, disorientation, nausea and vomiting, poor perfusion, headache, and thirst, with or without muscle cramps, occur after exposure to heat and humidity. Patients continue to sweat, but there should be no major CNS dysfunction. Treat with IV isotonic fluids, modified when electrolyte levels have been determined.

ALTERED MENTAL STATUS/COMA

Many important disease entities present with altered mental status (AMS) as the only clue to their etiology. Optimal outcome is dependent on stabilizing the ABCs and empirically treating for entities that have rational therapies. For example, if one has already empirically treated the AMS with IV dextrose, no excess morbidity will ensue even when it isn't possible to diagnose emergently the myriad etiologies that present with hypoglycemia.

Differential Diagnosis

A useful mnemonic is "AEIOU TIPS":

A: Alcohol
E: Electrolyte disorders (principally sodium)
Encephalopathies (eg, Reye's, infectious, progressive)
Endocrine (eg, DKA, thyrotoxicosis, adrenal crisis)
I: Inborn errors
Intussusception (lethargy may precede any gastrointestinal symptoms)
O: Overdose (sedative/hypnotics, barbiturates, cyclic antidepressants, narcotics, OTC medications, cyanide, many others)
U: Uremia
T: Trauma (head injury, hemorrhagic shock, cellular injury, non-accidental)
I: Insulin (hypo/hyperglycemia)
P: Psychogenic (malingering)
S: Sepsis, stroke, shock, seizures

Management

Even with known ingestions, care is largely supportive. (1) Strict attention to the ABCs is vital. (2) Give 100% oxygen, naloxone 1–2 mg IV, dextrose .5–1.0 g/kg (2–4 mL/kg D_{25}), the "AMS cocktail." (3) Obtain a bedside glucose determination as soon as possible. (4) Obtain the *history*: duration of symptoms, fever, trauma, possibility of ingestion and drugs in the home, history suggestive of seizures, headaches, chronic illnesses and symptoms thereof. (5) Conduct a *physical examination*: complete vital signs, which often give clues to ingestions; respiratory pattern, eg, hyperventilation, Cheyne-Stokes, etc; posturing; pupillary size and reactivity; eye movements, including brainstem testing; meningismus, other clues to etiology such as cutaneous lesions, odor on breath, rash. (6) *Lab and diagnostic imaging*: electrolytes, complete blood count, glucose, creatinine, liver function tests, ammonia, blood culture, tox screen, urinalysis.

Consider cranial CT if signs of mass lesion, cerebral edema, or meningitis are present. If CT is normal proceed with a lumbar puncture. (7) Frequently reassess and maintain vital functions. (8) Consider consultation with neurologists and toxicologists and as indicated.

29 | Pediatric Procedures

Nancy Carlson, MD, &
Dale William Steele, BA, MD

RESTRAINT & POSITIONING

The optimal care of children logically includes an understanding of specific procedures often required in diagnosis and management. In most cases of failure to complete a procedure successfully, the fault lies in undue haste in preparing a struggling or crying patient. The physician should therefore become acquainted with various methods of restraining pediatric patients. Before starting any procedure, all items of equipment that may be needed should be set out for immediate use as required.

If drapes cover the child, adequate monitoring of cardiorespiratory function is mandatory. In using total body restraint, be certain that cardiorespiratory function is not impaired. Adequate analgesia and sedation should be considered when appropriate.

Many of the following procedures require the use of an iodine solution; the solution must be carefully washed off to prevent severe burns in neonates.

VENIPUNCTURE

The antecubital and external jugular veins are the safest and most frequently used large vessels for venipuncture and withdrawal of blood. (The femoral vein should be employed only in emergencies.) Smaller vessels in the dorsa of the hands and feet and scalp veins may also be used for withdrawing blood samples. Applying negative pressure with a syringe attached to the needle may cause collapse of these vessels because of their small size. Therefore, for these vessels, a different technique should be employed to obtain blood (see below).

The skin should be cleansed thoroughly with alcohol or an iodine solution. The use of a "butterfly" (21- or 23-gauge) needle will facilitate entry into the vein and subsequent withdrawal of blood.

Antecubital Vein Puncture

After placing a proximal turniquet, palpation of the antecubital vein is often possible even if it is not visible.

External Jugular Vein Puncture

A. Preparation: Wrap the child firmly so that the arms and legs are adequately restrained. The wraps should not extend higher than the shoulder girdle. Place the child on a flat, firm table so that both shoulders are touching the table; the head is rotated fully to one side and extended partly over the end of the table so as to align the vein (Fig. 29–1). Adequate immobilization is essential.

B. Technique: Use a 21- or 23-gauge pediatric scalp vein infusion set ("butterfly"; ie, a needle attached to plastic wings and tubing) for withdrawing blood. The child should be crying and the vein distended when entered. Thrust the needle under the skin and apply gentle, constant negative pressure with the syringe as the vein is entered. This will prevent air embolism resulting from air being drawn into the vein when the child inspires. After removing the needle, exert firm pressure over the vein for 3–5 minutes while the child is in a sitting position.

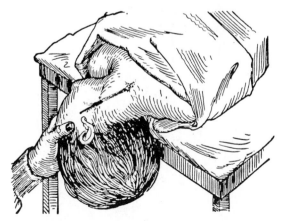

Figure 29–1. External jugular vein puncture.

Femoral Vein Puncture

Caution: This is a hazardous procedure, particularly in the neonate, and should be employed only in emergencies. Septic arthritis of the hip may complicate femoral vein puncture as a result of accidental penetration of the joint capsule. Arteriospasm with serious vascular compromise of the lower extremity may result from hematoma formation. Great care should be exercised in cleansing the skin prior to venipuncture so as to decrease the risk of infection.

A. Preparation: Place the child on a flat, firm table. Abduct the leg so as to expose the inguinal region. Use strict sterile precautions.

B. Technique: Locate the femoral artery by its pulsation. The left femoral vein is preferable because it lies medial to the artery throughout its course (Fig. 29–2). Be certain of the position of the femoral pulse at the time of puncture. Insert a short-beveled needle into the vein (perpendicularly to the skin) about 3 cm below the inguinal ligament; use the artery as a guide (Fig. 29–2). If blood does not enter the syringe immediately, withdraw the needle slowly, drawing gently on the barrel of the syringe;

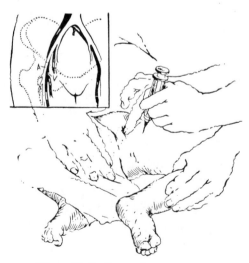

Figure 29–2. Femoral vein puncture.

the needle sometimes passes through both walls of the vein, and blood is obtained only when the needle is being withdrawn. After removing the needle, exert firm, steady pressure over the vein for 3–5 minutes. If the artery has been entered, check the limb periodically during the next hour. If blanching of the extremity occurs, the application of heat may be of value.

Small Vein Puncture

After cleansing the skin, securely grasp the child's hand or foot in a manner that allows milking of the extremity. Using a 21- or 23-gauge straight needle with a clear hub, pierce the skin and advance the needle until blood flows into the hub. Gently milk the extremity and allow blood to drip into the collection vial. This technique allows sampling from small vessels that would collapse with negative pressure from a syringe.

COLLECTION OF MULTIPLE SPECIMENS OF BLOOD

When a number of blood samples must be obtained over a short period of time (eg, when glucose and electrolyte determinations are needed for a diabetic patient with ketoacidosis), multiple venipunctures may be avoided by employing an indwelling 22-gauge or larger Teflon intravenous catheter. The catheter and stylet are inserted in an arm or hand vein in the usual manner (see below). When the stylet is removed, the catheter hub is attached by means of a male Luer adapter to a heparin lock filled with heparinized saline (2 units/mL). Blood may be withdrawn at intervals by applying a tourniquet to the extremity, inserting a needle attached to a syringe through the sterilely prepared rubber port, and drawing off and discarding a minimum of 3–5 mL. A second needle and syringe are then used to collect the blood specimen. The tourniquet is removed, and the buffalo cap and catheter are subsequently cleared by injecting heparinized saline through the rubber port.

INTRAVENOUS THERAPY

Venous Access

A. Sites: For small infants, a scalp, wrist, hand, foot, or arm vein will usually be most convenient. Any accessible vein may be used in an older child. In an emergency if the vein cannot be entered, fluids may be administered by intraosseous infusion. In children with poor peripheral perfusion, attempts should focus on the antecubital, saphenous, and external jugular veins. The saphenous vein has a predictable course, and cannulation by location alone is often successful.

B. Equipment: For scalp infusions use a 25-gauge butterfly. For peripheral veins in infants use a 24- or 22-gauge Teflon catheter. It is helpful to have a T-connector set-up with a 3-mL syringe of saline available. If an IV is being placed in an extremity, it is best to secure the extremity to a padded board prior to beginning the procedure.

C. Technique:

1. Insertion of the Butterfly–First flush the tubing with an isotonic solution. Insert the needle under the skin, and disconnect the syringe from the tubing so that blood return can occur when the needle tip enters the vein. Advance the needle until blood return is noted in the tubing. Holding the needle stationary, remove the tourniquet, reattach the syringe to the tubing, and attempt to flush solution into the vein. Watch carefully for evidence of fluid extravasation. Secure the needle and wings of the butterfly in place. Bolster the wings of the butterfly as needed with cotton to hold the needle at a proper angle. Coil the butterfly tubing and tape away from the needle entry site. Attach intravenous tubing.

2. Insertion of the Catheter–The catheter/stylet apparatus consists of an intravenous catheter with removable stylet. Insert the apparatus under the skin, and advance it until blood appears in the catheter hub. Flushing the catheter gently after the initial blood return may facilitate cannulation, especially in infants. Holding the stylet stationary, advance the catheter over the stylet into the vessel. Withdraw the stylet and attach intravenous tubing to the catheter hub. Secure the catheter in place carefully.

D. Precautions: The rate of flow should be checked frequently. An accurate record must be kept of the amount and type of fluid added. For small infants (particularly if premature), a pump system is preferable for careful control of the volume of intravenous fluid infused. Phlebitis usually develops after a few days. Dextrose concentrations greater than 12.5 gm% should not be infused peripherally. Inspect the limb at regular intervals for evidence of undue pressure circulatory embarrassment, or extravasation.

Intraosseous Infusion

Venous access in children is often a challenge. It may be excessively delayed or impossible in children with cardiac arrest or shock. Prolonged attempts to obtain venous access may delay life-saving therapy. However, fluids and drugs that are infused into the medullary space of long bones quickly enter the venous circulation.

A. Sites: The flat medial surface of the proximal tibia is usable up to 5 or 6 years (see technique below) (Fig. 29–3A.) Other options include the medial surface of the distal tibia, proximal to the medial *malleolus* which may be used in older children and adults or the medial aspect of the distal femur (Fig. 29–3B).

B. Equipment: Any large-bore needle may be used. However, a needle with a stylet is preferred to prevent plugging the lumen with bone fragments. Spinal needles are commonly available, but are long and subject to dislodgement. The Kormed/Jamshidi Illinois sternal/iliac needle is somewhat easier to use,

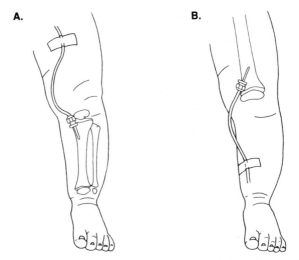

Figure 29–3. Sites for bone marrow infusion. **A.** Insertion site for an intraosseous tibial line. **B.** Insertion site for an intraosseous femoral line.

and more readily stabilized. Several commercially produced intraosseous needles are similarly useful. In children less than 18 months of age use an 18- to 20-gauge needle. In older children a 13- to 16-gauge needle may be used.

C. Technique: Palpate the tibial tuberosity with the index finger. Grasp the medial aspect of the tibia with the thumb. Insert the needle halfway between these two points 1 to 2 cm distal to the tibial tuberosity. Local anesthetic should be injected into the skin and periosteum before needle placement in the conscious patient. Advance the needle with a twisting motion until a slight decrease in resistance is met. The needle should be inserted pointing slightly away from the joint space in a caudal direction. It should remain firmly in place without support. Avoid advancing the needle through the opposite side of the bone by placing a finger on the needle approximately one cm from the bevel, or by using a preset depth indicator. It may not always be possible to aspirate blood and marrow with a syringe. If so, the needle may be flushed with saline. Minimal resistance to infusion with no evidence of extravasation indicates appropriate placement. Only a single attempt per tibia is possible, as fluid will exit from previous holes in the cortex of the bone. For volume resuscitation, fluid should be injected under pressure by syringe. Gravity may be used to infuse fluid once the patient is hemodynamically stable.

D. Complications: Extravasation occurs commonly around the puncture site, especially with pressure infusion and prolonged placement. Other potential complications are fracture, damage to the epiphyseal plate, and pulmonary fat embolus. Osteomyelitis is rare.

E. Clinical Uses: Intraosseous infusion is used for fluid resuscitation with saline, glucose, and blood. Infusion of various drugs including sodium bicarbonate, atropine, dopamine, isoproterenol, epinephrine, diazepam, antibiotics, phenytoin, pancuronium, and succinylcholine have been reported. The injection of 10 mL of saline solution following drug injection may improve transport of drugs from the marrow cavity. While this route is rapid and relatively safe, continued efforts to obtain venous access should always be made.

Venous Cutdown

Venous cutdown is indicated for small infants and for situations in which a seriously ill older child is in urgent need of fluids and difficulty is encountered in entering a vein. In these cases, expose a vein surgically and, under direct visualization, insert a Teflon catheter with an inner needle stylet.

A. Sites: The saphenous vein running anterior to the medial malleolus of the tibia will be found the most satisfactory. It can be entered at any point along its course. Hence, by starting at the ankle, the same vein can be used 2 or 3 times if necessary.

B. Equipment: A Teflon catheter with inner stylet is easiest to use. A pediatric cutdown tray containing scalpel, hemostats, forceps, and curved clamps should be available.

C. Preparation: Apply a tourniquet. Cleanse the skin and drape the leg as for a surgical procedure, using sterile precautions. The foot can be securely taped to a board splint (Fig. 29–4). Make a large wheal with 1 or 2% lidocaine solution (without epinephrine) in the skin over the vein.

D. Technique:

1. Incision–With a scalpel, make an incision just through the skin. The incision should be about 1 cm long and at a right angle to the direction of the vein. Using a fine curved clamp, spread the incision widely, dissecting through the subcutaneous fat in a direction parallel to the vein.

2. Identification of the Vein–Usually, the vein is seen lying on the fascia. Some dissection of subcutaneous fat may be necessary. Insert a curved clamp to the periosteum and bring the vein to the surface (Fig. 29–5). Be certain it is a vein, not a nerve or tendon, by noting the flow of blood. Pass 2 silk ties (No. 00)

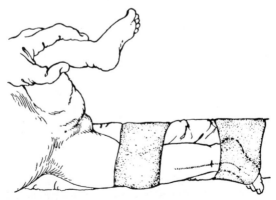

Figure 29–4. Position and taping of leg for venous cutdown.

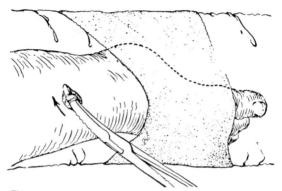

Figure 29–5. Isolation of vein for venous cutdown.

under the isolated vein. Using a hemostat, dissect the vein free for a length of 1–2 cm. Apply gentle traction on proximal and distal ties to maximally expose the vessel. In small infants, the vein is small and fragile; great care must be taken in handling it.

3. Insertion of the Catheter–Introduce the catheter with the stylet needle bevel-up. When the needle is in the vessel lumen, hold the stylet stationary and gently advance the catheter. Withdraw the stylet and release tension on the proximal tie so that the catheter may be threaded and blood return ascertained. If there is no blood flow, remove the tourniquet and attempt to inject a small amount of intravenous solution into the vein. Watch for a wheal or extravasation of fluid, indicating that the catheter is not in the vessel. If the catheter flushes easily, remove the proximal and distal ligatures and suture the plastic wings of the catheter hub to the skin. This can most easily be accomplished by placing a skin closure suture on either side of the catheter hub. Tie the suture, and then pass the free ends through holes provided in the wings of the plastic hub. Tie the suture again. This should hold the catheter securely in the vessel. Apply tape across the hub and tubing for further security.

Arterial Access

In a pediatric intensive care unit, intra-arterial access is often necessary to monitor blood pressure and permit frequent arterial blood sampling. Access through a "line" must be carefully monitored by experienced personnel to prevent hemorrhage from the access site. Arterial lines should not be used to administer large amounts of fluid or to give any medications. Patency of the line should be maintained by use of a solution of normal saline to which heparin, 2 units/mL, has been added. The saline solution may be given at a rate of 2–4 mL/h by mechanical pump to ensure continuous infusion.

A. Sites: The radial artery and posterior tibial artery are the most appropriate vessels for cannulation because of the presence of collateral circulation. Use of more proximal arteries is dangerous because of the possibility of vessel thrombosis resulting in distal ischemia. The location of the vessel should be determined by palpating the pulse. The radial artery usually lies just medial to the radial head. The posterior tibial artery can be palpated posterior to the medial malleolus. Use of a transilluminator or doppler device may aid in locating the artery.

B. Equipment: In addition to the equipment used for venous cutdown (see above), a transducer is needed for continuous monitoring of systolic, diastolic, and mean blood pressures.

C. Preparation: Secure the child's limb on a board splint to expose the desired vessel. When using the radial artery, position the wrist in a slightly dorsiflexed position. Cleanse the skin and drape as for a surgical procedure. Make a wheal with 1% lidocaine (without epineprine) in the skin over the artery. (For cannulation under direct visualization, proceed as for venous cutdown.)

D. Technique: Insert a 22-gauge Teflon catheter with the stylet needle bevel-up (no syringe attached) at a 45-degree angle to the skin surface. Advance the stylet until the arterial blood flow is obtained. If blood flow is not obtained pull the catheter back slowly, as it is not uncommon to pierce both walls of the artery. Adjust the position of the needle until blood return is maximal. Holding the stylet stationary, lower the catheter and stylet until they are flush with the skin and then advance the catheter. Remove the stylet and attached intravenous tubing to the hub of the catheter by use of a T-connector. Secure the catheter in place as for venous cutdown.

URINE COLLECTION

Voided Urine

A pediatric urine collector (a plastic bag with a round opening surrounded by an adhesive surface that binds to the skin) may be used.

If a specimen is to be used for culture, catheterization or percutaneous bladder aspiration is advised; these are the most reliable methods that decrease the chances of contamination of the specimen. Voided midstream collections are difficult to obtain from children and are subject to contamination.

Catheterization

A. Equipment: If the procedure is being performed to obtain a single specimen for culture, use an appropriately sized plastic feeding tube (No. 5 French feeding tube for infants). If the catheter is to remain in place for continuous monitoring of urine output, use a Foley catheter with balloon and a closed sterile collection system. Have ready gloves and drapes, iodine solution, urine cup for specimen collection, normal saline solution to inflate the Foley balloon, and lubricant for the catheter; these should all be sterile.

B. Technique: Have adequate personnel available to restrain the patient during the procedure.

1. Female Patients–Place the female patient in the frog-leg position to expose the urinary meatus. Separate the labia majora, and prepare and drape the patient as for a surgical procedure. Using sterile gloves, apply lubricant to the end of the catheter and pass the catheter through the urethral opening. Continue to thread the catheter gently until urine flow is obtained. Allow the first aliquot of urine to drain out of the catheter. Collect subsequent urine for culture. If a Foley catheter is used, inflate the balloon with the appropriate volume of normal saline solution (the volume is written on the catheter); inflation is through a one-way valve in the sidearm tubing. Pull back on the catheter to test that the balloon is in the bladder and that the catheter is secured. Tape the tubing to the thigh and attach the sterile collection unit and tubing.

2. Male Patients–Hold the male patient's legs in extension. Prepare the glans as for a surgical procedure, retracting the foreskin if present. Proceed as above, taking special care to advance the catheter gently while applying gentle traction on the penis, with the meatus pointed cephalad. If resistance is encountered, retract the catheter slightly, change the angle of entry, and attempt to pass the catheter again.

C. Follow-Up Measures: To prevent phimosis in male patients, remember to return the foreskin to its normal position after catheter insertion.

Suprapubic Percutaneous Bladder Aspiration

Suprapubic percutaneous bladder aspiration is preferable to catheterization when a sterile urine specimen is required for culture and bacterial count.

A. Preparation: The diaper should be dry for at least 45 to 60 minutes. This procedure should not be attempted in patients with abdominal distension, bleeding diathesis, or previous abdominal surgery. Place the patient in a supine position, with the lower extremities held in a frog-leg position. Prepare the skin carefully as for a surgical procedure.

B. Technique: Introduce a 22-gauge, 1.5-in straight needle (attached to a syringe) 1 cm above the pubis, with the needle perpendicular to the skin. With a quick, firm motion, advance the needle while applying gentle traction on the syringe. Stop when urine is aspirated. After urine has been obtained, withdraw the needle with a single, swift motion. If a second attempt is unsuccessful, further attempts are usually futile.

OBTAINING SPINAL FLUID BY LUMBAR PUNCTURE

Lumbar Puncture in Children & Older Infants

The procedure should be deferred in unstable patients, or in those in whom increased intracranial pressure is suspected.

A. Preparation: Have a helper restrain the patient in the flexed lateral position on a firm, flat table. Sterile gloves should be worn. Draw an imaginary line between the 2 iliac crests and use the intervertebral space immediately above or below this line (L3–4 interspace). Prepare the skin surrounding this area as for a surgical procedure, with iodine and alcohol. Drape the area with sterile towels. Infiltrate the skin and subcutaneous tissues with 1–2% lidocaine (not necessary in infants).

B. Technique: Use a short 23-gauge spinal needle for infants; use a long 21-gauge needle for older children. Insert the lumbar puncture needle, with the stylet bevel-up, just below the vertebral spine in the midline (Fig 29–6). Keep the needle perpendicular to both planes of the back or pointing slightly cephalad. A distinct "give" is usually felt when the dura is pierced; if in doubt, remove the stylet to watch for fluid. When fluid is obtained, a 3-way stopcock and manometer may be attached to measure opening pressure (at the beginning of collection) and closing pressure (at the end of collection). Cardiorespiratory function should be monitored throughout the procedure.

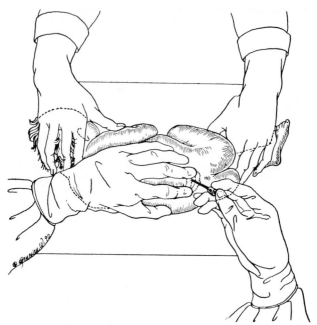

Figure 29-6. Lumbar puncture with assistance of nurse.

Lumbar Puncture in Small Infants

For small infants, lumbar puncture may be performed at the level of the superior iliac crests, with the patient in a sitting position and leaning forward. The stylet may be removed after the needle is firmly lodged in the subcutaneous tissues. The needle should then be advanced very slowly while watching the needle hub for cerebrospinal fluid. Cerebrospinal fluid may flow very slowly, and the "give" may not be felt in small infants. Gentle aspiration with a small syringe may be necessary.

BODY CAVITY PUNCTURES

Thoracentesis

Thoracentesis is used to remove pleural fluid or air for diagnosis or treatment.

Caution: Risks include introduction of a new infection; pneumothorax or hemothorax (or both) as a result of tearing of the lung; hemoptysis; syncope (pleuropulmonary reflex or air embolus); and pulmonary edema as a result of too rapid removal of large amounts of fluid. None of these are common if reasonable care is taken.

A. Sites: Locate the fluid or air by physical examination and by x-ray. Ultrasound examination prior to thoracentesis may aid in location of fluid and selection of an optimal site. If entering at the base, locate the bottom of the opposite uninvolved lung as a guide so the puncture will not be below the pleural cavity. Enter the dependent pleural cavity to remove fluid, or enter the superior chest (usually through the second interspace anteriorly, 1–2 cm lateral to the sternum on the right side, or just left of the midclavicular line on the left side when the patient is in a supine position) to relieve pneumothorax.

B. Equipment: For evacuation of a pneumothorax, use a 19- or 21-gauge needle (butterfly) with a 20–60 mL syringe attached to the tubing via a 3-way stopcock. For removal of pleural fluid, use an 18- to 19-gauge Teflon catheter (with inner removable stylet) attached to a 20-mL syringe via a 3-way stopcock. If a large amount of fluid is to be removed, it can be pumped through a rubber tube attached to the sidearm of the stopcock, thereby avoiding leakage of air into the pleural space.

C. Preparation: The patient should sit up, if possible, and lean forward with support. If too ill or too young to sit up, the patient should be held with the involved side (ie, lung with the effusion) in the most dependent position. Prepare skin as for a surgical procedure. Use a 1–2% lidocaine to infiltrate the skin and down to the pleura.

D. Technique: Insert the stylet and catheter in an interspace, passing just above the edge of the rib. The intercostal vessels lie immediately below each rib. Usually, it is not difficult to know when the pleura is pierced, but suction on the needle at any stage will show whether or not fluid has been reached. Remove the inner stylet, and quickly attach the stopcock and syringe to the hub of the catheter, thereby avoiding creation of a pneumothorax. In cases of long-standing infection, the pleura may be thick and the fluid loculated, necessitating more than one puncture site. If a large amount of fluid is present, it should be removed slowly at intervals, 100–500 mL each time, depending on the size of the patient. Pleural fluid is apt to coagulate unless it is frankly purulent; thus, to facilitate examination, an anticoagulant should be added to the fluid after it is removed.

BONE MARROW PUNCTURE

Bone marrow puncture is indicated for diagnosis of blood dyscrasias, neuroblastoma, and storage diseases. It is also used to obtain specimens for culture. The procedure should be done with great caution when a defect of the clotting mechanism is suspected.

A. Sites: In children, the posterior iliac crest is the preferred site. When the child is restrained in a prone position, the iliac crest can be located and a spot can be marked approximately 1 cm below the crest. Puncture of the sternal marrow is rarely indicated in children. The site between the tibial tubercle and the medial condyle over the anteromedial aspect is recommended by some for bone marrow puncture in infants.

B. Preparation: Prepare the skin surrounding the area as for a surgical procedure. Scrub and wear sterile gloves. Use 1% lidocaine solution to infiltrate the skin and tissues down to the periosteum.

C. Technique: Use a 21-gauge lumbar puncture needle for infants; use an 18- or 19-gauge special marrow needle with a short bevel for older children. Insert the needle with stylet in place, perpendicular to the skin, through the skin and tissues, down to the periosteum. Push the needle through the cortex, using a screwing motion with firm, steady, and well-controlled pressure. Generally some "give" is felt as the needle enters the marrow; the needle will then be firmly in place. Immediately fit a dry syringe (20- to 50-mL) into the needle and apply strong suction for a few seconds. A small amount of marrow will enter the syringe; this should be smeared on glass coverslips or slides for subsequent staining and counting. Remove the needle after withdrawing marrow, and exert local pressure for 3–5 minutes or until all evidence of bleeding has ceased. Apply a dry dressing.

UMBILICAL VESSEL CATHETERIZATION

Umbilical Artery Catheterization

Umbilical artery catheterization is indicated for those infants who require frequent sampling of blood. Complications of

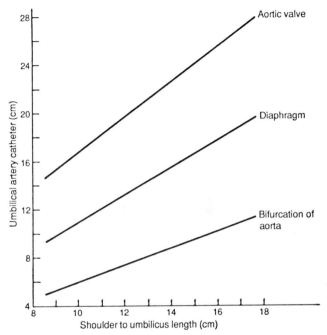

Figure 29–7. Relationship between length of umbilical artery catheter placed and shoulder-umbilicus length in an infant. (Adapted from Dunn P: *Arch Dis Child.* 1966:**41**:73.)

umbilical artery catheterization include thrombosis, embolism, vasospasm, and perforation of the vessel. There is no consensus regarding the ideal placement of the catheter.

A. Catheter Placement: Umbilical artery catheters can be placed in one of two positions: above the diaphragm in the thoracic aorta (T6–T9; high), or just below the aortic bifurcation (L3–L4; low). The graph in Figure 29–7 may be used to estimate the appropriate length of catheter to be inserted. As a general rule, it is best to overestimate, as the catheter can always be pulled back after confirming placement by x-ray.

To use the graph, measure the distance (in cm) from the shoulder down to a line perpendicular to the umbilicus, then add the length of the umbilical stump to the appropriate catheter length determined from the graph.

B. Equipment: For term infants use a 5.0 French umbilical artery catheter; use a 3.5 French for infants less than 32–34 weeks' gestation. Attach a 3-way stopcock to the catheter and flush the system with heparinized saline. Other equipment needed include a scalpel with a straight blade, umbilical tape, and 2 fine, curved, nontoothed forceps.

C. Preparation: The umbilicus and surrounding skin should be prepped and draped. As always, the infant should be monitored and placed under a radiant warmer. A snug tie of umbilical tape should be placed around the base of the cord and easily tightened if bleeding should occur.

D. Technique: The cord is cut with one slicing motion about one cm above the base preferably in a moist part of the cord. Identify the 2 (occasionally there is only one) arteries, which should be narrow, white, and thick-walled compared with the dilated, thin-walled vein. Using a fine, curved, toothless forceps, probe the artery gently; first using one tip and then inserting both tips and allowing the forceps to gently open within the vessel. This will allow adequate dilation of the vessel so that the catheter tip will easily pass into the lumen. Gentle retraction of the vessel wall will facilitate passage of the catheter. Insert the catheter to the desired distance. If resistance is met, try loosening the umbilical tape or changing the angle of the umbilical stump while applying gentle steady pressure. DO NOT FORCE THE CATHETER. If these attempts are unsuccessful, try the second artery.

Once the catheter is in place, attach a syringe to the stopcock; blood should be easily aspirated. The catheter can be sewn in place using a purse-string stitch in the Wharton's jelly and/or constructing a tape bridge. An x-ray should be taken to confirm the placement of the catheter tip.

Umbilical Vein Catheterization

An umbilical venous catheter is most commonly used for emergency intravenous access in the delivery room for the administration of fluids, glucose, and medications. Other uses include exchange transfusions and long-term intravenous access in the very-low-birth-weight infant. Complications of umbilical vein catheterization include thrombosis, embolism, vasospasm, and perforation of the vessel. Portal vein thrombosis with subse-

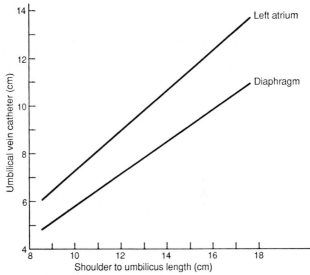

Figure 29–8. Relationship between length of umbilical venous catheter placed and shoulder–umbilicus length in an infant (Adapted from Dunn P: *Arch Dis Child.* 1966:**41**:71.)

quent development of presinusoidal portal hyertension has been associated with umbilical vein catheterization.

A. Catheter Placement: The catheter tip should be placed in a low position for use in emergencies, and exchange transfusions and in a high position for long-term use. For low position, insert the catheter only as far as is required to get good blood flow with aspiration. For a high position, the catheter tip should be placed in the inferior vena cava just above the level of the diaphragm and, therefore, above the ductus venosus, portal vein, and the hepatic veins. The graph in Figure 29–8 can be used to estimate the length of catheter needed. Measure the distance (in cm) from the shoulder to a line perpendicular to the umbilicus and add the length of the umbilical stump to the appropriate catheter length determined from the graph.

B. Equipment: Same as for umbilical artery catheterization.

C. Preparation: Same as for umbilical artery catheterization.

D. Technique: Identify the thin-walled, dilated vessel and remove any clots with a forceps. Insert the catheter to the desired length. When in place, blood should be easily aspirated. Unless it is an emergency, check catheter tip placement with an x-ray and secure with a suture and/or a tape bridge.

Poisons & Toxins | 30

Barry H. Rumack, MD, &
Richard C. Dart, MD, PhD

At least 1.2 million cases of poisoning were reported to the American Association of Poison Control Centers in 1987, and approximately 60% of those were children under 6 years of age. The most frequent causes of poisoning (each accounting for about 8–9% of the total) were cleaning substances, plants, and analgesics.

Accidents involving household poisons, especially in children under the age of 5, can be attributed to 4 main factors: improper storage, failure to return a poison to its proper place, failure to read the label properly, and failure to recognize the substance as poisonous. It is clearly the responsibility of a parent to create a safe environment for the child.

Although many common exposures do not result in serious symptoms, the child who survives the ingestion of a highly toxic poison may be permanently disabled. Disabilities may include esophageal stricture after ingestion of lye, permanent liver or kidney damage after ingestion of poisons such as chlorinated hydrocarbons, or bone marrow depression after benzene poisoning.

GENERAL MANAGEMENT OF POISONINGS

Prophylaxis

Instructions in poison prevention and poison-proofing of homes should be given to the parents prior to or during the child's 6-month checkup. As the child grows, further areas of discussion should be raised with the parents. For example, when the child begins climbing or walking, the danger of storing pharmaceuticals in the medicine cabinet should be discussed, and other areas of storage should also be investigated. Parents should be asked about the contents of such areas as under the sink (drain cleaners), kitchen pantries (cleaning supplies), bathroom cabinets (medicines, antiseptics), basements and utility rooms (paints, thinners, salt), garage (antifreeze, automotive supplies), storage sheds (pesticides, herbicides), and laundry rooms (detergents, ammonia, fabric softeners).

Other general concepts of poison-proofing the house should be discussed. Sample questions would include: Has there been ample provision for locked storage? How should medicines and products be disposed of safely? How should containers be labeled, especially if the product is taken from its original container? What are the best methods of dealing with a child's normal investigation of the environment that may lead to tasting or handling toxic substances?

Treatment issues should also be discussed. Do the parents know of the use of such substances as activated charcoal and syrup of ipecac? If possible, they should be given the phone number of the local poison control center, and urged to obtain any poison prevention literature that the center may be distributing. The physician should provide (or prescribe) a 1-oz bottle of syrup of ipecac for the parent.

Poison prevention is important. The peak age of accidental poisoning is 2 years. If a child ingests a poison, there is a 56% chance of a repeat poisoning in the family within 1 year, and a 25% chance of a repeat poisoning in the same child. If adequate prevention has been discussed, the risk of repeat poisonings is reduced. When repeated exposures to toxic substances occur, child battering or neglect should be considered.

Diagnosis

Most childhood exposures are not intentional ingestions. Rather, the child ''textures'' and ''tastes'' the poison using its mouth as a sensitive organ. Ninety-five percent of all childhood exposures do not result in serious symptoms, most probably because the amount ingested is quite small. In the absence of a definite history of ingestion or of contact with a toxic substance, the diagnosis of poisoning versus another childhood illness presents many difficulties. Most of the symptoms of poisoning are not diagnostic, but certain clues to the presence of an unsuspected poisoning are included below.

A. History: The child is frequently found near the source of the poison shortly after having eaten it. Product containers should be brought to the office or hospital, since the ingredients are often listed on the labels. The physician should call the nearest poison control center or manufacturer in cases of exposure, since product formulation and treatment may have changed since the time the label was printed. Poison centers can also be of help if the label does not have specific ingredients, or if it has been obliterated. Unfortunately, the initial history correlates with the actual agent ingested less than half the time. It is best to compare the clinical condition of the patient with the probable signs and symptoms of poisoning using a recognized reference, such as the computer-updated POISINDEX Information System.

B. Symptoms and Signs: The signs and symptoms may vary greatly, depending upon what toxic substances are involved in the exposure. Symptoms may be gastrointestinal, respiratory, cardiovascular, neurologic, or metabolic. Table 30–1 gives examples of common symptoms seen with various toxic agents.

Table 30–1. Symptoms and signs of acute poisoning by various substances.[1]

Symptoms and Signs	Substance or Other Cause
Albuminuria	Arsenic, mercury, phosphorus.
Alopecia	Thallium, arsenic, selenium, radiation sickness.
Blood changes Anemia	Lead, naphthalene, chlorates, favism, solanine and other plant poisons, snake venom.
Cherry-red blood	Cyanide. (The lips in carbon monoxide poisoning are usually dusky and not cherry-red.)
Hematuria or hemoglobinuria	Heavy metals, naphthalene, nitrates, chlorates, favism, solanine, and other plant poisons.
Hemorrhage	Warfarin, thallium, snake venom.
Methemoglobinemia	Nitrates, nitrites, aniline dyes, methylene blue, chlorates, pyridium.
Breath odors Bitter almond	Cyanide (Odor only detected by 40% of people.)
Garlic	Arsenic, phosphorus, organic phosphate, selenium.
Oysters	DMSO.

(*continued*)

Table 30–1. Symptoms and signs of acute poisoning by various substances.[1] (*continued*)

Symptoms and Signs	Substance or Other Cause
Burns of skin and mucous membranes	Lye, hypochlorite, phenol, sodium bisulfate, etc.
Cardiovascular collapse	Arsenic, boric acid, iron, phosphorus, food poisoning, nitrates.
Cyanosis	Barbiturates, opiates, nitrites, aniline dyes, chlorates.
Eye manifestations Lacrimation	Organic phosphates, nicotine, mushrooms, riot agents.
Ptosis	Botulism, thallium.
Pupillary constriction	Opiates, parathion and other organic phosphates, mushrooms and some other plant poisons.
Pupillary dilatation	Atropine, nicotine, antihistamines, phenylephrine, mushrooms, thallium, oleander.
Strabismus	Botulism, thallium.
Visual disturbances	Atropine, parathion and other organic phosphates, botulism.
Fever	Atropine, salicylates, food poisoning, antihistamines, tranquilizers, camphor.
Flushing	Atropine, antihistamines, tranquilizers.
Gastrointestinal tract symptoms Abdominal cramps	Corrosive substances, food poisoning, lead, arsenic, black widow spider bite, boric acid, carbon tetrachloride, organic phosphates, phosphorus, nicotine, castor beans, fluorides, thallium.
Diarrhea	Food poisoning, iron, organic phosphates, arsenic, napththalene, castor beans, mercury, boric acid, thallium, nicotine, nitrates, solanine and other plant poisons, mushrooms.
Dry mouth	Atropine, antihistamines, ephedrine, furosemide.
Hematemesis	Corrosive substances, warfarin, aminophyline, fluorides.

(*continued*)

Table 30–1. Symptoms and signs of acute poisoning by various substances.[1] (*continued*)

Symptoms and Signs	Substance or Other Cause
Stomatis	Corrosive substances, thallium.
Vomiting	Aminophyline, food poisoning, organic phosphates, nicotine, digitalis, arsenic, boric acid, lead, mercury, iron, phosphorus, thallium, DDT, dieldrin, nitrates, castor beans, mushrooms, oleander, naphthalene.
Headache	Carbon monoxide, organic phosphates, atropine, lead, dieldrin, carbon tetrachloride.
Heart abnormalities	
Bradycardia	Digitalis, mushrooms, organic phosphates.
Tachycardia	Atropine, tricyclic antidepressants.
Other irregularities of rhythm	Nitrates, oleander.
Jaundice	Phosphorus, chlordane, favism, mushrooms, acetaminophen.
Muscle involvement	
Cramps	Lead, black widow spider bite.
Spasm or dystonia	Phenothiazines.
Nervous system involvement	
Ataxia	Lead, organic phosphates, antihistamines, thallium.
Coma	Barbiturates, carbon monoxide, cyanide, opiates, ethyl alcohol, salicylates, hydrocarbons, parathion and other organic phosphates, lead, mercury, boric acid, antihistamines, digitalis, mushrooms.
Convulsions	Aminophyline, amphetamine and other stimulants, atropine, camphor, boric acid, lead mercury, parathion and other organic phosphates, nicotine, phenothiazines, antihistamines, arsenic, DDT, dieldrin, kerosene, fluorides, nitrates, barbiturates, digitalis, salicylates, solanine and other plant poisons, thallium.

(*continued*)

Table 30–1. Symptoms and signs of acute poisoning by various substances.[1] *(continued)*

Symptoms and Signs	Substance or Other Cause
Delirium	Aminophyline, antihistamines, atropine, salicylates, lead, barbiturates, boric acid.
Depression	Barbiturates, kerosene, tranquilizers, arsenic, lead, boric acid, DDT, naphthalene.
Mental confusion	Alcohol, barbiturates, atropine, nicotine, antihistamines, carbon tetrachloride, mercury, digitalis, mushrooms.
Paresthesias	Lead, thallium, DDT.
Weakness	Organic phosphates, arsenic, lead, nicotine, thallium, nitrates, fluorides, botulism.
Pallor	Lead, naphthalene, chlorates, favism, solanine and other plant poisons, fluorides.
Proteinuria	Arsenic, mercury, phosphorus.
Respiratory tract symptoms Aspiration pneumonia	Kerosene.
Cough	Hydrocarbons, mercury vapor.
Respiratory difficulty	Barbiturates, opiates, salicylates, ethyl alcohol, organic phosphates, dieldrin.
Respiratory failure	Cyanide, carbon monoxide, antihistamines, thallium, fluorides.
Respiratory stimulation	Salicylates, amphetamine and other stimulants, atropine, mushrooms.
Salivation and sweating	Parathion and other organic phosphates, muscarine and other mushroom poisoning, nicotine.
Shock	Food poisoning, iron, arsenic, fluorides.
Skin erythema	Boric acid.

[1] Adapted from Arana JM: The clinical diagnosis of poison. *Pediatr Clin North Am* 1970;**17**:477.

C. Laboratory Findings: Evidence may be obtained from the appearance, smell, or chemical analysis of blood, urine, vomitus, gastric washings, or fat obtained by biopsy. Occasionally, characteristic odors of poisons may be detected on the patient's breath. Blood in vomitus or stool may suggest the ingestion of a strong irritant or corrosive. Other specialized tests include urinary porphyrins (lead), red cell stippling (lead), cholinesterase levels (organophosphates), and salicylate levels. The use of ferric chloride or Phenistix may be helpful in initial urine testing for salicylates and phenothiazines, but should always be followed by more specific quantitative or qualitative laboratory tests.

D. X-Ray Findings: Various x-rays may be helpful in evaluating poison exposures. Just a few examples would include location of swallowed coins or other radiopaque pharmaceuticals and foreign objects, x-rays of bones to evaluate chronic lead and bismuth poisoning, and evaluation of pulmonary edema from aspiration of hydrocarbons.

EMERGENCY TREATMENT

(See Table 30–2.)

Emergency care should be supervised by a physician and not left to other office personnel. Much of this care is best done in a hospital, where complete facilities and antidotal substances are available. Consultation with a certified regional poison center is highly recommended for confusing or severe cases. The immediate management of acute poisoning in children should include the measures outlined below.

Ingested Poisons

Speed is essential for effective therapy. The choice of which method to use is not always clear. Induced vomiting is much more effective than lavage with a small-bore nasogastric tube; however, a large-bore nasogastric tube is more effective than emesis.

A. Emesis in the Home: Contraindications to emesis include absent gag reflex, coma, convulsions, and ingestion of strong acids or strong bases. Emesis should not be induced in patients who may develop alterations in mental status. Since the induction of emesis may be delayed 30 minutes or more, it is important

Table 30–2. Emergency treatment for poisoning.

Ingested Poisons
1. Syrup of ipecac may be useful in all cases except corrosives, (ongoing or impending) coma, or seizures.
2. Lavage only if semiconscious or in coma. Endotracheal tube is inserted in larger children.
3. Activated charcoal.
4. Dilute ingested chemicals with water. *Do not* give fluids to dilute ingested medications.

Inhaled Irritants
1. Oxygen therapy.
2. Mouth-to-mouth resuscitation.
3. Humidity.
4. Observe for pneumonitis and pulmonary edema.

Local Irritants
1. Copious water irrigation.
2. Careful eye examination.
3. No chemical "antidotes."

Available Consultants
1. Poison control centers.
2. State health departments.
3. Medical center consultants.
4. Pharmaceutical houses.
5. US agricultural office.
6. Medical examiner (coroner's office, toxicologist).

Specific "Antidote" Treatment Available
1. Amphetamines (see p 956).
2. Arsenic (see p 957).
3. Belladona derivatives (see p 959).
4. Carbon monoxide (see p 961).
5. Cyanide (see p 962).
6. Ferrous sulfate (see p 963).
7. Mercury (see p 967).
8. Narcotics (see p 971).
9. Nitrites and nitrates (see p 971).
10. Phosphates, organic (see p 974).
11. Snake bites (see p 977).
12. Spider bites (see p 978).
13. Tricyclic antidepressants (see p 979).

to instruct the parents on the use of ipecac as early as possible. Syrup of ipecac can be used to induce emesis at a dose of 30 mL for a child 40–45 kg or greater, 15 mL for a child 1–12 years old, and 5–10 mL in a child 6–12 months old (consider administering this dose in a health care facility only). After the dose has been given, the child should be encouraged to drink 4–6 oz of clear fluid, and then should be ambulated. This dose may be repeated once if emesis does not occur within the first 30 minutes. *Do not* administer more than 30 mL of syrup of ipecac to a young child. *Do not* use mustard water, salt water, or gag a child with a spoon. Consult your local poison control center to determine whether or not it is necessary to send the child to a health care facility after emesis. In many cases it will be important to send the child to the hospital whether or not vomiting has occurred. If vomiting has occurred, have the parents recover the regurgitated vomitus in a pan for later analysis.

B. Emesis in the Hospital: Administer syrup of ipecac as outlined above. The use of syrup of ipecac produces an average recovery of 30% of the ingested agent.

C. Lavage: The use of gastric lavage is recommended if performed soon after ingestion, or in comatose or convulsing patients. The patient's airway should be protected by placement in the Trendelenburg and left lateral decubitus position with suction available. In unconscious patients, cuffed, endotracheal intubation is recommended. In children over 5, lavage should be done with 150–200 mL of lukewarm tap water or saline per wash. In younger children, 50–100 mL of normal saline per wash is used. Lavage should continue until the return is clear. The amount of fluid returned in the lavage should approximate the amount of fluid given to avoid fluid-electrolyte imbalance.

D. Activated Charcoal: This adsorbent material has a large surface area on which to adsorb various toxins. Although additives such as cherry syrup, ice cream, milk, and cocoa powder or chocolate milk have been recommended to increase the palatability of activated charcoal, most of these decrease the adsorbing capacity somewhat, and should only be used when there is no other way of getting the child to take the charcoal. In patients with a nasogastric tube in place, using the tube to place the charcoal in the child's stomach is preferable to mixing with these other agents. Sorbitol and bentonite do not appear to alter the absorptive capacity of charcoal.

The most common use of activated charcoal is as a single dose. The optimum dose in children is 15–30 g, with some authors suggesting that 1–2 g/kg be used as a rough guideline, especially in infants. The FDA suggests a minimal dilution of 240 mL of water per 20–30 g of activated charcoal given as an aqueous slurry. A maximum dose has not been recommended. For some poisons, a repeated oral dose of charcoal may enhance total body clearance. A saline cathartic or sorbitol can be given with the first dose, but the safety of administering multiple cathartic doses with the charcoal has not been established. Multiple doses of cathartic have caused life-threatening complications. Occasionally, when large doses are required and the patient is unable to hold the charcoal down, continuous nasogastric infusion of 0.25–0.5 g/kg/h may be successful in ameliorating the vomiting associated with charcoal administration.

Activated charcoal is not absorbed orally, but adverse reactions have occurred, including black stools, vomiting (12–16%), constipation, gastrointestinal obstruction, aspiration pneumonitis, and emphysema.

There are certain classes of toxins in which activated charcoal may not be a standard recommendation. Small molecular weight agents such as ions (iron, lithium) are not adsorbed effectively. When given with a corrosive, it may cause vomiting, which could cause further damage to esophageal mucous membranes. In addition, many corrosives are not well adsorbed by charcoal. When given with hydrocarbons, charcoal may cause vomiting, which could lead to aspiration.

E. Catharsis: The dose of the saline cathartics magnesium of sodium sulfate is 250 mg/kg, and the dose of magnesium citrate is 4 mL/kg up to 300 mL per dose. Usually only one dose of a saline cathartic is administered. Sorbitol is also used as a cathartic, both alone and combined with activated charcoal. In a child over 1 year of age, 1–1.5 g/kg per dose as a 35% solution may be administered up to a maximum of 50 g per dose. It is best to administer sorbitol in a health care facility so fluids and electrolyte status can be monitored.

Surface Poisons

Remove poisons by washing the area with large volumes of water or soap and water. In cases involving water-insoluble substances, the solubility of that compound in various solvents should be checked before recommending large areas of the skin be washed with alcohol or various hydrocarbons. These substances may defat the skin, and may present more hazard than the toxin itself. *Caution: Do not* use chemical antidotes. Neutralization with liberated heat during the reaction may actually increase the extent of injury.

Inhaled Poisons

Patients exposed to toxic inhalants should be removed from exposure to these compounds, monitored for respiratory distress, and given emergency airway support, 100% humidified supplemental oxygen with assisted ventilation, or both, as required. An Ambu bag or other positive-pressure device may be required.

MANAGEMENT OF SPECIFIC COMMON TYPES OF POISONING IN CHILDREN

ACETAMINOPHEN

In large overdose, this commonly used analgesic-antipyretic may produce hepatotoxicity. Because of differences in metabolism, children under age 12 are unlikely to suffer hepatotoxicity even if plasma levels of the drug are in the toxic range. Children over age 12 may develop hepatotoxicity if untreated and if plasma levels are in the toxic range (Fig 30–1).

Initial symptoms during the first 24 hours may include nausea, vomiting, diaphoresis, and a feeling of general malaise. Coma and metabolic acidosis have been seen. If the patient is not treated, hepatotoxicity may be observed via laboratory tests at approximately 36 hours, with peak AST (SGOT), ALT (SGPT), bilirubin levels, and prothrombin time occurring by 3 days. This hepatotoxic event is transient, and even in children with AST levels as high as 20,000 IU/L, discharge from the hospital with no sequelae usually occurs by the seventh day.

The plasma drug level should be determined 4 or more hours after ingestion, when it will have reached its peak. This assumes there is no further absorption. If the level is in the toxic range, treatment with the antidote must be initiated.

Treatment

Emesis or lavage should be performed upon arrival at the emergency care facility. In general, activated charcoal should be administered in the first 4 hours to ensure the amount of acetaminophen absorbed is small. N-acetylcysteine (Mucomyst), which is antidotal for acetaminophen, does bind to charcoal; the degree of absorption is not clinically significant.

ACIDS, CORROSIVES

The strong mineral acids exert primarily a local corrosive effect on the skin and mucous membranes. Classically, acids

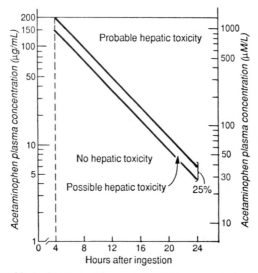

Figure 30–1. Semilogarithmic plot of plasma acetaminophen levels vs. time (Rumack-Matthew nomogram for acetaminophen poisoning). *Cautions for use of this chart:* (1) The time coordinates refer to time of ingestion. (2) Serum levels drawn before 4 hours may not represent peak levels. (3) The graph should be used only in relation to a single acute ingestion. (4) The lower solid line 25% below the standard nomogram is included to allow for possible errors in acetaminophen plasma assays and estimated time from ingestion of an overdose. (Adapted, with permission, from Rumack BH, Matthew H: Acetaminophen poisoning and toxicity. *Pediatrics* 1975;**55**:871. Copyright Midromedex Inc, 1974–1989.)

cause oral and gastric burns, but seldom produce esophageal damage. The majority of these burns resolve. However, pyloric constriction with obstruction and vomiting may occur at 3 weeks. This response is thought to be due to pylorospasm occurring immediately after ingestion, which traps the acid in this area and produces a more significant burn.

Symptoms include severe pain in the throat and upper gastrointestinal tract; marked thirst; bloody vomitus; difficulty in swallowing, breathing, and speaking; discoloration and destruction of skin and mucous membranes in and around the mouth; collapse; and shock. Milder burns may result in fewer symptoms but serious sequelae are still possible.

Eye contact may produce severe pain, swelling, corneal erosions, and in some severe cases, blindness. Normally, brief exposures to acidic solutions with a pH of greater than 2 produce no injury to the corneal epithelium. Inhalation of acidic agents may produce dyspnea, chest pain, and pulmonary edema. Bronchospasm and hypoxemia may result.

Treatment

Do not give emetics or lavage. Dilute the acid immediately with 4–8 oz (not over 15 mL/kg) of water or milk. Avoid carbonates or bicarbonates internally, since they may form gas and cause distension of a perhaps weakened stomach wall. Do not administer other alkaline or neutralizing agents. Diagnostic endoscopy may be performed as indicated within the first 12 to 24 hours. This procedure may help grade the extent of damage and predict the necessity of further treatment. The use of steroids is debatable. They are extensively used by some surgeons in the same way as for alkaline burns. The dose of prednisone recommended is 1–2 mg/kg/d for 21 days.

ALCOHOL, ETHYL

Incoordination, slow reaction time, blurred vision, staggering gait, slurred speech, hypoglycemia, convulsions, and coma are the potential manifestations of overdosage. The diagnosis of alcoholic intoxication is commonly overlooked in children.

Treatment

Supportive treatment and aggressive management of any degree of hypoglycemia are usually the only treatments required. Although naloxone may antagonize the depressant effects found in ethanol overdose, the effect is not predictable or consistent. Fructose has been advocated as an accelerator of ethanol metabolism, but it is not commonly used in children.

AMPHETAMINES

Acute ingestion results in initial hypertension, hyperpyrexia, and hyperactivity. Extreme, unmanageable hyperactivity and anxiety, as well as flushing, various cardiac arrhythmias, cardiac pain, convulsions, and eventual circulatory collapse may be seen. Gastrointestinal complaints include nausea, vomiting, diarrhea, and abdominal pain.

Treatment

Standard gastric decontamination should be performed. The immediate administration of charcoal may be more effective than syrup of ipecac for the awake but symptomatic patient. Gastric lavage, followed by activated charcoal, may be the optimal decontamination regimen for patients who are exhibiting CNS effects.

The hyperactivity is generally managed with diazepam (0.25–0.4 mg/kg, up to a maximum of 5 mg in children 30 days to 5 years old and a maximum of 10 mg in children over 5 years; given intravenously over 2–3 minutes) unless severe hallucinations and agitation are present. In these cases, intravenous haloperidol or droperidol may be more effective. Clorpromazine is generally not recommended. Acid diuresis is not recommended.

ANTIHISTAMINES

The effects of poisoning with these agents are variable, but anticholinergic or sympathomimetic effects are apparent in most cases. Atropinelike toxic effects such as dry mouth, fever, and dilated pupils may predominate. Signs of CNS toxicity include ataxia, hallucinations, and convulsions followed by coma and respiratory depression. Especially in older children, depression comparable to that seen with poisoning with tranquilizers may be prominent.

Prolonged toxic manifestations may be caused by sustained-action tablets. Most antihistamines are combined in products that also contain stimulants (phenylpropanolamine, ephedrine) and analgesics (aspirin, acetaminophen). These agents should be considered when treating antihistamines.

Treatment

Treatment consists of emesis or lavage, charcoal, and catharsis; the latter are important when sustained-action tablets have been ingested. Convulsions should be controlled with diazepam. Stimulants are contraindicated. Decrease fever with fluids and sponge baths as required. Avoid salicylates and acetaminophen, especially if found in a combination product. Physostigmine, 0.5–2 mg intravenously, slowly, will reverse coma, hallucinations, dysrhythmias, convulsions, and hypertension, but should only be used to reverse life-threatening manifestations. It may also be useful as a diagnostic test when the cause of symptoms is unclear. Repeat doses should be given only to reverse severe toxic manifestations.

ARSENIC

Acute arsenic ingestion usually produces symptoms in 30 minutes. It is characterized by severe gastrointestinal symptoms and may be accompanied by a metallic taste, hoarseness, dysphagia, renal damage, shock, and fever. Increased capillary permeability, dehydration, protein depletion, garlicy odor on the breath, and hypotension may be noted. Chronic toxicity is characterized by peripheral neuritis, weight loss, and, sometimes, involvement of the skin, kidneys, and gastrointestinal tract. Laboratory determination of arsenic levels in vomitus, urine, and tissues is confirmatory. Blood levels below 1 μg/100 mL are within the normal range. Blood levels are generally only useful after acute exposures.

Treatment
Treatment consists of antishock therapy and specific therapy with dimercaptosuccinic acid (DMSA, Chemet) 10 mg/kg/dose, tid for 5 days, followed by the same dose bid for 14 more days. Use of dimercaprol (BAL), 2.5 mg/kg intramuscularly immediately and then 2 mg/kg intramuscularly every 4 hours, may be indicated. After 4–8 injections, give BAL twice daily for 5–10 days or until recovery. BAL produces a reaction similar to serum sickness in over 80% of patients.

BARBITURATES

There are two categories of barbiturate poisoning: (1) intoxication with short-acting drugs (eg, pentobarbitol, secobarbitol), which are detoxified in the liver; and (2) intoxication with long-acting drugs (eg, phenobarbitol), which are cleared via the kidneys. The general symptoms are similar in both types and consist of drowsiness, ataxia, difficulty in thinking clearly, depression of

Table 30–3. Clinical classification of coma.[1]

Symptoms	Class
Asleep; can be aroused and can answer questions.	0
Comatose; does not withdraw from painful stimuli; reflexes intact.	1
Comatose; does not withdraw from painful stimuli; no respiratory or circulatory depression; most reflexes intact.	2
Comatose; no respiratory or circulatory depression; most or all reflexes absent.	3
Comatose; respiratory depression, with cyanosis; circulatory failure or shock (or both); reflexes absent.	4

[1] After Reed.

spinal reflexes, respiratory depression, hypotension, and coma. Coma should be classified by the Reed classification (Table 30–3).

Treatment

Since histories are usually unreliable, treatment decisions based on an estimate of the amount of barbiturate ingested may be risky. Any amount in excess of 10–15 mg/kg for long-acting agents or 5–8 mg/kg for short-acting agents may produce more than therapeutic depression. Treatment measures are based on the type of barbiturate ingested (ie, short-acting or long-acting). Following suspected ingestion, close observation should be continued for a minimum of 4–6 hours.

A. Short-Acting Drugs:

1. Emesis, lavage, charcoal, and cathartics should be administered as under Emergency Treatment (see p 154). Emesis may be contraindicated because of the short time to CNS depression.

2. Analeptic agents (eg, doxapram, nikethamide, caffeine) are contraindicated in all cases.

3. Respiratory assistance should be provided, by respirator if necessary.

4. Hypotension is common and should be treated with isotonic volume expansion. Vasopressors may be utilized if fluids are inadequate.

5. Shock lung with pulmonary edema may occur and may require positive end-expiratory pressure.

6. Forced diuresis is ineffective, since less than 3% of the drug is excreted via the kidneys. Fluids should be held to three-

fourths of maintenance, since cerebral edema may be a complication, especially following anoxia. Hemodialysis and hemoperfusion may be helpful but should be reserved for severe cases.

7. Vital signs should be monitored continuously until the patient has been free of symptoms for 24 hours and charcoal stools have been passed.

8. Coma lasts approximately 10 hours for each milligram of barbiturate above the therapeutic level of 0.5–2 mg/dL.

B. Long-Acting Drugs:

1–5. As above.

6. Forced alkaline diuresis improves clearance by 3 times. Urine output should be 3–6 mL/kg/h, preferably 6 mL/kg/h. If the urine pH is less than 7.5, alkalinization may be performed with sodium bicarbonate.

7. Hemodialysis or charcoal perfusion may be useful if the patient is not responsive to the above measures. These procedures are rarely needed, and their use should not be based on blood levels but rather on deteriorating clinical condition.

8. Therapeutic levels of long-acting barbiturates are 2–4 mg/dL, but patients with tolerance may have considerably higher levels without toxicity. Correlate levels with clinical status before using them to classify severity of toxicity.

BELLADONNA DERIVATIVES
(Atropine, Scopolamine, Jimson Weed)

The belladonna alkaloids are parasympathetic depressants with variable CNS effects. Symptoms are dryness of mouth, thirst, difficulty in swallowing, and blurring of vision. Physical signs include dilated pupils, flushed skin, tachycardia, fever, delirium, delusions, weakness, and stupor. Symptoms are rapid in onset but may last for long periods, because gastric emptying time is slowed.

Treatment
Induce emesis. Physostigmine, 0.5–2 mg intravenously slowly, dramatically reverses the central and peripheral effects of belladonna alkaloids. Physostigmine should be reserved for cases of severe toxicity. Owing to a short half-life, its effects usually end within an hour and the patient's symptoms recur. Seizures should respond to diazepam; if not, physostigmine may be used. Forced diuresis is ineffective with the synthetic alka-

loids. Peritoneal and hemodialysis are ineffective; exchange transfusions may be helpful if very high doses have been taken.

BIRTH-CONTROL PILLS

The only toxic effects noted are nausea, vomiting, and vaginal bleeding. These effects are rare. The only treatments are prevention, by keeping all medications out of the reach of children, and fluid replacement when necessary.

BORIC ACID

Toxicity can result from ingestion or absorption through inflamed skin. Manifestations include severe gastroenteritis, CNS signs such as irritability, restlessness, and seizures, and a fiery red rash, called toxic epidermal necrolysis. Shock, coma, and death may be seen in more serious ingestions.

Note: There is no justification for keeping boric acid solution or powder where infants and children can be accidentally exposed to it. The drug has no medicinal value.

Treatment

Gastric lavage or induced emesis (or both) is the immediate therapy. Although it is commonly stated that boric acid is not adsorbed by activated charcoal, one study showed that 90 g of activated charcoal did adsorb 38% of a 3-g dose of boric acid. Very large doses of charcoal may be required. Good supportive care includes maintenance of fluid and electrolyte balance and treatment of hypotension with isotonic fluids and vasopressors as needed. Seizures may be treated with intravenous diazepam. Excretion of ingested or absorbed boric acid can be facilitated with exchange transfusion, hemodialysis, or peritoneal dialysis. Hemodialysis is more effective than peritoneal dialysis and is probably indicated in severely symptomatic patients with impaired renal function, and in patients with severe fluid-electrolyte abnormalities not amenable to conventional therapy.

CARBON MONOXIDE

Carbon monoxide combines with hemoglobin to form carboxyhemoglobin, which cannot carry oxygen and may result in tissue hypoxia. The cellular cytochrome systems may also be affected. Levels of carboxyhemoglobin can be measured easily, and they correlate well with the degree of toxicity. In acute exposures, the patient is generally asymptomatic with levels of 10–20%; levels of 20–30% produce mild symptoms, 30–40% moderate symptoms, and 40–50% severe symptoms. Symptoms are more severe in patients who have exercised or taken alcohol or who reside at high altitudes. Symptoms range from mild flu-like symptoms of headache, nausea, vomiting, to lethargy, depressed sensorium, and occasionally seizures. The heart is particularly sensitive to the hypoxia caused by carbon monoxide and clinical effects including tachycardia, hypotension, peripheral vasodilatation, cyanosis, shock, and cardiac arrest may be seen. Early cardiac arrhythmias are thought to be rare. Severe carbon monoxide intoxication may result in pulmonary edema. After prolonged exposure, psychotic behavior may be noted. Residual or delayed neurologic effects may occur after acute carbon monoxide poisoning. The incidence of sequelae appears to correlate directly with the level of consciousness and the duration of initial coma. Patients with normal CT scans appear to do better than similar patients with abnormal scans.

Treatment

Therapy consists of removal from the source and administration of oxygen. The half-life of carboxyhemoglobin is 40–90 minutes in 100% oxygen and 180–360 minutes in room air. The half-life is somewhat dependent on respiratory rate, age, pulmonary health, and physical activity. Hyperbaric oxygen is now considered to be the treatment of choice for symptomatic patients. Hyperbaric oxygen increases the concentration of the oxygen dissolved in the plasma and displaces carbon monoxide from the hemoglobin. Severely symptomatic patients should be referred to a facility with a hyperbaric chamber. Severe symptoms include coma, dizziness, seizures, focal neurologic deficits, severe metabolic acidosis (pH less than 7.25), pulmonary edema, and other cardiovascular signs.

CYANIDE

Cyanide specifically inhibits the cytochrome oxidase system, causing cellular anoxia. The onset of symptoms after inhalation is rapid but may be delayed by minutes to hours after ingestion. Symptoms include giddiness, hyperpnea, headache, palpitation, and unconsciousness. The breath may smell of bitter almonds. Death usually occurs in 15 minutes unless treatment is immediate.

Treatment

Immediately begin 100% oxygen. Obtain the Lilly Cyanide Antidote Kit and prepare it for use. Note that most of the doses are for adults and need to be modified for children. A dosage chart for children is available on the POISINDEX Information System. Intravenous sodium nitrite 3% is given first, followed by intravenous sodium thiosulfate (25%). The amount of sodium nitrite should not exceed that listed in the chart. Fatal methemoglobinemia may result. As an approximation only, the average child with 12 g of hemoglobin would be given 0.33 mL/kg of the 3% sodium nitrite at a rate of 2–5 mL/min. This should produce approximately 30% methemoglobinemia. The initial dose of sodium thiosulfate 25% is 1.65 mL/kg. If clinical response is inadequate, additional sodium nitrite, at half the amount of the initial dose, may be administered 30 minutes following the first dose. These antidotes should only be used in significantly symptomatic patients such as those with seizures, unconsciousness, acidosis, or unstable vital signs. Supportive care is effective in less severe poisonings.

DETERGENTS

Fatalities due to poisoning with anionic and nonanionic detergents have not been reported. The primary symptoms associated with these agents alone include nausea, vomiting, and diarrhea. Occasionally, these detergents may contain alkaline irritants that have the potential for causing alkaline burns.

Cationic detergents may also be found in the home, in products such as antiseptics and antistatic agents. Acute poisoning from these agents may cause gastroenteritis, convulsions, burns, and strictures. Insufficient data are available to determine the nontoxic amount of a cationic detergent or noncorrosive concentration (approximately 7.5%). Extrapolating from one adult fatality, a serious amount of a 1% solution in a child weighing 10 kg would be about 1 oz. Burns may occur with benzalkonium chloride in concentrations of 10% or greater.

Treatment

Anionic and nonanionic detergents generally cause minimal effects and require only monitoring for excessive fluid loss if vomiting and diarrhea are extensive.

In cases involving cationic detergents, dilution with water or milk may be initiated first; there is some risk in inducing emesis or performing gastric lavage since many of these compounds are corrosive and if systemic effects occur, seizures and coma may be seen fairly rapidly. These agents are well adsorbed to charcoal and rapid administration of activated charcoal is recommended for large amounts of dilute solutions. With more concentrated solutions, esophagoscopy should be considered and performed within the first 24–48 hours. Definitive burn care may be required if burns are identified on esophagoscopy. Supportive care may be required for seizures, hypotension, and pulmonary edema.

FERROUS SULFATE

Accidental ingestion of ferrous sulfate (elemental iron) in amounts as low as 60 mg/kg may cause serious intoxication. Five phases of intoxication are described: (1) Hemorrhagic gastroenteritis occurs shortly after ingestion (30–120 minutes); shock due to blood loss may be present. (2) A recovery phase occurs and lasts from 2 to 12 hours after ingestion. (3) Delayed shock may occur 12–24 hours after ingestion and may be due to a vasodepressant action of ferritin or unbound ionic iron. (4) Liver damage occurs at 3–5 days. (5) Delayed gastric obstruction due to scarring of local corrosive injury may occur, usually at 3 weeks after ingestion.

The history is the most important diagnostic clue. X-rays of the abdomen may show the radiopaque tablets in the gastrointestinal tract. Patients with a serum iron level of over 500 μg/dL require chelation therapy.

Treatment

Remove ferrous sulfate by induced vomiting and lavage with a large-bore tube. Supportive measures (blood, plasma, saline, and vasopressors as indicated) are imperative. Exchange transfusion may be useful if the patient does not respond to standard measures. Deferoxamine (Desferal) is useful in cases of severe intoxication. The dose is 15 mg/kg/h as a drip—not a push—during the first 12–24 hours. Intramuscular deferoxamine should only be used if intravenous access cannot be established. In general, as long as chelation occurs, the urine shows a reddish "vin rosé" color.

FLUORIDES

Fluorides are found in high concentrations in agricultural poisons and insecticides. Lower concentrations are found in such things as toothpaste and fluoride tablets used for prevention of dental caries. Clinical reactions produced by fluorides include nausea, vomiting, colicky abdominal pain, diarrhea, cyanosis, excitement, and convulsions. In most instances, gastrointestinal signs and symptoms predominate, but in fatal poisonings, death is usually a result of cardiac failure or respiratory paralysis. In serious poisonings, degeneration of the kidney may occur, as may hypocalcemia, hyperkalemia, and a variable skin rash. In general, ingestion of fluoride tablets used for dental care does not result in severe symptoms owing to their low concentration (1 mg per tablet).

Treatment

Calcium salts (chloride, carbonate, lactate) have been used orally as lavage solutions in concentrations of 5 mL/L of water or a 0.15% calcium hydroxide (lime water) solution. Most household exposures are treated with milk in large quantities (10–15 mL/kg orally). Vomiting may be induced or gastric lavage performed with a large-bore tube. Activated charcoal is not generally of use with fluoride ingestion. For a cathartic, sodium sulfate, sodium citrate, or sorbitol may be used. Monitor serum calcium and observe for clinical signs of hypocalcemia. If necessary, administer calcium gluconate (10%) slowly intravenously, and repeat as necessary. After the initial correction of hypocalcemia, a calcium gluconate infusion at a rate of 15 g/m^2 for 24 hours may be required to compensate for the slow release of fluoride ion from the bone.

GLUE

Toluene was once the most common solvent used in glue, but it has largely been replaced in products by less toxic substances. The most frequent symptoms following glue "sniffing" include weakness, fatigue, confusion, lacrimation, euphoria, headache, dizziness, muscular weakness, nausea, and dilated pupils. Chronic inhalers may develop muscular weakness syndromes, gastrointestinal syndromes, or neuropsychiatric syndromes. Death may occur from respiratory failure.

Treatment

Eliminate exposure to the solvent. Conservative management is indicated, but fluid-electrolyte status should be monitored, as should hepatic, renal, and hematologic parameters. Chronic abusers should receive substance abuse counseling.

HALLUCINOGENS

Marijuana has stimulant, depressant, and hallucinogenic properties, but usually the depressant properties predominate. Euphoria, mood swings, and distortion of time and space commonly occur. Performance skills may be affected. Panic states or psychotic reactions are uncommon.

LSD (lysergic acid diethylamide) causes euphoria, mood swings, loss of inhibitions, and depersonalization. Flashbacks (recurrence of initial effects), panic states, and hallucinations occur in some individuals.

Mescaline typically produces mydriasis, salivation, tachypnea, headache, nausea and vomiting, flushing, and diaphoresis. Auditory, gustatory, olfactory, tactile, and visual hallucinations have all been seen with mescaline. These psychologic effects are generally mild in adults, but may be more pronounced in children; they rarely last longer than 6–12 hours.

PCP (phencyclidine) is a veterinary anesthetic that causes agitation, paranoid behavior, nystagmus, hypertension, muscle rigidity, respiratory depression, renal failure, "staring" coma, and occasionally self-destructive behavior. It is often mistakenly taken as or with LSD, mescaline, psilocybin, or marijuana.

Treatment

Treatment of hallucinogenic agents is primarily symptomatic and supportive. Patients should be placed in a low-stimulus environment and given reassurance by a parent, psychiatrist, or psychologist. Anxiety states can be reduced with diazepam (0.04–0.2 mg/kg per dose every 2–4 hours to a maximum of 0.6

mg over 8 hours). Seizures may also be treated with diazepam (0.2–0.5 mg/kg per dose, maximum 5 mg in children under 5 and 10 mg in children over 5). Management of PCP ingestion may include treatments for dystonias, renal failure due to rhabdomyolysis or myoglobinuria, hypoglycemia, and hypertension.

IBUPROFEN

Children who are exposed to mild overdoses of this agent generally don't have serious effects. One study states that children who ingest up to 2.4 grams remain asymptomatic. In cases where symptoms occur, abdominal pain, vomiting, drowsiness, and lethargy are seen most frequently. A few case reports, especially in young children, have reported apnea, seizures, metabolic acidosis, and CNS depression leading to coma.

Treatment

For children who have ingested less than 100 mg/kg, only dilution with milk or water, to soothe any potential gastrointestinal irritation, is required. Dilution should be with less than 4 oz of fluid in children. If more than 400 mg/kg have been ingested, there is a potential for seizures or CNS depression. In such cases, gastric lavage may be preferred to emesis. In cases where 100–400 mg/kg have been ingested, emesis may be of equal value. A cathartic combined with activated charcoal may also be of some use in adsorbing the material and removing it from the gastrointestinal tract. Multiple-dose activated charcoal has been suggested because of the possibility of enterohepatic circulation. Patients should be monitored for hypotension, seizures, acidosis, and gastrointestinal bleeding. Hemodialysis and alkalinization of the urine have not been shown effective in treatment of ibuprofen poisoning.

LYE & BLEACHES

Ingestion of lye and bleaches may result in ulceration and perforation of the gastrointestinal tract and in long-term complications (adult) as vomiting may occur with excessive fluids. Perform esophagoscopy after 12 hours but before 24 hours. Corticosteroids may be helpful and, if used, should be given early and continued for 3 weeks. Antibiotics are not indicated unless an infection is demonstrated. Give supportive therapy with sedation and analgesia as necessary. Intravenous nutrition and fluids may be necessary in the early stages of treatment. Early tracheostomy may be indicated in cases of severe ingestion.

MEPROBAMATE
(Equanil, Miltown)

Respiratory depression, coma, arrhythmias, lethargy, headache, hyperactive deep-tendon reflexes, increased heart rate, hypotension, and pulmonary edema may be noted. Death may occur from cardiac or respiratory failure.

Treatment

Emesis or gastric lavage with a large-bore tube may be performed. Although supportive treatment may be sufficient in mild intoxications, hemodialysis, hemoperfusion, or charcoal hemoperfusion may be indicated in severe cases. Forced diuresis is theoretically useful, but hypotension and the risk of pulmonary edema make this procedure difficult and potentially harmful. Peritoneal dialysis is not as effective as hemodialysis.

MERCURY

Acute symptoms of severe inorganic mercury poisoning include sudden, profound circulatory collapse, increased heart rate, peripheral vasoconstriction, vomiting, decreased blood pressure, and possibly bloody diarrhea. Kidney failure has been seen within 24 hours. Severe acidosis and leukocytosis may occur. Some symptoms may be delayed until after 12 hours, including a mercury gum line, lower nephron nephrosis, ulcerative colitis, hepatic damage, and shock. Chronic symptoms generally reported are those of gastrointestinal irritability, a blue-black gum line, salivation, stomatitis, nephrosis, and irritability. Acrodynia occurs in children following chronic exposure to small amounts of mercury, including topically applied mercury.

Treatment

For ingested mercury, consider emesis or gastric lavage. Inorganic mercury salts may produce gastric erosion, and the possibility of perforation should be considered before using emesis or lavage in patients presenting some time after an ingestion. Abdominal x-rays may be helpful in determining whether lavage or emesis is required. Good supportive and symptomatic care should be given for symptoms such as seizures and hypotension. A timed, 24-hour baseline urinary mercury level is a good index of total body burden. For acute poisoning, extrapolating a collection of 2–12 hours is a good initial index. This should be followed by a 24-hour collection. Chelation can be performed with several agents. The first choice is DMSA, 10 mg/kg tid for 5 days followed by the same dose bid for 14 days. Penicillamine, 100 mg/kg/d orally in children, may be given, up to a maximum of 1 g/d in divided doses for 3–10 days. The urine should be monitored daily for urinary excretion of mercury. If the urine mercury decreases rapidly, the body burden is probably small. After waiting 10 days, a repeat baseline collection should be performed to determine whether rebound has occurred and rechelation is necessary. For those individuals who are sensitive to penicillamine, or cannot take oral medications, BAL may be used in doses of 3–5 mg/kg per dose every 4 hours given deep IM for the first 2 days, 2.5–3 mg/kg per dose IM every 6 hours for the next 2 days, then 2.5–3 mg/kg per dose every 12 hours for a week after that. Again, urine mercury levels should be monitored to assess the effects of therapy.

MUSHROOMS

Mushrooms are responsible for rare deaths and common nonfatal poisonings. A history of mushroom ingestion always arouses concern, which is intensified because some toxins present in mushrooms may not show their effects until many hours after ingestion and because it is often not known exactly what kind of fungus was ingested.

The most common intoxicating American species are delineated below. Almost 90% of cases of childhood accidental ingestions involve nontoxic puffballs or nontoxic "little brown mushrooms." The services of a mycologist must be obtained through a botanical garden or poison control center to identify the species.

Clinical Findings & Treatment
Clinical findings and treatment vary according to the type of mushroom ingested (Table 30–4).

Table 30–4. Mushroom poisoning.

Class	Representatives	Clinical Effects	Treatment
Cyclopepides	Amanita verna Amanita phalloides Galerina species	Vomiting, diarrhea, delayed liver and kidney damage	Supportive care, penicillin, silibinin
Muscarinic	Boletus satanas Clitocybe dealbata Inocybe species	Salivation, bradycardia, miosis, increased peristalsis, hypotension, wheezing	If muscarinic, atropine, 50 µg/kg SC
Hydrazine	Gyromitra species	Vomiting, diarrhea, muscle cramps, fever, liver failure, seizures, coma	For CNS effects, pyridoxine
Psilocybin	Psilocybe species	Hallucinations	Treatment usually not necessary
Coprine	Coprinus atramentarius	Flushing, vomiting, tachycardia, vertigo	Usually symptomatic; for severe cases methylpyrazole (experimental)
Muscimol	Amanita muscarid Amanita patherina	Drowsiness, delirium, muscle spasms, seizures, coma	Supportive
Orellanine	Cortinarius species (some)	Delayed kidney damage	Supportive, hemoperfusion

A. Cyclopeptide-containing: Vomiting and severe diarrhea occur after a latent period of 6–20 hours, followed by liver and kidney damage.

B. Muscarinic-containing: These fungi may contain muscarine that may cause parasympathomimetic manifestations. Some may cause an anticholinergic syndrome (see Belladonna Derivatives, above). Hallucinations may occur with ingestion of either type of mushroom. If patients have severe atropinic signs, physostigmine may be tried (see above).

C. Hydrazine-containing: These are potentially toxic mushrooms that may cause nausea and vomiting, muscle cramps, abdominal pain, severe diarrhea, fever, liver failure, seizures, and coma. Hemolysis may be seen, as may methemoglobinemia. The toxin, which closely resembles monomethylhydrazine, may be removed or decreased by cooking or drying. Pyridoxine may be antidotal for neurologic symptoms, but there is limited experience with its use. The dose recommended in the literature is 25 mg/kg given as an infusion over 15–30 minutes. Repeat doses up to a maximum daily dose of 15–20 g may be administered for recurring neurologic signs such as seizures and coma. The maximum nontoxic dose of pyridoxine is unknown, but doses of 0.2–5 g/d for 2–40 months have caused neurologic symptoms such as ataxia and severe sensory nervous system dysfunctions. Methemoglobinemia can be treated with methylene blue in a dose of 1–2 mg/kg per dose (0.1–0.2 mL/kg per dose) given intravenously over a few minutes as needed every 4 hours. Additional doses may be required. Doses of greater than 15 mg/kg may cause hemolysis.

D. Psilocybin-containing: Psilocybin causes nausea, vomiting, headache, and hallucinations. Onset of symptoms is generally within 30–60 minutes, but may be as long as 3 hours. Most cases recover fully within 12 hours. Tonic-clonic seizures, usually intermittent, have occurred in children after ingestion of large quantities.

NARCOTICS
(Opiates)

Narcotic intoxication (eg, morphine, codeine, and diphenoxylate [in Lomotil]) produces respiratory depression, hypotension, pinpoint pupils, skeletal muscle relaxation, decreased urinary output, and, occasionally, shock. Propoxyphene (Darvon) has been associated with convulsions in a high percentage of cases of overdosage. Diphenoxylate is especially known for its delayed-onset CNS and respiratory depression.

Treatment

Acute overdosage is treated similarly to barbiturate intoxication. Respiratory assistance and maintenance of adequate blood pressure are mandatory. Naloxone (Narcan) is an effective narcotic antagonist that does not cause respiratory depression and has no known toxicity even in large doses. The dose of naloxone should be no less than 2.0 mg regardless of the patient's age. If there is no immediate response, the dose may be repeated several times. The use of doses based on a set ratio of dose per unit of weight (mg/kg) is frequently inaccurate, since the treatment goal of reversing binding cannot be achieved consistently with these doses. Patients who have had opiate reversal with naloxone should be observed carefully for recurrence of CNS and respiratory depression.

NITRITES & NITRATES

Methemoglobinemia is produced by the administration of a nitrite compound or a nitrate that is converted to the nitrite in the large bowel. Sodium nitrite, food preservatives, phenacetin, home remedies such as spirits of nitrite, a high concentration of nitrites in water, as well as various inhalants (amyl, butyl, and isobutyl nitrate) may produce these effects. The onset may be gradual and symptoms may be deceiving. Ingestion of as little as 10 mL of isobutyl or amyl nitrate has produced severe methemoglobinemia and death in both adults and children. Clinical signs include hypertension, tachycardia, respiratory depression, methemoglobinemia, headache, nausea, vomiting, and diarrhea, and in severe cases, seizures may be seen. Symptoms depend on the amount of available hemoglobin to carry oxygen, but generally do not occur until approximately 30% of the hemoglobin has been converted to methemoglobin. A drop of the patient's blood dried on filter paper may appear brown if levels are 15% or greater.

Treatment

Intravenous methylene blue allows electron transfer to reverse methemoglobinemia. A 1% solution is administered in the amount of 0.1 mL/kg and may be repeated 30 minutes later to reverse symptoms. Persistence of methemoglobinemia at high levels in a symptomatic patient is an indication for exchange transfusion. Laboratory determinations for methemoglobin are available.

PETROLEUM DISTILLATES
(Charcoal Starter, Kerosene, Paint Thinner, Turpentine, & Related Products)

The petroleum distillates are mixtures of saturated and unsaturated hydrocarbons of the aliphatic and aromatic series. The following products are common causes of poisoning: kerosene, lamp oils, turpentine, other pine products, gasoline, lighter fluid, insecticides with petroleum distillate bases, benzene, naphtha, and mineral spirits.

Ingestion of petroleum distillates causes local irritation with a burning sensation in the mouth, esophagus, and stomach. Vomiting and occasionally diarrhea with blood-tinged stools may occur. Kerosene and similar products are likely to cause spontaneous emesis in 1 hour in about 90% of patients. It is essential to remember that just a few drops aspirated into the pulmonary tree can cause a severe and fatal pneumonia, a complication to which infants and children are particularly prone. Pulmonary complications are reported with greater frequency among children who ingest kerosene or mineral seal oil than in those who ingest other petroleum distillate products with higher viscosity. Pulmonary involvement is usually indicated by cyanosis, rapid breathing, tachycardia, and fever. Basilar rales may progress rapidly to massive pulmonary edema or hemorrhage, infiltration, and secondary infection.

In general, ingestion of more than 30 mL (1 oz) of a petroleum distillate is associated with a higher incidence of CNS complications such as lethargy, coma, seizures, confusion, disorientation, and peripheral neuropathy. CNS involvement is reported most frequently among patients who ingest lamp oils and kerosene. In severe poisonings, there may be cardiac dilatation, hepatosplenomegaly, proteinuria, formed elements in the urine, and cardiac dysfunction associated with congestive heart failure. In fatal poisonings, death usually occurs in 2–24 hours.

Treatment

Although controversial, induced emesis is useful in cases where systemic toxicity is predicted. The American Academy of Pediatrics recommends emesis if more than 1 mL/kg has been ingested. Estimation of the amount ingested may be difficult in children. Gastric lavage should be performed only if a cuffed endotracheal tube is inserted, because there is no such thing as a "careful gastric lavage" in children. If the amount ingested is small, a saline cathartic is all that is necessary. For CNS depression, supportive care is indicated.

"Prophylactic" antibiotic therapy is of questionable value and does not speed resolution when pneumonia exists. Oxygen and mists are helpful. Corticosteroids have not been shown to be of benefit in treating hydrocarbon pneumonitis. Hospitalization is indicated only if the child has taken a large amount or is symptomatic. Fever and other symptoms may continue for as long as 10 days without infection, and pneumatoceles may develop 3–5 weeks after pneumonitis.

Withhold digestible fats, oils, and alcohol, which may promote absorption from the bowel or cause aspiration pneumonitis on their own.

The rapidity of recovery depends upon the degree of pulmonary involvement. Resolution may take as long as 4 weeks.

PHENOTHIAZINES

Phenothiazine compounds produce significant anticholinergic, alpha-adrenergic blocking, and extrapyramidal properties. The symptoms seen will depend on the class of the agent ingested, but may include extrapyramidal motor symptoms (opisthotonos, oculogyric crisis, torticollis, trismus, rigidity) and convulsions.

Treatment

Decontamination should be done either with emesis or gastric lavage depending on the potential for CNS depression and seizures. Activated charcoal and a cathartic will also be useful. Symptomatic measures should be used and blood pressure monitored. Phenytoin (2 mg/kg every 8 hours) may be useful in reversing the depressed intraventricular conductivity of the myocardium. Dystonic disorders may be treated with diphenhydramine at a dose of 1–2 mg/kg to a maximum of 50 mg intravenously. The malignant neuroleptic syndrome, sometimes seen with phenothiazines such as haloperidol and fluphenazine, may be treated successfully with oral dantrolene at a dose of 2.5 mg/kg intravenously followed by 2.5 mg/kg every six hours.

PHOSPHATES, ORGANIC
(Diazinon, Disyston, Malathion, Parathion, etc)

Many insecticides contain organic phosphates. All inhibit cholinesterases, resulting in parasympathetic and CNS stimulation. Symptoms include headache, dizziness, blurred vision, diarrhea, abdominal pain, dyspnea, chest pain, bronchial constriction, pulmonary edema, respiratory failure, convulsions, cyanosis, coma, loss of reflexes and sphincter control, sweating, salivation, miosis, tearing, muscle fasciculations, and even generalized collapse.

Lowered red cell cholinesterase activity helps to confirm the diagnosis.

Treatment

The patient who has been exposed dermally must be decontaminated with soap and water or tincture of green soap as soon as possible to prevent further absorption. For children who have ingested an organophosphate, lavage is probably safer than emesis because of the rapid onset of symptoms, Many organophosphates are dissolved in a hydrocarbon solvent, which could lead to aspiration. Atropine is useful for treatment of the muscarinic effects, but will not reverse nicotinic effects. Early, prompt, and adequate atropinization is of paramount importance in symptomatic patients. Begin with 50 μg/kg intravenously in a small child and 1–2 mg intravenously in an older child. Repeat every 15–30 minutes until dry mouth, mydriasis, and tachycardia appear. Severely poisoned patients may require exceedingly large doses of atropine to achieve adequate atropinization. If anticholinergic findings occur following a diagnostic dose of atropine, the patient is probably not seriously poisoned. In addition, pralidoxime (2-PAM), 500 mg intravenously injected slowly over 5 minutes, should be given if symptoms are severe.

Supportive measures include oxygen, artificial respiration, postural drainage of secretions, and measures to combat shock and seizures.

RAUWOLFIA DERIVATIVES

Rauwolfia derivatives produce parasympathetic effects: nasal congestion, salivation, sweating, bradycardia, abdominal cramps, and diarrhea. Parkinsonian symptoms occasionally develop.

Treatment

Give supportive treatment and remove the poison by emesis and lavage. The effects of parkinsonism may be alleviated with anticholinergic agents such as atropine. This treatment should be reserved for severe cases. Atropine may also be useful to reverse the gastrointestinal effects. Digitalis derivatives should not be used to reverse cardiac failure. The combination has shown evidence of enhancing cardiac dysrhythmias.

RIOT-CONTROL CHEMICALS

Riot-control chemicals consist of an agent in hydrocarbon solvent such as kerosene, and in some cases a propellant such as freon gas. There are a number of chloroacetophenone derivatives as well as chloropicrin agents, dibenzoxazepine compounds, orthochlorobenzylidene malononitrile agents, and capsicum. The chemical agent typically causes lacrimation, photophobia, and in some instances nausea and vomiting. In lower concentration, these materials cause lacrimation and pain but no tissue damage. Skin sensitization and corneal scarring can occur, particularly when the chemical is released close enough to the victim's face or skin to create a high local concentration.

Treatment

The most effective treatment is prompt removal from the sprayed area and careful decontamination of the patient. After removing all clothes, the patient should shower carefully, using copious amounts of soap and water. An ophthalmologist should examine the eyes for possible corneal damage. Medical personnel involved in decontamination should wear protective clothing.

SALICYLATES

Salicylates are still frequently involved in pediatric exposures. Acute salicylate poisoning involves vomiting, tinnitus, hyperpnea, acid-base disturbances such as respiratory alkalosis and metabolic acidosis, electrolyte imbalances such as hypokalemia, fever, dehydration, lowered cerebrospinal fluid glucose levels, and pulmonary edema. Severe cases may involve hallucinations, seizures, coma, cerebral edema, and mild hepatotoxicity.

Salicylates stimulate the respiratory center, a property that may cause respiratory alkalosis. Bases are then compensatorily excreted. Salicylates also interfere with intermediary metabolism and allow the accumulation of organic acids. The two processes together produce a metabolic acidosis that is difficult to treat. In chronic cases, the initial alkalosis may not be evident.

Treatment

Emesis and lavage are useful methods for eliminating salicylates that have not been absorbed. The method used depends on such factors as the patient's condition (coma, seizures), dosage form (liquid vs tablet), and time since ingestion. Activated charcoal and cathartics are also useful.

Adequate hydration is important, usually with a hypotonic glucose solution such as 0.2–0.45 normal saline. In acidotic patients, administration of sodium bicarbonate (3–6 mL/kg/h of a solution containing 88 mEq/L) should be given.

Potassium supplementation may be required because sodium or potassium is excreted with the bicarbonate during the respiratory alkalosis stage. Depletion may be present even with normal serum potassium. Potassium supplements may be at levels of 10–20 mEq/L of fluid, depending on the patient's condition.

Treatment of tetany may require intravenous calcium. The dose depends on serum calcium levels. The pulmonary edema is *not* responsive to digoxin, diuretics, or tourniquets.

Alkalinizing the urine to a pH of 7–8 will enhance salicylate excretion but without proper potassium supplementation may be difficult to maintain. Carbonic anhydrase inhibitors such as Diamox should *not* be used to alkalinize the urine because of negative acid-base reactions.

SCORPION STINGS

The toxin of the less venomous species of scorpions causes only local pain, and redness. That of the more venomous species causes generalized muscular pains, nausea, vomiting, opisthotonos and a distinctive movement disorder with variable CNS involvement.

Treatment

Keep the patient recumbent and quiet. If the species is known to be one of those that does not cause systemic reactions, stings can be treated much as bee or wasp stings. If absorption has occurred, and the patient is complaining of muscle spasms, consider administering 0.1 mg/kg of diazepam. Provide adequate sedation and institute supportive measures. Symptomatic measures should be used for control of seizures, hypertension, and supraventricular tachycardia. Antivenin is of some value in cases involving *Centruroides* species, but is only available in Arizona.

SNAKE BITES

In the United States nearly all snakebites are inflicted by members of the *Crotalidae* family (rattlesnakes, moccasins, copperhead). Bites by the *Elapidae* (coral snakes) are much less common and are not covered here.

Manifestations of crotalid envenomation include local pain, swelling and erythema, nausea and vomiting, abdominal cramps, and a metallic taste. Local wound manifestations usually develop promptly, but may be delayed for several hours. Systemic signs such as hypotension may develop early or late. Hypotension is caused by volume depletion secondary to diffuse capillary injury.

Treatment

Keep the patient recumbent and quiet. Immobilize bitten part below heart level and remove rings and other constrictive items. Transport to medical facility immediately. After arrival at medical facility, the injured part should be immobilized at or above heart level. Do not use ice. Treat shock and respiratory failure with standard resuscitation from shock. A band that occludes venous and lymphatic return from the limb may be applied, although its efficacy is unknown. Incision and suction are not useful. A high vacuum suction device is available that effectively removes venom through the puncture wound in an animal model. If a constrictive band of any type has been placed it should not be removed until intravenous access is secured.

The primary methods of treatment are volume resuscitation and Antivenin (*Crotalidae*) polyvalent. Resuscitation should be performed with an isotonic fluid. Antivenin should be given when progressive tissue injury, hemotological injury, or hypotension develop. Antivenin is most effective when given early. After 6–8 hours it is less helpful, but may still be indicated if injury is worsening. The package insert provides directions on its use. The dose ranges from 5 to 30 vials or more depending on the severity of the envenomation, the species of snake, and the patient's age. If the patient develops an allergic reaction, the antivenin should be discontinued immediately. If indicated, it may be cautiously restarted after treatment with epinephrine and antihistamines. Blood component therapy is rarely needed, but may be indicated for severe anemia, thrombocytopenia or coagulopathy. Steroids are not useful during the acute phase of poisoning. Tetanus prophylaxis and standard local wound care should be provided. Consultation with a physician experienced in the treatment of snakebite and antivenin use is highly recommended for all envenomations.

SPIDER BITES

Black Widow Spider

The bite of a female black widow spider (*Latrodectus mactans*) causes pain at the site of injection. Clinical manifestations include generalized muscle pains with severe abdominal cramps, irritability, nausea and vomiting, variable CNS symptoms, profuse perspiration, labored breathing, and collapse. Convulsions may rarely occur in children. Examination reveals small maculopapular erythema at the area of bite, board-like rigidity of the abdomen, restlessness, and hyperactive deep tendon reflexes.

Keep the patient recumbent and quiet with adequate sedation. No first aid measures have proven to be of value. Calcium gluconate in a dose of 50 mg/kg intravenously (up to 250 mg/kg per 24 hours) has been shown to be of some value in reducing the muscle spasms. Methocarbamol in a dose of 15 mg/kg every 6 hours has also been of some value. Antivenin (*Latrodectus mactans*) effectively reduces muscle cramping, CNS effects, and hypertension. This antivenin should be reserved for patients who display severe symptoms that are not relieved by other methods. Instructions for use are included in the package. Tetanus immunization status should be updated. Other methods to reduce muscle spasm and pain include diazepam and narcotics.

Brown Spider

The North American brown recluse spider (violin spider, *Loxosceles reclusa*) is most commonly seen in the central and Midwestern areas of the USA. Its bite characteristically produces a localized reaction with progressively more severe pain over 8 hours. The initial bleb on an erythematous ischemic base may occur before ulceration. Other symptoms may include cyanosis, a morbilliform rash, fever, shock, chills, malaise, weakness, nausea and vomiting, joint pains with hemoglobinuria, jaundice, and delirium.

Medical care is supportive, no specific antivenin is available. Many bites require little treatment other than local care and an antitetanus agent. If there is severe itching, diphenhydramine, 5 mg/kg/d orally (maximum dosage 25–50 mg 4 times a day) may be used. The use of steroids is questionable. A polymorphonucular leukocyte inhibitor such as dapsone or colchicine may be helpful. Dapsone may cause hemolysis, which is also a complication of *Loxosceles* envenomation. Surgical intervention should be delayed until 6 or more weeks after the bite. In rare cases, platelets may be needed when thrombocytopenia is present. Hyperbaric oxygen is being investigated for the treatment of bites rated as class 3 or 4 (severe). Therapy was instituted 2–6 days after envenomations, and all cases healed properly without hospitalization, surgery, serious skin slough, or significant scarring.

TRICYCLIC ANTIDEPRESSANTS
(Amitriptyline, Doxepin, Imipramine, Nortriptyline, etc)

Amitriptyline (Elavil), doxepin (Sinequan), imipramine (Tofranil), nortriptyline (Aventyl), and other tricyclic antidepressants characteristically cause cardiac dysrhythmias, CNS abnormalities (agitation, hallucinations, seizures, and coma), and other signs of atropinism such as dilated pupils, malar flushing, dry mouth, hyperpyrexia, and urinary retention. Some of the newer cyclic antidepressants such as amoxapine have less cardiovascular toxicity but still cause CNS toxicity, with subsequent convulsions.

Treatment

Emesis is not indicated after overdose since rapid neurologic deterioration may occur. Gastric lavage and activated charcoal and a cathartic may be of use. Multiple-dose activated charcoal may be effective with these agents. Prolonged PR intervals may respond to phenytoin. Lidocaine may be of some use as well. Use of sodium bicarbonate is also helpful in correcting and preventing recurrence of cardiac dysrhythmias. The blood pH should be kept at 7.5–7.6. Good supportive care is required for control of seizures, hypertension, hypotension, respiratory depression, and pulmonary edema. Cardiac monitoring should continue until 24 hours after signs of toxicity have resolved.

Drug Therapy (Formulary) | 31

Wendy Frieling, MD, Alan K. Kamada, PharmD,
& Stanley J. Szefler, MD

The complexity of drug therapy in children has evolved over the years; not only must the appropriate "drug of choice" be selected, an individualized dosing scheme that includes dose and frequency of dosing must be chosen to ensure safety and obtain optimum efficacy. Thus, a basic knowledge of each drug by the prescriber is essential. A number of factors influence the selection of dose and dosing interval, including patient differences in absorption, distribution, metabolism, and excretion of drugs. Concomitant disease states and physiologic conditions that may vary with age can also influence drug disposition. Because of this, it is not appropriate to simply scale down adult doses when administering medications to children. The following chapter will provide a brief overview of the major factors involved in selecting medication doses in children, followed by a Formulary of medications commonly used in pediatric practice.

DETERMINATION OF DOSE & DOSING INTERVAL

Factors Influencing Dose & Dosing Interval
In the pediatric patient, a number of physiologic factors will influence the absorption, distribution, metabolism, and/or excretion of medications, and thus may alter the doses and frequency of dosing required. These are outlined in Table 31–1.

Calculation of Dose
Standard doses are readily available when treating adult patients, however because of the individualization required, choosing the appropriate dose for a child is somewhat more complex. In the past, pediatric drug doses have been based on age, however it is more appropriate to determine doses based either on

Table 31-1. Physiologic factors influencing drug disposition.[1]

Disposition Parameter	Physiologic Variable	Affected Age Group(s)	Pharmacokinetic Result	Example Drug
Absorption	Increased gastric pH	Neonates, infants, young children	Increased bioavailability of basic drugs Decreased bioavailability of acidic drugs	Phenobarbital
	Decreased gastric and intestinal motility	Neonates, infants		
	Increased gastric and intestinal motility	Older infants, children	Unpredictable bioavailability	Digoxin
	Decreased bile acids	Neonates	Decreased bioavailability	Vitamin E
Distribution	Increased total body water and extracellular water	Neonates, infants	Increased volume of distribution	Theophylline, aminoglycosides
	Decreased albumin and protein binding	Neonates, infants	Increased volume and increased free drug concentration	Phenytoin
Metabolism	Decreased enzyme capacity	Neonates, infants	Increased elimination half-life and decreased clearance	Phenobarbital
	Increased enzyme capacity	Young children	Decreased elimination half-life and increased clearance	Theophylline
Excretion	Decreased glomerular function	Neonates, infants	Increased elimination half-life	Aminoglycosides
	Decreased tubular function	Neonates, infants	Increased elimination half-life	Penicillins, sulfonamides

[1] Reprinted with permission, from *Applied Pharmacokinetics: Principles of Therapeutic Drug Monitoring*, 3rd ed. Evans WF, Schentag JJ, Jusko WJ (editors). Applied Therapeutics, Inc., 1992.

body weight (ie, mg/kg) or body surface area (ie, mg/m^2). The Formulary following this chapter includes pediatric doses on a mg/kg basis. For some medications it is better to dose by body surface area (BSA). The following formula is used:

$$\text{pediatric dose} = \text{adult dose} \times \frac{\text{BSA}}{1.73 \text{ m}^2}$$

Body surface area is determined from Fig. 31–1 using the patient's height and weight.

For intravenous medications, loading doses are often employed to allow the medication to distribute to the various tissue "compartments." Loading doses may also be appropriate for oral medications with long elimination half-lives. To calculate loading doses the volume of distribution (Vd), a theoretical parameter indicative of the space to which the drug distributes, must be known. The calculation of a loading dose is as follows:

loading dose (mg/kg)
   = desired plasma concentration (mg/L) × Vd (L/kg)

Volumes of distribution may also be calculated for medications administered by the oral or other routes provided bioavailability is relatively complete. For calculation of maintenance doses, the clearance or rate of elimination of the drug must be known. To calculate maintenance infusions, the following equation is used:

maintenance dose (mg/kg/hour)

   = desired plasma concentration (mg/L)

   × clearance (L/kg/hour)

In general practice, population averages are used for the initial calculation of loading and maintenance doses. Guidelines for loading doses and maintenance doses are included in the Formulary following this chapter. Further dosage individualization is then based on measured plasma drug concentrations. A special consideration which may cause some confusion when dosing drugs in pediatric patients is the removal of drugs by dialysis. Those drugs which are significantly removed by dialysis are listed in Table 31–2.

When calculating pediatric doses the maximum adult doses should not be exceeded, unless clinical situations known to alter

Table 31–2. Percentage of drugs removed by dialysis.

Drug	Hemodialysis (%)	Peritoneal Dialysis (%)	Drug	Hemodialysis (%)	Peritoneal Dialysis (%)
Acetaminophen	20–50	0–5	Ethosuximide	20–100	
Acetazolamide	20–50		Flecainide	0–5	
Acetohexamide		0–5	Flucytosine	50–100	20–50
Acyclovir	50–100		Flurazepam	0–5	
Amantadine	5–20	5–20	Gentamicin	50–100	20–50
Amikacin	50–100	20–50	Glutethimide	0–20	
Amoxicillin	20–50		Heparin	0–5	0–5
Amphotericin B	0–5		Imipenem/cilastatin	20–50	
Ampicillin	20–50	0–5	Isoniazid	50–100	
Aspirin	50–100	50–100	Kanamycin	50–100	20–50
Atenolol	20–50		Ketoconazole	0–5	0–5
Azathioprine	5–50		Lidocaine	0–5	
Azlocillin	20–50		Lithium	50–100	50–100
Aztreonam	20–50	5–20	Lorazepam	0–5	
Bretylium	20–50		Mebendazole	0–5	
Captopril	20–50		Meprobamate	20–50	5–20
Carbenicillin	20–50		Methicillin	0–5	
Cefaclor	20–50		Methyldopa	5–20	5–20
Cefamandole	20–50		Methylprednisolone	5–20	
Cefazolin	20–50	5–20	Metoclopramide	0–5	
Cefonicid	5–20		Metronidazole	0–5	
Cefoperazone	5–20	0–5	Mexiletine		5–20
Ceforanide	20–50		Mezlocillin		0–5
Cefotaxime	20–50	5–20	Minocycline	0–5	20–50
Cefotetan	5–20		Moxalactam	50–100	0–5
Cefoxitin	20–50	5–20	Nadolol	5–50	5–20
Ceftazidime	50–100	5–20	Nafcillin	0–5	

Drug		
Ceftizoxime	20–50	5–20
Ceftriaxone	0–5	
Cefuroxime	20–50	5–20
Cefalexin	20–50	5–20
Cephalothin	20–50	
Chloral hydrate	50–100	
Chloramphenicol	5–20	0–5
Chlordiazepoxide	0–20	
Chlorpropamide		0–5
Cimetidine		5–20
Ciprofloxacin	5–20	
Clavulanic acid	50–100	
Clindamycin	0–5	0–5
Clonidine	0–5	
Cloxacillin	0–5	
Colchicine	0–5	
Cyclophosphamide	20–50	
Diazepam	0–5	
Dicloxacillin	0–5	
Digitoxin	0–5	
Digoxin	0–5	0–5
Disopyramide	0–5	
Doxycycline	0–5	
Enalapril	20–50	
Erythromycin	5–20	
Ethambutol	0–5	
Ethanol	50–100	
Ethchlorvinol	0–20	0–5

Drug		
Neomycin	50–100	
Netilmicin	50–100	
Oxacillin	0–5	
Oxazepam	0–5	
Penicillin G	5–50	
Pentobarbital	5–20	0–20
Phenobarbital	20–100	5–50
Phenothiazines	0–5	
Phenytoin	0–5	0–5
Piperacillin	20–50	
Primidone	20–50	
Procainamide/N-acetyl-procainamide	5–50	
Propoxyphene	0–5	
Propranolol	0–5	
Quinidine	5–20	5–20
Ranitidine	5–20	
Secobarbital	5–20	0–20
Sulfamethoxazole	5–20	
Tetracycline	5–20	
Ticarcillin	20–50	
Tobramycin	50–100	20–50
Tocainide	20–50	
Tolbutamide	0–5	
Trimethoprim	5–50	
Valproic acid	0–5	0–5
Vancomycin	0–5	5–20
Verapamil	0–5	

[1] Adapted with permission, from Gambertoglio JG, Rodondi LC. Dialysis of drugs. In: Knoben JE, Anderson PO, (editor): *Handbook of Clinical Data*. Drug Intelligence Publications. 1988.

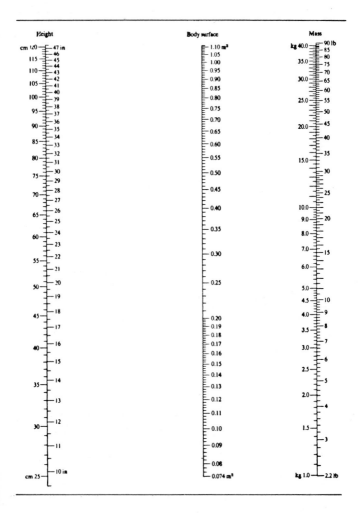

Figure 31–1. Body surface area: Children. To determine the body surface area in a child, use a straight edge to connect the height and mass. The point of intersection on the body surface line gives the area in m². (Reproduced with permission, from *Geigy Scientific Tables,* 8th ed. Vol 1. Lentner C [editor]. CIBA-GEIGY, Basle, 1981.)

Table 31–3. Suggested therapeutic plasma drug concentrations.[1]

Drug	Concentration
Amikacin[2]	Peak: 20–25 µg/mL
	Trough: 1–4 µg/mL
Caffeine	5–15 µg/mL
Carbamazepine	5–10 µ/mL
Chloramphenicol	10–20 µg/mL
Digoxin	0.5–2.0 µg/L
Gentamicin[b]	Peak: 6–8 µg/mL
	Trough: 0.5–1.0 µg/mL
Phenobarbital	10–30 µg/mL
Phenytoin	10–20 µg/mL
Primidone	5–15 µg/mL
Procainamide	4–6 µg/mL
Quinidine	3–5 µg/mL
Theophylline	Asthma: 5–15µg/mL
	Apnea: 5–10 µg/mL
Tobramycin[2]	Peak: 6–8 µg/mL
	Trough: 0.5–1.0 µg/mL
Valproic acid	50–100 µg/mL
Vancomycin	Peak: 25–35 µg/mL
	Trough: 5–10 µg/mL

[1] References: Yaffe SJ, Aranda JV. *Pediatric Pharmacology: Therapeutic Principles in Practice.* Saunders, 1992; Evans WE, Schentag JJ, Jusko WJ. *Applied Pharmacokinetics; Principles of Therapeutic Drug Monitoring.* Applied Therapeutics, 1992.

[2] range for serious infections; slightly higher concentrations desired for life-threatening infections.

drug disposition are present or as indicated by drug monitoring. Clinical situations which may alter the disposition of some medications (and may require dosage adjustments) include liver and kidney disease, altered fluid status, obesity, and significant drug interactions.

Monitoring Drug Therapy

For some medications plasma concentrations have been well correlated to their therapeutic activity. Therapeutic ranges, determined from both efficacy and safety data, have been developed for a number of medications and are listed in Table 31–3.

Thus for these particular medications, therapeutic drug monitoring is useful in titrating doses to obtain optimum efficacy while ensuring safety from toxicities. It should be kept in mind that a number of factors, including timing of the last dose and blood samples, bioavailability, distribution, and rate of elimination can all affect the measured plasma drug concentrations and should be considered when unexpected or seemingly erroneous plasma concentrations are measured. Also, specific laboratories and institutions will usually have their own normal reference ranges.

BREAST-FEEDING & DRUG THERAPY

Drug exposure to the neonate and infant may also occur through breast feeding, although generally in very low concentrations. Nevertheless, a number of questions should be considered when using medications in mothers who are breast feeding. These include:

1. Is maternal drug therapy actually necessary?
2. If so, what is the least toxic drug that can be used?
3. Can the dosing schedule be altered to minimize drug exposure to the infant?
4. Are there known adverse effects, and would they be easily identified in the infant?
5. Are idiosyncratic or allergic reactions of particular concern to the infant?
6. Are there any physiologic factors present which would result in accumulation of the drug in the infant?
7. Will the amount of drug delivered via breast milk approximate a therapeutic dose to the infant?

While drug overdose via breast milk exposure is rare, it should be kept in mind that idiosyncratic or allergic reactions generally are not dose related. Of special concern are radiolabelled compounds and chemotherapeutic agents; these should generally not be given to a mother if breast-feeding is continued. Drugs which are contraindicated in the breast-feeding mother are listed in Table 31–4.

CONCLUSIONS

There are a number of varying factors that alter the disposition of drugs in pediatric patients. Awareness of these factors when prescribing medications to children will minimize toxicities

Table 31–4. Drugs contraindicated during breast-feeding.[1]

Contraindicated	Relative Contraindication
Amantadine	Alcohol
Amiodarone	Anti-thyroid drugs
Bromocriptine	Clonidine
Clemastine	Dapsone
Cocaine	Diazepam
Cimetidine	Ethosuximide
Chloramphenicol	Iodides
Cyclophosphamide	Isoniazid
Cyclosporin	Methadone
Doxorubicin	Nicotine
Ergotamine	Nitrofurantoin
Gold salts	Phenobarbital
Isotretinoin	Procainamide
Lithium	Sulfonamides
Methotrexate	
Metronidazole	
Phencyclidine (PCP)	
Phenindione	
Radioactive compounds	
Thiouracil	

[1] References: Anderson PO. Drugs and breast feeding. In: Knoben JE, Anderson PO, (editors). *Handbook of Clinical Drug Data.* Drug Intelligence Publications, 1988; Niebyl JR. Teratology and drugs in pregnancy and lactation. In: Scott JR, DiSaia PJ, Hammond CB, Spellacy WN. *Danforth's Obstetrics and Gynecology.* Lippencott, 1990.

while maximizing the drug's efficacy. The Formulary following this chapter includes suggested doses for children, and in some cases adult doses are also included. Neonatal doses are not always included; other sources should be consulted for specific drug dosing in the neonate. Note that not all cautions and contraindications are listed for each medication. Other sources are recommended for complete prescribing information.

RECOMMENDED RESOURCES

For a more comprehensive discussion of relevant topics related to individualization of treatment regimens in pediatric patients, the following resources are recommended:

1. Roberts RJ. *Drug Therapy in Infants. Pharmacologic Principles and Clinical Experience.* Saunders, 1984.
2. Yaffe SJ, Aranda JV. *Pediatric Pharmacology. Therapeutic Principles in Practice.* Saunders, 1992.
3. Evans WE, Schentag JJ, Jusko WJ. *Applied Pharmacokinetics. Principles of Therapeutic Drug Monitoring.* Applied Therapeutics, 1992.
4. Knoben JE, Anderson PO. *Handbook of Clinical Drug Data.* Drug Intelligence Publications, 1988.
5. Briggs GG, Freeman RK, Yaffe SJ. *Drugs in Pregnancy and Lactation.* Williams & Wilkins, 1990.

FORMULARY

Acetaminophen (many trade names) How supplied: tabs: 80, 325, 500 mg; caplets: 160 mg; liquid: 50 mg/15 mL; syrup; 160 mg/5 mL; drops: 80 mg/0.8 mL; suppository: 120, 125, 130, 300, 325, 500, 600, 650 mg. Dose: base on wt: 10–15 mg/kg/dose PO, PR Q4-6H; based on age: 1–2 yrs, 120 mg/dose; 2–3 yrs, 160 mg/dose; 4–5 yrs, 240 mg/dose; 6–8 yrs, 320 mg/dose; 9–10 yrs, 400 mg/dose; 11–12 yrs, 480 mg/dose; adult, 325–1000 mg/dose.

Acetazolamide (Diamox) How supplied: tabs: 125, 250 mg; caps (sustained release): 500 mg; injection: 500 mg/5 mL. Dose: 1) glaucoma: Oral: 8–30 mg/kg/day divided every 6–8 h; IM, IV: 5–10 mg/kg/dose every 6 h. 2) edema: Oral, IV, IM: 5 mg/kg or 150 mg/m^2/day or every other day. 3) epilepsy: Oral: 8–30 mg/kg/day in 1–4 divided doses. 4) urine alkalinization: 5 mg/kg/dose repeated 2–3 times per 24 h. 5–30 mg/kg/day PO or IV Q6–8H; adult: 250–1000 mg/day PO or IV Q6H–QOD. *Note:* Safety and efficacy in children has not been established.

Acetylcysteine (Mucomyst) How supplied: vials: 10% and 20% in 4, 10, and 30 mL vials. Dose: nebulization: Infants: 2 mL of 5% solution nebulized 3–4 times per day; Children: 3–5 mL of 5–10% solution 3–4 times per day; Adolescents: 5–10 mL of 5–10% solution 3–4 times per day. Acetaminophen overdose: 140 mg/kg loading dose PO or NG, then 70 mg/

* The following sources were used to compile information for this section: *Physicians Desk Reference.* Medical Economics Data, 1992; *Formulary of Accepted Drugs and Drug Dosing Handbook.* The Children's Hospital, 1992.

kg/dose PO or NG Q4H for a total of 17 doses (dilute 1:4 in water or soft drink).

ACTH (Acthar, Cortrophin-Zinc, Cortrosyn, HP-Acthar) How supplied: gel: 40, 80 USP/mL in 1, 5 mL vials; aqueous: 25, 40 USP/vial. Dose: infantile spasms: IM: 20–40 units/day or 80 units (gel) every other day.

Albumin How supplied: injection: 5% in 50, 250, 500, 1000 mL vials; 25% in 20, 50, 100 mL vials. Dose: 0.5–1.0 g/kg/dose IV as needed. *Note:* Maximum of 6 g/kg/24h for hypovolemia.

Albuterol (Proventil, Ventolin) How supplied: tabs: 2,4 mg; syrup: 2 mg/5 mL; solution for nebulization: 5 mg/mL; inhaler: 90 μg/puff, approx 200 puffs/inhaler. Dose: oral: children, 0.1 mg/kg/dose Q8H; adult, 2–4 mg Q8H; inhalation: 1–2 puffs Q4–6H; nebulization: 0.1 mg/kg/dose; max 5 mg/dose, diluted in 2–3 mL of NS, usually 2–4 times daily but may be repeated prn.

Allopurinol (Lopurin, Zyloprim) How supplied: tabs: 100, 300 mg. Dose: hyperuricemia: <6 yr: 150 mg/d PO Q8H; 6–10 yr: 300 mg/d PO Q8H; adult: 200–600 mg/d PO Q8H (max dose 800 mg/d).

Aluminum Hydroxide (Amphojel, AlternaGel, others) How supplied: tabs: 320, 640 mg; suspension: 320, 600 mg/5 mL. Dose: hyperacidity: 1–2 tsp PO 4–6 times/day. hyperphosphatemia: 50–150 mg/kg/day divided every 4–6 hours.

Aminocaproic Acid (Amicar) How supplied: tabs: 500 mg; syrup: 250 mg/1 mL; injections: 250 mg/1 mL. Dose: excessive bleeding: adult: initial dose of 5 g PO or IV once, then 1.0–1.25 g PO or IV Q1H (max dose 30 g in 24 hr). *Note:* Safety and efficacy in children has not been established.

Aminophylline How supplied: (see also theophylline) tabs: 100, 200 mg (79% theo); syrup: 105 mg/5 mL (86% theo, 90 mg theo/5 mL; injection: 25 mg/1 mL (79% theo, 20 mg theo/1 mL). Dose: oral: see theophyline; intravenous: loading: 2–6 mg/kg IV; maintenance (IV drip): neonates, 0.2 mg/kg/h; 1 mo–1 yr, 0.2–0.9 mg/kg/h; 1–9 yr, 1.0–1.2 mg/kg/h; 9–16 yr, 0.8–1.0 mg/kg/h; young adult smokers, 0.8–1.0 mg/kg/h; nonsmoking adults, 0.5–0.7 mg/kg/h.

Amitriptyline (Elavil, Endep, others) How supplied: tabs: 10, 25, 50, 75, 100, 150 mg; injection: 10 mg/1 mL. Dose: Adolescents: 10 mg PO TID plus 20 mg PO at night; Adults: 75–150 mg PO every day in divided doses. *Note:* Not recommended for children under 12 year of age.

Ammonium Chloride How supplied: tabs: 300, 500, 1000 mg; caps: 300, 500 mg; syrup: 500 mg/5 mL; injection: 0.4, 4.0, 5.0 mEq/1 mL. Dose: urine acidification: 60–75 mg/kg/day PO or IV Q6H (max dose 4–6 g/d).

Aspirin How supplied: tabs: 65, 75, 200, 300, 325, 500, 600, 650 mg; caps: 325 mg; suppositories: 60, 65, 130, 150, 195, 200, 300, 325, 600, 1200 mg. Dose: antipyretic, analgesic: 10–15 mg/kg/dose PO or PR Q4h; adult, 325–650 mg/dose Q4H (max 4–6 doses/d); antirheumatic: 65–100 mg/kg/d PO Q4H; Kawasaki disease: 100 mg/kg/day PO divided every 6 hours.

Atropine Sulfate How supplied: tabs: 0.3, 0.4, 0.6 mg; injection: 0.1, 0.4, 1.0 mg/1 mL. Dose: bradycardia: Children; 0.01–0.03 mg/kg/dose IV, IM, SC (max 2.5 mg); Adults: 0.5–1.0 mg/dose IV, IM, SC (max 2 mg); nebulization: 0.05 mg/kg/dose in 2 mL of NS (max dose 1.0–2.5 mg) given TID, BID; cardiac arrest: 0.01–0.03 mg/kg/dose ET or IV Q2–5 min (min dose 0.1 mg); adult, 0.5–2.0 mg/dose.

Azathioprine (Imuran) How supplied: tabs: 50 mg; injection: 100 mg/20 mL. Dose: renal transplant: 1–5 mg/kg/d PO or IV. Dose: rheumatoid arthritis: 1 mg/kg/day PO, work up to 2.5 mg/kg/day PO.

Baclofen (Lioresal) How supplied: tabs: 10, 20 mg. Dose: reversible spasticity: 5 mg/dose PO TID and gradually increase as needed to max dose of 20 mg/dose QID.

Beclomethasone (Beclovent, Beconase, Vanceril) How supplied: oral inhaler: 42 μg/puff, approx 200 puffs/inhaler; nasal inhaler: 42 μg/puff; nasal spray: 42 μg/spray. Dose: 6–12 yr, 1–2 inhalations Q6–12H (max 10 inhalations/d); >12 yr, 2 inhalations Q6–12H (max 20 inhalations/d).

Bethanechol (Urecholine, others) How supplied: tabs: 5, 10, 25, 50 mg; vials: 5 mg/1 mL. Dose: abdominal distention/urinary retention: 0.6 mg/kg/d PO Q6–8H; adult, 30–120 mg/d TID–QID; 0.15–0.2 mg/kg/d SC Q6–8H; adult, 2.5–5.0 mg/d SC Q6–8H. *Note:* Safety and effectiveness in children has not been established.

Bisacodyl (Dulcolax) How supplied: tabs: 5 mg; suppository: 10 mg. Dose: oral: 0.3 mg/kg/dose; adult, 1–15 mg/dose; rectally: <2 yr, 5 mg/dose; >2 yr, 10 mg/dose (max one dose per day).

Caffeine How supplied: (as citrate) solution: 10 mg/1 mL; injection: 10 mg/1 mL. Dose: 20 mg/kg/dose PO or IV loading dose, then 10 mg/kg/d PO or IV QD.

- **Calcium Chloride** How supplied: 10% or 100 mg/1 mL solution (1.4 mEq Ca^{2+}/1 mL). Dose: hypocalcemia: Children: 70–300 mg/kg/day IV in 4 divided doses or as a continuous infusion IV; cardiac arrest: Children: 20–50 mg/kg/dose IV.
- **Calcium Gluconate** How supplied (as per text). Dose: hypocalcemia: Children: 200–1000 mg/kg/day IV in 4 divided doses or as a continuous infusion. Dose: Maintenance: Children: 200–500 mg/kg/day PO divided every 6 hours; Maintenance: Adults: 5–15 g/day PO divided every 6 hours.
- **Calcium Lactate (13% calcium)** How supplied: tabs: 325, 650 mg. Dose: children, 400–500 mg/kg/d PO Q6–8H; adult, 1.5–3 g/kg/d PO TID.
- **Captopril (Capoten)** How supplied: 12.5, 25, 50, 100 mg. Dose: Infants (<2 mos): 0.1–0.25 mg/kg/dose every 8–24 h, titrate up to 0.5 mg/kg/dose every 6–24 h; Infants (>2 mos) and children: Initial staring dose of 0.3 mg/kg/24 h, titrate in 2-fold increments to a max of 6 mg/kg/day in 1–4 divided doses of 75 mg/day; Adult: 25 mg/dose PO Q8–12H initially and increase as tolerated up to max of 450 mg/d. *Note:* Safety and efficacy in children has not been established.
- **Carbamazepine (Tegretol)** How supplied: tabs: 200 mg; chewable tabs: 100 mg; suspension: 100 mg/5 mL. Dose: 6–12 yr, initial: 100 mg/dose PO BID; increment: weekly increases of 100 mg/d PO TID–QID; maintenance: 400–800 mg/d PO TID–QID (max dose 1000 mg/d); >12 yr, initial: 200 mg/dose PO BID; increment: weekly increases of 200 mg/d PO TID–QID; maintenance: 800–120 mg/d PO TID–QID (max dose 1200 mg/d). *Note:* Safety and efficacy in children <6 years old has not been established.
- **Charcoal, activated** How supplied: 25, 50 g bottles. Dose: 1 g/kg/dose PO or NG Q4H PRN (usual adult dose 50 g).
- **Chloral Hydrate** How supplied: tabs: 250, 500 mg; syrup: 500 mg/10 mL, 1000 mg/10 mL; suppository: 325, 500, 650 mg. Dose: children: 25–100 mg/kg/dose PO, NG, PR; adult: 250–2000 mg/dose PO, NG, PR.
- **Chlordiazepoxide (Librium)** How supplied: tabs: 5, 10, 25 mg; caps: 5, 10, 25 mg; injection: 100 mg/5 mL. Dose: oral: >6 yr, 5 mg/dose PO BID–QID; adult, 5–25 mg/dose PO BID–QID; injection: >12 yr, 25–100 mg/dose IM or IV Q2–4H PRN.
- **Chlorothiazide (Diuril)** How supplied: tabs: 250, 500 mg; suspension: 250 mg/5 mL; injection: 500 mg/20 mL. Dose: oral:

children, 20 mg/kg/d PO Q12H; adult, 500–2000 mg/d PO
Q12–24H; intravenous: adult, 500–2000 mg/d IV Q12–24H.

Chlorpheniramine (many trade names) How supplied: tabs: 4 mg;
caps, timed release: 8, 12 mg; syrup: 2 mg/5 mL; injection:
10 mg/1 mL. Dose: 0.35 mg/kg/d PO or SC QID; adult, 2–4
mg/dose TID–QID.

Chlorpromazine (Thorazine) How supplied: tabs: 10, 25, 50, 100,
200 mg; caps: 30, 75, 150, 200, 300 mg; syrup: 10 mg/5 mL;
suppository: 25, 100 mg; injection: 25 mg/1 mL. Dose: oral:
0.5 mg/kg/dose PO Q4–6H; adult, 10–50 mg/dose; rectal:
1–2 mg/kg/dose PR Q6–8H; adult, 10–50 mg/dose; injection:
0.5 mg/kg/dose IM or IV Q6–8H; adult, 25–100 mg/dose
(maximum doses: <5 yr, 40 mg/d; 5–12 yr, 75 mg/d; adult,
1–2 g/d).

Cholestyramine (Questran) How supplied: powder: 9 g/packet, 9
g/tin. Dose: >6 yr, 240 mg/kg/d PO TID; adult, 4 g/dose PO
TID–QID.

Cimetidine (Tagamet) How supplied: tabs: 200, 300, 400, 800 mg;
syrup: 300 mg/5 mL; injection: 150 mg/1 mL. Dose: 20–40
mg/kg/d PO or IV Q6H; adult, 300 mg/dose PO or IV Q6H.

Citrate (Polycitra, Polycitra K, Bicitra) How supplied: Polycitra:
1 mEq Na, 1 mEq K, 2 mEq bicarbonate/1 mL; Polycitra
K: 0 mEq Na, 2 mEq K, 2 mEq bicarbonate/1 mL; Bicitra:
1 mEq Na, 0 mEq K, 1 mEq bicarbonate/1 mL. Dose: 5–15
mL/dose PO Q6–8H; adult, 10–30 mL/dose PO Q6–8H.

Clemastine (Tavist) How supplied: tabs: 1.34, 2.68 mg; syrup:
0.5 mg/5 mL. Dose: 6–12 yr: 0.5–1.0 mg/dose PO BID (max
dose 3 mg/d); >12 yr: 1–2 mg/dose PO BID (max dose 6
mg/d).

Clonazepam (Clonopin) How supplied: tabs: 0.5, 1.0, 2.0 mg.
Dose: <10 yr: initial 0.01–0.03 mg/kg/d PO Q8–12H; increments of 0.25–0.50 mg every 3rd day to max maintenance
dose of 0.1–0.2 mg/kg/d Q8–12H; adult: initial 1.5 mg/day
PO TID; increments of 0.5–1.0 mg every 3rd day to max
maintenance dose of 20 mg/d PO TID.

Codeine How supplied: tabs: 15, 30, 60 mg (sulfate); injection:
20, 60 mg/1 mL (phosphate). Dose: analgesic: children,
0.5–1.0 mg/kg/dose PO or IV Q4–6H; adult, 30–60 mg/dose
PO or IV Q4–6H; antitussive: children, 0.2–0.5 mg/kg/dose
PO Q4–6H; adult, 15–30 mg/kg/dose PO Q4–6H.

Cortisone Acetate (Cortone) How supplied: tabs: 25 mg; injection: 25, 50 mg/1 mL. Dose: physiologic replacement: oral,

approx 25 mg/m^2/day PO TID; IM, approx 15 mg/m^2/d QD; stress: 2–4 times physiologic replacement dose.

Cromolyn Sodium (Intal, Nasalcrom, Opticrom) How supplied: inhaler: 800 μg/puff, approx 200 puffs/inhaler; liquid for nebulization: 20 mg/2 mL; nasal spray: 5.2 mg/spray, 100 sprays/13 mL container; eye drops: 40 mg/1 mL (4%), 10 mL container. Dose: inhalation: 2 puffs QID; nebulization: 20 mg/dose TID–QID; nasal: 1 spray each nostril 3–4 times/d; eyes: 1–2 drops each eye 4–6 times/d.

Cyproheptadine (Periactin) How supplied: tabs: 4 mg; syrup: 2 mg/5 mL. Dose: 0.25 mg/kg/d PO Q8–12H (max dose 0.5 mg/kg/d).

Dantrolene (Dantrium) How supplied: caps: 25, 50, 100 mg; injection: 20 mg/70 mL. Dose: malignant hyperthermia: prophylaxis, 4–8 mg/kg/d PO Q6–8H starting 1–2 days before anesthesia; treatment, 1 mg/kg IV repeated prn up to max of 10 mg/kg. Dose: spasticity: Oral: Initial 0.5 mg/kg/dose BID, increase frequency to TID/QID at 4–7 day intervals, then increase dose by 0.5 mg/kg to max of 3 mg/kg/dose 2–4 times per day up to 400 mg/day.

Deferoxamine Mesylate (Desferal) How supplied: 500 mg/vial. Dose: diagnostic challenge: 1 g IM once; therapeutic: acute iron intoxication: 15 mg/kg/h IV by continuous infusion; 50 mg/kg/dose IM Q6H (max 500 mg/dose except 1000 mg/dose for first dose only).

Desmopressin Acetate (DDAVP) How supplied: nasal solution: 0.1 mg/1 mL; injection: 4 μg/1 mL. Dose: diabetes insipidus: children, 5–30 μg/d Q12–24H intranasally; adult, 10–40 μg/d Q8–24H intranasally; *or* 2–4 μg/day IV or SC Q12–24 H; coagulopathy: 0.3 μg/kg/dose IV.

Dexamethasone (Decadron, others) How supplied: tabs: 0.25, 0.5, 0.75, 1.5, 4, 6 mg; elixir: 0.5 mg/5 mL; injection: 4, 24 mg/1 mL. Dose: increased intracranial pressure: initial: 0.5–1.5 mg/kg/dose IV or IM; adults, 10 mg/dose IV or IM; maintenance: 0.2–0.5 mg/kg/d IV or IM Q6H; adults, 4 mg/dose IV or IM Q6H, then taper slowly; airway edema: 0.25–0.5 mg/kg/dose PO, IV, or IM Q6H for 4–6 doses.

Dextroamphetamine (Dexedrine, others) How supplied: tabs: 5, 10 mg; caps: 5, 10, 15 mg; elixir: 5 mg/5 mL. Dose: attention deficit disorder: 3–5 yr: 2.5 mg/d PO initially then increments of 2.5 mg at weekly intervals; daily dose BID–TID; >5 yr: 5.0 mg/d PO initially then increments of 5.0 mg at weekly intervals; daily dose BID–TID, max dose 40 mg/d.

Dextromethorphan (many trade names) How supplied: available in many preparations. Dose: 0.5–1 mg/kg/d PO Q6–24H.

Diazepam (Valium) How supplied: tabs: 2, 5, 10 mg; injection: 5 mg/1 mL. Dose: sedation: children, oral: 0.1–0.8 mg/kg/d PO Q6–8H; injection: 0.04–0.2 mg/kg/dose IV Q2–4H; adult, oral: 2–10 mg/dose PO Q6–8H; injection: 2–10 mg/dose IV Q3–4H; seizures: children: <5 yr, 0.2–0.5 mg/kg/dose IV Q15–30 min; total max 5 mg; >5 yr, 1 mg/dose IV Q15–50 min; total max 10 mg, repeat Q2–4H prn.

Diazoxide (Hyperstat, Proglycem) How supplied: caps: 50 mg; liquid: 50 mg/1 mL; injection: 15 mg/1 mL. Dose: hypertension: children and adults, 1–3 mg/kg/dose IV rapid bolus, repeat Q5–15 min, then Q4–24H; hypoglycemia: infants, 8–15 mg/kg/d PO or IV Q8–12H; children and adults, 3–8 mg/kg/d PO or IV Q8–12H.

Digoxin How supplied: tabs: 125, 250, 500 μg (bioavailability 60–80%); caps: 50, 100, 200 μg (bioavailability 90–100%); elixir: 50 μg/1 mL (bioavailability 70–85%); injection: 100, 250 mg/1 mL (IV bioavailability 100%). Dose: tabs or elixir: premature, 20–30 μg/kg PO digitalizing dose; maintenance dose is 20–30% of oral digitalizing dose, BID; full term, 25–35 μg/kg PO digitalizing dose*; 1–24 mo, 35–60 μg/kg PO digitalizing dose*; 2–5 yr, 30–40 μg/kg PO digitalizing dose*; 5–10 yr, 20–35 μg/kg PO digitalizing dose*; >10 yr, 10–15 μg/kg PO digitalizing dose*; then maintenance dose is 25–35% of oral digitalizing dose, divided BID*; in <10 yr digitalizing doses given as ½ the total digitalizing dose initially then ¼ the total digitalizing dose Q8–18H × 2.

Dimenhydrinate (Dramamine, others) How supplied: tabs: 50 mg; syrup: 15 mg/5 mL; injection: 50 mg/1 mL. Dose: <12 yr: 5 mg/kg/d PO or IM Q6H (max 300 mg/d); >12 yr: 50–100 mg/dose PO or IM Q4H (max 400 mg/d).

Dimercaprol (BAL) How supplied: oil for injection 100 mg/1 mL. Dose: lead poisoning: 3–4 mg/kg/dose IM Q4H for 2–7 days; arsenic poisoning: 2.5 mg/kg/dose IM Q4–6H for 2 days then decrease dose over next few days.

Diphenhydramine (Benadryl, others) How supplied: tabs: 50; caps: 25, 50 mg; elixir: 12.5 mg/5 mL; injection: 10, 50 mg/1 mL. Dose: children, 5 mg/kg/d PO, IV, or IM Q6–8H

---

* IV: digitalizing doses are 80% of the oral digitalizing doses. Maintenance doses are based on the same percentages of the loading doses as above and divided BID.

(max dose 300 mg/d); adult, 10–50 mg/kg/dose PO, IV, or IM Q6–8H (max dose 400 mg/d).

Diphenoxylate (Lomotil) How supplied: tabs: 2.5 mg; liquid: 2.5 mg/5 mL. Dose: >2 yr, 0.3–0.4 mg/kg/d PO QID; adult, 5 mg/dose PO TID–QID.

Dobutamine (Dobutrex) How supplied: injection: 12.5 mg/1 mL. Dose: IV infusion: 2.5–15 µg/kg/min (max dose 40 µg/kg/min).

Docusate Sodium (Colace, others) How supplied: caps: 50, 100, 150 mg; liquid: 10 mg/1 mL; syrup: 20 mg/5 mL, 50 mg/15 mL. Dose: <3 yr, 10–40 mg/d PO QD–QID; 3–6 yr, 20–60 mg/d PO QD–QID; 6–12 yr, 40–120 mg/d PO QD-QID; >12 yr, 50–200 mg/d PO QD–QID.

Dopamine (Intropin) How supplied: injection: 40, 80, 160 mg/1 mL. Dose: IV infusion: 2–20 µg/kg/min (max dose 20–50 µg/kg/min).

Edrophonium (Tensilon) How supplied: injection: 10 mg/1 mL. Dose: use in the diagnosis of myasthenia gravis; Infants: initial 0.1 mg, followed by 0.4 mg if no response: 0.5 mg total dose. Children: initial 0.04 mg/kg followed by 0.16 mg/kg if no response, to max of 10 mg; total dose 0.2 mg/kg.

Enalapril Maleate (Vasotec) How supplied: tabs: 2.5, 5, 10, 20 mg. Dose: adult, 5 mg/dose PO QD initially then increase up to 40 mg/day PO QD–BID. *Note:* Safety and efficacy in children has not been established.

Epinephrine Dose: 1) bronchospasm (1:200 or sus-phrine): children: (1:1000 dilution) 0.005 mL/kg SC, not more than every 6 hours; adults: (1:1000) 0.1–0.3 mL not more than every 6 hours. 2) Refractory hypotension: start infusion 0.1 µg/kg/min, titrate to desired effect. 3) Cardiac arrest: (1:10,000) 0.1–0.3 mL/kg IV, intra-osseus, ET, Q3–5 min PRN. 4) Anaphylaxis: Children (1:1000) 0.01 mL/kg SC (max 0.5 mL) Q15 min times two doses, then Q4H PRN; Adults (1:1000) 0.1–0.3 mL/dose SC (max 0.3 mL) Q15–20 min up to 4 hours.

Epinephrine, racemic Dose: >2 years: 0.5 mL diluted with 3 mL NS as nebulization; may repeat Q2H. <2 years: 0.25 mL (as above).

Ethacrynic Acid (Edecrin) Dose: difficult to control edema, CHF, hepatic or renal disease: older children, 25 mg/dose PO initially then slowly increase in 25 mg/dose increments Q2–3 days (max 3 mg/kg/day divided every 12h) (contraindicated in infants).

Ethosuximide (Zarontin) Dose: (optimal dose usually 20 mg/kg/ d) 3–6 yr, 250 mg/d PO initially then increase slowly by 250 mg/d increments Q4–7 days, daily dose divided Q12–24H; >6 yr, 500 mg/day PO initially then increase slowly by 250 mg/d increments Q4–7 days, daily dose divided Q12–24H (max dose 1.5 g/d).

Fentanyl (Sublimaze) How supplied: injection: 50 μg/1 mL. Dose: 1–3 μg/kg/dose IV or IM.

Flunisolide (Nasalide, Aerobid) How supplied: nasal spray (0.25%): 25 μg/spray, 200 sprays/bottle. Dose: seasonal or perennial rhinitis: nasal inhalent: 6–14 yrs, 1 spray each nostril TID or 2 sprays each nostril BID (max dose 4 sprays/ nostril/day); adult, 2 sprays each nostril BID–TID (max dose 8 sprays/nostril/d). Asthma: oral inhalation: children >6 yrs: oral inhalation BID (max 4 inhal/24h); Adults: 2 inhalations twice daily (max 8 inhal/24 h).

Fluoride How supplied: tabs: 0.25, 0.5, 1.0 mg; liquid; 0.5, 2, 4 mg/1 mL. Dose: 2 wk–2 yr, 0.25 mg/d; 2–3 yr, 0.25–0.5 mg/ d; 3–16 yr, 0.5–1.0 mg/d.

9-alpha Fluorocortisol (Florinef) How supplied: tabs: 0.1 mg. Dose: 0.05–0.15 mg/d PO.

Flurazepam (Dalmane) How supplied: caps: 15, 30 mg. Dose: >15 yr, 15–30 mg/dose PO QHS.

Folic Acid How supplied: tabs: 1 mg. Dose: 0.2–1.0 mg/d PO; adult, 1 mg/day PO.

Furosemide (Lasix, others) How supplied: tabs: 20, 40, 80 mg; syrup: 10 mg/1 mL; injection: 10 mg/1 mL. Dose: children, 1–2 mg/kg/dose PO, IV, or IM Q6–12H; adult, 20–80 mg/ dose PO, IV, or IM Q12–24H (max 600 mg/d).

Gamma Benzene Hexachloride (Kwell, Scabene) How supplied: 1% cream, lotion, and shampoo. Dose: skin: a thin layer applied from the neck down, left on the skin for 8–12H then washed off, usually only one treatment is necessary, an adult usually uses 60 mL; hair: 30–60 mL per application, worked thoroughly into dry hair, stand for 4 mins, lather with water, rinse thoroughly, remove nits with comb pro- vided. Repeat treatment in 7 days if lice or nits are still present.

Glucagon How supplied: injection: 1 mg/1 mL. Dose: 0.5–1.0 mg/dose SC, IM, or IV Q10–25 min (max 2 mg/dose).

Haloperidol (Haldol) How supplied: tabs: 0.5, 1, 2, 5, 10, 20 mg; syrup: 2 mg/1 mL; injection: 5 mg/1 mL. Dose: psychotic disorders: 0.05–0.15 mg/kg/day to divided PO BID–TID;

non-psychotic behavior disorders and Tourette's: 0.05–0.075 mg/kg/day.

Heparin Sodium How supplied: injection: 10, 100, 1,000, 2,500, 5,000, 7,500, 10,000, 15,000, 20,000, 40,000 U/1 mL. Dose: children, 50 U/kg IV bolus once, then 10–25 U/kg/hr as continuous infusion; adult 10,000 U/dose IV bolus once, then 5,000–10,000 U/dose IV Q4–6H.

Hydralazine (Apresoline) How supplied: tabs: 10, 25, 50, 100 mg; injection: 20 mg/1 mL. Dose: chronic hypertension: oral: children, 0.75–3.0 mg/kg/d PO Q6–12H; adult, 10–50 mg/dose PO QID; Hypertensive crisis: injection: children, 0.1–0.2 mg/kg/dose IM or IV Q4–6H; adult, 20–40 mg/dose IM or IV Q4–6H.

Hydrochlorothiazide (Esidrix, HydroDiuril, others) How supplied: tabs: 25, 50, 100 mg. Dose: children, 2–3 mg/kg/d PO BID; adult, 26–100 mg/dose PO QD–BID (max 200 mg/d).

Hydrocortisone (Solu-cortef) Dose: physiologic replacement: approx. 12.5 mg/m^2/d IM or IV QD; asthma: children, initial dose 4–8 mg/kg/dose IV once then 8 mg/kg/d IV Q6H; adult, 100–500 mg/dose IV Q2–6H.

Hydroxyzine (Atarax, Vistaril) Dose: oral: children, 1–2 mg/kg/d PO TID–QID; adult, 25–100 mg/dose PO QID; injection: children, 1 mg/kg/dose, IM; adult, 25–100 mg/dose IM. Antipyretic and analgesic: children: 5–10 mg/kg/dose Q6–8H; Adults: 1200–3200 mg/day PO divided Q4–6H.

Imipramine (Tofranil) How supplied: tabs: 10, 25, 50 mg; caps: 75, 100, 125, 150 mg; injection: 12.5 mg/1 mL. Dose: depression: adolescents, initially 30–40 mg/d PO BID–TID, then gradually increase to maintenance of max 100 mg/d PO QD–BID; adult, initially 75–100 mg/d PO BID then gradually increase to maintenance of 50–300 mg/d PO QD–BID; enuresis: >6 yrs: 25 mg/dose 1 hr before bedtime may increase to 50 mg/dose for 6–12 yr; 75 mg/dose for >12 yr (max dose 2.5 mg/kg/d).

Indomethacin (Indocin) How supplied: caps: 25, 50 mg; suspension: 25 mg/5 mL; injection: 1 mg/vial. Dose: patent ductus closure:

age at first dose	dose:	(dose in mg/kg) #1	#2	#3
<48 hr		0.2	0.1	0.1
2–7 d		0.2	0.2	0.2
>7 d		0.2	0.25	0.25

doses given 12–24 hr apart, total of 3 doses antiinflammatory: <14 yr, 1–3 mg/kg/d PO TID–QID; adult, 50–200 mg/
d PO BID–QID.

Insulin How supplied: many formulations are available including
human, pork, and beef products; some are rapid-onset (regular, Semilente), intermediate-onset (Lente, NPH) and delayed-onset (Ultralente); there are many considerations in
deciding which type of insulin is optimal. Dose: DKA: usual
dose 0.1 U/kg/hr IV of regular insulin given as continuous
IV infusion; maintenance: usual dose range is 0.5–1.0 U/kg/
d given in divided doses SC.

Ipecac Syrup How supplied: 7% syrup in 15 and 30 mL bottles.
Dose: 6–12 mos: 10 mL PO once, followed by clear liquids;
1–12 yrs: 15–30 mL PO once, followed by clear liquids; >12
yr: 30–60 mL PO once, followed by clear liquids; may repeat
dose once if no emesis occurs within 20 min.

Iron Dextran How supplied: injection: 50 mg of elemental
iron/1 mL. Dose: iron deficiency anemia: calculated using
the following formulas: dose in mL: wt (kg) $\times$ 0.0476 $\times$
(normal Hgb—patient Hgb); dose in mg of iron: wt (kg) $\times$
2.4 $\times$ (normal Hgb—patient Hgb); add 1 mL/5 kg (50
mg iron/5 kg) of body weight to the dose calculated
above to replenish ironstores, up to max 14 mL total;
max IV dose is 2 mL/d; max IM daily dose is based on
weight:

<5 kg	0.5 mL
5–10 kg	1.0 mL
>10 kg	2.0 mL
adult	5.0 mL

Note: Prior to receiving iron dextron therapy, all individuals
should receive a test dose, either 0.5 mL IV or IM.

Iron Supplements How supplied: ferrous sulfate (Fer-In-Sol):

	ferrous sulfate	elemental iron
caps:	190 mg	60 mg
drops:	75 mg/0.6 mL	15 mg/0.6 mL
syrup:	90 mg/5 mL	18 mg/5 mL

ferrous gluconate (Fergon):

	ferrous gluconate	elemental iron
tabs:	320 mg	35 mg
caps:	435 mg	50 mg
elixir:	300 mg/5 mL	34 mg/5 mL

Dose: dietary supplement (in mg of elemental iron): premature infant, 1–2 mg/kg/d PO QD–TID: term infants, 1 mg/kg/d PO QD–TID: (US RDA for >4 yr = 18 mg/d); iron deficiency (in mg of elemental iron): 6 mg/kg/d PO TID.

Isoproterenol (Isuprel) How supplied: injection (1:5000): 0.2 mg/1 mL. Dose: cardiac arrest, severe bronchospasm: 0.1–1.0 μg/kg/min as continuous IV infusion.

Isotretinoin (Accutane) How supplied: caps: 10, 20, 40 mg. Dose: severe cystic acne: 0.5–1.0 mg/kg/d PO BID (max dose 2 mg/kg/d). *Note:* Contraindicated in pregnancy.

Lactulose (Cephulac, others) How supplied: syrup: 10 g/15 mL. Dose: infants: 2.5–10 mL/d PO TID–QID; older children and adolescents: 40–90 mL/d PO TID–QID; adult: 30–45 mL/dose PO TID–QID.

Levothyroxine (Synthroid) How supplied: tabs: 25, 50, 75, 100, 112, 125, 150, 175, 200, 300 μg; injection: 20, 50 μg/1 mL. Dose: children, 0–6 mo: 8–10 μg/kg/d PO (25–50 μg/d); 6–12 mo: 6–8 μg/kg/d PO (50–75 μg/d); 1–5 yr: 5–6 μg/kg/d PO (75–100 μg/d); 6–12 yr: 4–5 μg/kg/d PO (100–150 μg/d); adult, initially 25–50 μg/d PO then increase in increments of 25 μg Q2–3 wks to maintenance of 100–200 μg/d. (IV dose is approx 50% of PO dose.)

Lidocaine (Xylocaine) How supplied: (1% = 10 mg/1 mL); injection: 0.5%, 1.0%, 1.5%, 2.0% and also 50 mg/5 mL, 100 mg/5 mL prefilled syringes; ointment: 2.5%, 5.0%; oral spray: 10%; viscous: 2%. Dose: local anesthesia: 3–4.5 mg/kg max total dose; intravenous for cardiac arrhythmias: 1 mg/kg IV bolus Q5 min × 3, may be given as continuous IV infusion of 20–50 μg/kg/min.

Lindane (see Gamma Benzene Hexachloride)

Loperamide (Imodium, Imodium A-D) How supplied: caps: 2 mg: syrup: 1 mg/5 mL. Dose: initial daily dose: 2–5 yr: 1 mg/dose PO TID (3 mg/d); 6–8 yr: 2 mg/dose PO BID (4 mg/d); 8–12 yr: 2 mg/dose PO TID (6 mg/d); subsequent daily dose: 1 mg/10 kg weight/dose with each subsequent loose stool, max daily dose as listed above; adult: 4 mg/dose PO once, then 2 mg/dose with each subsequent loose stool (max 16 mg/d).

Lorazepam (Ativan) How supplied: tabs: 0.5, 1, 2 mg; injection: 2, 4 mg/1 mL. Dose: intravenous: 0.05–0.1 mg/kg/dose IV Q6H (adults 2–4 mg/dose max); oral: adults 2–6 mg/d PO Q8–12H (max 10 mg/d).

Lypressin (Diapid) How supplied: nasal spray: 2 USP/spray, 50 USP/1 mL, 8 mL bottle. Dose: diabetes insipidus: 1–2 sprays in each nostril QID, a QHS dose may be needed also.

Magnesium Citrate How supplied: solution: 300 mL bottles. Dose: 4 mL/kg/dose PO, max 200 mL dose.

Magnesium Hydroxide (Milk of Magnesia) How supplied: tabs; 311 mg; suspension: 405 mg/5 mL. Dose: children <2 yrs: 0.5–1.0 mL/kg/dose PO prn; children 2–5 yrs: 5–15 mL/day as a single or divided dose; children 6–11 yrs: 15–30 mL/day; adult: 15–60 mL/dose PO prn (1 mL = approx 80 mg).

Magnesium Sulfate How supplied: solution: 50% (500 mg/1 mL). Dose: cathartic: child, 250 mg/kg/dose PO; adult, 10–30 g/day PO.

Mannitol How supplied: injection: 50, 100, 150, 200, 250 mg/1 mL. Dose: cerebral edema: 0.5–1.0 g/kg/dose IV prn.

Meclizine (Antivert, Bonine) How supplied: tabs: 12.5, 25, 50 mg. Dose: vertigo: 25–100 mg/d PO Q6–12H; motion sickness: 25–50 mg/d PO 1 h prior to travel. *Note:* Not recommended in children <12 yrs.

Meperidine (Demerol) How supplied: tabs: 50, 100 mg; syrup: 50 mg/5 mL; injection: 25, 50, 75, 100 mg/1 mL. Dose: children: 1–1.5 mg/kg/dose PO, SC, or IM Q3–4H prn; adult: 50–150 mg/dose PO, SC, or IM Q3–4H prn.

Metaproterenol (Alupent, Metaprel) How supplied: tabs: 10, 20 mg; syrup: 10 mg/5 mL; inhaler: 0.65 mg/puff, 300 puffs/inhaler; solution for nebulization: 5% (50 mg/1 mL). Dose: oral: <6 yr, 1.3–2.6 mg/kg/d PO TID–QID; 6–9 yr, 10 mg/dose PO TID–QID; >9 yr, 20 mg/dose PO TID–QID; inhalation (not recommended for children <12 yrs): 2–3 puffs at Q3–4H, max 12 puffs/d; nebulization: 0.2–0.5 mL/dose in 2.5 mL NS Q1–6H prn.

Methadone How supplied: tabs: 5, 10 mg; liquid: 5, 10 mg/5 mL; injection: 10 mg/1 mL. Dose: analgesic: adult, 2.5–10 mg/dose PO, SC, or IM Q3–4H. *Note:* Not recommended for use in children.

Methimazole (Tapazole) How supplied: tabs: 5, 10 mg. Dose: hyperthyroidism: children, initially 0.4 mg/kg/d PO Q8H then 50% of initial dose as maintenance; adult, initially 15–60 mg/d PO Q8H then 5–30 mg/d PO TID.

Methsuximide (Celontin) How supplied: caps: 150, 300 mg. Dose: Adults: 300 mg/d PO for 1 wk, then increase by 300 mg/d every 1 wk for 3 wk up to max 1200 mg/d, usual maintenance dose is 10–20 mg/kg/d PO; Children; 10–20 mg/kg/day divided BID/QID.

Methyldopa (Aldomet) How supplied: tabs: 125, 250, 500 mg; suspension: 250 mg/5 mL; injection: 50 mg/1 mL. Dose: children, oral: 10 mg/kg/d PO Q6–12H, increase at 2-day intervals to max 65 mg/kg/day or 3 g/d, whichever is less: intravenous (for hypertensive crisis): 20–40 mg/kg/day IV Q6H (max 65 mg/kg/d or 3 g/d, whichever is less); adult, oral: 250 mg/dose PO BID–TID, increase at 2-day intervals to max 3 g/d, usual maintenance dose is 500–2000 mg/d PO BID–QID; intravenous (for hypertensive crisis): 250–500 mg/dose IV Q6H, max 1 gm Q6H.

Methylene Blue How supplied: solution: 1% (10 mg/1 mL). Dose: antidote for cyanide poisoning and drug-induced methemoglobinemia: 1–2 mg/kg/dose slowly IV.

Methylphenidate (Ritalin) How supplied: tabs: 5, 10, 20 mg; slow-release caps: 20 mg. Dose (>6 yr): 5 mg/dose PO BID (before breakfast and lunch), increase gradually 5–10 mg/wk to max 60 mg/d.

Methylprednisolone (DepoMedrol, Medrol, Solumedrol) How supplied: tabs: 2, 4, 8, 16, 24, 32 mg; injection (SoluMedrol, as succinate for IV, IM): 40, 125, 500, 1000, 2000 mg/vials; injection (Depo-Medrol, as acetate for IM repository): 20, 40, 80 mg/1 mL. Dose: asthma: initially 1–2 mg/kg/dose IV once, then 0.5–1.0 mg/kg/dose IV Q6H; anti-inflammatory: 0.16–1.0 mg/kg/day PO or IV Q6–12H.

Metoclopramide (Reglan) How supplied: tabs: 5, 10 mg; syrup: 5 mg/5 mL; injection: 5, 10 mg/1 mL. Dose: GE reflux: 1–6 yr, 0.1 mg/kg/dose PO or IV QID; 6–12 yr, 2.5–5 mg/dose PO or IV QID; adult, 10–15 mg/dose PO or IV QID; antiemetic: 1–2 mg/kg/dose IV Q2–3H prn.

Midazolam (Versed) How supplied: injection: 1, 5 mg/1 mL. Dose: conscious sedation: 0.07–0.08 mg/kg/dose IM, usual adult dose 5 mg/dose; 0.1–0.2 mg/kg/dose IV, usual adult dose 1–5 mg/dose; 0.3 mg/kg/dose intranasal.

Mineral Oil How supplied: plain and flavored preparations, 4.2

g mineral oil/15 mL. Dose: children >6 yrs: 5–30 mL PO QD given as single or divided dose. Not recommended for children <6 yrs. Adults 16–30 mL/dose, titrate dose based on stools.

Morphine Sulfate How supplied: tabs: 10, 15, 30 mg; elixir: 2, 4, 20 mg/1 mL; suppository: 5, 10, 20 mg; injection: 8, 10, 15 mg/1 mL. Dose: children, 0.1–0.2 mg/kg/dose SC, IM, or IV Q2–4H prn; adult, 10–30 mg/dose PO Q4H prn, or 2–10 mg/dose IV Q2–4H prn.

Naloxone (Narcan) How supplied: injection: 0.02, 0.4, 1.0 mg/1 mL. Dose: children, 0.01–0.1 mg/kg/dose IV once, may repeat dose of 0.1 mg/kg if needed, SC and IM route acceptable; adult, 0.4–2 mg/dose IV once, may repeat Q2–3 min; max dose 4 mg.

Neomycin Sulfate How supplied: tabs: 500 mg; suspension: 500 mg/5 mL. Dose: hepatic encephalopathy: initially 2.5–7 g/m^2/d PO Q6H for 5–7 days, then 2.5 g/m^2/day PO Q6H.

Neostigmine (Prostigmin) How supplied: tabs: 15 mg; injection: 0.25, 0.5, 1 mg/1 mL. Dose: myasthenia gravis: test dose: children, 0.04 mg/kg/dose IM, 0.02 mg/kg/dose IV; adult, 0.02 mg/kg/dose IM; treatment: children: 0.01–0.04 mg/kg/dose SC, IM, or IV Q2–3H prn; adult: 0.5 mg/dose SC, IM, or IV Q3–4H prn (max 10 mg/day); 15–375 mg/d PO prn. *Note:* Safety and efficacy in children has not been established.

Nifedipine (Adalat, Procardia) How supplied: caps: 10, 20 mg. Dose: hypertension: children (not FDA approved): 0.25–0.5 mg/kg/dose PO or sublingual Q6–8H, not to exceed adult doses; adult: 10–20 mg/dose PO TID, max 30 mg/dose and 180 mg/d.

Nitroglycerine How supplied: injection: 0.8, 5, 10 mg/1 mL. Dose: 0.25–10 µg/kg/min as continuous IV infusion.

Nitroprusside (Nipride) How supplied: injection: 50 mg/5 mL. Dose: hypertensive crisis: 0.5–10 µg/kg/min as continuous IV infusion.

Norepinephrine (Levophed) How supplied: injection: 1 mg/1 mL. Dose: shock: 0.05–0.1 µg/kg/min as continuous IV infusion.

Pancreatic Enzymes (Cotazym, Creon, Pancrease, Viokase, others) How supplied: powder: Cotazym (in caps), Viokase; enteric-coated spheres: Cotazym-S, Creon, Pancrease; non-enteric coated tabs: Viokase. Dose: 1–3 caps or tabs, or ¼ tsp of powder, with each meal, adjusted for each patient prn.

Pancuronium (Pavulon) How supplied: injection: 1, 2 mg/1 mL. Dose: 0.03–0.1 mg/kg/dose IV Q½–2H prn, titrate dose based on patient's response.

Paraldehyde How supplied: solution: 1 g/1 mL; injection 1 g/1 mL. Dose: seizures: rectal or oral, 0.3 mL/kg/dose in oil Q4–6H (adult 16–32 mL). For rectal dosage, mix paraldehyde 2:1 with oil (peanut, cottonseed, or olive); for oral dosage, dilute in milk or fruit juice.

Paregoric How supplied: solution: 0.4 mg morphine/1 mL. Dose: opiate withdrawal in newborns: 0.2–0.5 mL/dose PO Q3–4H prn, max 0.7 mL/kg/dose; analgesia: 0.25–0.5 mL/kg/dose PO QD–QID, max 10 mL/dose.

Pemoline (Cylert) How supplied: tabs: 18.75, 37.5, 75 mg; chewable tabs: 37.5 mg. Dose: treatment of ADHD: children ≥6 yrs: initially 37.5 mg/d PO QAM, increase by 18.75 mg/d at weekly intervals prn (max dose 112.5 mg/d).

Penicillamine (Cuprimine) Dose: Wilson's Disease: children: 20 mg/kg/day divided QID oral; adult: 0.75–1.5 g/day divided QID oral, adjust dose to result in an initial 24-hour cupriuresis of >2 mg for 3 months; Cystinuria: children: 30 mg/kg/day divided QID oral; adult: 1–4 g/day divided QID oral, adjust dose to limit cystine excretion to 100–200 mg/day if no history of stones and <100 mg/day with history of stones; Rheumatoid arthritis: children: efficacy has not been established; Adults, 125–250 mg/day, may increase at 1–3 month intervals by 125–250 mg (max = 1500 mg/day); Arsenic poisoning: 100 mg/kg/day PO divided QID (max = 1 g/day); Lead poisoning: children: 25–40 mg/kg/day oral divided BID–TID; Adults: 1–1.5 g/day for 1–2 months, continue until blood lead level is <60 μg/dL.

Pentobarbital (Nembutal) How supplied: caps: 50, 100; suppository: 30, 60, 120, 200 mg; injection: 50 mg/1 mL. Dose: sedation: 2–6 mg/kg/dose PO, max 100 mg/dose.

Phenazopyridine (Pyridium) How supplied: tabs: 100, 200 mg. Dose: symptomatic relief of urinary tract infection: children >6 yrs: 100 mg/dose PO TID after meals; adult, 200 mg/dose PO TID after meals.

Phenobarbital How supplied: tabs: 15, 30, 60, 100 mg; elixir: 20 mg/5 mL; injection: 65, 130 mg/1 mL. Dose: sedation: 2–3 mg/kg/dose PO or IM Q6–8H prn; seizures; 10–25 mg/kg/dose IM or IV initially, then 4–6 mg/kg/d PO Q12H (adults 150–250 mg/d).

Phenytoin (Dilantin) How supplied: tabs: 50 mg; caps: 30, 100 mg; suspension: 30, 125 mg/5 mL; injection: 50 mg/1 mL. Dose: seizures: 10–20 mg/kg/dose slow IV initially, not to exceed 1 mg/kg/min, then 4–8 mg/kg/d PO or IV QD–TID; adult, 300–600 mg/d PO or IV QD–TID.

Physostigmine Salicylate (Antilirium) How supplied: injection: 1 mg/1 mL. Dose: reversal of CNS effects caused by anticholinergics: 0.02 mg/kg/dose IM or IV, no more than 0.5 mg/min, repeat Q5–10 min up to max total dose of 2 mg.

Potassium Iodide How supplied: syrup: 325 mg/5 mL; solution: 1 g/mL. Dose: expectorant: children, 100–300 mg/d PO BID–TID; adult, 300–900 mg/d PO TID.

Potassium Supplement How supplied: potassium chloride: effervescent tabs: 25, 50 mEq; caps: 4, 8, 10 mEq: liquid: 5%, 10%, 20% (5% = 10 mEq/15 mL); powder: 15, 20 mEq/packet, 25 mEq/scoop; injection: 2 mEq/1 mL. Dose: maintenance: approx 1–2 mEq/kg/d PO QD–QID (40–80 mEq/d for adults); hypokalemia: 0.5–1.0 mEq/kg/dose slow IV.

Pralidoxime (Protopam) How supplied: tabs: 500 mg; injection: 1 g/20 mL. Dose: reversal of paralysis due to organophosphates: 20–40 mg/kg/dose slow IV, as 5% solution, repeat Q1H prn; adult 1–2 g/dose slow IV, dose may be given SC, IM, or PO if necessary.

Prazosin (Minipress) How supplied: tabs: 1, 2, 5 mg. Dose: hypertension: NOT APPROVED FOR USE IN CHILDREN; adult: initial 1 mg/dose PO BID–TID, slowly increase to a total daily dose of 20 mg; usual dose 6–15 mg/d.

Prednisone How supplied: tabs: 1, 2.5, 5, 10, 20, 25, 50 mg; syrup: 5 mg/5 mL. Dose: physiologic replacement: 4–5 mg/m²/d PO BID; asthma: 1–2 mg/kg/d PO QD–BID, max 20–40 mg/d for 3–5 days; anti-inflammatory: 0.5–2 mg/kg/d PO BID–QID.

Primidone (Mysoline) How supplied: tabs: 50, 250 mg; suspension: 250 mg/5 mL. Dose: seizures: <8 yr, days 1–3; 50 mg/dose PO QHS: days 4–6: 50 mg/dose PO BID; days 7–9: 100 mg/dose PO BID; day 10 on: 125–250 mg/dose PO TID; usual maintenance dose 10–25 mg/kg/d PO TID; >8 yr, days 1–3: 100–125 mg/dose PO QHS: days 4–6: 100–125 mg/dose PO BID; days 7–9: 100–125 mg/dose PO TID; day 10 on: 250 mg/dose PO TID, slowly increased to max 750–1500 mg/d TID–QID.

Probenecid (Benemid) How supplied: tabs: 500 mg. Dose: hyperuricemia: >2 yr: 25 mg/kg/dose PO once, then 40 mg/kg/d PO QID; >14 yr: 1–2 g/dose PO once, then 2 g/d PO QID.

Procainamide (Pronestyl) How supplied: tabs: 250, 375, 500 mg; sustained-release tabs: 500 mg; caps: 250, 375, 500 mg; injection: 100, 500 mg/1 mL. Dose: cardiac arrhythmias: children, oral: 15–50 mg/kg/d PO Q3–6H, max 4 g/d; IV: 10–15 mg/kg/dose IV over 30 min, then 20–80 µg/kg/min continuous IV infusion; adult, oral: approx 50 mg/kg/d PO Q3–6H, usually 250–500 mg/dose Q3–6H, max 4 g/d; IV: 100–200 mg IV over 30 min, max 1 g, then 2–6 mg/min continuous IV infusion.

Prochlorperazine (Compazine) How supplied: tabs: 5, 10, 25 mg; sustained-release caps: 10, 15, 30 mg; syrup: 5 mg/5 mL; suppository: 2.5, 25 mg; injection: 5 mg/1 mL. Contraindicated in children <2 yrs. Dose: antiemetic: oral 9–13 kg: 2.5 mg/dose PO or PR QD–BID; 14–18 kg: 2.5 mg/dose PO or PR BID–TID; 19–40 kg: 2.5–5 mg/dose PO or PR BID–TID; adult: 5–10 mg/dose PO TID–QID, or 25 mg PR BID: IM: children: 0.13 mg/kg/dose; adult: 5–10 mg/dose TID–QID (max 40 mg/d).

Promethazine (Phenergan) How supplied: tabs: 12.5, 25, 50 mg; syrup: 6.25, 25 mg/5 mL; suppository: 12.5, 25, 50 mg; injection: 25, 50 mg/1 mL. Dose: antihistamine: children, 0.1 mg/kg/dose PO TID and 0.5 mg/kg/dose PO QHS; adult, 12.5–25 mg/dose PO TID and QHS; nausea: children, 0.25–0.5 mg/kg/dose PO, PR, or IM Q4–6H prn; adult, 12.5–25 mg/dose PO, PR, or IM Q4–6H prn; sedation: children, 0.5–1 mg/kg/dose PO, PR, or IM Q6H prn; adult, 25–50 mg/dose PO, PR, or IM Q6H prn; motion sickness: children, 0.5 mg/kg/dose PO, or PR BID prn; adult, 25 mg PO or PR BID prn.

Propranolol (Inderal) How supplied: tabs: 10, 20, 40, 60, 80, 90 mg; extended-release caps: 80, 120, 160 mg; injection: 1 mg/1 mL. Dose: hypertension: children: initial 1 mg/kg/d PO BID, maintenance 2–4 mg/kg/d PO BID; adult: initial 40 mg/dose PO BID, then increase slowly to maintenance dose of 120–240 mg/d PO Q8–12H (max dose 640 mg/d); arrhythmias: children: 0.01–0.1 mg/kg/dose slow IV (max 1 mg/dose), then 0.5–4 mg/kg/d; adult: 1–3 mg/dose slow IV, then 10–30 mg/d PO TID–QID; tetralogy spells: 0.15–0.25 mg/kg/dose slow IV, may repeat once, max 10 mg/dose, then 1–2 mg/kg/dose PO Q6H; migraine prophylaxis: <35 kg: 10–20 mg/dose PO TID; >35 kg: 20–40 mg/dose PO TID; adult: sustained-release 60–160 mg/dose QD.

Propylthiouracil (PTU) How supplied: tabs: 50 mg. Dose: hyperthyroidism: initial 6–7 mg/kg/d PO Q8H, then maintenance usually $\frac{1}{3}$–$\frac{1}{2}$ of initial dose; initial adult dose usually 300 mg/d PO Q8H.

Prostaglandin E$_1$ (Prostin) How supplied: injection: 500 µg/1 mL. Dose: to maintain patency of ductus arteriosus dose is 0.05–0.1 µg/kg/min as continuous IV infusion.

Protamine sulfate How supplied: injection: 5, 10 mg/1 mL. Dose: 1 mg will neutralize approx 100 U of heparin (max dose is 50 mg per 10-min period).

Pseudoephedrine (Sudafed, Novafed, others) How supplied: tabs: 30, 60 mg; syrup: 30 mg/5 mL. Dose: 4 mg/kg/d PO QID; adult, 30–60 mg/dose PO Q6–8H.

Pyridostigmine (Mestinon) How supplied: tabs: 60 mg; extended-release tabs: 180 mg; syrup: 60 mg/5 mL; injection: 5 mg/1 mL. Dose: symptomatic treatment of myasthenia gravis: children, 7 mg/kg/d PO Q4–6H, adjust prn; adult: usual dose 600 mg/d PO prn.

Quinidine How supplied: gluconate (62% quinidine base): tabs: 324 mg (202 mg base); extended-release tabs: 324 mg (202 mg base); sulfate (83% quinidine base): tabs: 100, 200, 300 mg (88, 176, 264 mg base). Dose: (as base) children, test dose: 2 mg/kg/dose PO once; maintenance dose: 15–60 mg/kg/d PO Q6H; adult, test dose: 1 tab PO; maintenance: 100–600 mg/dose PO Q6–8H.

Ranitidine (Zantac) How supplied: tabs: 150, 300 mg; injection: 25 mg/1 mL. Dose: children, oral: 2–4 mg/kg/d PO BID; parenteral: 1–2 mg/kg/d IM or IV Q6–8H; adults, oral: 150–300 mg/d PO QD–BID; parenteral: 50 mg/dose IM or IV Q6–8H.

Scopolamine Hydrobromide (Transderm Scōp, others) How supplied: tabs: 400, 600 mg; transderm patch: releases 1.5 mg over 3 days. Dose: motion sickness: transderm patch 1 per 3 days (apply 4 hours prior to travel).

Secobarbital (Seconal) How supplied: tabs: 50, 100 mg; caps: 50, 100 mg; elixir: 22 mg/5 mL; suppository: 30, 60, 120, 200 mg; injection: 50 mg/1 mL. Dose: sedation: 6 mg/kg/d PO or PR Q8H; adult 20–40 mg/dose PO or PR BID–TID.

Sodium Polystyrene Sulfonate (Kayexalate) How supplied: powder: 3.6 g/tsp (exchanges approx 1 mEq K/g). Dose: treatment of hyperkalemia: children, oral: 1 g/kg/dose PO Q6H; rectal: 1 g/kg/dose PR Q2–6H; adult, oral: 15 g/dose PO QD–QID; rectal: 30–50 g/dose PR Q6H.

Spironolactone (Aldactone) How supplied: tabs: 25, 50, 100 mg. Dose: edema associated with aldosterone excretion: 1–3.3 mg/kg/d PO QD–BID; adults 25–200 mg/d PO QD–BID.

Succinylcholine (Anectine) How supplied: injection: 20 mg/1 mL. Dose: infants, small children: 2 mg/kg/dose IV; adolescents and older children: 1 mg/kg/dose IV; adult: 0.3–1.1 mg/kg/dose IV; may be given IM if necessary, 3–4 mg/kg/dose IM (max 150 mg/dose).

Sucralfate (Carafate) How supplied: tabs: 1 g. Dose: short-term treatment of duodenal ulcers: >12 yr: 1 g/dose PO QID.

Sulfasalazine (Azulfidine) How supplied: tabs: 500 mg; enteric-coated tabs: 500 mg; suspension: 250 mg/5 mL. Dose: management of ulcerative colitis: >2 yr: initial 40–100 mg/kg/d PO Q4–8H, then 30 mg/kg/d PO QID; adult: initial 3–4 g/d PO Q4–8H, then 2 g/d PO QID, max 6 g/d.

Terbutaline (Brethine) How supplied: tabs: 2.5, 5 mg; inhaler: 200 µg/puff, approx 300 puffs/inhaler; injection: 1 mg/1 mL (may be used for nebulization). Dose: oral: <12 yr: 0.05–0.1 mg/kg/dose PO TID; >12 yr: 2.5–5 mg/dose PO TID; inhalation: children >12 yrs: 2 puffs Q4–6H prn; nebulization: (not FDA approved for this use) 0.1 mg/kg/dose Q1H prn, max 2.5 mg/dose; subcutaneous: 0.005–0.1 mg/kg/dose SC Q15–30 min × 2 (max 0.25 mg/dose).

Terfenadine (Seldane) How supplied: tabs: 60 mg. Dose: perennial and seasonal allergic rhinitis and other allergic symptoms. >12 yr, 60 mg/dose PO BID. *Note:* Safety and efficacy in children <12 yrs has not been established.

Theophylline (many trade names) How supplied: (see also Aminophylline) tabs: 100, 200, 300 mg; syrup: 80 mg/15 mL; sustained-release tabs: 100, 200, 300, 450 mg; sustained release caps: Slo-Bid gyrocaps: 50, 100, 200, 300 mg; Slo-Phyllin gyrocaps: 60, 125, 250 mg; Theo-Dur sprinkles: 50, 75, 125, 200 mg. Dose: neonatal apnea: loading dose 5 mg/kg/dose PO once; maintenance: <36 wk: 1–2 mg/kg/d PO Q8–12H; >36 wk: 2–4 mg/kg/day PO Q8–12H; asthma: loading dose of 1 mg/kg will raise serum level approx 2 µg/mL; children <1 yr: dose in mg/kg/d = (0.2) (age in wks) + 5; children >1 yr: 12–14 mg/kg/d up to 300 mg/day times 3 days, then if tolerated, 400 mg/day (adult, ≥45 kg) or 16 mg/kg/d up to 400 mg/day (<45 kg) times 3 days, then if tolerated, 600 mg/day (adults ≥45 kg) or 20 mg/kg/d up to 600 mg/day (<45 kg). Further dosage adjustments based on symptoms, adverse effects and serum concentrations.

Thioridazine (Mellaril) How supplied: tabs: 10, 15, 25, 50, 100, 150, 200 mg; liquid: 30, 100 mg/1 mL; suspension: 25, 100 mg/5 mL. Dose: psychotic disorders and severe behavioral problems: 2–12 yr: 0.5–3 mg/kg/d PO BID–QID; adult: initial 50–100 mg/dose PO TID, then gradually increase to 200–800 mg/day PO BID–QID.

Tolazoline (Priscoline) How supplied: injection: 25 mg/1 mL. Dose: persistent pulmonary vasoconstriction and hypertension of the newborn: initial 1–2 mg/kg/dose IV, then 1–2 mg/kg/hr as continuous IV infusion.

Tolmetin Sodium (Tolectin) How supplied: tabs: 200 mg; caps: 400 mg. Dose: relief of signs and symptoms of rheumatoid arthritis and osteoarthritis: >2 yr: 15–30 mg/kg/d PO TID–QID; adult: 600–1800 mg/d PO TID–QID.

Trimethobenzamide (Tigan) How supplied: caps: 100, 250 mg; suppository: 100, 200 mg; injection: 100 mg/1 mL. Dose: antiemetic: <15 kg: 100 mg/dose PR TID–QID; 15–40 kg: 100–200 mg/dose PO or PR TID–QID; adult: 200–250 mg/dose PO or PR TID–QID; 200 mg/dose IM TID–QID.

Valproic Acid (Depakene, Depakote) How supplied: tabs: 250 mg; enteric-coated tabs: 125, 250, 500 mg; syrup: 250 mg/5 mL. Dose: simple and complex absence seizures: initial 15 mg/kg/d PO BID, then increments every week of 5–10 mg/kg/d, max 60 mg/kg/d.

Vasopressin (Pitressin) 2 U/spray, 50 U/1 mL; injection: aqueous: 20 U/1 mL; in oil: 5 U/1 mL. Dose: postoperative abdominal distention: 5–10 U IM BID–TID prn (decrease for children); injection aqueous: 5–10 U SC or IM BID–TID prn.

Vecuronium (Norcuron) How supplied: injection: 1, 2 mg/1 mL. Dose: to facilitate endotracheal intubation and to provide skeletal muscle relaxation during surgery or mechanical ventilation. 0.08–0.1 mg/kg/dose IV repeated Q30–60 min prn.

Verapamil (Calan, Isoptin) How supplied: tabs: 40, 80, 120 mg; sustained-release caplets: 240 mg; injection: 2.5 mg/1 mL. Dose: supraventricular tachyarrythmias IV: children >1 yr: 0.1–0.5 mg/kg/dose slow IV (max 5 mg/dose), may repeat once Q30 min; adult: 5–10 mg/dose slow IV, may repeat once Q30 min. Dose: hypertension: children: safety and efficacy in children <18 yrs has not been established; Adults: 240–480 mg/day divided TID.

Vitamin K (AquaMEPHYTON, Konakion) How supplied: (as phytonadione) tabs: 5 mg; injection: 2, 10 mg/1 mL. Dose: neonatal prophylaxis: 0.5–1 mg/dose IM, once within 1 h of birth; anticoagulant overdose: 2.5–10 mg/dose PO, SC, IM, or IV, may repeat once, up to 25 mg/dose; hypoprothrombinemia: 2.5–25 mg/dose PO, SC, IM, or IV, up to 50 mg/dose.

FORMULARY OF ANTI-INFECTIVES AND ANTIBIOTICS

Note: Where specific doses for premature infants and neonates are not listed, consult other sources.

Acyclovir (Zovirax) How supplied: ointment: 5%; caps: 200 mg; injection: 500 mg. Dose: topical: Q3H; 200 mg PO 5 times/day; 30 mg/kg/d IV Q8H. Coverage: herpes simplex; varicella-zoster. Comments: Ointment is efficacious only in initial herpes genitalis. Capsules are efficacious in suppression and treatment of initial and recurrent herpes genitalis. Decrease dose in renal failure.

Amantadine (Symmetrel) How supplied: syrup: 50 mg/5 mL; caps: 100 mg. Dose: children 1–9 yrs: 4.4–8.8 mg/kg/d PO divided Q12H (max 150 mg/d); children >9 and adults: 200 mg/d PO divided BID. Coverage: influenza A. Comments: Must be started within 24–48 hr of onset of symptoms.

Amikacin (Amikin) How supplied: injection: 100 mg/2 mL; 500 mg/2 mL; 1 mg/4 mL. Dose: Adults, children and older infants: 15 mg/kg/d IV or IM Q8H; max 1.5 g/d. Newborns: loading dose of 10 mg/kg followed by 7.5 mg/kg IV Q12H. Coverage: gram-negatives. Toxicity: renal, VIII nerve. Comments: Peak 15–30 μg/mL, trough <5 μg/mL. Adjust dose in renal failure.

Amoxicillin (Amoxil, Polymox, Trimon, Wymox) How supplied: caps: 250, 500 mg; suspension: 125, 250 mg/5 mL; chewable tabs: 125, 250 mg. Dose: 40 mg/kg/d PO Q8H. Coverage: non-penicillinase producing gram-positive cocci *Listeria, E Coli, Salmonella, Shigella.*

Amoxicillin and potassium clavulanate (Augmentin) How supplied: suspension: 125 mg amox + 31.25 mg clav/5 mL, 250 mg amox + 62.5 mg clav/5 mL; chewable tabs: 125 mg amox + 31.25 mg clav, 250 mg amox + 62.5 mg clav/5 mL; tabs: 250 mg amox + 125 mg clav, 500 mg amox + 125 mg clav. Dose: same as amoxicillin. Coverage: β-lactamase-producing gram negatives and gram positives.

Amphotericin B (Fungizone) How supplied: injection: 50 mg. Dose: 0.25–1 mg/kg/d IV over 2–6 h Q24H. Coverage: *Aspergillus; Candida; Cryptococcus; Blastomyces; Sporotrichum; Coccidioides; Histoplasma; mucormycoses.* Toxicity: renal. Use for severe fungal infections only. *Note:* Safety and efficacy in pediatric patients is not well established.

Ampicillin (Omnipen, Polycillin, Principen) How supplied: suspension: 125, 250, 500 mg/5 mL; chewable tabs: 125 mg; drops: 100 mg/mL; caps: 240, 500 mg; injection: 0.125, 0.25, 0.5, 1, 2, 43 g. Dose: 50 mg/kg/d PO Q6H; 100–400 mg/kg/d IV or IM Q4–6 H. Coverage: same as Amoxicillin.

Aztreonam (Azactam) How supplied: injection: 0.5, 1, 2 g. Dose: 90–120 mg/kg/d IV or IM Q6–8H. Coverage: gram negatives including *Pseudomonas aeruginosa*.

Carbenicillin (Geocillin, Geopen) How supplied: tabs: 382 mg; injection: 2, 5g. Dose: 30–50 mg/kg/d PO Q6H. Coverage: gram negatives except *Klebsiella*. Toxicity: platelet dysfunction. Comments: Some *Serratia* and *Pseudomonas* are resistant.

Cefaclor (Ceclor) How supplied: suspension: 125, 250 mg/5 mL; caps 250, 500 mg. Dose: 40 mg/kg/d PO Q8–12H. Coverage: streptococci; some *H influenzae;* some *S aureus.*

Cefamandole (Mandol) How supplied: injection: 0.5, 1, 2 g. Dose: 50–100 mg/kg/d IV or IM Q4–8H. Coverage: same as cefaclor; some *Klebsiella* and *Proteus;* anaerobes.

Cefazolin (Ancef, Kefzol) How supplied: injection: 0.25, 0.5, 1 g. Dose: 50–100 mg/kg/d IM or IV Q8H. Coverage: gram-positive cocci; some gram negatives.

Cefixime (Suprax) How supplied: suspension: 100 mg/5 mL; tabs: 400 mg. Dose: 8 mg/kg/d PO Q24H. Coverage: gram negatives including *H influenzae;* gram positives except staphylococci and enterococci. Comments: only oral third-generation cephalosporin.

Cefoperazone (Cefobid) How supplied: injection: 1, 2 g. Dose: NOT APPROVED FOR USE IN CHILDREN; Adults: 2–4 g/day divided Q12H IV or IM. Coverage: same as Cefixime.

Cefotaxime (Claforan) How supplied: injection: 1, 2 g. Dose: 100–200 mg/kg/d IM or IV Q6–8H; meningitis, 200 mg/kg/d IM or IV Q6H. Coverage: same as Cefixime; dose not cover *Listeria.*

Cefoxitin (Mefoxin) How supplied: injection: 1, 2 g. Dose: children >3 mos: 80–160 mg/kg/d IM or IV Q4–6H; Adults: 1–2 g Q6–8H IV or IM (max 12 g/d). Coverage: same as Cefazolin plus anaerobes.

Ceftazidime (Fortaz, Tazicef, Tazidime) How supplied: injection: 0.5, 1, 2 g. Dose: children: 30–50 mg/kg IV Q8H (max 6 g/

d); Adults: 1 g Q8–12H IV or IM. Coverage: same as Cefotaxime: most *Pseudomonas*.

Ceftriaxone (Rocephin) How supplied: injection: 1.25, 0.5, 1, 2 g. Dose: children: 50–100 mg/kg/d IM or IV Q12–24H; meningitis, 100 mg/kg/d IM or IV Q12H; Adults: 1–2 g Q12–24H IV (max 4 g/24h) Coverage: same as Cefotaxime.

Cefuroxime (Ceftin, Kefurox, Zinacef) How supplied: injection: 0.75, 1.5 g. Dose: children <2 yrs: 125 mg/dose BID PO; children >2 yrs: 250 mg/dose BID PO; Adults: 250–500 mg/dose BID PO. Coverage: streptococci; some staphylococci, some gram negatives. Comments: May result in delayed CSF sterilization.

Cephalexin (Keflet, Keflex, Keftab) How supplied: drops: 100 mg/mL; suspension: 125, 250 mg/5 mL; tabs/caps: 0.25, 0.5, 1 g. Dose: 25–50 mg/kg/d PO Q6H. Coverage: gram-positive cocci.

Cephapirin (Cefadyl) How supplied: injection: 0.5, 1, 2, 4 g. Dose: 40–80 mg/kg/d IM or IV Q6H; Adults: .5–1 g/dose Q4–6H (max 12g/24h). Coverage: gram-positive cocci.

Cephradine (Anspor, Velosef) How supplied: suspension: 125, 250 mg/5 mL; caps: 250, 500 mg; Dose: 25–50 mg/kg/d PO Q6H. Coverage: same as Cephalexin.

Chloramphenicol (Chloromycetin) How supplied: suspension: 150 mg/5 mL; caps: 250 mg; injection: 1 g. Dose: 50–75 mg/kg/d PO or IV Q6H; meningitis, 75–100 mg/kg/d IV divided Q6H. Coverage: gram positives and gram negatives; *Rickettsiae; Chlamydiae*. Comments: Peak 10–25 μg/mL, trough 5–10 μg/mL.

Chloroquine (Aralen PO₄, Plaquenil, Aralen HC1) How supplied: tabs: 500 mg (300 mg base); tabs: 200 mg (155 mg base); injection: 250 mg (200 mg base). Dose: malaria: suppression: 5 mg/kg base QWK (max 310 mg base QWK) acute treatment: 10 mg/kg base; 6 hr later, 5 mg/kg base; 18 hr later, 5 mg/kg base; 24 hr later, 5 mg/kg base. Coverage: *Plasmodium* sp (some *P falciparum* resistant); *Entameoba histolytica* (extraintestinal). Toxicity: retinal. Comments: Suppressive therapy should begin 2 weeks prior to potential exposure.

Ciprofloxacin (Cipro) How supplied: tabs: 250, 500, 750 mg. Dose: NOT APPROVED FOR USE IN CHILDREN; Adults: 250–500 mg PO Q12H. Coverage: gram negatives including *Pseudomonas*.

Clindamycin (Cleocin) How supplied: solution: 75 mg/5 mL;

caps: 75, 100 mg; injection: 150, 300, 600 mg. Dose: children: 20–30 mg/kg/d PO Q6H; 25–40 mg/kg/d IM or IV Q6–8H; Adults: 150–450 mg/dose Q6–8H PO (max 1.8 g/d); 1.2–1.8 g/24h divided BID–TID, IV or IM (max 4.8 g/24h). Coverage: anaerobes and some gram-positive cocci.

Colistin (Coly-Mycin) How supplied: suspension: 125 mg/5 mL. Dose: 5–15 mg/kg/d PO Q8H. Coverage: enteropathogenic *E coli; Shigella.*

Dicloxacillin (Dycill, Dynapen, Pathocil) How supplied: suspension: 62.5 mg/5 mL; caps: 125, 250, 500 mg. Dose: 12–25 mg/kg/d PO Q6H; Adults: 125–500 mg PO Q6H. Coverage: penicillin-resistant staphylococci.

Doxycycline (Doryx, Vibramycin, Vibra-Tabs) How supplied: suspension: 25 mg/mL; syrup: 50 mg/mL; caps: 50, 100 mg; injection: 100, 200 mg. Dose: children >8 yr: 4 mg/kg/d PO Q12H for 24 hr then 2 mg/kg/d PO Q24H; 2–4 mg/kg/d IV over 2 hr Q24H. Adults: 200 mg/dose Q12H on day 1, followed by 100 mg/dose Q12H maintenance. Coverage: gram positives; *Rickettsiae; Chlamydiae; Mycoplasma; Brucella; Bacteroides.* Toxicity: permanent tooth discoloration when given during tooth development.

Erythromycin (E.E.S, E-mycin, EryPed, Ery-Tab, Ethril, others) How supplied: drops: 100 mg/mL, 100 mg/2.5 mL; suspension: 125, 200, 250, 400 mg/5 mL; chewable tabs: 125, 200, 250 mg; tabs: 250, 330, 400, 500 mg; caps: 125, 250 mg; topical solution: 2% ophthalmic solution: 0.5%; amps: 0.25, 0.5, 1 g; injection: 1.5, 1g. Dose: 20–40 mg/kg/d PO Q6–8H; 20–50 mg/kg/d IV Q6H; acne: topical; eye: topical. Coverage: same as Doxycycline: *Legionella; Bordetella pertussis; Corynebacterium diphtheriae; Clostridia.*

Erythromycin and sulfisoxazole (Pediazole) How supplied: suspension: 200 mg ery + 600 mg sulf/5 mL. Dose: 40 mg/kg of ery PO Q6–8H. Coverage: same as erythromycin: *H influenzae.*

Ethambutol (Myambutol) How supplied: tabs: 100, 400 mg. Dose: 15 mg/kg/d PO Q24H. Coverage: *M tuberculosis.* Toxicity: optic neuritis.

Flucytosine (Ancobon) How supplied: caps: 250, 500 mg. Dose: Adult: 50–150 mg/kg/d PO Q6H. Coverage: *Candida; Cryptococcus.* Toxicity: Bone marrow suppression. Comments: Check sensitivities; many candida species are resistant. *Note:* Safety and efficacy in children has not been established.

Furazolidine (Furoxone) How supplied: suspension: 50 mg/15 mL; tabs: 100 mg. Dose: children >1 month: 5–8 mg/kg/d PO Q6H; Adults: 100 mg/dose QID PO. Coverage: *Vibrio cholerae; Giardia*. Comments: Turns urine brownish color. *Notes:* Do not combine with alcohol. Do not give to children <1 month old.

Gentamicin (Garamycin) How supplied: injection: 20, 60, 80 mg; ophthalmic solution; ophthalmic ointment. Dose: children: 6.7–7.5 mg/kg/d IM or IV divided Q8H; eye: topical solution, Q4H; ointment, Q6H; Adults: 3–5 mg/kg/d IM or IV divided Q8H. Coverage: same as Amikacin. Toxicity: same as Amikacin. Comments: Peak 8–10 μg/mL, trough <2 μg/mL.

Griseofulvin (Fulvicin P/G, Fulvicin U/F, Grifulvin, others) How supplied: suspension: 125 mg/5 mL; tabs: 125, 165, 250, 330, 500 mg; caps: 125, 250, 500 mg. Dose: children: 10–15 mg/kg/d PO Q24H; Adults: 500 mg PO QD. Coverage: *Trichophyton* sp; *Microsporum* sp; *Epidermophyton floccosum*. Comments: Contraindicated in patients with porphyria or hepatocellular failure.

Imipenem-Cilastatin (Primaxin) How supplied: injection: 250, 500 mg. Dose: NOT APPROVED FOR USE IN CHILDREN; Adult: 500–750 mg Q12H IM, or 250–500 mg Q6–8H IV. Dose is based on imipenem. Coverage: gram negatives and positives including *Pseudomonas; Serratia; Enterobacter; Proteus*.

Iodoquinol (Yodoxin) How supplied: tabs: 210, 650 mg. Dose: children <6 yrs: (210-mg tabs) one tablet per 15 pounds body weight; children 6–12 yrs: (210-mg tabs) 2 tablets TID; Adults: (210-mg tabs) 3 tablets TID. Coverage: *Entamoeba histolytica* (intestinal).

Isoniazid (INH, Laniazid) How supplied: syrup: 50 mg/5 mL; tabs: 50, 100, 300 mg. Dose: children: 10–20 mg/kg/d PO Q24H; Adults: 5 mg/kg/d PO (usual dose 300 mg PO QD). Coverage: *M tuberculosis*. Toxicity: hepatic; neuro due to pyridoxine deficiency. Comments: Supplement with pyridoxine; use <10 mg/kg/d when given with rifampin.

Kanamycin (Kantrex) How supplied: injection: 75, 500 mg, 1 g; caps: 500 mg. Dose: 15 mg/kg/d IM or IV Q8–12H; 50–100 mg/kg/d PO Q6H. Coverage: same as Amikacin; *Vibrio, Salmonella, Shigella*. Toxicity: same as Amikacin. Comments: Oral dosing not absorbed—used for bowel sterilization. Peak 15–30 μg/mL, trough <10 μg/mL.

Ketoconazole (Nizoral) How supplied: cream: 2% in 15, 30, 60 g tubes; tabs: 200 mg. Dose: topical: to affected area Q24H; children >2 yrs: 3.6–6.6 mg/kg/d PO Q24H; Adults: 200 mg/24 h (max 400 mg/24h). Coverage: some dermatophytes; *Candida; Blastomyces, Coccidioides, Histplasma*. Toxicity: hepatic. *Note:* Should not be used in children <2 yrs and not in children of any age unless potential benefit outweighs risk.

Mebendazole (Vermox) How supplied: chewable tabs: 100 mg. Dose: pinworms: 100 mg PO; one dose; other nematodes: 100 mg Q12H for 3 days. Coverage: *Trichuris; Enterobius; Ascaris; Ancylostoma; Necator.*

Metronidazole (Flagyl, Metric-12, Protostat) How supplied: tabs: 250, 500 mg; injection: 500 mg. Dose: anaerobic infections: adults: 1.5 mg/kg one time, then 7.5 mg/kg Q6H IV. Amebiasis: children: 30–50 mg/kg/d divided TID; adults: 750 mg PO TID. Trichomoniasis: 2 g PO as a single dose or 250 mg TID for 7 days. Coverage: anaerobes; *Giardia; Entamoeba histolytica;* trichomoniases. *Note:* Safety and efficacy for IV use in children has not been established.

Mezlocillin (Mezlin) How supplied: injection: 1, 2, 3, 4 g. Dose: children 1 mo–12 yrs: 200–300 mg/kg/d IV Q4–6H; Adults: 1.5–4 g/dose Q4–6H IV (max 24 g/24h). Coverage: gram negatives.

Miconazole (Monistat) How supplied: cream, lotion: 2%; vaginal cream: 2%; vaginal suppository: 100, 200 mg; injection: 200 mg. Dose: children: topical: to affected area Q12H; vaginal: 1 applicator QHS; vaginal: 100–200 mg QHS or for systemic fungal infection; 20–40 mg/kg/d IV Q8H (max 60 mg/kg/infusion); Adults: 200–3600 mg/day divided TID IV. Coverage: some dermatophytes; *Candida; Cryptococcus; Coccidioides*. Comments: May also be administered intrathecally.

Mupirocin (Bactroban) How supplied: ointment: 2% in 15 g tube. Dose: topical Q8H. Coverage: Impetigo due to *S aureus,* B-hemolytip strep, *S pyogenes.*

Nafcillin (Nafcil, Unipen) How supplied: solution: 250 mg/5 mL; caps: 250 mg; tabs: 500 mg; injection: 0.5, 1, 2 g. Dose: children: 50–200 mg/kg/d IM or IV Q6H; Adults: 500 mg IV or IM Q6H. Coverage: penicillinase-producing staphylococci.

Niclosomide (Niclocide) How supplied: tabs: 500 mg. Dose: *Taenia saginasa and Diphyllobothrium latum:* 11–34 kg; 1 g PO single dose; 34–59 kg: 1.5 g PO single dose; >59 kg: 2 g PO single dose; for *H nana,* as above, then: 11–34 kg; 0.5 g PO Q24H; 34–59 kg: 1 g PO Q24H; >59 kg: 2 g PO Q24H. Coverage: *Taenia saginata; Diphyllobothrium latum; Hymenolepis nana. Note:* Safety and efficacy has not been established in children <2 yrs.

Nitrofurantoin (Furadantin, Macrodantin) How supplied: suspension: 25 mg/5 mL; caps: 25, 50, 100 mg; tabs: 50, 100 mg. Dose: children: 5–7 mg/kg/d PO Q6H; Adults: 50–100 mg/dose Q6H. Coverage: gram negatives. Toxicity: primaquine-sensitive hemolytic anemia. Comments: Used only for UTI.

Nystatin (Mycostatin, Milstat, Nystex) How supplied: cream, ointment, powder: 100,000 U/g; suspension: 100,000 U/mL; tabs: 500,000 U. Dose: topical: to affected area Q12H; for oral thrush: infants: 2 mL/dose Q6H; children: 4–6 mL/dose or 1 tab/dose Q6H applied directly to areas of thrush. Coverage: *Candida.* Comments: Also comes in vaginal preparations.

Oxacillin (Bactocill, Prostaphlin) How supplied: suspension: 250 mg/5 mL; caps: 250, 500 mg; injection: 0.25, 0.5, 1, 2, 4 g. Dose: children: 150–200 mg/kg/d IM or IV Q6H; Adults: 250–2000 mg/dose Q4–6H IV or IM. Coverage: penicillinase-resistant staphylococci.

Oxytetracycline (Terramycin) How supplied: caps: 250 mg; injection: 50, 100, 250 mg. Dose: children > 8 yr: 20–50 mg/kg/d PO Q6H; 15–25 mg/kg/d IM Q12H; Adults: 1–2 g divided QID PO or 250 mg IM Q24H or 300 mg IM divided Q8–12H. Coverage: same as Doxycycline. Toxicity: same as Doxycycline.

Penicillin G (Pentids, Prizerpen G) How supplied: suspension: 125, 250, 500 mg/5 mL; tabs: 125, 150, 250, 500 mg; injection: 1, 2, 5, 10, 20 million U. Dose: 25–50 mg/kg/d PO Q6–8H; 0.1–0.25 million U/kg/d divided Q4–6H IM or IV. Coverage: some gram-positive cocci; some gram-negative cocci; oral anaerobes.

Penicillin G, benzathine (Bicillin) How supplied: injection: 0.6, 0.9, 1.2, 3 million U. Dose: 25,000–50,000 U/kg IM single dose. Coverage: Streptococci groups A, C, G, H, L, M.

Penicillin G, procaine (Wycillin) How supplied: injection: 0.3, 0.6, 1.2, 2.4 million U. Dose: 25,000–50,000 U/kg/d IM. Coverage: same as penicillin G; spirochetes.

Penicillin V (Betapen-VK, Ledercillin VK, Pen VEE VK, Vee-tids) How supplied: solution: 125, 250 mg/5 mL; tabs: 125, 250,

500 mg. Dose: 25–50 mg/kg/d PO divided Q6–8H. Coverage: streptococci groups A, C, G, H, L, M; oral anerobes.

Pentamidine (Pentam 300) How supplied: injection: 300 mg. Dose: 4 mg/kg/d IM or IV. Coverage: *Pneumocystis carinii.* Toxicity: hypotension.

Piperacillin (Pipracil) How supplied: injection: 2, 3, 4, g. Dose: NOT APPROVED FOR USE IN CHILDREN; 200–300 mg/kg/d IV divided Q4–6H; Adults: 2–4 g/dose Q4–8H (max 24 g/24h). Coverage: gram negatives; anaerobes.

Praziquantel (Biltricide) How supplied: tabs: 600 mg. Dose: schistosomiasis: 60 mg/kg/d PO Q8H for 3 doses; clonorchiasis and opisthorchiasis: 75 mg/kg/d PO Q8H for 3 doses. Coverage: *Schistosoma* sp. *Note:* Safety in children <4 yrs has not been established.

Pyrantel (Antiminth) How supplied: suspension: 250 mg/5 mL. Dose: children and adults: 11 mg/kg PO as single dose; repeat in 2 wks (max 1 g/dose). Coverage: *Enterobius; Ascaris.*

Pyrimethamine (Daraprim) How supplied: tabs: 25 mg. Dose: For prophylaxis of malaria: children <4 yr: ¼ tab PO QWK; 4–10 yr: ½ tab PO QWK; >10 yr: 1 tab PO QWK. For *T gondii:* 1 mg/kg/d PO Q12H with a sulfa; Adults: 50–75 mg PO QD. Coverage: *Plasmodium* sp; *Toxoplasma gondii.*

Quinacrine (Atabrine) How supplied: tabs: 100 mg. Dose: 6 mg/kg/d PO Q8H. coverage: *Giardia.* Toxicity: hepatic; hemolysis in G6PD deficiency. Comments: Turns skin yellow.

Ribavirin (Virazole) How supplied: vial: 6 g. Dose: 6 g aerosolized over 12–18 hr Q24H. Coverage: Respiratory syncytial virus. Comments: Must be started within the first 3 days of RSV lower respiratory tract infection.

Rifampin (Rifadin, Rimactane) How supplied: caps: 150, 300 mg. Dose: 10–20 mg/kg/d PO Q12–24H, max 600 mg/dose. For *H influenzae* prophylaxis: 20 mg/kg/d Q12H for 4 doses. For *N meningitidis* prophylaxis: 20 mg/kg/d Q24H for 4 doses. Coverage: *Mycobacterium; Neisseria; H influenzae.* Toxicity: hepatic. Comments: All body secretions may be colored red-orange.

Spectinomycin (Trobicin) How supplied: injection: 2, 4 g. Dose: Adults: 2 g in single dose; max 2 g IM. Coverage: *N gonorrhoeae.* *Note:* Safety and efficacy in children has not been shown.

Streptomycin How supplied: injection: 1, 5 g. Dose: tuberculosis: children: 20–30 mg/kg/d IM Q12H (max 2 g/day); Adults:

15 mg/kg/day divided Q12H IM. Coverage: *M tuberculosis:* some gram negatives. Toxicity: vestibular.

Sulfadoxine and pyrimethamine (Fansidar) How supplied: tabs: 500 mg SDX/25 mg PMA. Dose: For prophylaxis: <4 yr: ½ tab PO Q2WK; 4–8 yr: 1 tab PO Q2WK; 9–14 yr: 1½ tab PO Q2WK; >14 yr: 2 tab PO Q2WK; *or* half the above doses QWK. Same quantity may be used as a single dose for an acute attack. Coverage: *Plasmodium* sp including chloroquine-resistant *P falciparum*. Toxicity: hemolysis in G6PD deficiency; Stevens-Johnson syndrome. Comments: Fansidar-resistant *P falciparum* now exist. *Note:* Do not use in infants <2 mos.

Sulfamethizole (Thiosulfil) How supplied: tabs: 500 mg. Dose: CONTRAINDICATED IN INFANTS <2 MO; 30–45 mg/kg/d PO Q6H; Adults: 500–1000 mg/dose TID–QID. Coverage: *E coli; Klebsiella; Enterobacter; S aureus; Proteus; H influenzae*. Comments: Used only for UTI.

Sulfamethoxazole (Gantanol) How supplied: suspension: 500 mg/5 mL; tabs: 500 mg. Dose: CONTRAINDICATED IN INFANTS <2 MO; 50–60 mg/kg/d PO Q12H; Adults: 2 g PO divided Q12H. Coverage: same as sulfamethizole; malaria. Comments: Primarily used for UTI.

Sulfisoxazole (Gantrisin) How supplied: suspension: 500 mg/5 mL; tabs: 500 mg. Dose: CONTRAINDICATED IN INFANTS <2 MO; 150 mg/kg/d PO Q6H; max 6 g/d; Adults: 4–8 g/24h divided Q6H PO. Coverage: same as sulfamethizole. Comments: Use in half daily dose for prophylaxis of otitis media.

Tetracycline (Achromycin, Sumycin) How supplied: syrup: 125 mg/5 mL; suspension: 125 mg/5 mL; caps: 250, 500 mg; tabs: 250, 500 mg; injection: 100, 250, 500 mg. Dose: children >8 yr: 25–50 mg/kg/d PO Q6H; Adults: 250–500 mg/dose PO Q6H. Coverage same as Doxycycline. Toxicity: same as Doxycycline.

Thiabendazole (Mintezol) How supplied: suspension: 500 mg/5 mL; chewable tabs: 500 mg. Dose: 50 mg/kg/d PO Q12H; max 3 g/d. Coverage: strongyloidiasis; cutaneous larva migrans; visceral larva migrans; trichinosis. *Note:* Safety and efficacy in children <30 lbs has not been established.

Ticarcillin (Ticar) How supplied: injection: 1, 3, 6 g. Dose: 200–300 mg/kg/d IV Q4–6H. Coverage: same as Carbenicillin. Toxicity: Platelet dysfunction.

Ticarcillin and clavulanate (Timentin) How supplied: injection: 3/0.1, 3/0.2 g. Dose: NOT APPROVED FOR USE IN CHILDREN; same as Ticarcillin. Coverage: same as Ticarcillin; *Klebsiella; S aureus, H influenzae.*

Tobramycin (Nebcin) How supplied: injection: 20, 80 mg, **1.2** g. Dose: 6–7.5 mg/kg/d IM or IV Q6–8H. Coverage: gram negatives including *Pseudomonas.* Toxicity: same as Amikacin. Comments: May need higher doses in patients with cystic fibrosis; peak 6–8 µg/mL, trough 0.5–1.0 µg/mL.

Trifluridine (Viroptic) How supplied: ophthalmic solutions: 1%. Dose: 1 drop Q2H to affected eye. Coverage: herpes simplex.

Trimethoprim (Proloprim, Trimpex) How supplied: tabs: 100, 200 mg. Dose: Adults: 100 mg/dose PO Q12H. Coverage: *E coli, Proteus mirabilis, Klebsiella pneumoniae, Enterobacter,* coagulase-negative staphylococci. *Note:* Effectiveness in children <12 yrs has not been established.

Trimethoprim-sulfamethoxazole (Bactrim, Septra) How supplied: suspension: 40 mg TMP/200 mg SMX/5 mL; tabs: 80 mg TMP/400 mg SMX, 160 mg TMP/800 mg SMX; injection: 400 mg TMP/2000 mg SMX. Dose: CONTRAINDICATED IN INFANTS <2 MO; children: 6–12 mg TMP/kg/d PO Q12H: 10–20 mg TMP/kg/d IV Q6H; Adults: 160 mg TMP Q12H. Coverage: gram positives and gram negatives; *Salmonella; Shigella, P carinii.*

Vancomycin (Vancocin, Vancoled, Vancor) How supplied: pulvules: 125, 250 mg; bottle: 1, 10 g; injection: 0.5, 1 g. Dose: pseudomembranous colitis: 20–40 mg/kg/d PO Q6H; max 2 g/d. Staphylococcal infection: 40 mg/kg/d IV Q8H. Coverage: *Clostridium difficile;* gram-positive cocci including methicillin-resistant. Toxicity: rash, hypotension, renal, 8th cranial nerve.

Vidarabine (Vira-A) How supplied: ophthalmic ointment: 3%; injection: 1 g. Dose: topical: ½ in. to affected eye 5 times/day; 10–15 mg/kg/d IV over 12–24 hr Q24H. Coverage: herpes simplex.

Zidovudine (AZT) (Retrovir) How supplied: solution: 150 mg/5 mL; caps: 100 mg. Dose: 720 mg/m^2/d Q6H (max 200 mg Q6H). Coverage: HIV. Toxicity: granulocytopenia; anemia.

Appendix

NORMAL BLOOD CHEMISTRY VALUES & OTHER HEMATOLOGIC VALUES*
(Values may vary with the procedure employed.)

The following is a compilation of normal values for some commonly used laboratory tests. Where values differ with age, tables have been provided. Some laboratory values that are often ordered together are arranged in tables. It is important to note that the methodology used for various laboratory tests and the units in which they are reported, may vary significantly between different laboratories. If any doubt exists, consult your laboratory for normal ranges.

Determinations for:
(S) = Serum
(B) = Whole blood

(P) = Plasma
(RBC) = Red blood cells

Acid-Base Measurements (B)
pH: 7.30–7.46: 1 day
  7.32–7.46: 2 days–1 month
  7.34–7.43: >1 month
Pao_2: 65–76 mm Hg (8.66–10.13 kPa).
$Paco_2$: 36–38 mm Hg (4.8–5.07 kPa).
Base excess: -2 to $+2$ meq/L, except in newborns (range, -4 to -0).

Alanine Aminotransferase (ALT, SGPT) (S)
Newborns (1–3 days): 1–25 IU/L at 37°C.
Adult males: 7–46 IU/L at 37°C.
Adult females: 4–35 IU/L at 37°C.

Albumin
Birth–3 months: 3.2–4.8 g/dL.
Over 1 year: 3.7–5.7 g/dL.

Alkaline Phosphate (S)
(See Table, below.)

Ammonia (P)
Newborns: 90–150 μg/dL (53–88 μmol/L: higher in premature and jaundiced infants.
Thereafter: 0–60 μg/dL (0–35 μmol/L).

Alkaline phosphatase in serum.

Values at 37°C using *p*-nitrophenyl phosphate buffered with AMP (kinetic).		
Group	**Males (IU/L)**	**Females (IU/L)**
Newborns (1–3 days)	95–368	95–368
2–24 months	115–460	115–460
2–5 years	115–391	115–391
6–7 years	115–460	115–460
8–9 years	115–345	115–345
10–11 years	115–336	115–437
12–13 years	127–403	92–336
14–15 years	79–446	78–212
16–18 years	58–331	35–124
Adults	41–137	39–118

Amylase (S)
Neonates: 5–81 IU/L.
2–12 months: Levels increase slowly to adult levels.
Adults: 28–108 IU/L at 37°C.

α₁-Antitrypsin (S)
1–3 months: 127–404 mg/dL.
3–12 months: 145–362 mg/dL.
1–2 years: 160–382 mg/dL.
2–15 years: 148–394 mg/dL.

* Adapted from Meites S (editor): *Pediatric Clinical Chemistry*, 3rd ed. American Association for Clinical Chemistry, 1989, The Childrens Hospital of Denver Clinical Laboratory, and many other sources.

Ascorbic Acid:
See Vitamin C.

Aspartate Aminotransferase (AST, SGOT) (S)
Newborns (1–3 days): 16–74 IU/L at 37°C.
Adult males: 8–46 IU/L at 37°C.
Adult females: 7–34 IU/L at 37°C.

Base Excess:
See Acid-Base Measurements.

Bicarbonate, Actual (P)
Calculated from pH and $Paco_2$.
Newborns: 17.2–23.6 mmol/L.
2 months–2 years: 19–24 mmol/L.
Children: 18–25 mmol/L.
Adult males: 20.1–28.9 mmol/L.
Adult females: 18.4–28.8 mmol/L.

Bilirubin (S)
Levels after 1 month are as follows:
Conjugated: 0–0.3 mg/dL (0–5 μmol/L).
Unconjugated: 0.1–0.7 mg/dL (2–12 μmol/L).
For peak newborn levels, see figure (below).

Bleeding Time
See Coagulation Factor Table.

BUN:
See Urea Nitrogen.

C Peptide (S)
5–15 years (8:00 AM fasting): 1–4 ng/mL.
Adults (8:00 AM fasting): <4 ng/mL.
Adults (nonfasting): <8 ng/mL.

Calcium (S)
Premature infants (first week): 3.5–4.5 meq/L. (1.7–2.3 mmol/L).
Full-term infants (first week): 4–5 meq/L (2–2.5 mmol/L).
Thereafter: 4.4–5.3 meq/L (2.2–2.7 mmol/L).

Calcium (Ionized)
At pH 7.4: 3.9–4.5 mg/dL (0.9–1.12 mmol/L).

Carotene (S, P)
0–6 months: 0–40 μg/dL (0–0.75 μmol/L).
6 mos–adult: 40–180 μg/dL (0.75–3.4 μmol/L)

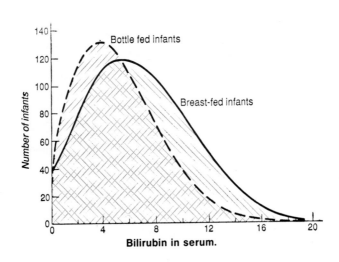

Bilirubin in serum.

Coagulation factors and tests.[1]

Factor	Level
II (Prothrombin)	0.5–1.5 U/mL
V (Proaccelerin)	0.5–1.5 U/mL
VII (Proconvertin)	0.5–1.5 U/mL
VIII (Antihemophilic globulin)	0.5–1.5 U/mL
IX (Christmas factor)	0.5–1.5 U/mL
Fibrinogen	182–368 mg/dL
Bleeding time	3–9 min
Partial Thromboplastin Time (PTT)	25.3–33.1 sec
Prothrombin Time (PT)	11.3–13.2 sec
Thrombin Time (TT)	8.5–13.5 sec

[1] All values are for children.

Cation-Anion Gap (S, P)
5–15 mmol/L.

Ceruloplasmin (Copper Oxidase) (S, P)
21–43 mg/dL (1.3–2.7 μmol/L).

Chloride (S, P)
Premature infants: 95–110 mmol/L.
Full-term infants: 96–116 mmol/L.
Children: 98–105 mmol/L.
Adults: 98–108 mmol/L.

Cholesterol (S, P)
See Lipid Profile Table.

Complement (S)
C3: 0–6 mos: 53–166 mg/dL.
6 mos–adult: 75–195 mg/dL.
C4: 0–6 mos: 7–42 mg/dL.
6 mos–adult: 9.5–45 mg/dL.

Copper (S)
Newborns: 15–45 μg/dL (2.36–7.08 μmol/L).
1 month: 56–92 μg/dL (8.81–14.48 μmol/L).
3 months: 93–124 μg/dL (14.64–19.52 μmol/L).
1 year: 95–147 μg/dL (14.95–23.14 μmol/L).
8 years: 85–121 μg/dL (13.38–19.04 μmol/L).

Creatine (S, P)
0.2–0.8 mg/dL (15.2–61 μmol/L).

Creatine Kinase (Creatine Phosphokinase) (S, P)
Newborns (1–3 days): 40–474 IU/L at 37°C.
Adult males: 30–210 IU/L at 37°C.
Adult females: 20–128 IU/L at 37°C.

Creatinine (S, P)
(See Table, next page.)

Creatinine Clearance
Values show great variability and depend on specificity of analytical methods used.
Newborns (1 day): 5–50 mL/min/1.73 m² (mean, 18 mL/min/1.73 m²).
Newborns (6 days): 15–90 mL/min/1.73 m² (mean, 36 mL/min/1.73 m²).
Adult males: 85–125 mL/min/1.73 m².

Ferritin (S)
Newborns: 20–200 ng/mL (mean, 117 ng/mL).
1 month: 60–550 ng/mL (mean, 350 ng/mL).
1–15 years: 7–140 ng/mL (mean, 31 ng/mL).
Adult males: 50–225 ng/mL (mean, 140 ng/mL).
Adult females: 10–150 ng/mL (mean, 40 ng/mL).

Creatinine in serum and plasma.

Group	Males mg/dL (μmol/L)	Females mg/dL (μmol/L)
Newborns (1–3 days)*	0.2–1.0 (17.7–88.4)	0.2–1.0 (17.7–88.4)
1 year	0.2–0.6 (17.7–53.0)	0.2–0.5 (17.7–44.2)
2–3 years	0.2–0.7 (17.7–61.9)	0.3–0.6 (26.5–53.0)
4–7 years	0.2–0.8 (17.7–70.7)	0.2–0.7 (17.7–61.9)
8–10 years	0.3–0.9 (26.5–79.6)	0.3–0.8 (26.5–70.7)
11–12 years	0.3–1.0 (26.5–88.4)	0.3–0.9 (26.5–79.6)
13–17 years	0.3–1.2 (26.5–106.1)	0.3–1.1 (26.5–97.2)
18–20 years	0.5–1.3 (44.2–115.0)	0.3–1.1 (26.5–97.2)

* Values may be higher in premature newborns.

Fibrinogen (P)
See Coagulation Factor Table.

Folate (S)
Prepubertal children: Mean folic acid values are reported to be slightly higher than mean adult values but remain within the normal range.
Adults: 3–21 ng/mL.

Galactose (S, P)
1.1–2.1 mg/dL (0.06–0.12 mmol/L).

Glucose (S, P)
Premature infants: 40–80 mg/dL (2.22–4.44 mmol/L).
Full-term infants: 40–100 mg/dL (2.22–5.56 mmol/L).
Children and adults (fasting): 60–105 mg/dL (3.33–5.88 mmol/L).

γ-Glutamyl Transpeptidase (S)
0–1 month: 12–271 IU/L 37°C (kinetic).

1–2 months: 9–159 IU/L 37°C (kinetic).
2–4 months: 7–98 IU/L 37°C (kinetic).
4–7 months: 5–45 IU/L 37°C (kinetic).
7–12 months: 4–27 IU/L 37°C (kinetic).
1–15 years: 3–30 IU/L 37°C (kinetic).
Adult males: 9–69 IU/L 37°C (kinetic).
Adult females: 3–33 IU/L 37°C (kinetic).

Glycohemoglobin (Hemoglobin A$_{1c}$) (B)
Normal: 6.3–8.2% of total hemoglobin. Diabetic patients in good control of their condition ordinarily have levels <10%.
Values tend to be lower during pregnancy.

Immunoglobins (S)
(See Table, next page.)

Hematologic values.

	Hct (%)	MCV (fL)	HgB (g/dL)
Birth	44–64	85–125	14–24
2 weeks–3 months	30–49	80–102	10–17
6 months–1 year	30–40	78	11–15
4 years–10 years	31–43	80–82	12.5–15

Immunoglobulins in serum.

Group	IgG (mg/dL)	IgA (mg/dL)	IgM (mg/dL)
Cord blood	766–1693	0.04–9	4–26
2 weeks–3 months	299–852	3–66	15–149
3–6 months	142–988	4–90	18–118
6–12 months	418–1142	14–95	43–223
1–2 years	356–1204	13–118	37–239
2–3 years	492–1269	23–137	49–204
3–6 years	564–1381	35–209	51–214
6–9 years	658–1535	29–384	50–228
9–12 years	625–1598	60–294	64–278
12–16 years	660–1548	81–252	45–256

Iron (S, P)
Newborns: 20–157 µg/dL (3.6–28.1 µmol/L).
6 weeks–3 years: 20–115 µg/dL (3.6–20.6 µmol/L).
3–9 years: 20–141 µg/dL (3.6–25.2 µmol/L).
9–14 years: 21–151 µg/dL (3.8–27 µmol/L).
14–16 years: 20–181 µg/dL (3.6–32.4 µmol/L).
Adults: 40–175 µg/dL (7.2–31.3 µmol/L).

Iron-Binding Capacity (S, P)
Newborns: 59–175 µg/dL (10.6–31.3 µmol/L).
Children and adults: 250–400 µg/dL (45–75 µmol/L).

Lactate (B)
Venous blood: 5–18 mg/dL (0.5–2 mmol/L).
Arterial blood: 3–7 mg/dL (0.3–0.8 mmol/L).

Lactate Dehydrogenase (LDH) (S, P)
Values using lactate substrate (kinetic).
Newborns (1–3 days): 30–348 IU/L at 37°C.
1 month–5 years: 150–360 IU/L at 37°C.
5–8 years: 150–300 IU/L at 37°C.
8–12 years: 130–300 IU/L at 37°C.

12–14 years: 130–280 IU/L at 37°C.
14–16 years: 130–230 IU/L at 37°C.
Adult males: 70–178 IU/L at 37°C.
Adult females: 42–166 IU/L at 37°C.

Lead (B)
<20 µg/dL (1.07 µmol/L).

LH:
See Luteinizing Hormone.

Lipase (S, P)
20–136 IU/L based on 4-hour incubation.

Magnesium (S, P)
Newborns: 1.5–2.3 meq/L (0.75–1.15 mmol/L).
Adults: 1.4–2 meq/L (0.7–1 mmol/L).

Manganese (S)
Newborns: 2.4–9.6 µg/dL (0.44–1.75 µmol/L).
2–18 years: 0.8–2.1 µg/dL (0.15–0.38 µmol/L).

Methemoglobin (B)
0–0.3 g/dL (0–186) µmol/L).

Osmolality (S, P)
285–295 mos m/kg.

Oxygen Capacity (B)
1.34 mL/g of hemoglobin.

Lipid profile.

	Triglycerides (mg/dL)*	Cholesterol (mg/dL)	HDL (mg/dL)	LDL (mg/dL)	VLDL (mg/dL)
<1 year	*	112–203	‡	‡	‡
2–20 years	10–130	120–205	37–73	66–145	6–15
20–29 years		120–240	37–73	66–145	6–15

* = 12–14 hr fast

‡ Values not determined in age range.

Partial Thromboplastin Time (P)
See Coagulation Factor Table.

Phenylalanine (S, P)
0.7–3.5 mg/dL (0.04–0.21 mmol/L).

Phosphorus, Inorganic (S, P)
Premature infants:
At birth: 5.6–8 mg/dL (1.18–2.58 mmol/L).
6–10 days: 6.1–11.7 mg/dL (1.97–3.78 mmol/L).
20–25 days: 6.6–9.4 mg/dL (2.13–3.04 mmol/L).
Full-term infants:
At birth: 5–7.8 mg/dL (1.61–2.52 mmol/L).
3 days: 5.8–9 mg/dL (1.87–2.91 mmol/L).
6–12 days: 4.9–8.9 mg/dL (1.58–2.87 mmol/L).
Children:
1 year: 3.8–6.2 mg/dL (1.23–2 mmol/L).
10 years: 3.6–5.6 mg/dL (1.16–1.81 mmol/L).

Adults: 3.1–5.1 mg/dL (1–1.65 mmol/L).
(See also Glucose Tolerance Test.)

Potassium (S, P)
Premature infants: 4.5–7.2 mmol/L.
Full-term infants: 3.7–5.2 mmol/L.
Children: 3.5–5.5 mmol/L.
Adults: 3.5–5.3 mmol/L.

Proteins (S)
(See Table, below.)

Prothrombin (Factor II) (P)
See Coagulation Factor Table.

Prothrombin Time (P)
See Coagulation Factor Table.

Protoporphyrin, "Free" (FET, ZPP) (B)
Values for free erythrocyte protoporphyrin (FEP) and zinc protoporphyrin (ZPP) are 1.2–2.7 μg/g of hemoglobin.

Proteins in serum.

Values are for cellulose acetate electrophoresis and are in g/dL. SI conversion factor: g/dL × 10 = g/L.

Group	Total Protein	Albumin	α₁- Globulin	α₂- Globulin	β- Globulin	γ- Globulin
At birth	4.6–7.0	3.2–4.8	0.1–0.3	0.2–0.3	0.3–0.6	0.6–1.2
3 months	4.5–6.5	3.2–4.8	0.1–0.3	0.3–0.7	0.3–0.7	0.2–0.7
1 year	5.4–7.5	3.7–5.7	0.1–0.3	0.5–1.1	0.4–1.0	0.2–0.9
>4 years	5.9–8.0	3.8–5.4	0.1–0.3	0.4–0.8	0.5–1.0	0.4–1.3

Pyruvate (B)
Resting adult males (arterial blood): 50.5–60.1 μmol/L.
Adults (venous blood): 34–102 μmol/L.

Pyruvate Kinase (RBC)
7.4–15.7 units/g of hemoglobin.

Sedimentation Rate (Micro) (B)
<2 years: 1–5 mm/h.
>2 years: 1–8 mm/h.

SGOT:
See Aspartate Aminotransferase.

SGPT:
See Alanine Aminotransferase.

Sodium (S, P)
Children and adults: 135–148 mmol/L.

Thrombin Time (P)
See Coagulation Factor Table.

Thyroid-Stimulating Hormone (TSH) (S)
See Thyroid Function Table.

Thyroxine (T₄) (S)
See Thyroid Function Table.

Thyroxine, "Free" (Free T₄) (S)
See Thyroid Function Table.

α-Tocopherol:
See Vitamin E.

Transaminase:
See Alanine Aminotransferase and Aspartate Aminotransferase.

Triglycerides (S, P)
See Lipid Profile Table.

Triiodothyronine (T₃) (S)
See Thyroid Function Table.

Trypsinogen, Immunoreactive (S, P)
Newborns: 5–97 ng/mL.
99.5th percentile: 136 ng/mL.
99.8th percentile: 162 ng/mL.

Tyrosine (S, P)
Premature infants: 3–30.2 mg/dL (0.17–1.67 mmol/L).
Full-term infants: 1.7–4.7 mg/dL (0.09–0.26 mmol/L).
1–12 years: 1.4–3.4 mg/dL (0.08–0.19 mmol/L).
Adults: 0.6–1.6 mg/dL (0.03–0.09 mmol/L).

Urea Nitrogen (S, P)
1–2 years: 5–15 mg/dL (1.8–5.4 mmol/L).
Thereafter: 10–20 mg/dL (3.5–7.1 mmol/L).

Uric Acid (S, P)
Males: 0–14 years: 2–7 mg/dL (119–416 μmol/L).
>14 years: 3–8 mg/dL (178–476 μmol/L).
Females: 0–14 years: 2–7 mg/dL (119–416 μmol/L).
>14 years: 2–7 mg/dL (119–416 μmol/L).

Vitamin A (S, P)
19–77 μg/dL (0.66–2.70 μmol/L).

Vitamin B₁₂ (S, P)
330–1025 pg/mL (243–756 pmol/L).

Thyroid Function Tests

Total T4 (μg/dL)	Total T3 (ng/dL)	TSH (μU/ml)
1–3 days: 11.8–22.6	32–216	62.5–13.3
1–2 wk: 9.8–16.6	250	
2–4 wk: 7.0–15.0	160–240	0.6–10
1–12 mo: 7.2–16.5	110–280	0.6–6.3
1–10 y: 6.4–15.0	94–269	0.6–6.3
10–15 y: 5.6–11.7	83–213	0.6–6.3

Vitamin C (Ascorbic Acid) (S, P)
0.2–2 mg/dL (11–114 μmol/L).

Vitamin D (S)
1.25-Dihydroxycholecalciferol: 25–49 pg/mL.
25-Hydroxycholecalciferol: 26–31 ng/mL.

Vitamin E (α-Tocopherol) (S, P)
Premature infants: 0.05–0.35 mg/dL (1.2–8.4 μmol/L).
Full-term infants: 0.10–0.35 mg/dL (2.4–8.4 μmol/L).
2–5 months: 0.2–0.6 mg/dL (4.8–14.4 μmol/L).
6–24 months: 0.35–0.8 mg/dL (8.4–19.2 μmol/L).

2–12 years: 0.55–0.9 mg/dL (13.2–21.6 μmol/L).
Breast-fed infants: 0.6–1.1 mg/dL (14.4–26.4 μmol/L).

Zinc (S)
Males: 83–88 μg/dL (12.7–13.5 μmol/L).
Females: 85–91 μg/dL (13–13.9 μmol/L).
Females taking oral contraceptives: 86–93 μg/dL (13.2–14.2 μmol/L).
At 16 weeks of gestation: 66–70 μg/dL (10.1–10.7 μmol/L).
At 38 weeks of gestation: 54–58 μg/dL (8.3–8.9 μmol/L).

NORMAL VALUES: URINE, SWEAT, & CSF*

URINE

Calcium
5–15 μg/24 h (2.5–7.5 mmol/24 h.

Catecholamines (Norepinephrine, Epinephrine)
(See Table, next page.)

Chloride
Infants: 1.7–8.5 mmol/24 h.
Children: 17–34 mmol/24 h.
Adults: 140–240 mmol/24 h.

Coproporphyrin:
See Porphyrins.

Epinephrine:
See Catecholamines.

Metanephrine & Normetanephrine
<2 years: <4.6 μg/mg of creatinine (23.3 nmol).

2–10 years: <3 μg/mg of creatinine (15.2 nmol).
10–15 years: <2 μg/mg of creatinine (10.3 nmol).
>15 years: <1 μg/mg of creatinine (5.1 nmol).

Norepinephrine:
See Catecholamines.

Normetanephrine:
See Metanephrine & Normetanephrine.

Osmolality
Infants: 50–600 mosm/kg.
Older children: 50–1400 mosm/kg.

Porphobilinogen:
See Porphyrins.

* Adapted from Meites S (editor): *Pediatric Clinical Chemistry*, 3rd ed. American Association for Clinical Chemistry, 1989, The Childrens Hospital of Denver Clinical Laboratory, and many other sources.

Catecholamines in urine.

Group	Norepinephrine µg/24 h (nmol/24 h)		Epinephrine µg/24 h (nmol/24 h)	
<1 year	5.4–15.9	(32–94)	0.1–4.3	(0.5–23.5)
1–5 years	8.1–30.8	(48–182)	0.8–9.1	(4.4–49.7)
6–15 years	19.0–71.1	(112–421)	1.3–10.5	(7.1–57.3)
>15 years	34.4–87.0	(203–514)	3.5–13.2	(19.1–72.1)

Porphyrins
δ-Aminolevulinic acid: 0–7 mg/24 h (0–53.4 µmol/24 h).
Porphobilinogen: 0–2 mg/24 h (0–8.8 µmol/24 h).
Coproporphyrin: 0–160 µg/24 h (0–244 nmol/24 h).
Uroporphyrin: 0–26 µg/24 h (0–31 nmol/24 h).

Potassium
26–123 mmol/L.

Sodium
Infants: 0.3–3.5 nmol/24 h (6–10 mmol/m²).
Children and adults: 5.6–17 mmol/24 h.

Uroporphyrin:
See Porphyrins.

Vanilmandelic Acid (VMA)
Because of the difficulty in obtaining an accurately timed 24-hour collection, values based on microgram per milligram of creatinine are the most reliable indications of VMA excretion in young children.
1–12 months: 1–35 µg/mg of creatinine (31–135 µg/kg/24 h).
1–2 years: 1–30 µg/mg of creatinine.
2–5 years: 1–15 µg/mg of creatinine.
5–10 years: 1–14 µg/mg of creatinine.
10–15 years: 1–10 µg/mg of creatinine.
Adults: 1–7 µg/mg of creatinine (1–7 mg/24 h: 5–35 µmol/24 h).

SWEAT

Electrolytes
Values for sodium or chloride or both. Elevated values in the presence of a family history or clinical findings of cystic fibrosis are diagnostic of cystic fibrosis.
Normal: <55 mmol/L.
Borderline: 55–70 mmol/L.
Elevated: >70 mmol/L.

CSF VALUES

Appearance
clear, colorless

Cells
White blood cells
Birth: 0–30
>3 months: 0–5
Red blood cells
Birth: 2–50
>3 months: 0

Glucose (mg/dL):
50–80 (two-thirds of blood glucose)

Protein (mg/dL)
Birth: 40–150
1–6 months: 20–65
>6 months: 15–35

BEDSIDE LABORATORY TESTS

1. Apt test—used to distinguish maternal from fetal blood. Mix specimen (vomitus, stool) with an equal amount of tap water; centrifuge. Proceed only if supernatant is pink. To 5 parts supernatant add 1 part 0.25 N (1%) NaOH. If the pink color persists >2 minutes it means fetal Hgb is present. If the pink turns yellow it means adult Hgb is present (denatured by NaOH).

2. Clinitest—used to detect reducing substances in stool; reflects carbohydrate malabsorption.
Mix 1 part stool with 2 parts water (use 1N HCl if testing for sucrose). Add 15 drops of this mixture to one Clinitest tablet. Compare color of suspension with chart for percentage of reducing substances. Abnormal if $\geq \frac{1}{2}\%$.

3. Cold agglutinins—present in *Mycoplasma* disease. Collect 4–5 drops of blood in small purple-top tube (0.2 mL EDTA). Place tube in ice water for 30–60 seconds. Rotate tube and look for clumping. Agglutination that occurs when cold and resolves with warming is interpreted as a cold agglutinin titer >1:64.

4. Fecal leukocytes—present in inflammatory enterocolitis. Place stool mucus on microscope slide. Add 2 drops 0.5% methylene blue. Wait 2–3 minutes. Examine under microscope.

Table 1. Normal peripheral blood values at various age levels.

Value	1st d	2nd d	6th d	2 wk	1 mo	2 mo
Red blood cells[1] (million/µL)	5.9 (4.1–7.5)	6 (4.0–7.3)	5.4 (3.9–6.8)	5 (4.5–5.5)	4.7 (4.2–5.2)	4.1 (3.6–4.6)
Hemoglobin (g/dL)	19 (14–24)	19 (15–23)	18 (13–23)	16.5 (15–20)	14 (11–17)	12 (11–14)
White blood cells[1] (per µL)	17,000 (8–38)		13,500 (6–17)	12,000	11,500	11,000
PMNs (%)	57	55	50	34	34	33
Eosinophils[1] (total) (per µL)	20–1,000				150–1,150	
Lymphocytes (%)	20	20	37	55	56	56
Monocytes (%)	10	15	9	8	7	7
Immature white blood cells (%)	10	5	0–1	0	0	0

Platelets (per µL)	350,000	325,000	300,000		
Nucleated red blood cells/100 white blood cells[1]	0–10	0.0–0.3	0	0	0
Reticulocytes (%)	3 (2–8)	1 (0.5–5.0)	0.4 (0.0–2.0)	0.2 (0.0–0.5)	0.5 (0.2–2.0)
Mean diameter of red blood cells (µm)	8.6			8.1	
MCV[2] (fl)	85–125	89–101	94–102	90	
MCHC[2] (%)	36	35	34		
MCH[2] (pg)	35–40	36	31	30	
Hematocrit (%)	54 ± 10	51	50	35–50	

[1] Total nucleated red blood cells: first day, <1000/µL.

[2] MCV = mean corpuscular volume. MCHC = mean corpuscular hemoglobin concentration. MCH = mean corpuscular hemoglobin.

Table 1 (cont'd.). Normal peripheral blood values at various age levels.

Value	3 mo	6 mo	1 yr	2 yr	5 yr	8–12 yr	Adults Males	Adults Females
Red blood cells[1] (million/μL)	4 (3.5–4.5)	4.5 (4–5)	4.6 (4.1–5.1)	4.7 (4.2–5.2)	4.7 (4.2–5.2)	5 (4.5–5.4)	5.4 (4.6–6.2)	4.8 (4.2–5.4)
Hemoglobin (g/dL)	11 (10–13)	11.5 (10.5–14.5)	12 (11–15)	13 (12–15)	13.5 (12.5–15.0)	14 (13.0–15.5)	16 (13–18)	14 (11–16)
White blood cells[1] (per μL)	10,500	10,500	10,000	9,500	8,000	8,000	7,000 (5–10)	7,000 (5–10)
PMNs (%)	33	36	39	42	55	60	57–58	57–58
Eosinophils[1] (total) (per μL)	70–550	70–550					100–400	100–400
Lymphocytes (%)	57	55	53	49	36	31	25–33	25–33
Monocytes (%)	7	6	6	7	7	7	3–7	3–7
Immature white blood cells (%)	0	0	0	0	0	0	0	0

Platelets (per µL)	260,000			260,000		260,000	260,000
Nucleated red blood cells/100 white blood cells[1]	0	0	0	0	0	0	0
Reticulocytes (%)	2 (0.5–4.0)	0.8 (0.2–1.5)	1 (0.4–1.8)	1 (0.4–1.8)	1 (0.4–1.8)	1 (0.4–1.8)	1 (0.5–2.0)
Mean diameter of red blood cells (µm)	7.7		7.4		7.4		7.5
MCV[2] (fl)	80	78	78	80	80	82	82–92
MCHC[2] (%)		33		32	34	34	34
MCH[2] (pg)	27	26	25	26	27	28	27–31
Hematocrit (%)	35	30–40	36	37	31–43	40	40–54 / 37–47

[1] Total nucleated red blood cells: first day, <1000/µL.
[2] MCV = mean corpuscular volume. MCHC = mean corpuscular hemoglobin concentration. MCH = mean corpuscular hemoglobin.

Table 2. Body surface area: Adults.

Height	Body surface	Mass
cm 200 — 79 in	2.80 m²	kg 150 — 330 lb
	78	145 — 320
195 — 77	2.70	140 — 310
	76	135 — 300
190 — 75	2.60	130 — 290
	74	125 — 280
185 — 73	2.50	120 — 270
	72	2.40	260
180 — 71		115 — 250
	70	2.30	110 — 240
175 — 69		105 — 230
	68	2.20	100 — 220
170 — 67	2.10	
	66		95 — 210
165 — 65		
	64	2.00	90 — 200
160 — 63	1.95	85 — 190
	62	1.90	
155 — 61	1.85	80 — 180
	60	1.80	
150 — 59	1.75	75 — 170
	58	1.70	70 — 160
145 — 57	1.65	
	56	1.60	65 — 150
140 — 55	1.55	
	54	1.50	60 — 140
135 — 53	1.45	
	52	1.40	55 — 130
130 — 51	1.35	
	50	1.30	50 — 120
125 — 49	1.25	
	48	1.20	45 — 110
120 — 47	1.15	105
	46	1.10	100
115 — 45		40 — 95
	44	1.05	90
110 — 43	1.00	85
	42		35 — 80
105 — 41	0.95	75
	40	0.90	70
cm 100 — 39 in	0.86 m²	kg 30 — 66 lb

To determine the body surface area in an adult, use a straight edge to connect the height and mass. The point of intersection on the body surface line gives the area in m².

From Lentner C (ed): *Geigy Scientific Tables*, ed. 8. Basle, CIBA-GEIGY, 1981, vol. 1, p. 226.

Index